RHEUMATOLOGY

Diagnosis and Therapeutics
2nd Edition

RHEUMATOLOGY

Diagnosis and Therapeutics

2nd Edition

John J. Cush, MD
Chief, Rheumatology and Clinical Immunology
Presbyterian Hospital of Dallas
Clinical Professor of Internal Medicine
The University of Texas Southwestern Medical School
Dallas, Texas

Arthur Kavanaugh, MD
Professor of Medicine
Director, Center for Innovative Therapy
Division of Rheumatology, Allergy, and Immunology
University of California at San Diego
San Diego, California

C. Michael Stein, MD
Associate Professor of Medicine and Pharmacology
Division of Rheumatology and Clinical Pharmacology
Vanderbilt University School of Medicine
Nashville, Tennessee

Cover Illustration by Vincent Perez

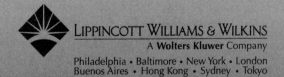

LIPPINCOTT WILLIAMS & WILKINS
A **Wolters Kluwer** Company
Philadelphia • Baltimore • New York • London
Buenos Aires • Hong Kong • Sydney • Tokyo

Acquisitions Editor: Danette Somers
Project Manager: Bridgett Dougherty
Manufacturing Manager: Benjamin Rivera
Marketing Manager: Kathy Neely
Cover Designer: Larry Didona
Compositor: Graphic World Publishing Service
Printer: RR Donnelley, Crawfordsville

Printed in the USA

Library of Congress Cataloging-in-Publication Data
ISBN: 0-7817-5732-0

Care has been taken to confirm the accuracy of the information presented and to describe generally accepted practices. However, the authors, editors, and publisher are not responsible for errors or omissions or for any consequences from application of the information in this book and
make no warranty, expressed or implied, with respect to the currency, completeness, or accuracy
of the contents of the publication. Application of this information in a particular situation remains the professional responsibility of the practitioner.

The authors, editors, and publisher have exerted every effort to ensure that drug selection and
dosage set forth in this text are in accordance with current recommendations and practice at the
time of publication. However, in view of ongoing research, changes in government regulations,
and the constant flow of information relating to drug therapy and drug reactions, the reader is
urged to check the package insert for each drug for any change in indications and dosage and
for added warnings and precautions. This is particularly important when the recommended agent
is a new or infrequently employed drug.

Some drugs and medical devices presented in this publication have Food and Drug Administration (FDA) clearance for limited use in restricted research settings. It is the responsibility of the
health care provider to ascertain the FDA status of each drug or device planned for use in their
clinical practice. Neither the editor nor the publisher nor any other party who has been involved
in the preparation of publication of this work warrants that the information contained herein is
in every respect accurate or complete, and they are not responsible for any errors or omissions
or the results obtained from the use of such information.

10 9 8 7 6 5 4 3 2

Dedication

We are forever grateful for the undying support of Floyd, Ming, Pepper, and Stout.

Contents

SECTION II. RHEUMATIC DISEASES / 105

SECTION III. PHARMACOPEIA FOR THE RHEUMATIC DISEASES / 397

SECTION VII. APPENDICES / 525

Foreword to the 1st Edition

When I entered the field of rheumatology in 1950, clinical practice in this budding area of specialization was relatively straightforward, but at the same time it had its difficulties. Take rheumatoid arthritis as an example. The diagnosis was made essentially on the basis of the history, physical examination, and sedimentation rate. Sensitized sheep cell agglutination tests for rheumatoid factor were being done, but practitioners sneered at them, proclaiming that in those patients in whom the test was positive, they could make the diagnosis from the history and physical alone. The difficult part of treating the patient with rheumatoid arthritis came at the end of the examination. One had two drugs to offer—aspirin and gold salts. Gold salts were thought to be toxic and to be reserved for people with severe disease. So, one faced the inevitable embarrassment of telling the patient to take aspirin. Thus, a patient visit that started with a bang ended with a whimper. This period of limited treatment options has dramatically changed in the last half century.

When I started in rheumatology in 1950, laboratory investigation was centered on the composition of the connective tissue and how it became abnormal in disease. This was a natural consequence of the state of knowledge at the time. Investigation of connective tissue biochemistry had made good progress: the amino acid composition of collagen had been worked out, and the proteoglycan constituents, hyaluronic acid and chondroitin sulfate, had been isolated and characterized by Karl Meyer. A phenomenon called "fibrinoid degeneration" occupied people's minds. It was supposed to be so characteristic of the rheumatic diseases that Robert Good used to call them the "fibrinoid diseases." Observing the diffuse deposition of fibrinoid in the collagen of the connective tissue in systemic lupus erythematosus, Klemperer and coworkers in 1942 coined the name "collagen diseases." However, the rediscovery of the rheumatoid factor by Rose and Ragan and the discovery of the L.E. cell factor by Hargraves in 1948 sparked an explosion of research on the role of the immune response in the etiology and pathogenesis of this group of diseases. This, in turn, has lead to a massive growth in our knowledge of these diseases and, consequently, the number of outlets for dissemination of this knowledge.

There are journals of rheumatology in every major country, three large textbooks of rheumatology, and, inevitably, a half-dozen "condensed" texts. The present book, Rheumatology: Diagnosis and Therapeutics is unique among these condensed texts. Its uniqueness lies in the fact that it is essentially a compendium of the rheumatic diseases helpfully organized into three sections: (1) tests and procedures utilized in the diagnosis of the rheumatic diseases; (2) clinical information about the individual diseases, including their diagnosis and treatment; and (3) drugs used in treatment, with pertinent information about each drug. This format makes it possible for the reader to focus rapidly on the information he or she needs. In each of the three sections, the amount of information provided for each item listed is substantial.

As mentioned above, a vast amount of knowledge has accumulated in the field of rheumatology in the last fifty years. The amount of information has grown sufficiently large for the health professional to profit from having this "compendium" readily at hand.

Morris Ziff, PhD, MD
Ashbel Smith Professor Emeritus of Internal Medicine
Morris Ziff Professor of Rheumatology
The University of Texas Southwestern Medical Center
Dallas, Texas

Preface

Rheumatology: Diagnosis and Therapeutics was originally designed and written for busy residents and fellows. However, in the course of its original compilation and subsequent revision, the authors also wrote a book for themselves and their colleagues. The book includes concise, comprehensive and organized factual information relevant to both the trainee and rheumatologist. The content, design and easy retrieval of information have made this textbook attractive to trainees, internists, family practitioners, nurse practitioners, orthopedists, and rheumatologists alike. Comments from those who purchased the first edition extolled the completeness and brevity of this well-organized handbook of rheumatology. Many stated this was an invaluable addition to their library, office, clinic exam room, or coat pocket. The 2nd edition holds true to this formula, yet expands its topics and treatments to include the latest advances in rheumatology.

Rheumatology is a branch of medicine that focuses on the biology, cause, diagnosis and treatment of a variety of musculoskeletal and other systemic disorders. These diverse diseases may be idiopathic, infectious, reactive, inflammatory, autoimmune, degenerative, and mechanical in origin. These disorders range from the common (tendonitis, bursitis, osteoarthritis, fibromyalgia) to the very uncommon (polymyositis, reactive arthritis, Lyme disease, and osteonecrosis). Confusion may arise as distinctly different conditions target the same anatomic structures via common pathogenic mechanisms and thus may share common symptoms and findings. For the non-rheumatologist, it may be difficult to distinguish and diagnose the more than 100 causes of arthritis. The authors teach that many of these conditions can be easily recognized, diagnosed and treated by any clinician who is armed with the necessary information and resources; whether that is a laboratory test, pathognomic feature, diagnostic criteria, or choice of therapy.

Most clinicians have a basic understanding of common disorders, yet they are often challenged with specific questions regarding the optimal diagnosis and care of patients with musculoskeletal complaints. This text provides an ideal resource that meets the needs of daily practice by having easily retrievable, template-driven information.

This 2nd edition retains the primary strength of the original text by being divided into 3 main sections (Diagnosis, Rheumatic Diseases, and Drugs), each of which has succinct information presented alphabetically in an organized fashion. The net result is a text that is written to complement the manner in which it will be used – for rapid answers to questions about specific tests, examination maneuvers, joint injections, disease definitions, ICD-9 codes, complications of disease, diagnostic criteria, approach to treatment, drug use, doses, and side effects. This edition has updated and stream-lined the first edition and added more than 50 new entries on tests, diseases, and drugs. New entries under the Diagnosis section include CCP antibodies, sialography, anti-LKM antibodies, ischemic forearm testing, and ultrasound. The Rheumatic Diseases section includes several new entries on pediatric disorders (Kawasaki's disease, toxic synovitis of the hip, Osgood-Schlatter disease, slipped capital femoral epiphysis, Legg-Calvé-Perthes disease). Other new topics include urticaria, periodic febrile syndromes, enthesopathy, calcinosis, thrombotic thrombocytopenic purpura, hypermobility syndrome, Kikuchi's disease, saturnine gout, palindromic rheumatism, osteoid osteoma, osteochondromatosis, parasite arthritis, McArdle's disease, and other inherited myopathies. The Pharmacopeia (drug) section was revamped to allow for the addition of many new agents including celecoxib, rofecoxib, meloxicam, valdecoxib, leflunomide, infliximab, etanercept, anakinra, adalimumab, mycophenolate, rituximab, bosentan, risedronate, raloxifene, teriparatide, cevimeline, hyaluronan, and glucosamine, to name a few.

The authors of the 2nd edition wish to express their gratitude to the co-authors who contributed to the first edition: Drs. Nancy Olsen, Ken Saag, and Salihuddin Kazi, whose influence remains felt in these pages. The ability of these educators to teach is valued by those who carry their efforts forward. The authors also wish to acknowledge the skill, insight and support of our editor, Danette Somers in the rewriting of this edition.

This textbook will significantly enhance a physician's diagnostic accuracy, clinical acumen, and ability to care for patients with musculoskeletal disorders. The design and content of this improved and updated second edition was strongly influenced by feedback from trainees and practitioners, especially while using it in the clinic. We continue to invite your comments and suggestions to enhance future editions of *Rheumatology: Diagnosis and Therapeutics*.

John J. Cush, MD
Arthur Kavanaugh, MD
C. Michael Stein, MD

Abbreviations

$	see key on page 400
a	alpha
b	beta
g	gamma
AAU	acute anterior uveitis
Ab	antibody
AC	acromioclavicular
ACD	anemia chronic disease
ACE	angiotensin converting enzyme
ACH	acetylcholine
ACL	anticardiolipin
ACR	American College of Rheumatology
AIDS	acquired immunodeficiency syndrome
AIMS	arthritis impact measurement scale
AL	amyloidosis
ALD	aldolase
ALT	alanine aminotransferase
AMA	antimitochondrial antibody
ANA	antinuclear antibodies
ANCA	antineutrophil cytoplasmic antibody
AOSD	adult-onset Still's disease
APL	antiphospholipid
APS	anti-phospholipid syndrome
ARF	acute rheumatic fever
AS	ankylosing spondylitis
ASA	acetylsalicylic acid (aspirin)
ASMA	anti–smooth muscle antibody
ASO	anti-streptolysin-O
AST	aspartate aminotransferase
ATLL	adult T cell lymphoma
AVN	avascular necrosis (osteonecrosis)
AZA	azathioprine
AZT	zidovudine
BAL	bronchoalveolar lavage
BCP	basic calcium phosphate crystals
BFP-STS	biologic false-positive serologic tests for syphilis
BM	bone marrow
BMD	bone mineral density
C	cervical
C3, C4	complement
CAH	chronic active hepatitis
CBC	complete blood count

CDC	Center for Disease Control
CHF	congestive heart failure
CK	creatine kinase
CLL	chronic lymphocytic leukemia
CMC	carpometacarpal
CML	chronic myelogenous leukemia
CMV	cytomegalovirus
CNS	central nervous system
COPD	chronic obstructive pulmonary disease
COX	cyclooxygenase
CPK	creatine kinase
CPPD	calcium pyrophosphate dihydrate
CREST	calcinosis, Raynaud's, esophageal dysmotility, sclerodactyly, telangiectasias
CRP	C-reactive protein
CSF	cerebrospinal fluid
CT	computerized tomography
CTS	carpal tunnel syndrome
CTX	cyclophosphamide
CVID	common variable immunodeficiency
CXR	chest x-ray
CYA	cyclosporine
DEXA	dual-energy x-ray absorptiometry
DFA	direct fluorescent antibody
DIC	disseminated intravascular coagulation
DIL	drug-induced lupus
DILS	diffuse infiltrative lymphocytosis syndrome
DIP	distal interphalangeal
DISH	diffuse idiopathic skeletal hyperostosis
DJD	degenerative joint disease (osteoarthritis)
DLE	discoid lupus erythematosus
DM	dermatomyositis
DMARD	disease-modifying antirheumatic drug
DNA	deoxyribonucleic acid
DRVVT	dilute Russell viper venom time
dsDNA	double-stranded DNA
DU	duodenal ulcer
EA	early antigen
EBNA	Epstein-Barr
EBV	Epstein-Barr virus
ECHO	echocardiogram
ECM	erythema chronicum migrans
EDTA	ethylenediaminetetraacetic acid
EEG	electroencephalogram
EIA	enzyme immunoassay
ELISA	enzyme-linked immunosorbent assay
EM	electron microscopy
EMG	electromyography

EMS	eosinophil-myalgia syndrome
ENA	extractable nuclear antigen
ESR	erythrocyte sedimentation rate
ESRD	end-stage renal disease
FDA	Food and Drug Administration
FMF	familial Mediterranean fever
G6PD	glucose-6-phosphate dehydrogenase
GBM	glomerular basement membrane
GC	gonococcus
GCA	giant cell arteritis
GCSF	granulocyte colony-stimulating factor
GI	gastrointestinal
GU	genitourinary
GU	gastric ulcer
GYN	gynecologic
h	hour
HAQ	health assessment questionnaire
HAV	hepatitis A virus
HBV	hepatitis B virus
HCQ	hydroxychloroquine
HCT	hematocrit
HCV	hepatitis C virus
Hgb	hemoglobin
HIV	human immunodeficiency virus
HLA	human leukocyte antigen
HSP	Henoch-Schönlein purpura
HTLV	human T-lymphotropic virus
IA	intraarticular
IBD	inflammatory bowel disease
IBM	inclusion body myositis
IC	immune complex
IDA	iron deficiency anemia
IEP	immunoelectrophoresis
IFA	immune fluorescent assay
IFN	interferon
Ig	immunoglobulin
IIF	indirect immunofluorescence
IIM	idiopathic inflammatory myopathy
IL	interleukin
ILD	interstitial lung disease
IM	infectious mononucleosis
ITP	idiopathic thrombocytopenic purpura
IU	international unit
IV	intravenous
IVDA	intravenous drug abuse
JA	juvenile arthritis
JRA	juvenile rheumatoid arthritis
KCS	keratoconjunctivitis sicca

KOH	potassium hydroxide
L	lumbar
LAC	lupus anticoagulant
LD	Lyme disease
LDH	lactate dehydrogenase
LE	lupus erythematosus
LFT	liver function test
LGL	large granular lymphocytes
LS	lumbosacral
LSD	lysergic acid diethylamide
MCP	metacarpophalangeal
MCTD	mixed connective tissue disease
MCV	mean corpuscular volume
MG	myasthenia gravis
MHC	major histocompatibility complex
MPA	microscopic polyangiitis
MPO	myeloperoxidase
MRA	magnetic resonance angiography
MRH	multicentric reticulohistiocytosis
MRI	magnetic resonance imaging
MS	multiple sclerosis
MSA	myositis-specific antibodies
MSU	monosodium urate
MTP	metatarsophalangeal
MTX	methotrexate
NA	not applicable (not available)
NCV	nerve conduction velocity
NMR	nuclear magnetic resonance
NPO	nothing by mouth
NSAID	nonsteroidal antiinflammatory drug
OA	osteoarthritis
OSHA	Occupational Safety and Health Administration
PAN	polyarteritis nodosa
PAS	periodic acid–Schiff
PBC	primary biliary cirrhosis
PCM	penicillamine
PCR	polymerase chain reaction
PIP	proximal interphalangeal
PM	polymyositis
PM/DM	polymyositis/dermatomyositis
PMR	polymyalgia rheumatica
PNS	peripheral nervous system
PR3	proteinase 3
PSA	psoriatic arthritis
PSS	progressive systemic sclerosis
PT	prothrombin time
PTT	partial thromboplastin time

PUD	peptic ulcer disease
PVNS	pigmented villonodular synovitis
RA	rheumatoid arthritis
RAST	radioallergosorbent test
RBC	red blood cell
RDW	red cell distribution width
RF	rheumatoid factor
RHD	rheumatic heart disease
RIA	radioimmunoassay
RNA	ribonucleic acid
ROM	range of motion
ROS	review of systems
RPGN	rapidly progressive glomerulonephritis
RPR	rapid plasma reagin test
RSD	reflex sympathetic dystrophy
S	sacral
SAA	serum amyloid A
SAARD	slow-acting antirheumatic drug
SAPHO	synovitis, acne, pustular lesions, hyperostosis, osteitis
SC	sternoclavicular
SCAT	sheep cell agglutination test
SCID	severe combined immunodeficiency
SCLE	subacute cutaneous lupus
SF	synovial fluid
SF-36	short form 36
SI	sacroiliac
SIEP	serum immunoelectrophoresis
SLAM	systemic lupus activity measure
SLE	systemic lupus erythematosus
SLEDAI	SLE disease activity index
SPA	spondyloarthropathy
SPEP	serum protein electrophoresis
SRP	signal-recognition particle
SSZ	sulfasalazine
STS	soft tissue swelling
T4	thyroxine
TA	temporal arteritis
TB	tuberculosis
TIBC	total iron-binding capacity
TMJ	temporomandibular joint
TNF	tumor necrosis factor
TSH	thyroid-stimulating hormone
TTP	thrombotic thrombocytopenic purpura
UCTD	undifferentiated connective tissue disease
UPEP	urine protein electrophoresis
VCA	viral capsid antigen
WBC	white blood cell
XRAY	radiograph

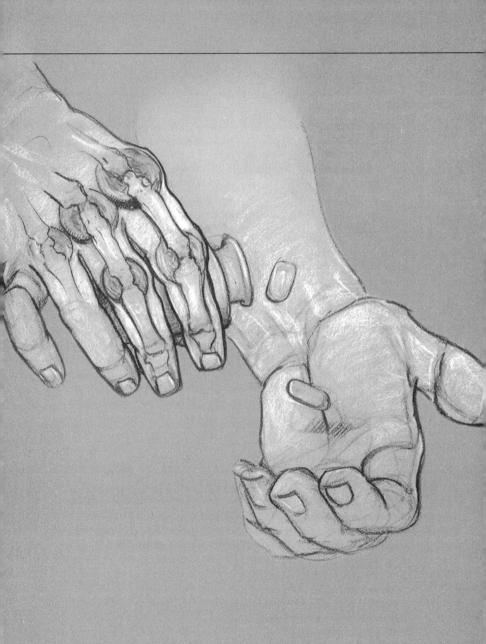

SECTION I

DIAGNOSIS

Diagnosis: A User's Guide

The first section of this guide focuses on the diagnosis of rheumatic complaints. An accurate diagnosis is obtained with the aid of a skillful clinical history and physical examination, with or without the aid of synovial fluid analysis, diagnostic tests, or musculoskeletal imaging. This section includes the chapters "Evaluation of Musculoskeletal Complaints," "Synovial Fluid Analysis and Arthrocentesis," and "Diagnostic Tests."

Evaluation of Musculoskeletal Complaints

This chapter presents the essential elements of clinical history and musculoskeletal examination. Proper categorization of the patient's complaints will aid in formulating a differential diagnosis. A detailed rheumatic review of symptoms is listed along with their associated rheumatic diagnoses. The musculoskeletal examination, demonstrated with specific maneuvers and signs, will refine the diagnosis and identify the patient's functional capacities.

Synovial Fluid Analysis and Arthrocentesis

This chapter focuses on synovial fluid analysis and interpretation of synovial fluid findings. Arthrocentesis of selected joints (knee, shoulder, wrist, ankle) is described, along with the indications, contraindications, precautions, procedures, complications, and use of intraarticular corticosteroids.

Diagnostic Tests

This chapter alphabetically catalogs the range of laboratory tests, diagnostic procedures, imaging methods, and disease assessment tools commonly used to evaluate patients with musculoskeletal conditions. Each topic describes the diagnostic test or procedure, methodology, background information, interpretation of results, guidelines for appropriate use, and information on confounding factors. Information is organized by a template of headings that may include "Synonyms," "Description," "Method," "Normal Values," "Abnormal Values," "Increased In," "Decreased In," "Interpretation," "Confounding Factors," "Complications," "Indications," "Contraindications," "Alternative Procedures," "Cost," and "Comment." The range of cost for select tests or procedures is based on 2004 costs gathered from several sources in the United States. The actual cost may vary according to method, availability, and geographic site.

CHAPTER 1.1

EVALUATION OF MUSCULOSKELETAL COMPLAINTS

Musculoskeletal complaints account for more than one-third of all adult outpatient evaluations in the primary care setting. A focused rheumatologic evaluation should be considered for those who manifest physical and functional limitations, focal or widespread musculoskeletal complaints, multisystem findings with rheumatic features, or (possibly) those found to have abnormal laboratory or imaging results suggesting a rheumatic disorder. Although an accurate and early diagnosis is pivotal, many musculoskeletal complaints and conditions are self-limited and may only require symptomatic therapy. Others may take several visits and observation over time before the clinical features necessary to establish a firm diagnosis are fully manifested.

General Approach

Evaluation of musculoskeletal complaints should include a comprehensive medical history and physical examination, with particular emphasis on features that might indicate a rheumatologic process. The primary goals of the patient's evaluation are to discern whether the complaint reflects an underlying urgent or "red flag" condition that merits a prompt diagnosis. Only a few rheumatologic disorders are urgent and require a prompt diagnosis and therapeutic intervention to minimize pain or serious morbid sequelae. These red flag conditions include fracture, septic arthritis/bursitis, and crystal-induced arthritis. These conditions are unified in that they often present as acute monarthritis. In the absence of a red flag condition, the patient evaluation should disclose if the nature of the complaint is

- Inflammatory or noninflammatory
- Articular or periarticular in origin
- Acute or chronic
- Mono/oligoarticular or polyarticular

By determining the nature of the complaint, the clinician can then categorize the complaint (e.g., acute inflammatory monarthritis or chronic noninflammatory polyarthritis) and begin to establish a differential diagnosis (Table 1). Identification of other distinctive articular and extraarticular features (see "Essential Clinical History" section) often provides the necessary clues to make a timely and accurate diagnosis. Finally, the clinician should remember to consider common conditions first. Low back pain, fracture, fibromyalgia, overuse syndromes (bursitis, tendinitis), and gout are far more common than systemic lupus, scleroderma, Lyme disease, or septic arthritis.

Table 1
Differential Diagnosis of Musculoskeletal Complaints

DURATION	Articular Mono/Oligoarticular		Periarticular Focal	
	Inflammatory	Noninflammatory	Inflammatory	Noninflammatory
ACUTE	Septic arthritis Gout Pseudogout Viral arthritis[a] Reiter's syndrome Lyme disease Acute rheumatic fever Hemarthrosis Palindromic rheumatism	Fracture Trauma Mechanical derangement Sickle cell crisis	Bursitis Septic bursitis Tendinitis Tenosynovitis Costochondritis Enthesitis Periostitis	Carpal tunnel syndrome Sickle cell crisis Reflex sympathetic dystrophy
CHRONIC	Tuberculous arthritis Fungal arthritis Psoriatic arthritis Spondyloarthropathy Pseudogout Sarcoidosis Juvenile arthritis	Osteoarthritis Osteonecrosis Neuropathic arthritis Hemarthrosis Pigmented villonodular synovitis Foreign body synovitis	Tendinitis Costochondritis Enthesitis Periostitis	Carpal tunnel syndrome Myofascial pain syndrome Raynaud's phenomenon Osteoid osteoma

DURATION	Polyarticular		Widespread	
ACUTE	Viral arthritis[a] Septic arthritis Acute rheumatic fever Serum sickness Reiter's syndrome	Sickle cell crisis	Enthesitis Polymyalgia rheumatica Relapsing polychondritis	Sickle cell crisis
CHRONIC	Rheumatoid arthritis Psoriatic arthritis Enteropathic arthritis Crystal-induced arthritis Juvenile arthritis Lyme disease SLE Scleroderma MCTD	Osteoarthritis Hemochromatosis Hypertrophy osteoarthropathy	Polymyalgia rheumatica Polymyositis Myasthenis gravis Eosinophilic fasciitis Enthesitis	Fibromyalgia Chronic fatigue syndrome Myxedema Osteoporosis Paget disease Psychogenic rheumatism

[a]Viral arthritis includes Epstein-Barr virus, Parvovirus B19, hepatitis B or C, rubella, human immunodeficiency virus.

SLE, systemic lupus erythematosus; MCTD, mixed connective tissue disease.

Inflammatory versus Noninflammatory

Musculoskeletal disorders are often classified as having inflammatory or non-inflammatory symptoms or signs that reflect the nature of the underlying pathologic process. Inflammatory disorders include a variety of infectious (e.g., tuberculosis), crystal-induced (e.g., gout), immunologic [e.g., systemic lupus erythematosus (SLE)], and reactive (e.g., Reiter's syndrome) disorders. Noninflammatory disorders may be traumatic (e.g., fracture), degenerative (e.g., osteoarthritis), neoplastic (e.g., osteoid osteoma), or functional (e.g., psychogenic) in origin.

Inflammatory and noninflammatory features can be identified during the history and physical examination and may be supported by laboratory data (Table 2). The cardinal signs of inflammation—erythema, warmth, pain, or swelling—should be sought. Inflammatory pain is often maximal in the morning, improved by activity and time, and almost always associated with prolonged morning stiffness (>1 hour) or systemic symptoms. Swelling of soft tissue (i.e., synovium or tenosynovium) with or without synovial effusion should suggest an inflammatory process. Laboratory evidence of inflammation (i.e., elevated erythrocyte sedimentation rate, C-reactive protein, or thrombocytosis) may be seen with inflammation and should not be elevated in uncomplicated noninflammatory disorders.

Articular stiffness commonly accompanies musculoskeletal disorders. Morning stiffness is ascertained by asking, "upon arising from a nights sleep, how long (minutes or hours) does it take for your stiffness to go away or get as good as it is going to get?" Rheumatologists often emphasize the importance of morning stiffness in distinguishing inflammatory and noninflammatory states. Unfortunately, the specificity of this feature is poor because common

Table 2
Distinguishing Inflammatory and Noninflammatory Findings

Feature	Inflammatory	Noninflammatory
Pain (worse when?)	Yes (morning)	Yes (night)
Swelling	Soft tissue (± effusion)	Bony
Erythema	Sometimes present	Absent
Warmth	Sometimes present	Absent
Morning stiffness	Prominent (>1 h)	Minor (<45 min)
Systemic features[a]	Sometimes present	Absent
Elevated ESR or CRP	Frequent	Uncommon
Synovial fluid WBCs	WBCs >2,000/mm^3	WBCs <2,000/mm^3
Examples	Septic arthritis, RA, gout, polymyalgia, rheumatica	OA, adhesive capsulitis, osteonecrosis

[a]Fever, rash, weight loss, anorexia, anemia.

ESR, erythrocyte sedimentation rate; CRP, C-reactive protein; WBCs, white blood cells; RA, rheumatoid arthritis; OA, osteoarthritis.

noninflammatory diseases such as fibromyalgia and osteoarthritis (OA) may also be accompanied by more than 1 hour of morning stiffness. Stiffness brought on by brief periods of rest, lasting minutes rather than hours, is called gel phenomenon. Gel phenomenon is common with noninflammatory conditions such as osteoarthritis, adhesive capsulitis, and fibromyalgia. Noninflammatory disorders are typically worsened by activity. Thus, patients typically complain of maximal pain in the evening or at night. Bony swelling and a lack of systemic features are characteristic of noninflammatory conditions.

Articular versus Periarticular

During the musculoskeletal evaluation, the examiner must determine whether the complaint originates from articular or periarticular structures because the two are commonly confused. A careful history and examination using knowledge of local anatomy and specific maneuvers are necessary to distinguish between the two. Articular structures include the synovium, synovial fluid, articular cartilage, and joint capsule. The extent of articular involvement is defined as monarticular (one joint), oligoarticular or pauciarticular (two to four joints), or polyarticular (more than four joints). The differential causes of monarticular and oligoarticular complaints are similar, hence they are typically considered together (i.e., mono/oligoarticular) (Table 1).

Periarticular structures include tendon, bursa, ligament, muscle, bone, fascia, nerve, or overlying skin. Periarticular complaints may be described as focal or widespread. Arthralgia (complaint of joint pain) may actually arise from articular or periarticular sites. Periarticular complaints are often misconstrued as articular pain because of their proximity. Table 3 details several distinguishing features useful in discriminating between articular and periarticular joint pain. The approach to evaluating articular and periarticular pain involving the hand, shoulder, neck, low back, hip, or knee is discussed individually in Section II: Rheumatic Diseases.

Table 3
Distinguishing Articular and Periarticular Joint Pain

Clinical Feature	Articular	Periarticular
Anatomic structures	Synovium, synovial fluid, articular cartilage, joint capsule	Tendon, bursa, ligament, muscle, bone, fascia, nerve, skin
Painful site	Diffuse, deep tenderness	Focal or "point" tenderness
Pain on movement	Pain on active and passive motion in all planes	Pain on active motion in a few, specific planes
Swelling	Common (bony or soft tissue)	Uncommon

Essential Clinical History

The differential diagnosis may be narrowed further by reviewing key historical information. Because some types of arthritis may affect one population more than others, important diagnostic clues can be obtained from basic demographic information such as gender, race, and family history (Table 4). Some disorders preferentially affect particular racial groups; polymyalgia rheumatica, giant cell arteritis, and Wegener granulomatosis are most common in whites, whereas sarcoid and SLE are commonly seen in African Americans.

On presentation, the clinician should determine whether the complaint is acute or chronic, based on whether the complaint has been present 6 weeks or less (acute) or longer than 6 weeks (chronic). The presentation of fracture, gonococcal arthritis, and gout is typically acute; fibromyalgia, OA, and rheumatoid arthritis (RA) are chronic by history. Other aspects of the onset and chronology often provide useful clues (Table 4). For example, intermittent complaints (with disease-free intervals) may indicate a crystal-induced arthropathy (e.g., gout, pseudogout). Incremental involvement of new joints describes an additive pattern characteristic of OA and RA. Migratory arthritis is defined as a rapidly changing pattern in which new joint complaints appear, resolve in days, and reappear at another site(s). A migratory pattern may be seen in rheumatic fever and viral (i.e., hepatitis B) or gonococcal arthritis. The number and distribution of involved joints also provide useful information (Table 4). Complaints may be described as monarticular, oligoarticular (or pauciarticular), polyarticular, focal, or widespread (Table 1). Symmetric joint involvement in the upper extremity is typical of RA, whereas OA, Reiter's syndrome, and gout often demonstrate asymmetric, lower extremity disease. Axial (spinal) involvement is common in OA and ankylosing spondylitis. Finally, the clinician should be aware that drug-induced musculoskeletal side effects or rheumatic disorders are a common and often overlooked cause of musculoskeletal complaints (Table 4).

A comprehensive rheumatic review of systems may disclose extraarticular features indicating particular rheumatic disorders. Table 5 details a suggested review of systems and possible clinical associations. For example, the examiner may narrow the diagnostic possibilities by questioning about the presence of fever (suggesting SLE, septic arthritis, or gout), ocular inflammation (Reiter's syndrome, sarcoid, Behçet's disease), rash (dermatomyositis, SLE, psoriatic arthritis), mucosal ulceration (Behçet's disease, drug induced), nail abnormalities (psoriasis, Reiter's syndrome), myalgias (myositis, fibromyalgia, viral arthritis), heel pain (HLA-B27 spondyloarthropathies, fasciitis), nodules (RA, gout, hyperlipidemia), dysphagia (scleroderma, myositis, Sjögren's syndrome), paresthesias (carpal tunnel syndrome, vasculitis, Lyme disease), and sleep disturbance (fibromyalgia, rotator cuff dysfunction).

Physical Examination

The physical examination should confirm or expand on the differential diagnosis established during the medical history. In addition, the physical exami-

Table 4
Clinical Associations Based on History and Physical Examination

Age
  Young (<25 y): JRA, SLE, Reiter's syndrome, gonococcal arthritis, hypermobility
  Middle (25–65 y): Fibromyalgia, tendinitis, bursitis, low back pain, RA
  Elderly (>65 y): OA, crystal arthritis, polymyalgia rheumatica, septic arthritis, osteo-
    porosis, drug-induced syndromes
Gender
  Males: Gout, ankylosing spondylitis, reactive arthritis, OA of the hip
  Females: Fibrositis, RA, SLE, OA
Race
  White: PMR, giant cell arteritis, Wegener granulomatosis
  African American: SLE, sarcoidosis
  Asian: RA, SLE, Takayasu arteritis, Behçet's disease, SAPHO syndrome, Kikuchi's
    disease
  Mediterranean: FMF, Takayasu arteritis
Family history
  Ankylosing spondylitis, gout, Heberden nodes of OA
Onset and chronology
  Acute: Fracture, septic arthritis, gout, rheumatic fever, Reiter's syndrome
  Chronic: OA, RA, SLE, psoriatic arthritis, fibromyalgia
  Intermittent: Gout, pseudogout, Lyme disease, palindromic rheumatism, Behçet's
    disease, FMF
  Additive: OA, RA, Reiter's syndrome, psoriatic arthritis
  Migratory: Viral arthritis (hepatitis B), rheumatic fever, SLE, gonococcal arthritis
Number of joints involved
  Monarthritis (1 joint): Septic arthritis, gout, pseudogout, fracture, OA, osteonecrosis,
    Reiter's syndrome
  Oligoarthritis (2–4): OA, psoriatic, Reiter's syndrome, pseudogout, gout, Lyme dis-
    ease, sarcoid
  Polyarthritis (>4): RA, SLE, OA, viral arthritis, psoriatic arthritis
Joint distribution [disorders to consider based on distribution or site(s) of involvement]
  Symmetric: RA, OA, psoriasis, tophaceous gout, viral arthritis
  Asymmetric: OA, Reiter's syndrome, psoriasis, early gout, sarcoid, spondyloarthropa-
    thy
  Axial: OA, ankylosing spondylitis, fibromyalgia, spinal stenosis, diffuse idiopathic
    skeletal hyperostosis
  Lower extremity: Reiter's syndrome, gout, sarcoid, OA, diabetes (Charcot disease)
  Upper extremity: RA, OA, psoriatic arthritis
  Sternoclavicular: Septic arthritis (especially with substance abuse), RA, trauma
  Distal interphalangeal: OA (Heberden node), psoriatic arthritis, swan-neck deformity
  Proximal interphalangeal: RA, OA (Bouchard node), psoriatic, SLE, viral arthritis, bou-
    tonnière deformity
  Metacarpophalangeal: RA, pseudogout, hemochromatosis, psoriatic arthritis
  Wrist: RA, psoriatic arthritis, septic (e.g., gonococcal) arthritis, deQuervain's tenosy-
    novitis, carpal tunnel syndrome, ganglion cyst
  Elbow: RA, gout, olecranon bursitis, septic arthritis or bursitis, epicondylitis
  Shoulder: Rotator cuff tear, subacromial bursitis, bicipital tendinitis, OA, osteonecro-
    sis, septic arthritis
  Hip: OA, RA, osteonecrosis, osteoid osteoma, fracture, iliopsoas bursitis,
    trochanteric bursitis

Table 4 (continued)
Clinical Associations Based on History and Physical Examination

---

Knee: OA, RA, pseudogout, gout, septic arthritis, sarcoid, Lyme disease, popliteal cyst, anserine bursitis, meniscal tear, chondromalacia patella, hemophilia, sickle cell, osteonecrosis

Ankle/tarsus: Gout, septic arthritis, RA, sarcoid, hemophilia, diabetes

Metatarsophalangeal: RA, OA, gout, Reiter's syndrome

Toes: RA, psoriatic arthritis, Reiter's syndrome, trauma

Drug-induced syndromes

Arthralgias: Quinidine, cimetidine, quinolones, chronic acyclovir, interferon, interleukin-2, nicardipine, Bacille Calmette Guérin vaccines (BCG), human immunodeficiency virus protease inhibitors

Myalgias/myopathy: Steroids, penicillamine, hydroxychloroquine, zidovudine, statins, clofibrate, interferon, interleukin-2, alcohol, cocaine, taxol, colchicine, tryptophan, cyclosporine

Gout: Diuretics, aspirin, cytotoxics, cyclosporine, alcohol, moonshine, ethambutol

Drug-induced lupus: Hydralazine, procainamide, quinidine, methyldopa, phenytoin, isoniazid, chlorpromazine, lithium, penicillamine, minocycline, tumor necrosis factor or angiotensin-converting enzyme inhibitors

Osteonecrosis: Steroids, alcohol, radiation therapy, trauma

Osteopenia: Steroids, chronic heparin, phenytoin, methotrexate

Scleroderma/tight skin: Vinyl chloride, bleomycin, pentazocine, solvents, carbidopa, tryptophan, rapeseed oil

Vasculitis: Allopurinol, amphetamines, cocaine, thiazide, penicillamine, propylthiouracil, montelukast, hepatitis B vaccine, tumor necrosis factor inhibitor, trimethoprim/sulfamethoxazole

---

JRA, juvenile rheumatoid arthritis; SLE, systemic lupus erythematosus; RA, rheumatoid arthritis; OA, osteoarthritis; PMR, polymyalgia rheumatica; FMF, familial Mediterranean fever.

nation will further establish whether the complaint is articular or periarticular, inflammatory or noninflammatory, focal or widespread, monarticular or polyarticular, or associated with systemic findings. Demonstration of particular physical signs and knowledge of anatomy will distinguish articular from periarticular conditions (Table 3). After a general physical examination, the musculoskeletal examination can be performed by careful inspection, palpation, and a variety of physical maneuvers to elicit diagnostic findings.

In each patient, specific aspects of the musculoskeletal examination should be addressed (Table 6). Examination of involved and uninvolved joints should reveal the extent or presence of inflammation, indicated by warmth, erythema, or swelling. Joints should be examined from all sides and the range of motion passively assessed in all planes. The examination should discern whether the joint complaint involves articular or periarticular structures. Joint swelling may be caused by a synovial effusion, proliferation of the synovial membrane (synovitis), or bony hypertrophy and can be identified by palpation and specific maneuvers. Synovial fluid often produces fluctuant or ballottable soft tissue enlargement. In large joints such as the knee, synovial effusion may be suggested by a "bulge" sign or ballottable patella (Table 7). Proliferation of

Table 5
Rheumatic Review of Symptoms

Symptom	Clinical Associations
Fever	Septic arthritis, gout, pseudogout, SLE, viral arthritis, MCTD, Reiter's syndrome, RA, vasculitis, rheumatic fever, adult Still's disease, drug-fever, Sweet's syndrome, osteomyelitis, Brucella, enteropathic arthritis, Behçet's disease
Weight loss	Uncontrolled inflammatory disorders (SLE, RA, polymyalgia rheumatica), vasculitis (temporal arteritis, polyarteritis), nonsteroidal antiinflammatory drug–induced peptic ulcer disease, enteropathic arthritis
Morning stiffness >1 h	RA, polymyalgia rheumatica, psoriatic arthritis, ankylosing spondylitis, Reiter's syndrome, fibromyalgia
Ocular involvement	Sjögren's syndrome, Behçet's disease, Reiter's syndrome, spondyloarthropathies, juvenile arthritis, sarcoid, RA, Wegener granulomatosis, Kawasaki syndrome, enteropathic arthritis, temporal arteritis, relapsing polychondritis, hydroxychloroquine therapy
Oral ulcers (painful?)	SLE (−), Reiter's syndrome (−), enteropathic arthritis (−), lues (−), Behçet's disease (+), herpes (+), methotrexate (+), gold (+)
Genital lesions (pain?)	Gonococcal (+), Behçet's disease (+), Reiter's syndrome (−), psoriasis (−), lues (−)
Rash	SLE, psoriasis, dermatomyositis, vasculitis, cryoglobulinemia, Lyme disease, viral arthritis, rheumatic fever, adult Still's disease, Sweet's syndrome, sarcoid, erythema nodosum
Tight skin	Scleroderma, CREST syndrome, morphea, MCTD, eosinophilic fasciitis, eosinophilia myalgia syndrome, calcinosis, pseudosclerodactyly (e.g., diabetes, hypothyroidism), drugs (bleomycin, vinyl chloride)
Nail abnormalities	Psoriasis, Reiter's syndrome, onychomycosis, vasculitis, endocarditis, hypertrophic osteoarthropathy
Periungual erythema	Dermatomyositis, SLE, scleroderma, MCTD, psoriasis, Reiter's syndrome
Raynaud phenomenon	Scleroderma, MCTD, SLE, RA, inflammatory myositis, Buerger's disease, vasculitis, antiphospholipid syndrome, primary Raynaud's phenomenon
Sausage digits (dactylitis)	Reiter's syndrome, MCTD, scleroderma, psoriasis, juvenile arthritis, sarcoid, sickle cell disease
Myalgias	Fibromyalgia, polymyositis, rhabdomyolysis, vasculitis, SLE, drug-induced lupus, RA, serum sickness, adult Still's disease, hypothyroidism, viral syndromes, drugs (statins, other lipid-lowering agents)
Spinal pain	Lumbosacral strain, degenerative disc disease, spondylitis (AS, psoriatic, enteropathic, Reiter's syndrome), OA, diffuse idiopathic skeletal hyperostosis, fibromyalgia, septic disciitis, vertebral compression fracture, osteomyelitis, metastases, spinal stenosis, tuberculosis, brucellosis

Table 5 (continued)
Rheumatic Review of Symptoms

Heel pain	Spondyloarthropathies (AS, Reiter's syndrome, psoriatic, enteropathic), osteoarthritis, plantar fasciitis, Achilles tendinitis, calcaneal fracture, fluorosis, retinoid therapy
Subcutaneous nodules	RA, gout (tophi), rheumatic fever, hyperlipidemia (xanthomas), panniculitis, erythema nodosum, sarcoid, MCTD, polyarteritis, calcinosis, leprosy, multicentric reticulohistiocytosis, ganglion
Dysphagia	Lower (substernal esophageal): scleroderma, CREST syndrome, MCTD, Crohn's disease
	Upper (pharyngeal): inflammatory myositis, Sjögren's syndrome (due to xerostomia)
Gastrointestinal involvement	Scleroderma, MCTD, enteropathic arthritis, vasculitis, Behçet's disease, Whipple's disease, SLE, hepatitis, familial Mediterranean fever, intestinal bypass syndrome, primary biliary cirrhosis, cryoglobulinemia
Serositis	SLE, RA, MCTD, drug-induced lupus, rheumatic fever, adult Still's disease, familial Mediterranean fever, Whipple's disease
Pulmonary involvement	Wegener's granulomatosis, Churg-Strauss angiitis, polymyositis, SLE, scleroderma, MCTD, Sjögren's syndrome, sarcoid, RA, ankylosing spondylitis, Goodpasture's syndrome, drug-induced lupus
Neuropathy	Carpal or tarsal tunnel syndrome, SLE, vasculitis, Lyme disease, RA, amyloidosis, cryoglobulinemia, amyloidosis, drug-induced
Sleep disturbance	Fibromyalgia, osteoarthritis, rotator cuff dysfunction, AS, steroid therapy, depression, osteoid osteoma

SLE, systemic lupus erythematosus; MCTD, mixed connective tissue disease; RA, rheumatoid arthritis; AS, ankylosing spondylitis.

Table 6
Musculoskeletal Examination Checklist

The examiner should assess for
  Signs of inflammation
  Articular or periarticular structures involved
  Joint swelling
  Range of motion
  Crepitus
  Contracture or deformity
  Joint stability, subluxation, dislocation
  Muscle strength
  Gait abnormalities
  Extraarticular manifestations

Table 7
Physical Examination: Specific Signs and Maneuvers

Sign/Maneuver	Joint	Use and Description
Bulge sign	Knee	Identifies a slight to moderate synovial effusion; the examiner should manually push or "milk" joint fluid downward and laterally from the suprapatellar pouch; a visible "bulge" (or shift in fluid) may be seen medially after applying pressure lateral to the knee
Drawer sign (Lachman test)	Knee	Identifies joint instability and possible anterior cruciate tear; with the patient supine and the leg at a 90-degree angle, the examiner pulls the proximal tibia forward; excessive laxity or forward excursion may indicate an anterior cruciate tear
McMurray test	Knee	Identifies meniscal cartilage tear; with the patient supine, the hip and knee flexed and internally rotated, the limb is extended while maintaining internal torque to detect a palpable or audible snap or "pop" or intraarticular pain; the procedure should be repeated in external rotation and torque
Patrick test (FABERE test)	Hip/SI	Identifies hip and SI abnormalities (FABERE stands for flexion, abduction, external rotation, and extension); with the patient lying supine, place the foot on the contralateral knee and externally rotate at the hip by moving the knee down and out; pain in the inguinal region may indicate hip disease; the SI joint may be compressed by simultaneously pushing the flexed ipsilateral knee and contralateral superior iliac crest downward
Straight leg raising test	Lumbar/sciatic nerve	Identifies abnormalities of the lumbar nerve roots and/or sciatic nerve; with the patient lying supine and the leg straight, elevate (flex) the limb upward by grabbing the heel; normally, the leg can be raised to an angle >80 degrees before discomfort is noted; if pain is noted before this point, lower slightly and dorsiflex the foot to put stretch on the sciatic nerve; dorsiflexion-induced pain suggests sciatic nerve or lumbar nerve root abnormalities; if dorsiflexion of the foot does not cause pain, then limitation of motion may be from tight hamstring tendons

Table 7
Physical Examination: Specific Signs and Maneuvers

Schober test	SI/lumbar	Identifies limited motion in the SI or lumbar spine; with the patient standing upright, place pen marks at L5 and then 10 cm cephalad; ask the patient to bend as far forward as possible (without flexing the knees) and measure the distance between marks; normally the distance between marks will increase by >5 cm; changes of <5 cm indicate limited SI and lumbar mobility
Drop arm test	Rotator cuff	Identifies complete tear of the rotator cuff; with the patient standing or sitting upright, abduct the arm fully (90 degrees); ask the patient to slowly lower the arm to his or her side; those with a complete tear of the rotator cuff will suddenly drop the arm down in pain or will be unable to lower the arm smoothly
Finkelstein sign	Wrist	Identifies deQuervain's tenosynovitis (involving the abductor pollicus longus and extensor pollicis brevis); place the flexed thumb inside a clenched fist; ulnar deviation of the wrist will produce pain over the involved tendons on the radial aspect of the joint (positive test)
Tinel sign	Wrist, ankle	Identifies carpal tunnel syndrome (median nerve entrapment) by repetitively tapping (thumping) the volar aspect of the wrist to produce an electric-like sensation or numbness in the first lateral 3 and 1/2 digits; tarsal tunnel syndrome may be diagnosed if symptoms are elicited by thumping over the flexor retinaculum (posterior to the medial malleolus) of the ankle

SI, sacroiliac.

synovial tissue can be felt as a supple, compressible, squishy soft tissue enlargement within the margins of the joint capsule. Bursitis (i.e., olecranon, prepatellar) may manifest as a localized pain, with or without a well-defined, fluctuant, subcutaneous swelling occurring over bony extensor surfaces and lying adjacent to the joint capsule. Swelling may also be caused by bony hypertrophy that may accompany OA, neuropathic arthritis, or trauma. Such hypertrophied joints often present as asymmetric, bony-hard enlargements of juxtaarticular bone that may or may not be painful.

Range of motion should be assessed with active (patient-initiated) and passive (examiner-assisted) movement in all planes and be quantified using a goniometer or contralateral comparison. Range of motion may include flexion, extension, rotation, abduction, adduction, lateral bending, inversion, eversion,

Table 8
Joint Range of Motion

Joint	Flexion (deg)	Extension (deg)	Other
Neck	45°	>50°	Lateral bend 45°, rotation >60°
Shoulder	180°	>40°	Abduction 90°, rotation 90°
Elbow	>150°	0–5°	Pronation 80°, supination 90°
Wrist	>80°	>60°	Ulnara 60°, radial[a] 25°
MCP	>80°	>25°	
PIP	>110°	0°	
DIP	>75°	0°	
Lumbosacral	90°	30°	Lateral bend 40°, rotation 45°
Hip	120°	>15°	Abduction >45°, IR/ER[b] >45°
Knee	>135°	0–15°	Inversion 30°, eversion 20°
MTP	30°	80°	

[a]Refers to radial or ulnar deviation.

[b]IR/ER, inversion and eversion.

MCP, metacarpophalangeal; PIP, proximal interphalangeal; DIP, distal interphalangeal; MTP, metatarsophalangeal.

supination, pronation, and ulnar or radial deviation. The expected range of motion for individual joints is shown in Table 8. Findings may be recorded as either the arc of movement (in degrees) or that which is lacking (e.g., the shoulder lacked 30 degrees of full abduction).

Joint crepitus may be felt during these maneuvers. Whereas fine crepitus is common and insignificant in most large joints, coarse crepitus indicates advanced cartilaginous and degenerative changes. Joint motion may be limited by effusion, pain, deformity, or contracture.

Contractures often indicate antecedent synovial inflammation or trauma. Joint deformity suggests chronic joint pathology that may result from ligamentous destruction, soft tissue contracture, bony enlargement, ankylosis, erosive disease, or subluxation.

Joint stability can be assessed by palpation and by application of manual stress, and maneuvers such as the "drawer" sign may be used to diagnose cruciate ligament damage (Table 7). Subluxation or dislocation can be assessed by inspection and palpation.

The muscle examination will document strength and the presence of atrophy and also will elicit pain or spasm. Muscle strength testing should assess the musculature of the neck, trunk, and distal and proximal extremities and be quantified as shown in Table 9. The clinician should observe the patient rising from the chair. The gait should be observed and recorded if abnormal.

The examiner should carefully seek periarticular involvement, especially when articular complaints are not supported by objective findings referable to the joint capsule. Identification of periarticular pain helps prevent unwarranted and often expensive additional evaluations. Examples of periarticular

Table 9
Medical Research Council Scale for Grading Muscle Strength

0 = No movement
1 = Trace (flicker) movement
2 = Able to move with gravity eliminated
3 = Able to move against gravity, but not resistance
4 = Able to oppose gravity and resistance
5 = Normal strength

abnormalities include olecranon bursitis, epicondylitis (i.e., tennis elbow), enthesitis (i.e., Achilles tendinitis), and trigger points associated with fibromyalgia. In selected instances, specific maneuvers may be used (Table 7) to identify extraarticular abnormalities, such as a carpal tunnel syndrome (identified by the Tinel sign).

Further Investigations

The vast majority of rheumatic conditions can be easily diagnosed by a complete history and physical examination. Further investigations are infrequently required to establish the correct diagnosis. The clinician should avoid the temptation to use screening tests or broad batteries (rheumatic panels) of tests as an aid to diagnosis. Indiscriminate testing is expensive and often yields results with low predictive value. The utility and predictive value of rheumatic tests are disappointingly low when the pretest probability of a specific diagnosis is low. Primary indications for further testing include any monarticular presentation (consider arthrocentesis), systemic features (e.g., fever, rash), neurologic manifestations, antecedent trauma (consider radiographs, imaging), or chronic symptoms that are undiagnosed after an appropriate evaluation, symptomatic therapy, and observation over time (> 6 weeks).

Any history of recent trauma should prompt a careful examination and consideration of an appropriate imaging procedure. If necessary, laboratory investigations may include a complete blood count, selected chemistries, an acute-phase reactant (e.g., erythrocyte sedimentation rate or C-reactive protein), and possibly a serum uric acid level if gout is clinically suspected. Routine serologic testing for antinuclear antibodies or rheumatoid factor should be discouraged unless warranted by the clinical picture. Advanced serologic testing (e.g., anti-neutrophil cytoplasmic antibody, HLA-B27, anti-streptolysin [ASO]) is only indicated in selected clinical situations. Finally, arthrocentesis and synovial fluid analysis should be considered for patients with monarthritis, suspected infection, or crystal-induced arthritis or when the diagnosis is uncertain. The following chapters review the use, indications, and interpretation of synovial fluid testing, arthrocentesis, and commonly used diagnostic tests and imaging modalities.

BIBLIOGRAPHY

Cush JJ, Lipsky PE. Approach to articular and musculoskeletal disorders. In: Fauci AS, Braunwald E, Isselbacher KJ, et al., eds. Harrison's Principles of Internal Medicine, 14th ed. New York: McGraw-Hill, 1998:1928–1935.

Fries JF, Mitchell DM. Joint pain or arthritis. *JAMA* 1976;253:199–204.

Lipsky PE, Alarcon GS, Bombardier C, et al. Algorithms for the diagnosis and management of musculoskeletal complaints. *Am J Med* 1997;103:49S–85S.

Pincus T. A pragmatic approach to cost-effective use of laboratory tests and imaging procedures in patients with musculoskeletal symptoms. *Prim Care* 1993;20:795–814.

Wernick R. Avoiding laboratory test misinterpretation. *Geriatrics* 1989;44:61.

CHAPTER 1.2

SYNOVIAL FLUID ANALYSIS AND ARTHROCENTESIS

SYNOVIAL FLUID (SF) ANALYSIS

Description: SF analysis is often used to aid differential diagnosis and therapy. SF, the transudative product of type B synoviocytes, serves as a local lubricant and medium for nutrient replenishment to cartilage and other intraarticular structures. The primary goal of SF analysis is to discern whether a synovial effusion is noninflammatory, inflammatory, septic, or hemorrhagic.

Method: SF is primarily obtained by needle aspiration. A stepwise approach to joint aspiration and injection is detailed in Table 1. Joint fluid may also be obtained during other diagnostic and therapeutic procedures (i.e., arthrogram, arthroscopy, arthroplasty). SF usually will not clot but may with high fibrinogen levels (inflammatory states). Aspirated SF should be promptly divided among plain (red top) tubes (for glucose, if necessary), sodium (not lithium) heparin tubes (for crystals), EDTA (for cell count, differential, complement), or sterile culture tubes. If gonococcal arthritis is suspected, immediate inoculation on Thayer-Martin media is recommended. Delay in SF analysis may lower white blood cell (WBC) counts and increase the number of birefringent artifacts. Whereas the number of calcium pyrophosphate dihydrate (CPPD) crystals may decrease over time (i.e., weeks), monosodium urate (MSU) crystals will not. If the sample cannot be promptly analyzed, refrigerate at 4°C.

Crystal Analysis: A wet preparation requires only a few drops of SF. Glass slides and coverslips should be clean and free of dust and other potentially birefringent debris. Crystals can been seen under plain light microscopy but are best seen under the polarizing microscope.

—Gout: MSU crystals, seen in gouty effusions, are long, needle shaped, and negatively birefringent; they are usually intracellular during acute attacks.

—Pseudogout: CPPD crystals, found in pseudogout and chondrocalcinosis, are usually shorter, rhomboid or needle shaped, and positively birefringent.

—Cholesterol crystals: These appear as translucent "stacked panes of glass."

—Calcium oxalate crystals: These are positively birefringent and bipyramidal in shape.

—Hydroxyapatite crystals: These are not routinely seen and may only be identified by electron microscopy or by staining with alizarin red.

Table 1
Procedure for Arthrocentesis and Joint Injection

- Inform patient of purpose, expected benefits, and side effects of the procedure
- Document an informed consent to the procedure (verbal or written)
- Check for allergies: iodine, lidocaine, or adhesives?
- Position patient to maximize patient comfort and joint exposure
- Identify bony landmarks with pen
- Identify puncture site with imprint from retracted end of ballpoint pen
- Wash hands before procedure and wear gloves (required by Occupational Safety Health Administration)
- Prepare and lay out syringes, needles, corticosteroid, and anesthetic to be used
- Cleanse injection site with povidone iodine solution
- Begin with topical anesthetic (i.e., ethyl chloride) and spray until a light frost appears
- Swab site with alcohol preparation
- Keep the injection site sterile
- Speak to patient and inform of each step; pain may be felt while lidocaine is instilled (described as "burning") or when needle penetrates an inflamed joint capsule or bursa (described as "sharp")
- Use 22-, 23-, or 25-gauge needle for local anesthesia and joint injection
- Slowly infiltrate anesthetic (lidocaine), pausing before each advance of the needle
- With each advance, draw back on the plunger before injecting
- Switch to an 18-gauge needle (or largest possible) if aspirating joint fluid
- Use hemostat to clamp and stabilize needle while changing syringes
- Use a 5- or 10-mL syringe to aspirate joint fluid; reposition needle if necessary
- Synovial fluid may not always be obtained once inside the joint; if large amount of fluid remains, leave needle in place, use 20- or 30-mL syringes to withdraw
- Once "tapped dry," a corticosteroid preparation, with or without a small amount of lidocaine, may be instilled by leaving the needle in place, stabilizing it with a hemostat, and changing syringes
- Remove needle and apply local pressure for 2–4 min (longer if patients are on nonsteroidal antiinflammatory drugs, anticoagulant, or antiplatelet therapy)
- Process synovial fluid specimen promptly (i.e., laboratory workup, cultures, polarized microscopy)
- Advise home (bed/chair) rest and ice the injected site (ice packs every 2–3 h for 20 min) for the 24–36 h after injection
- Immobilization for 24–72 h after injection may improve outcome
- Counsel patient to call or return if fever or local pain/erythema develops
- Record volume withdrawn, color, appearance, viscosity, microscopic findings, and tests ordered on patient's chart

—Negative birefringence (i.e., MSU crystals): Present if the crystal appears yellow when parallel to the axis of the compensator and blue when perpendicular.

—Positive birefringence (i.e., CPPD crystals): Present if the crystal appears blue when parallel to the axis of the compensator and yellow when perpendicular.

Normal Values: Normal SF is transparent, clear, and colorless or pale straw colored. It is normally viscous, owing to high levels of hyaluronate. Expression of a drop of fluid from the syringe tip will produce a long, viscous, string-like tail ("string" sign). Viscosity, hyaluronate, and string sign are lost with inflammatory states. Normal SF WBC counts are <200 cells/mm³, with a predominance of mononuclear cells. Normally, small amounts (5 mL) of joint fluid are present in large (i.e., knee) joints and may also be obtained from small (i.e., finger) joints. When available, SF should be examined for appearance, viscosity, and WBC count and differential. The clinician should determine the need for polarized microscopy, bacteriologic cultures, fungal cultures, and cytology. Whenever infection is suspected, SF should be Gram stained and cultured appropriately.

Not Recommended: SF protein, albumin, glucose, lactate dehydrogenase, complement, and serologic tests are of no diagnostic value in the analysis of SF. Nonetheless, protein, albumin, and complement levels are lower than serum values; the glucose concentration is normal and usually within 10 to 15 mg/dL of serum values.

Abnormal SF: SF is abnormal in a variety of conditions, including osteoarthritis, meniscal and cruciate tears, inflammatory arthritis (i.e., rheumatoid arthritis), crystal arthritis (i.e., gout), and hemorrhagic conditions. Table 2 details SF abnormalities and their disease associations. In noninflammatory conditions, SF WBC counts are between 200 and 2,000 cells/mm³. In inflammatory states, SF WBC counts range from 2,000 to 75,000 cells/mm³ and show a predominance of neutrophils. Septic effusions often have WBC counts ranging from 60,000 to 500,000 cells/mm³, with an even greater percentage of neutrophils. In most bacterially induced septic arthritides, SF has >90% neu-

Table 2
Synovial Fluid Analysis

	Noninflammatory Type I	Inflammatory Type II	Septic Type III	Hemorrhagic Type IV
Appearance	Yellow	Yellow	Purulent	Bloody
Clarity	Clear	Cloudy	Opaque	Opaque
Viscosity	High	Decreased	Decreased	Variable
Cell count	200–2,000	2,000–75,000	>60,000	RBCs >>
(% PMNs)	(<25% PMNs)	(>50% PMNs)	(>80% PMNs)	WBCs
Example	Osteoarthritis, trauma, osteonecrosis, SLE	RA, Reiter's syndrome crystal arthritis SLE, viral arthritis, fungal arthritis, TB arthritis	Bacterial arthritis, crystal arthritis,	Trauma, fracture, ligament tear, hemophilia, Charcot arthritis, PVNS

RBCs, red blood cells; WBCs, white blood cells; PMNs, polymorphonuclear leukocyte; RA, rheumatoid arthritis; SLE, systemic lupus erythematosus; TB, tuberculosis; PVNS, pigmented villonodular synovitis.

trophils. SF WBC counts between 20,000 and 60,000 cells/mm³ may be seen in some infectious arthritides (i.e., gonococcal, fungal, tuberculous) or previously treated (i.e., antibiotics) septic arthritis. Gouty effusions occasionally yield SF WBC counts >60,000 cells/mm³.

Indications: SF should be analyzed when available. Indications for arthrocentesis are given below.

Comment: With only a few drops of SF, the examiner can do a visual inspection, assess viscosity, and perform SF culture, polarized microscopy, and a peripheral smear to gauge the number and type of cells present. Crystal arthritis may coexist with septic arthritis or other inflammatory arthritides; however, coexistence of gout and rheumatoid arthritis is very rare.

BIBLIOGRAPHY

Schmerling RH, Delbanco ML, Tosteson ANA, et al. Synovial fluid test: what should be ordered? JAMA 1990;264:1009–1014.
Siva C, Velazquez C, Mody A, et al. Diagnosing acute monoarthritis in adults: a practical approach for the family physician. Am Fam Physician 2003;68:83–90.

ARTHROCENTESIS

Description: Techniques for needle aspiration and injection of joints.

Indications: Indications for needle aspiration and injection of joints include (a) any undiagnosed acute or chronic monarthritis with effusion, (b) suspected infection or crystal-induced arthritis, (c) unexplained exacerbation of preexisting polyarthritis, (d) joint effusion after trauma, (e) intraarticular treatment (e.g., corticosteroids), (f) injection of contrast media for diagnostic arthrography, and (g) uncertain diagnosis. Clinical situations in which joint aspiration and injection with corticosteroids may be beneficial include painful monarticular osteoarthritis, focal pain/swelling in rheumatoid arthritis, acute gout or pseudogout, acute bursitis or tendinitis, early adhesive capsulitis, and possibly reflex sympathetic dystrophy.

Contraindications: Relative contraindications for intraarticular injection include suspected septic arthritis or bursitis (do not inject steroids!), overlying cellulitis, known bacteremia, neuropathic (Charcot disease) joint, joint pain secondary to referred pain, thrombocytopenia (platelet count <50,000/mm³), coagulopathy, anticoagulant therapy, uncontrolled diabetes, lack of response to previous injection, prosthetic joints, and inaccessible joints (i.e., hip, sacroiliac).

Method: Access to periarticular structures (i.e., bursae), joint cavity, or SF is best achieved by percutaneous needle aspiration. Table 1 details the steps involved in arthrocentesis. Preparation of commonly used materials into an "arthrocentesis tray" facilitates the process (Table 3). Many large (i.e., knee, shoulder) and small (i.e., metacarpophalangeal, sternoclavicular) joints are eas-

Table 3
Contents of Arthrocentesis Tray

Gloves (nonsterile)
Povidone iodine solution
Alcohol preparations
Gauze
Ethyl chloride spray (topical anesthetic)
Hemostat
1.5-in. sterile needles (18, 22, 23 g)
1-in. sterile needles (21, 23, 25 g)
Syringes
   3 mL (to inject steroid or lidocaine)
   5 mL (to instill lidocaine)
   10 mL (for initial synovial fluid withdrawal)
   20 or 30 mL (withdraw large amount of synovial fluid)
Tubes
   EDTA acid/lavender (cell count)
   Heparin/green (crystals, in vitro studies)
Single-dose vials of 1% lidocaine (without epinephrine)
Single-dose vials of corticosteroid preparation
Sterile container, culture media
Glass slides/coverslips
Band-Aids
Ballpoint pen
Cup or basin (for waste)

ily aspirated. Difficult or inaccessible joints should not be attempted by routine needle aspiration. Thus, fluoroscopically guided arthrocentesis is best suited for the hip, sacroiliac, apophyseal, toe interphalangeal, and temporomandibular joints. The operator should select an injection site after identifying anatomic landmarks and the point of maximal fluctuance or tenderness. Prepare all syringes before starting. Povidone iodine solution and alcohol swabs should be used to maintain a sterile field. (See below for methods used in arthrocentesis of selected joints.)

Precautions: Occupational Safety and Health Administration guidelines state that gloves (sterile or nonsterile) should be worn by the clinician and assistant(s) throughout the procedure and that sterile technique should be observed when handling needles, syringes, and joint fluid. Gloves and all materials contaminated by blood or SF should be disposed of in appropriate "sharps" or biohazard containers. Patients with a history of valvular heart disease should receive appropriate antibiotic prophylaxis before the procedure. Hand washing before and after arthrocentesis is advised.

Record: When applicable, the volume withdrawn, color, appearance, viscosity, cell count and differential; crystal appearance by light or polarized microscopy; Gram stain, culture, and sensitivity results; culture for acid-fast bacilli or fungi; and cytology should be recorded.

Avoid: SF protein or glucose; SF urate, lactate dehydrogenase, autoantibodies (i.e., rheumatoid factor, antinuclear antibody, lupus erythematosus cells); mucin clot test; pH; or complement testing should not be done. A low SF glucose level (50% of serum value) may be seen in rheumatoid arthritis, tuberculosis, and other forms of septic arthritis but is infrequent and not specific.

Complications: Although infrequent, the most common complications include allergic reactions (to iodine, adhesive, lidocaine), vasovagal episodes, local ecchymoses, and exacerbation of hyperglycemia in diabetics. Uncommonly, postinjection flares, corticosteroid crystal–induced synovitis, depigmentation of overlying skin, and subcutaneous atrophy are seen. Skin or joint infection, hemarthrosis, and calcification or rupture of periarticular structures are rare events with proper technique.

Therapy: Corticosteroid injection may provide significant relief as the sole therapy or as adjunctive therapy in many conditions. Steroid preparations vary in equivalent potency and diluent. (See Table 4 for a comparison of common parenteral steroid preparations.) Ideally, single-dose vials or ampules of steroids and lidocaine should be used to avoid medication sharing between patients. Whereas water-soluble steroids tend to be absorbed rapidly and have shorter durations of action, the converse is true for the insoluble steroid preparations (Table 4). The needle size and volume of steroid to be instilled depend on the relative size of the joint (Table 5). Lidocaine (1% solution) without epinephrine may be used for local anesthesia during the procedure. Depending on the size of the joint, 0.5 to 3 mL of lidocaine may be used for soft tissue anesthesia. Soft tissue anesthesia is recommended if aspiration of SF or difficulty with joint access is anticipated. Intraarticular steroid may be mixed with 0.25 to 0.5 mL (depending on size of joint/bursa) of 1% lidocaine to provide immediate pain relief, improve range of motion, and confirm the adequacy of injection. Corticosteroids should not be instilled into joints that are potentially

Table 4

Comparison of Commonly Used Intraarticular Corticosteroids Preparations

Trade Name	Generic Name	Concentration (mg/mL)	Equivalent Doses	Range of Water Solubility	Dosing (mg/mL)
Depo-Medrol	Methylprednisolone acetate	20, 40, 80	4	Insoluble	10–80
Aristospan	Triamcinolone hexacetonide	20	4	Insoluble	5–40
Kenalog, Aristocort	Triamcinolone acetonide	20	4	Soluble	5–40
Celestone	Betamethasone acetate	6	0.6	Insoluble	1.5–6
Hydeltra	Prednisolone tebutate	20	5	Soluble	5–50

Table 5
Materials and Doses for Joint Injections

Joint	Needle Length (gauge)[a]	Volume of Intraarticular Injection (mL)	Dose of Depo-Medrol (mg)
Knee	1.5 in. (22/18)	1–3	40–80
Shoulder	1.5 in. (22/18 or 19)	1–3	40–60
Wrist	1–1.5 in. (22/19)	0.5–2	20–40
Ankle	1.5 in. (22/19)	0.5–2	20–40
Elbow	1.5 in. (22/18)	0.5–2	20–40
MCP	5/8–1 in. (25/21)	0.25–0.5	5–10
PIP	5/8–1 in. (25/23)	0.25–0.5	5–10
MTP	5/8–1 in. (25/21)	0.25–0.5	5–10

[a] Sizes suggested apply to needle gauge during instillation only or aspiration/instillation, respectively.

septic, unstable, or neuropathic. Bed/home rest for 24 to 36 hours is recommended, with immobilization and local application of ice every 2 to 3 hours. An extended period of immobilization may enhance the outcome of the procedure but should be combined with nontraumatic, non–weight-bearing range-of-motion exercises.

Comment: The maximum number of steroid injections per site is not known but should kept to a minimum. A safe recommendation is to limit intraarticular/periarticular steroid injections to three or less per year per site, not to be repeated in consecutive years. Repetitive injections may become less effective, may adversely affect cartilage, and may increase the risk of infection or tendon rupture.

BIBLIOGRAPHY

Dooley P, Martin R. Corticosteroid injections and arthrocentesis. Can Fam Physician 2002;48:285–292.

Pfenninger JL. Injections of joints and soft tissue: part I. General guidelines. Am Fam Physician 1991;44:1196–1202.

Pfenninger JL. Injections of joints and soft tissue: part II. Guidelines for specific joints. Am Fam Physician 1991;44:1690–1702.

KNEE (PATELLOFEMORAL) ARTHROCENTESIS

Patient Position: Patient should lie supine and be made comfortable with the head supported and slightly inclined. If a flexion contracture exists, use pillows to support and position the knee so that the quadriceps is relaxed during the procedure.

Limb Position: The leg should be parallel to the ground and the knee may be slightly flexed. Remove the shoe and position the foot perpendicular to the ground so that the leg is neither externally nor internally rotated.

DIAGNOSIS

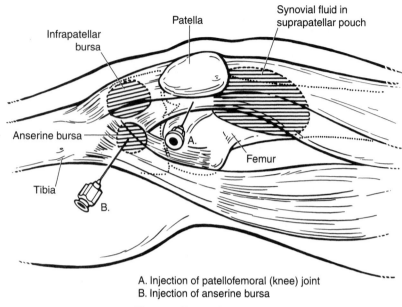

A. Injection of patellofemoral (knee) joint
B. Injection of anserine bursa

Figure 1. Knee arthrocentesis.

Bony Landmarks: Mark the medial, lateral, superior, and inferior borders of the patella (Fig. 1).

Site/Angle of Entry: Use a medial or lateral approach. Site selection should be based on maximum fluctuance (for aspiration) or tenderness (for injection). The needle should be placed between the midpoint and superior pole, 1 cm below the edge of the patella. The axis of entry is perpendicular to the leg, with a 20- to 25-degree downward tilt to avoid the underside of the patella. The needle should be advanced more than 3 cm to enter the joint space. Aspirate before injecting.

Amount of Injection: Use 40 to 80 mg of Depo-Medrol (methylprednisolone) (or equivalent), with or without 0.5 mL of 1% lidocaine, in a total volume of 1 to 3 mL.

Other Injectable Sites: With anserine bursitis, the bursae may be injected with the patient seated or supine. The bursa may be entered from the medial side, tangentially, at a 30-degree angle, injecting 20 to 40 mg Depo-Medrol (Fig. 1).

Comment: SF aspiration may be facilitated by manually compressing fluid downward ("milking") from the suprapatellar pouch into the joint space.

SHOULDER (GLENOHUMERAL) ARTHROCENTESIS

Patient Position: The patient should be seated upright with the shoulder joint fully exposed.

Limb Position: Place the patient's arms at the side, with hands on lap and palms facing upward so that the glenohumeral joint is partially externally rotated.

Bony Landmarks: Palpate the acromion (laterally), humeral head and coracoid process (anteriorly), bicipital tendon and groove (anterolaterally), and the acromioclavicular joint (superiorly). The humeral head is best palpated by placing the thumb over the joint anteriorly and having the patient internally and externally rotate the humerus.

Site/Angle of Entry: The entry site is anterior to where the humeral head can be felt to rotate inward (under the thumb) during rotation. This site is just inferior and lateral to the coracoid process (Fig. 2). The axis of entry is parallel to the ground, directly into the shoulder but angled (10–15 degrees) toward the midscapula. The needle should be fully advanced (>3 cm) to enter the joint. Aspirate before injecting.

Amount of Injection: Use 20 to 40 mg Depo-Medrol (or equivalent), with or without 0.5 mL of 1% lidocaine, in a total volume of 1 to 3 mL.

Other Injectable Sites: The subacromial (subdeltoid) bursa may be injected using the same patient/limb position (Fig. 2). Use 20 to 40 mg Depo-Medrol (or equivalent) with 0.5 mL of 1% lidocaine. After locating the point of maximal tenderness, enter laterally 1 cm beneath the acromion, with the needle axis parallel to the ground. The bicipital tendon may be injected tangentially after palpating the tendon, bicipital groove, and point of maximal tenderness. Do not inject into the tendon but instead inject close to the tendon sheath by advancing the needle until the tendon is felt, then withdrawing 1 to 2 mm.

Comment: Concomitant use of lidocaine allows the operator to gauge the adequacy of injection because many patients can "suddenly" move the shoulder more freely and without pain at the completion of the procedure.

WRIST (RADIOCARPAL) ARTHROCENTESIS

Patient Position: The patient may be seated or lying supine.

Limb Position: The wrist, hand, and forearm should be comfortable and parallel to the ground. A small towel can be rolled into a 3- to 4-cm elevation and put under the wrist, leaving it slightly flexed (10 degrees).

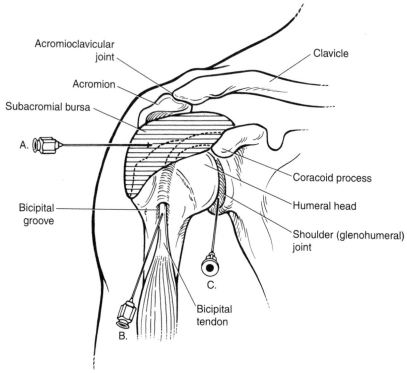

Figure 2. Shoulder arthrocentesis.

Bony Landmarks: Medially, palpate the tip of the ulnar styloid; laterally, the tip of the radial styloid; and dorsally, the extensor pollicis longus tendon. Draw a line (visually) from the tip of the ulnar to radial styloid (Fig. 3). Ask the patient to fully extend the thumb and note where the extensor pollicis longus tendon rises to bisect this line. The injection site is to the ulnar side of this intersection. Confirm this site by palpating along the radius, moving distally until the depression of the radiocarpal joint is felt.

Site/Entry Angle: Using a dorsal (extensor) approach, enter downward at a 90-degree angle to the ulnar side of the extensor pollicis longus tendon (away from the anatomic "snuff box"). The needle should be advanced more than 2 cm into the joint space. Aspirate before injecting.

Amount of Injection: Use 10 to 40 mg Depo-Medrol (or equivalent), with or without 0.25 mL of 1% lidocaine, in a total volume of 0.5 to 2 mL.

Other Injectable Sites: De Quervain tenosynovitis, affecting the extensor pollicis brevis and abductor pollicis longus tendons, may be injected with the

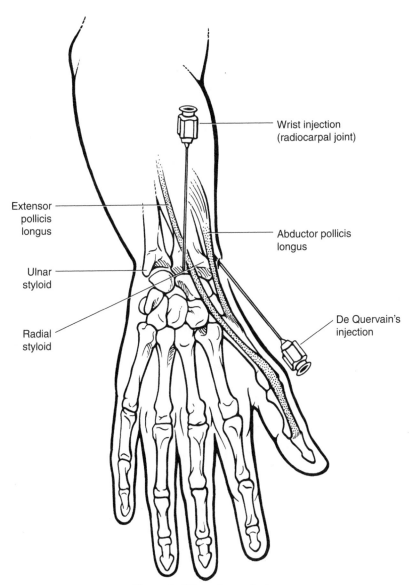

Wrist injection
(radiocarpal joint)

Extensor
pollicis
longus

Abductor pollicis
longus

Ulnar
styloid

De Quervain's
injection

Radial
styloid

Figure 3. Wrist arthrocentesis.

same amount of steroid preparation. Rotate the hand 90 degrees (thumb up) and place the wrist in slight ulnar deviation. Locate the point of maximal tenderness over the affected tendon. Enter tangentially at a 30-degree angle. Do not inject into the tendon but close to the tendon sheath.

ANKLE ARTHROCENTESIS

Patient Position: The patient should lie supine (or be seated) on the examination table.

Limb Position: In a lying position, the patient's foot should be positioned perpendicular to the floor and partially plantar flexed (75 degrees).

Bony Landmarks: Medially, palpate the tip of the medial malleolus; laterally, the tip of the lateral malleolus; and anteriorly, the extensor hallucis longus tendon. Draw a line (visually) from medial to lateral malleoli. Ask the patient to dorsiflex the big toe and note where the extensor hallucis longus tendon rises to bisect this line (Fig. 4). The injection site is medial to the tendon intersection.

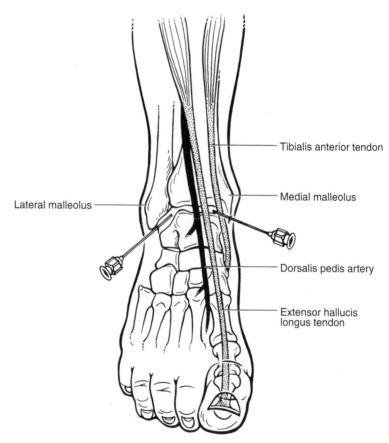

Figure 4. Ankle arthrocentesis.

Site/Angle of Entry: To inject the true ankle joint, use an anteromedial approach and place the needle at the injection site described above. Enter at a 90-degree angle (perpendicular to the floor) and direct the needle slightly laterally (toward the Achilles tendon). The needle should be advanced more than 3 cm into the joint space. The ankle may also be approached laterally (adjacent to the subtalar joint) using the same positioning, but entering just anterior to and beneath the lateral malleolus, with a slight inward angle. Aspirate before injecting.

Amount of Injection: Use 20 to 40 mg Depo-Medrol (or equivalent), with or without 0.25 mL of 1% lidocaine, in a total volume of 0.5 to 3 mL.

TROCHANTERIC BURSAL INJECTION

Patient Position: The patient should lie on his or her side, with the painful trochanter ("hip") facing up.

Limb Position: The legs should be comfortably extended, side by side.

Bony Landmarks: Usually the greater trochanter is the most elevated point over the hip curvature. Using one finger, identify the point of maximal tenderness over the bony greater trochanter.

Entry Angle: The needle should be directed downward at a 90-degree angle and slowly advanced until the tip pierces the painful bursa or touches the trochanter. Aspirate before injecting.

Amount of Injection: Use 40 to 60 mg Depo-Medrol (or equivalent) and 0.5 mL of 1% lidocaine in a total volume of 0.5 to 1.5 mL.

Comment: When entering an inflamed bursa, the operator may feel a "pop" or the patient may note a sudden sharp pain. Rarely is there sufficient bursal fluid to aspirate.

DIAGNOSTIC TESTS

ANGIOTENSIN-CONVERTING ENZYME (ACE)

Description: ACE catalyzes the conversion of angiotensin I to the potent vasopressor angiotensin II. ACE also inactivates the vasodilator bradykinin. Although it is produced primarily by endothelial and epithelial cells, ACE may also be synthesized in substantial quantities by activated macrophages in some pathologic conditions such as sarcoidosis.

Method: ACE is measured by bioassay; for example, an inhibitor-binding assay. Normal values may vary, and results must be interpreted according to laboratory standards.

Increased in: Elevated serum ACE levels are often associated with sarcoidosis and may be found in approximately 80% of patients with sarcoidosis, primarily in those with lung involvement. However, increased serum ACE levels are not specific for sarcoidosis and may also be found in conditions such as interstitial lung disease of various etiologies (e.g., asbestosis, silicosis), hematologic malignancies (e.g., Hodgkin's disease), endocrine diseases (e.g., hyperthyroidism and diabetes mellitus), and infections (e.g., leprosy). Moreover, patients with sarcoidosis may have normal serum ACE levels, depending on the organ involvement and extent and activity of disease. Also, although ACE levels have been reported to decrease after successful treatment of patients with sarcoidosis, this is not universally true. Thus, serum ACE levels must be interpreted carefully in sarcoidosis. Decreased serum levels of ACE have been suggested to indicate endothelial injury (e.g., in patients with scleroderma).

ACE has also been measured in fluids other than serum, including cerebrospinal fluid (CSF) and bronchoalveolar lavage fluid. Although suggested to be of diagnostic utility (e.g., increased ACE levels in the CSF suggesting neurosarcoidosis), interpretation of results of these tests is somewhat controversial. Until their utility is established, they are probably most appropriately considered research tools.

Confounding Factors: Factors that affect ACE levels include storage temperature, and samples kept frozen overnight or longer may have spuriously high values when tested.

Cost: $40–90.

BIBLIOGRAPHY

Lawrence EC. Serial changes in markers of disease activity with corticosteroid treatment in sarcoidosis. *Am J Med* 1983;74:747–756.

ACUTE-PHASE REACTANTS (ERYTHROCYTE SEDIMENTATION RATE, C-REACTIVE PROTEIN)

Description: Acute-phase reactants are a group of plasma proteins normally produced by the liver. Synthesis of these diverse proteins increases greatly in response to inflammatory stimuli in both acute and chronic settings. Examples of acute-phase reactants include (a) coagulation proteins (fibrinogen, prothrombin), (b) transport proteins (haptoglobin, transferrin, ceruloplasmin), (c) complement components (C3, C4), and (d) miscellaneous proteins [fibronectin, serum amyloid A, C-reactive protein (CRP), ferritin].

Acute-phase reactants are commonly used as an indirect measure of the extent of inflammation. For rheumatic diseases, the most commonly used acute-phase reactants are the CRP and the erythrocyte sedimentation rate (ESR). The ESR measures the rate of gravitational settling of erythrocytes and rouleaux formation, which is accelerated by a variety of factors, the most important of which is fibrinogen that lessens the negative charge between red blood cells (RBCs).

Method: In practice, the two most often used clinical tests for the acute-phase reactants are the ESR and CRP. The CRP is most often (and accurately) measured by rate nephelometry (an automated antigen/antibody-mediated reaction). The ESR is performed by the Westergren method (recommended by the International Committee for Standardization in Hematology) and uses anticoagulated venous blood, diluted 4:1 with sodium citrate and placed in a 200-mm glass tube with a 2.5-mm internal diameter. At the end of 1 hour, the distance (in millimeters) from the meniscus (plasma and sodium citrate) to the top of the column of erythrocytes is recorded as the ESR. The modified Westergren method substitutes ethylenediaminetetraacetic acid (EDTA) for sodium citrate and enables the same sample of blood to be used for other tests. Both methods yield identical results.

Normal Values: CRP is normally <0.8 mg/dL and is less affected by age or gender than the ESR. In young men, the ESR ranges from 0 to 13 mm/h and from 0 to 20 mm/h in women. Importantly, the ESR increases with advancing age. Rough formulas for age-adjusted estimates of ESR are as follows: men: ESR = age in years/2; women: ESR = (age in years + 10)/2.

Increased in: The ESR and CRP are increased in a variety of disorders including

—*Acute or chronic inflammatory disorders:* Gout, rheumatoid arthritis (RA), rheumatic fever, spondyloarthropathies, polymyalgia rheumatica, giant cell arteritis and other forms of vasculitis, inflammatory bowel disease, etc.

—*Tissue injury/necrosis:* Acute myocardial infarction, tissue ischemia or infarction, transplant rejection, malignant tumors, after surgery, burns, and trauma
—*Infections:* Bacterial (e.g., endocarditis, osteomyelitis, intraabdominal infections) and some viral infections (e.g., acute viral hepatitis)
—*Miscellaneous:* May also be elevated in late pregnancy and postpartum, hyper- and hypothyroidism, azotemia, nephrotic syndrome. *Note:* More than 10% of very high ESR (>75 mm/h) values lack an identifiable cause. This is particularly true in the elderly. The physician should wait and repeat the test in 3 to 6 months and not routinely embark on an exhaustive, expensive, or invasive search for an occult neoplastic, infectious, or inflammatory process.

Decreased in: The ESR may be low with RBC abnormalities (polycythemia, microcytosis, spherocytosis, sickle cell, other hemoglobinopathies), hypofibrinogenemia, congestive heart failure, and cachexia and in those on high-dose corticosteroids or tumor necrosis factor inhibitors. The ESR and CRP may be normal in patients with systemic lupus erythematosus (SLE), polymyositis, scleroderma, pregnancy, osteoarthritis, and most viral infections.

Confounding Factors: The ESR may be increased by macrocytosis, hypercholesterolemia, increased fibrinogen, and high ambient temperatures. The ESR may be decreased by disorders of RBC morphology (see above), high leukocyte counts, hyperviscosity states, or a delay (>2 hours) in testing.

Indications: The acute-phase reactants may be used in to distinguish inflammatory from noninflammatory disorders. Although nonspecific, they may be diagnostically or therapeutically useful. The American College of Physicians recommends that the ESR be used in the diagnosis and monitoring of polymyalgia rheumatica, temporal arteritis, and Hodgkin disease. With inflammatory disorders such as RA, the ESR should primarily be used to resolve conflicting clinical data (e.g., the patient whose examination improves but subjective complaints do not). Nonetheless, there is a long history of experience with the ESR in diagnosis and monitoring of inflammatory disorders such as RA.

The CRP is useful in monitoring disease activity and response to therapy in chronic inflammatory disorders (e.g., RA). Some prefer the CRP to the ESR in monitoring inflammatory disease because changes are more acute. The CRP increases rapidly after an inflammatory stimulus and returns to normal within days; the ESR may take days to increase and may return to normal values over weeks. Also, the CRP is more dynamic (the difference between the levels seen in inflammatory and normal states is greater). Surgeons sometimes prefer to monitor the CRP and use very high elevations in CRP to indicate postoperative infection because the ESR may be elevated owing to the surgery itself. In inflammatory conditions associated with protein-losing nephropathy, such as SLE, the ESR may always be elevated, and the CRP may be a better indicator of superimposed infection.

Cost: ESR, $19–36; CRP, $25–55; ferritin, $45–65.

Table 1
Comparison of the CRP and ESR

Acute-Phase Reactant	Advantages	Disadvantages
CRP	Rises and falls early less age dependent Few confounding factors Uninfluenced by RBC shape Fewer technical errors	Results may take longer Physicians less familiar Not well studied in diseases other than RA (e.g., SLE) Slightly more expensive than ESR
ESR	Simple to perform Readily available Greater familiarity Inexpensive	Rises and falls slowly Age and gender dependent Potential confounding factors Influenced by RBC morphology Technical errors can give false results

CRP, C-reactive protein; RA, rheumatoid arthritis; RBC, red blood cell; SLE, systemic lupus erythematosus; ESR, erythrocyte sedimentation rate.

Comments: Although the CRP generally parallels the ESR, it increases earlier than the ESR (4–6 hours) and returns to normal first. It is especially useful in situations in which the ESR results may be affected by confounding variables (anemia, polycythemia, abnormal RBC morphology, hypergammaglobulinemia, and congestive heart failure). The CRP is superior to the ESR in assessing disease activity and therapy in RA (Table 1).

The ESR is never diagnostic of a single disease, and trends may be more valuable than a single result. Extreme elevations (>100 mm/h) may suggest cancer, vasculitis (e.g., giant cell arteritis), adult-onset Still disease, spondyloarthropathy, or serious infections. Normal values do not exclude disease. It is not useful as a screening test in asymptomatic individuals.

BIBLIOGRAPHY

Otterness IG. The value of C-reactive protein measurement in rheumatoid arthritis. *Semin Arthritis Rheum* 1994;24:91–104.
Pepys MB, Hirschfield GM. C-reactive protein: a critical update. *Clin Invest* 2003;111:1805–1812.
Sox HC, Liang MW. The erythrocyte sedimentation rate: guidelines for rational use. *Ann Intern Med* 1986;104:515–523.

ALDOLASE

Synonyms: Fructose biphosphate aldolase.

Description: Aldolase is an enzyme that is elevated in some forms of muscle disease. Aldolase can be found in many tissues including skeletal muscle, liver, erythrocytes, and brain.

Method: Aldolase determinations are not routine in most laboratories. Several automated methods have been used including ultraviolet and coupled enzymatic determinations. Serum should be collected in a red-top tube.

Normal Values: Reference values are age related and may vary among laboratories. Newborns may have values as high as four times the adult value. Adult values usually range from 1.7 to 4.9 U/L.

Increased in: Levels are increased in polymyositis, dermatomyositis, inclusion body myositis, eosinophilia-myalgia syndrome, progressive Duchenne muscular dystrophy, limb-girdle and facioscapulohumeral muscular dystrophy, and muscle damage induced by infection (e.g., trichinosis, toxoplasmosis) or drug toxicity (e.g., cocaine). Levels are elevated in hepatitis (hepatitis B and C) but not cirrhosis or biliary obstruction. Aldolase may also be elevated in pancreatitis, myocardial infarction, delirium tremens, gangrene, myelogenous leukemia, renal cell carcinoma, eosinophilic fasciitis, measles, malignant hyperthermia, muscle trauma, and strenuous exercise.

Confounding Factors: Erythrocytes contain aldolase, which thus may be falsely elevated with hemolysis. Aldolase values are proportional to muscle mass and may decline with muscle wasting.

Indications: Aldolase determinations are useful in evaluating patients with muscle disease, especially when wasting or weakness is present. Aldolase is less sensitive than creatinine phosphokinase (CPK) in evaluating muscle disease. With the inflammatory myopathies, it may be useful in gauging response to corticosteroid therapy.

Cost: $30–48.

ANGIOGRAM

Description: Angiography is a radiographic imaging technique that uses intravenous or intraarterial contrast media to visualize the vasculature.

Indications: Arteriography is most useful in supporting a diagnosis of vascular occlusion. It is particularly helpful in diagnosing the vasculitides, such as polyarteritis nodosa (mesenteric and renal vessels imaged), isolated central nervous system (CNS) angiitis (brain), Takayasu arteritis (aortic arch and subclavian vessels), and, rarely, giant cell arteritis (aortic arch and its proximal branches). Irregularities of the vascular lumen (taperings and dilatations), aneurysms, and nonatherogenic-appearing occlusions may help establish a vasculitic diagnosis. Characteristic arteriographic findings in the distal extremities are also seen in thromboangiitis obliterans (Buerger disease). Pulmonary angiography may help diagnose pulmonary embolisms and allow concurrent measurement of right-sided intracardiac pressure, useful in establishing the diagnosis of pulmonary hypertension. Venography is occasionally needed as a follow-up procedure to noninvasive vascular studies when a deep venous thrombosis is suspected [such as in the antiphospholipid (APL) antibody syndrome].

Cost: Depending on the procedure, $500–1,500.

Comment: Angiography is a moderately safe approach to vascular imaging that may provide considerable assistance in substantiating some diagnoses. All patients should be questioned about hypersensitivity to intravenous contrast agents. Newer digital subtraction techniques minimize contrast load. Careful monitoring of renal function and volume status is needed after all intravascular radiographic contrast procedures.

ANTI-CCP ANTIBODIES

Description: Anti-CCP antibodies bind to cyclic citrullinated peptides (CCPs). Beginning in the 1960s, various autoantibodies distinct from rheumatoid factor (RF) have been described in the sera of patients with RA. These autoantibodies, including antiperinuclear factor, antifilaggrin, antikeratin, and anti-Sa, were suggested to be more specific than RF. In 1998, it was recognized that these antibodies all targeted citrullinated peptides. Citrulline is a nonstandard amino acid created by the deamination, by the enzyme peptidylarginine deiminase, of arginine residues on proteins. Citrullinated synovial proteins, such as fibrin and filaggrin, may be relevant to the immunopathogenesis of RA.

Methods: Anti-CCP antibodies are detected using enzyme-linked immunosorbent assay (ELISA). Cyclization of citrullinated peptides in the ELISA was found to more closely mimic natural conformational epitopes and thereby optimized performance characteristics of the assay. Currently, the second generation of the assay (CCP-2) is used around the world.

Clinical Associations: Compared with RF, anti-CCP antibodies may have higher specificity for the diagnosis of RA (90%–95%) with similar sensitivity (75%–85%). It has been noted that patients who ultimately have gone on to develop RA may develop anti-CCP antibodies before, in some cases years, symptoms. Therefore, anti-CCP antibodies have been suggested to be useful in the diagnosis of patients with early RA, among groups of patients with undifferentiated polyarthritis. Similar to RF, patients with RA with high titers of anti-CCP antibodies are more likely to have aggressive disease and with a greater likelihood of poor outcomes, such as radiographic joint damage. The use of anti-CCP antibodies may complement the use of RF.

Cost: Approximately $80–95.

BIBLIOGRAPHY

Vossenaar ER, VanVenrooij WJ. Citrullinated proteins sparks that may ignite the fire in rheumatoid arthritis. *Arthritis Res* 2004;6:107–111.

Wiik A, van Venrooij WJ. ACR Hotline (available at www.rheumatology.org/publications/hotline/1003anticcp.asp).

ANTIGLOMERULAR BASEMENT MEMBRANE (GBM) ANTIBODY

Synonyms: Anti-GBM.

Description: Autoantibodies that react with components of the alveolar and glomerular basement membranes are known as GBM antibodies or anti-GBM antibodies. Recently, the specific antigenic epitopes recognized by GBM antibodies have been demonstrated on the α_3 chain of type IV collagen.

Method: GBM antibodies, as well as antibodies specific to type IV collagen, are measured by ELISA.

Increased in: Anti-GBM antibodies are found in Goodpasture syndrome, which is characterized by pulmonary hemorrhage and rapidly progressive glomerulonephritis (see p. 186). In addition to being a marker for Goodpasture syndrome, anti-GBM antibodies may also play a pathogenic role in causing the pulmonary and renal damage in this disease.

Indications: GBM antibodies are a sensitive test for Goodpasture syndrome because they occur in >95% of patients. Moreover, they are specific and are rarely seen in normal persons or patients with other pulmonary-renal syndromes.

Cost: The test is typically performed in a specialized reference laboratory and costs approximately $170 (range, $110–190).

ANTI–LIVER-KIDNEY-MICROSOME (LKM) ANTIBODIES

Description: Anti–LKM antibodies are a series of autoantibodies directed against enzymes in the endoplasmic reticulum of hepatocytes and other cells that are mainly associated with various liver diseases. Anti–LKM-1 antibodies bind to cytochrome P-450IID6 (CYP2D6). Although once considered to be restricted to patients with type 2 idiopathic autoimmune hepatitis (AIH), anti–LKM-1 antibodies have also been found in some patients with hepatitis C. Anti-LKM-2 antibodies bind to a distinct cytochrome P-450 enzyme and have been associated with hepatitis induced by some medications. Anti–LKM-3 antibodies bind to the enzyme UDP-glucuronosyltransferase and are associated with hepatitis D infection. Infection with hepatitis D occurs in approximately 5% of hepatitis B–infected persons and is associated with a worse prognosis.

Methods: Anti-LKM antibodies are measured using ELISA.

Indications: Anti–LKM-1 antibodies are used in the assessment of patients suspected of having AIH. Different subtypes of AIH are classified according to autoantibody reactivity. Type 1 AIH (the most common, constituting approximately 80% of AIH cases) is associated with antinuclear antibodies (ANAs) and anti–smooth muscle antibodies. Type 2 AIH, which often occurs in children, is characterized by anti–LKM-1 antibodies. Type 3 AIH is characterized by antibodies to soluble liver antigen (also known as liver-pancreas antigen).

Cost: $80.

BIBLIOGRAPHY

Al-Khalodi JA, Czaka A. Current concepts in the diagnosis, pathogenesis, and treatment of autoimmune hepatitis. *Mayo Clin Proc* 2001;76:1237–1252.

ANTIMITOCHONDRIAL ANTIBODIES (AMAs)

Description: AMAs are antibodies to a variety of mitochondrial autoantigen complexes, designated M1–M9; M2 is the best characterized.

Method: Methods of detecting AMAs include indirect immunofluorescence (IIF) using rat kidney tissue substrate. Other methods include complement fixation, ELISA, and radioimmunoassays.

Normal Values: Negative (titers = 1:20).

Abnormal in: AMA is not specific and may be seen in a variety of disorders.
—*Primary biliary cirrhosis (PBC):* Antibodies to M2 are sensitive for PBC because they are detected in >90% of patients with this disorder and rarely seen in other diseases or normal persons. Titers in PBC typically exceed 1:160.
—*Autoimmune chronic active hepatitis:* AMAs are found in 5%.
—*Scleroderma:* Subsets of patients with scleroderma (diffuse and limited) may have an overlap with PBC. In such patients, the AMA may be positive.
—*Mitochondrial myopathy:* A rare subset of patients demonstrate mild PBC and severe progressive myopathy and are positive for AMA.
—*Other diseases:* AMAs have been detected in some patients with SLE, Sjögren syndrome, autoimmune thyroiditis, and myasthenia gravis.

Indications: AMA is most useful in the diagnosis of PBC and its differentiation from sclerosing cholangitis, a disease that can be clinically similar. It may be useful in distinguishing between PBC and extrahepatic biliary obstruction.

Cost: $50–80.

ANTINEUTROPHIL CYTOPLASMIC ANTIBODY (ANCA)

Synonyms: Cytoplasmic ANCA (C-ANCA), perinuclear ANCA (P-ANCA), myeloperoxidase, proteinase-3.

Description: ANCAs comprise a group of antibodies that bind to enzymes present in the cytoplasm of neutrophils. ANCAs are found in patients with several types of vasculitis and other conditions. These ANCAs may be of diagnostic and prognostic value.

Method: ANCAs are assayed using human neutrophils (or monocytes) fixed on a glass slide. Patient serum is added to the slide, and the presence of antibodies binding to the neutrophil cytoplasm is ascertained. ANCAs are cytoplasm determined by IIF. Because of an artifact that occurs during fixation of slides with ethanol, distinct staining patterns are observed (Table 2). With C-ANCA, a granular, diffuse, cytoplasmic staining pattern is observed. By contrast, P-ANCA exhibits perinuclear staining. An atypical perinuclear pattern, sometimes referred to as A-ANCA or X-ANCA, may also be observed. The different staining patterns are associated with binding to different antigens.

Abnormal Results

C-ANCA: The antigen associated with C-ANCA is proteinase-3; antibody testing specifically for this enzyme can confirm C-ANCA. Positive C-ANCA is associated with Wegener's granulomatosis, particularly in patients with active

Table 2
Antineutrophil Cytoplasmic Antibodies

	Staining Pattern	Target Antigen	Clinical Association
C-ANCA	Granular, diffuse cytoplasmic	Proteinase-3	Wegener's granulomatosis
P-ANCA	Perinuclear	MPO, lactoferrin, elastase, cathepsin, other antigens	Microscopic PAN, Churg-Strauss syndrome, idiopathic crescentic GN, inflammatory bowel disease, Felty's syndrome
A-ANCA or X-ANCA	Atypical perinuclear	Unknown	HIV, endocarditis, inflammatory bowel disease

C-ANCA, cytoplasmic antineutrophil cytoplasmic antibody; P-ANCA, perinuclear antineutrophil cytoplasmic antibody; MPO, myeloperoxidase; PAN, polyarteritis nodosa; GN, glomerulonephritis; HIV, human immunodeficiency virus.

disease. Depending on the extent and activity of disease, C-ANCA has approximately a 50% to 90% sensitivity for Wegener's granulomatosis. Moreover, although C-ANCA may be seen rarely in some other vasculitides (e.g., Churg-Strauss's, polyarteritis nodosa), it is relatively specific for Wegener's granulomatosis with a specificity >90%. In some, but not all patients with Wegener granulomatosis, the titer of C-ANCA may correlate with disease activity. In addition to being a diagnostic marker, C-ANCA may play an etiopathogenic role in Wegener granulomatosis.

P-ANCA: P-ANCA is associated with binding to various enzymes, including myeloperoxidase, lactoferrin, cathepsin, elastase, and others. P-ANCA and particularly myeloperoxidase antibodies are seen in approximately 60% of patients with microscopic polyarteritis and Churg-Strauss syndrome. P-ANCA may also be observed in a variety of other conditions, including inflammatory bowel disease, polyarteritis, and idiopathic crescentic glomerulonephritis.

Indications: A serum ANCA, myeloperoxidase, or proteinase-3 assay may be useful in evaluating patients with suspected Wegener's granulomatosis (see p. 388), pulmonary-renal syndromes, or systemic vasculitis. A positive ANCA assay should not supplant the use of biopsy or angiography in the diagnosis of Wegener's granulomatosis or vasculitis. In selected patients, serial ANCA testing may be useful in assessing disease activity or the success of therapy.

Cost: ANCA screen, $220–260; individual tests for proteinase-3, myeloperoxidase, and elastase range from $10–220.

BIBLIOGRAPHY

Tervaert JW, Heeringa P. Pathophysiology of ANCA-associated vasculitides: are ANCA really pathogenic? *Neth J Med* 2003;61:404–407.
Wiik A. Autoantibodies in vasculitis. *Arthritis Res Ther* 2003;5:147–152.

ANTINUCLEAR ANTIBODIES (ANAs)

Synonyms: ANAs, Fluorescent ANA (FANA), LE preparation.

Description: Autoantibodies that react with various components of the cell nucleus are called ANAs. ANA is the characteristic laboratory finding of SLE. However, ANA may be found in patients with a variety of other autoimmune conditions as well as in normal persons. The ANA test defines a population of autoantibodies that react with specific intracellular constituents (Table 3). This is clinically relevant because the presence of specific autoantibodies may correlate with particular organ involvement and prognosis. Some manifestations are more typical of patients possessing particular autoantibodies, such as the presence of renal disease in patients with anti-DNA antibodies.

Method: The ANA test was superseded by the discovery of the LE cell (a leukocyte that phagocytizes a nucleus) in 1948 as the first diagnostic test for

Table 3
Autoantibodies

Specificity	Antigen Recognized	Frequency in SLE	Frequency in Other Diseases	Clinical Associations
DNA	dsDNA	50%–60%	Very Uncommon	Associated with lupus nephritis, severe disease
Sm	U1, U2, U4–6 snRNP	30%–40%	Very uncommon	Interstitial lung disease
snRNP	U1 snRNP	30%–40%	100% in patients with MCTD	Symptoms are an overlap of SLE, DM/PM, PSS
Ro (SS-A)	60-kd RNA-binding	25%–30%	70% Sjögren's	Subacute cutaneous lupus, neonatal lupus
La (SS-B)	50-kd RNA-binding protein	10%–15%	60% Sjögren's	
Histone	Histone proteins H1, H2A, H2B, H3, H4	50%–70%	≥95% drug-induced lupus	Also common in idiopathic SLE
Scl-70	Topoisomerase I	<5%	40%–70% PSS (diffuse)	
Centromere/ kinetochore (staining pattern)	70/13-kd nuclear proteins	<5%	70%–85% in limited scleroderma (CREST)	Raynaud's phenomenon
Jo-1	Histidyl tRNA synthetase	<5%	20% PM/DM	Myositis, interstitial lung disease, arthritis

SLE, systemic lupus erythematosus; dsDNA, double-stranded DNA; snRNP, small nuclear ribonuclear proteins; MCTD, mixed connective tissue disease (see p. 243); DM, dermatomyositis; PM, polymyositis; PSS, progressive systemic sclerosis.

SLE. When it was later realized that the LE cell phenomenon was mediated by high titers of antinuclear antibodies, the LE cell test was replaced by more sensitive immunofluorescent tests specific for antibodies capable of binding various nuclear constituents. Hence, the LE cell preparation is seldom performed any more, but LE cells may be coincidentally found in body fluids (e.g., pleural fluid).

Initially, ANA tests were performed on rodent tissue sections. Of note, some nuclear antigens (e.g., Ro) are absent in rodents, and some organelles (e.g., nucleoli, centromeres) are present in limited numbers in normal tissue. Thus, before the mid-1980s, there were patients who had clinical manifestations characteristic of SLE and anti-Ro antibodies but a negative ANA test. With replacement of rodent tissues by the human HEp2 tumor cell as the standard substrate for ANAs, the concept of ANA-negative lupus has largely disappeared. The generic ANA test is now universally performed by IIF, using an HEp2 substrate.

Tests for the antigens to which specific ANAs react (e.g., Sm, RNP, Ro, La) can be performed by several methods, including ELISA.

Interpretation: In addition to being positive or negative, the ANA test is quantitatively reported as a titer. The clinical significance of the ANA test often parallels the strength of the titer reported. Typically, positive ANA results are reported in terms of both titer and pattern. Higher titers are more consistent with, but not diagnostic of, SLE. Typically, titers of ≥1:160 are considered positive, whereas titers of ≤1:80 are equivocal and often nonspecific.

The ANA test is also interpreted according to the pattern of nuclear staining observed. These patterns may correlate with different antigen reactivity (Table 3). A speckled pattern of immunofluorescence is most commonly seen with the HEp2 substrate but is perhaps least specific. A speckled ANA result is associated with various so-called extractable nuclear antigens (so named because they can be extracted from the nucleus by saline). These include Ro (SS-A), La (SS-B), Sm (anti-Smith), RNP, Scl-70, Jo-1, and many others. Anti-Ro and anti-La antibodies are also observed in patients with Sjögren's syndrome (hence the designations SS-A and SS-B). Anti-Ro may also be seen in neonatal lupus and subacute cutaneous lupus erythematosus. Anti-Sm is relatively specific for the diagnosis of SLE because it is infrequent in other diseases or in normal persons. Along with anti-RNP antibodies, patients with SLE with anti-Sm may be more prone to develop interstitial lung disease. Anti-RNP antibodies were also previously associated with mixed connective tissue disease (now better termed *undifferentiated connective tissue disease*). Anti–Scl-70 antibodies are associated with the diffuse form of systemic sclerosis. A nucleolar pattern of the ANA test is also seen in systemic sclerosis, SLE, and inflammatory myositis. A centromere pattern is associated with the limited form of systemic sclerosis (previously referred to as CREST syndrome). The homogeneous (or diffuse) ANA is also very nonspecific and often associated with antibodies to histones. Such antibodies are seen in SLE, and reactivity to specific histone proteins is characteristic of drug-induced lupus. A rim (or peripheral) pattern of immunofluorescence is associated with antibodies to "native" or double-stranded DNA (dsDNA). Anti-dsDNA antibodies are useful for the diagnosis of SLE because they are uncommon in other diseases. In addition, patients with high titers of anti-dsDNA antibodies are more prone to develop proliferative lupus nephritis. The titer of anti-dsDNA antibodies may vary with the activity of disease, particularly lupus nephritis, and sequential anti-DNA determination is sometimes used to follow the activity of SLE. Anti-DNA antibodies may be specifically determined by several assays, including the *Crithidia luciliae* assay and the Farr test. Results from these various tests are reported in different units, and it is important to be familiar with the laboratory performing these tests.

Normal Values: Local laboratories should establish positive and negative titers such that <5% of normal individuals have a positive result. For most clinical laboratories, an ANA result is said to be negative when the titer is ≤1:160.

Increased in: ANAs are found in patients with SLE and a variety of autoimmune diseases (e.g., Hashimoto thyroiditis, inflammatory myositis). A positive ANA result may be seen in patients with chronic liver disease (e.g., chronic active hepatitis, primary biliary cirrhosis), chronic renal disease, chronic interstitial lung disease, and drug-induced lupus and among intravenous drug abusers. The incidence of positive ANA results is threefold higher (15%) in the elderly. In addition, first-degree relatives of patients with autoimmune disease and normal persons (particularly women and older persons) may have a positive ANA result with no associated autoimmune disease.

ANA titers do not generally correlate with disease activity, and there is little value in repeating an ANA test in a patient known to be positive.

Indications: The ANA test is most commonly used in the diagnosis of SLE. It is almost 100% sensitive because virtually all patients with SLE have a positive ANA result. However, ANAs are not specific at all because they may be seen in other connective tissue diseases such as drug-induced lupus (>95% of patients are ANA positive), scleroderma (70%–90%), inflammatory myositis (40%–60%), and Sjögren's syndrome (75%–90%). Moreover, even some healthy persons have positive ANA results, particularly at low titer. The ANA test should not be used to screen patients with joint pain or presumed systemic illness.

Cost: Performed by indirect immunofluorescence on an HEp2 substrate, but are also available by ELISA. ANA tests are widely available and typically cost $50–75.

BIBLIOGRAPHY
Egner W. The use of laboratory tests in the diagnosis of SLE. *J Clin Pathol* 2000;53:424–432.

ANTIPHOSPHOLIPID ANTIBODIES/LUPUS ANTICOAGULANT (LAC)

Synonyms: APL or anticardiolipin (ACL) antibodies, LAC, biologic false-positive test for syphilis.

Description: APLs are antibodies that bind to negatively charged phospholipids, including cardiolipin. LAC is a functional description of abnormalities in several hematologic tests often found in patients with APL antibodies. Patients may possess all or only one of these laboratory abnormalities in clinical association with APL syndrome (see p. 119).

Method: APL antibodies are detected by ELISA. Such tests may be used to detect antibodies not only to cardiolipin but also to phosphatidylcholine and other negatively charged phospholipids. Although several antibody isotypes [e.g., immunoglobulin (Ig) G, IgA, IgM] can have ACL activity, high-titer IgG ACL most strongly correlates with the clinical APL syndrome. It has been demonstrated that most pathogenic ACL antibodies have binding activity only in the presence of another serum protein, β_2-glycoprotein-I (β_2GP-I). Antibodies that react with β_2GP-I may be important to the thrombotic tendency in patients with APL syndrome because they are not seen among patients with non-pathogenic ACL (i.e., ACLs not associated with clinical APL syndrome). Moreover, some patients with clinical APL syndrome may have antibodies that bind β_2GP-I (which are also detected by ELISA) and do not bind cardiolipin at all.

LAC refers to abnormalities in several hematologic laboratory clotting tests. The name is derived from observations that blood from some patients with SLE clotted more slowly than normal *in vitro,* suggesting an anticoagulant factor. This was a misnomer because not only did many of the patients not have lupus, but this laboratory finding was associated clinically with thrombosis rather than a bleeding tendency. To understand this phenomenon, recall that several *in vitro* clotting assays require the addition of negatively charged phospholipids to potentiate clot formation. APL antibodies bind to these phospholipids, interfering with their ability to promote clotting in the test tube. Thus, despite their association with thrombosis in patients, these antibodies demonstrate anticoagulant properties in the laboratory. Currently, several laboratory tests are widely performed that define the presence of an LAC. A prolonged partial thromboplastin time (PTT) with a normal prothrombin time is often the first suggestion of such an abnormality. If the PTT does not correct with a 1:1 dilution with normal serum (as expected with a deficiency of clotting factors), the presence of an inhibitor such as the LAC is suggested.

A variety of other dynamic clotting tests are available that are more phospholipid dependent than the PTT. Such tests are also used to confirm the presence of the LAC and include the dilute Russell viper venom time (DRVVT) and kaolin clot time. Finally, correction of a prolonged PTT by the addition of excess phospholipid, as is done in the platelet neutralization test and the hexagonal phospholipid test, suggests the LAC.

Tests for RPR (rapid plasma reagin) and VDRL (venereal disease research laboratory) also identify ACL.

Increased Values: APL antibodies are uncommon in normal persons. Normal values on the ELISA for APL antibodies are defined with abnormal values being >5 standard deviations above the mean. This value is designated 10 PL units (these units are known as GPL for IgG antibodies, MPL for IgM, and APL for IgA). APL antibodies are elevated in most patients with APL syndrome. High-titer IgG APL antibodies are most strongly correlated with clinical syndromes. Uncommonly, patients with clinical APL syndrome may have abnormalities only on LAC testing or antibodies only to β_2GP-I.

Elevated levels of APL antibodies are seen in patients with SLE. The reported prevalence of IgG or IgM APL antibodies varies from 17% to 60%, with most studies reporting >30%. The prevalence of APL is also elevated in patients with RA, being found in approximately 17% of patients (range, 4%–49%). In other autoimmune diseases, the prevalence of APL antibodies is not substantially above normal. APL antibodies may also be found in a variety of infectious diseases, including syphilis, tuberculosis, and human immunodeficiency virus and other viral infections. They may also be found in patients with cancers. In these nonautoimmune conditions, APL antibodies are rarely associated with APL syndrome (e.g., thrombotic events).

Abnormal LAC test results are not common in autoimmune diseases. They may be abnormal in patients with dysfibrinogenemia or with other types of clotting inhibitors.

Indications: APL antibodies may be sought in patients with symptoms suggesting APL syndrome, such as recurrent arterial or venous thromboses, fetal wastage, and thrombocytopenia. Testing for LAC and a false-positive RPR may also help secure such a diagnosis.

Cost: LAC panel, $35–220; cardiolipin antibodies, $300–500.

BIBLIOGRAPHY

Carreras LO, Forastiero RR, Martinuzzo ME. Which are the best biological markers of the antiphospholipid syndrome? *J Autoimmun* 2000;15:163–172.
Merkel PA, Chang Y, Pierangeli SS, et al. The prevalence and clinical associations of anticardiolipin antibodies in a large inception cohort of patients with connective tissue diseases. *Am J Med* 1996;101:576–583.

ANTI–SMOOTH MUSCLE ANTIBODY (ASMA)

Description: ASMA is autoantibody to cytoskeletal components of smooth muscle (principally actin). The etiology and function of these antibodies are unknown.

Method: ASMA is detected by IIF using smooth muscle tissue as substrate.

Normal Values: A negative result has a titer <1:20.

Abnormal in:
—*Autoimmune chronic active hepatitis:* Titers are >1:160 in >95% of cases.
—*PBC:* ASMA may be seen in as many as 30% of patients.

—*Other conditions:* Acute viral infections (e.g., mononucleosis), chronic viral hepatitis (especially hepatitis C), other autoimmune diseases.

Indications: ASMA assay may be useful in diagnosing autoimmune chronic active hepatitis and distinguishing it from PBC. The lack of specificity lowers its clinical usefulness.

Cost: $70–100.

Comment: Identification of specific cytoskeletal antigens and their antibodies may improve the usefulness of ASMA tests.

ANTISTREPTOLYSIN O (ASO)

Description: ASO is antibody to an extracellular streptococcal product, hemolysin O.

Method: A rapid latex-agglutination slide test is currently used most commonly. Older methods used tube dilutions with RBC hemolysis. Todd units are expressed as the reciprocal of the last tube showing hemolysis. International units (IU) using newer rapid latex are equivalent to Todd units.

Normal Values: Normal values are <200 to 240 IU (varies by laboratory) using the latex method. With the older methodology, normal values are <240 Todd units in adults and 320 Todd units in children.

Increased in: With streptococcal infection, titers peak 4 to 5 weeks after infection (this is usually the second or third week after the onset of acute rheumatic fever). Titers are elevated in 80% of patients with acute rheumatic fever and are usually not increased after streptococcal skin infection. ASO may be non-specifically elevated in patients with hypergammaglobulinemia or with heightened immunologic activity.

Confounding Factors: Titers of ASO vary with age, season, and geography. Higher values are seen in children and in those living in crowded living conditions and in temperate climates. Serum contamination and cross-reactivity with muscle sarcolemma can rarely yield false-positive results.

Indications: ASO is useful along with other antistreptococcal antibodies such as anti-DNAse B, anti-NAse, antistreptokinase, and antihyaluronidase to demonstrate evidence of recent streptococcal infection.

Cost: ASO, $40–75; DNAse B, $50–75.

Comments: There is a 90% to 95% likelihood that at least one of three anti-streptococcal antibodies will be elevated in the setting of acute rheumatic fever.

BIOPSY

Overview: Tissue biopsy is often a useful means of establishing the diagnosis or degree of disease activity in selected rheumatic disorders (Table 4). Tissue samples may reveal histologic evidence of inflammation, vasculitis, fibrosis, atrophy, necrosis, or infection. For all sites, one must determine how the tissue must be processed before obtaining the sample. This can be accomplished by contacting the pathologist beforehand. Specimens for culture, for example, cannot be put in fixative, and samples that are to undergo immunofluorescent analysis may require freezing rather than fixation. The most useful biopsy sites are skin, muscle, blood vessels, synovium, and nerves, as described below.

Skin: Histologic examination of skin using light or immunofluorescent microscopy may be helpful in the diagnosis of SLE, discoid lupus, dermatomyositis, scleroderma, cutaneous vasculitis, or panniculitis. The lupus band test uses skin biopsy to detect deposition of immunoglobulins at the dermal-epidermal junction of uninvolved skin. Although useful in the diagnosis of SLE, the lupus band test is seldom necessary. Inflammation in the walls of small cutaneous blood vessels can be used to diagnose cutaneous vasculitis, which is usually of the leukocytoclastic type. Although many issues can be successfully addressed using a 4-mm punch biopsy specimen, a deeper, incision wedge biopsy specimen may be required to evaluate some problems such as

Table 4
Indications for Tissue Biopsy in the Rheumatic Diseases

Biopsy Site	Suspected Diagnosis
Skin	Systemic lupus erythematosus
	Dermatomyositis
	Cutaneous vasculitis
	Panniculitis
Muscle	Inflammatory myopathies
	Metabolic myopathies
	Muscular dystrophy
Blood vessel	Temporal arteritis
Synovium	Rheumatoid arthritis
	Mycobacterial or fungal arthritis
	Neoplasms
	Pigmented villonodular synovitis
Nerve	Systemic vasculitis
Kidney	Systemic lupus erythematosus
	Acute renal failure
	Progressive nephrotic syndrome
	Acute nephritic syndrome
	Renal allograft rejection

eosinophilic fasciitis and panniculitis. Tissue samples should be taken from fresh new lesions, with an edge of normal skin included. Both punch and wedge biopsies are usually performed by dermatologists.

Muscle: Biopsy of involved muscle is often required to diagnose inflammatory myositis, metabolic myopathies, muscular dystrophies, or vasculitis. The biopsy site should be the most symptomatic area. End-stage or atrophic areas should be avoided. Also, muscles previously used for injection or electromyography should be avoided as they may yield false-positive results. Needle aspiration of muscle is useful for histologic evaluation, and the diagnostic yield may be improved by taking as many as four samples from the same cutaneous puncture site. Open surgical biopsies are usually required to obtain sufficient tissue to measure functional enzyme levels for evaluation of metabolic disorders. Contraction of the biopsied muscle should be avoided (as this causes artifact) by using a surgical muscle clamp. The biopsy specimen should be delivered to the pathologist immediately (within 30 minutes) after collection for proper specimen handling for histology by light microscopy, electron microscopy, and enzyme analysis.

Blood Vessels: Histologic analysis of the vasculature is routinely done whenever tissue biopsies are obtained. Blind tissue biopsies (i.e., muscle, skin, testes) are uncommonly useful in identifying significant vascular pathology. Hypersensitivity (also known as leukocytoclastic) vasculitis (inflammation of venules) is one of the most common vascular abnormalities seen on skin biopsy. Temporal artery biopsy is useful in establishing a diagnosis of giant cell arteritis. The diagnostic yield of the procedure is maximized by taking a large section of vessel (at least 3 cm in length) and examining at least 20 to 25 cross-sections. Multiple section analysis is required because "skip" vascular lesions may be missed. This procedure is usually done in the operating room under local anesthesia.

Synovium: Because synovial fluid often reflects processes active within the synovium, synovial fluid analysis is often attempted before considering synovial biopsy. Although synovial histology was once used as a diagnostic criterion for RA, this diagnosis is now easily made on clinical grounds without synovial biopsy. However, synovial tissue biopsy is essential for the diagnosis of synovial neoplasias or chronic joint infections such as those caused by mycobacteria or evaluation of chronic undiagnosed monarthritis. Synovial biopsy may be necessary when synovial fluid is unrevealing or not accessible. Synovial tissue culture is more often positive for mycobacterial or fungal infection than synovial fluid culture. Blind needle or arthroscopically guided biopsies usually yield sufficient tissue for histologic analyses and cultures; open surgical biopsies are only rarely required. Tissue samples are usually fixed in formalin or in alcohol if gout is suspected.

Nerve: Biopsy of the sural nerve is useful for evaluating suspected vasculitis. The yield of such a procedure is likely to be enhanced in the setting of a foot drop or lower extremity neuropathy. Thus, an abnormal nerve conduction study is likely to improve the diagnostic yield of a sural nerve biopsy. Usually, the biopsy is performed under local anesthesia, at the bedside, or in the clinic. There may be residual local hypesthesia present after the procedure.

Kidney: Renal biopsies are occasionally necessary to determine the underlying pathology in acute renal failure, progressive nephrotic syndrome, SLE, acute nephritic syndrome (hematuria, red cell casts, proteinuria, hypertension), and undiagnosed hematuria and to assess renal allograft and possible rejection. Kidney biopsy is not necessarily indicated in all patients with SLE with renal or urine abnormalities. It is most helpful in determining whether current renal abnormalities are owing to coexistent conditions [e.g., diabetes, hypertension, nonsteroidal antiinflammatory drug (NSAID) therapy] or if lupus renal lesions are reversible (high activity score) or irreversible (high chronicity score). Before the procedure, the patient's complete blood count (CBC), prothrombin time, PTT, and bleeding time should be checked. Relative contraindications for biopsy may include active infection, uncontrolled hypertension, thrombocytopenia, bleeding diathesis, and pregnancy. Biopsy is usually percutaneous, with ultrasound guidance. The most common complication, gross hematuria, occurs in 5% to 10% of patients and usually resolves in 2 to 3 days.

Cost: Depending on whether done as an outpatient or inpatient/operating room procedure; skin, $150; muscle, $250–350; kidney, $325–625 (plus hospital costs).

BIBLIOGRAPHY

Velthuis PJ, Kater L, van der Tweel I, et al. Immunofluorescence microscopy of healthy skin from patients with systemic lupus erythematosus: more than just the lupus band. *Ann Rheum Dis* 1992;51:720–725.

BONE SCAN

Synonyms: Bone scintigraphy, radionuclide scintigraphy.

Description: Bone scanning is an imaging method used to detect metabolic, inflammatory, or osseous skeletal abnormalities.

Method: Scintigraphy requires intravenous administration of technetium-99m diphosphate. ^{99m}Tc diphosphate is a bone-seeking radionuclide whose uptake is enhanced by blood flow and bone turnover/remodeling or proliferative bone formation. Patients are assessed immediately post-radionuclide (measures blood flow) and 2 to 3 hours later (bone uptake). The procedure takes 3 to 4 hours to complete, and patients need not fast or be NPO (nothing by mouth).

Normal Results: Normally there is a low level of homogeneous, symmetric tracer uptake in bone. Tracer normally concentrates in the bladder. Normal bone scan is seen in multiple myeloma.

Increased Uptake: Paget disease, reflex sympathetic dystrophy, osteomyelitis, septic arthritis, infected prosthetic joints, inflammatory arthritis, sacroiliitis, enthesitis, osteoarthritis, metastasis to bone, osteoid osteoma, and osteonecrosis show increased uptake. Although early (infarctive stage) osteonecrosis shows no uptake, later (reparative) stages may demonstrate increased uptake. Increased uptake is seen with inflammatory, degenerative, infectious, and neoplastic spinal disease. Occult fractures (including compression or stress fractures) may be found with delayed imaging (72 hours). Osteomyelitis is suggested by focal hyperperfusion, hyperemia, and increased bone uptake.

Complications: Allergic reaction to radionuclide is uncommon.

Indications: Bone scans may be used in the diagnosis of the previously noted conditions. It may provide useful information regarding the metabolic status of bone or for detecting infectious or neoplastic involvement of bone and periarticular structures. It may be indicated in total-body skeletal assessments of musculoskeletal disease. Scintigraphy may be useful in the serial evaluation of Paget disease or neoplastic disease or response to treatment in osteomyelitis. Infrequently, a bone scan may be used to assess patients with persistent polyarthralgia and repeatedly normal joint examinations or radiographs.

Cost: $400–800.

BIBLIOGRAPHY

Love C, Din AS, Tomas MB, et al. Radionuclide bone imaging: an illustrative review. *Radiographics* 2003;23:341–358.

COMPLETE BLOOD COUNT (CBC)

Synonyms: Hemogram, blood count, hematology profile.

Description: CBC is a profile of tests providing quantitative measures of RBC, white blood cell, and platelet indices. The CBC is useful for the diagnosis of anemia, bleeding disorders, infection, connective tissue disorders, and neoplasia and to monitor clinical status or response to medication.

Method: Most clinical laboratories use an automated electronic multichannel analyzer with aperture impedance or laser beam to estimate cell counts, size, and complexity. Venous blood should be collected in a lavender-top tube (containing the anticoagulant EDTA) and gently inverted several times to prevent coagulation. A peripheral smear of anticoagulated blood may be examined with Wright stain to evaluate RBC, white blood cell, and platelet morphology and relative cell number.

Normal Values: Consult local reference laboratory values.

RBC Abnormalities: See Table 5. RBC indices and abnormalities are defined as follows:

—*Mean corpuscular volume:* Useful in the diagnosis of microcytic or macrocytic anemias, drug effects (i.e., methotrexate, sulfasalazine, and dapsone increase mean corpuscular volume), or occult alcohol abuse.

—*RBC distribution width:* Measures anisocytosis (variation in RBC size); increased in iron deficiency and macrocytic anemias.

—*Heinz bodies (owing to precipitated hemoglobin):* Seen in thalassemia, glucose-6-phosphate or pyruvate kinase deficiency, postsplenectomy, drug-induced RBC injury (e.g., antimalarials, sulfonamides).

—*Schistocytes (fragmented RBCs):* Caused by microangiopathic hemolytic anemia, disseminated intravascular coagulation, thrombotic thrombocytopenic purpura, prosthetic heart valves, hemolysis, severe burn, and snake bite.

—*Acanthocytes (spiculated RBCs from abnormal membrane lipids):* Seen with hyposplenism, abetalipoproteinemia, severe liver or renal disease, and hereditary acanthocytosis.

—*Target cells (increase in cell membrane in relation to cell volume):* May be artifactual or caused by hemoglobin C and S, thalassemia minor, iron deficiency, or liver disease or post-splenectomy.

—*Howell-Jolly bodies (precipitated DNA in mature RBC):* Seen post-splenectomy and in hyposplenism, megaloblastic anemia (pernicious anemia), sickle cell, hemolytic anemia, and hereditary spherocytosis.

—*Burr cells (regularly scalloped, crenated RBCs):* May be artifactual or owing to uremia, gastrointestinal bleeding, or gastric carcinoma.

—*Elliptocytes (ovalocytes, oval-shaped RBCs):* May be hereditary or seen with iron deficiency anemia.

—*Sickle cells (caused by polymerization of hemoglobin S):* Seen in sickle cell syndromes (not in S trait)

—*Teardrop RBCs:* Consider polycythemia, myelofibrosis, thalassemia.

—*Basophilic stippling:* May be seen in heavy metal poisoning (e.g., lead), severe hemorrhage, or hemolysis.

Anemia: Anemia in patients with rheumatic disease may be owing to rheumatic disease, coexistent disorders, or the adverse effects of medication.

—*Anemia of chronic disease (ACD):* With ACD, the hematocrit seldom drops below 27%. RBC morphology is normal or hypochromic. ACD results from ineffective erythropoiesis owing to an inability to mobilize and use bone marrow iron stores. Bone marrow iron content is normal. ACD may be present in patients with chronic infection, neoplasia, or active inflammatory disorders such as RA or SLE. ACD does not accompany noninflammatory disorders such as osteoarthritis or fibromyalgia. Therapy should be primarily directed at the underlying disorder. Supplemental iron is of little value.

—*Iron deficiency anemia:* Commonly caused by gastrointestinal (especially with NSAID use) or menstrual blood loss. Morphology reveals hypochromic and microcytic RBCs and low serum ferritin levels. However, normal ferritin lev-

Table 5
Diagnostic Clues from Hemogram Components

Test	Increased in	Decreased in	Comment
Hgb/Hct	Polycythemia, hemoconcentration	Iron deficiency anemia, anemia of chronic disease, hemolysis	Hgb may be falsely elevated with lipemic plasma or with WBC > 50K
MCV	Drugs (MTX, SSZ, dapsone, Dilantin, estrogen), megaloblastic anemia, liver disease, alcoholism, myxedema, cold agglutinin disease	Microcytic anemia, iron deficiency, thalassemia, sideroblastic anemia, lead poisoning	May be increased (with marked leukocytosis, reticulocytosis, or hyperglycemia) or decreased (with hemolysis or fragmented RBCs)
RDW	IDA, sideroblastic, B_{12}/folate deficiency, alcoholism, liver disease	Thalassemia or ACD (normal or low RDW)	Usually normal or low in ACD; more sensitive in microcytic anemias
Reticulocyte count	Acute blood loss, hemolysis, sickle cell, RBC sequestration; Rx of IDA	SLE, BM aplasia, pancytopenia, megaloblastic anemia, alcoholism, liver disease, chronic renal failure, myxedema	Reticulocytes indicate effective erythropoiesis; useful in gauging response to iron, B_{12}, folate therapy or bloodloss
WBC neutrophils	Corticosteroids, epinephrine, lithium, acute infection, seizures, stress, myeloproliferative disorders, leukemia, vasculitis (PAN), Reiter's syndrome, acute gout, septic arthritis, rheumatic fever, adult Still disease, Sweet's syndrome, Kawasaki disease, familial Mediterranean fever	MTX, azathioprine, chlorambucil, cyclophosphamide, gold salts, NSAIDs (rare), SLE, drug-induced lupus, MCTD, overlap syndrome, RA, Sjögren syndrome, Felty's syndrome, cyclic neutropenia, bacterial sepsis, viral infection, hypersplenism, aplastic anemia, radiation, CLL, hemodialysis, nutritional deficiency (folate, copper, etc.)	Falsely elevated WBC may be due to clumping associated with monoclonal gammopathy, cryoglobulins, cold agglutinins, or nucleated RBCs; African Americans may manifest lower WBC counts than whites
Lymphocytes	Mononucleosis, viral (EBV, CMV, mumps), pertussis, Crohn disease, ulcerative colitis, hypersensitivity drug reactions, serum sickness vasculitis	Chemotherapy (azathioprine, cyclophosphamide, chlorambucil), corticosteroids, radiation, SLE, MCTD, renal failure, myasthenia gravis	Absolute lymphocyte counts may be helpful in diagnosing certain disorders (e.g., SLE) or gauging response to chemotherapy

	Increased	Decreased	Comments
Monocytes	RA, SLE, sarcoidosis, inflammatory bowel disease, myeloproliferative disorders, postsplenectomy, SBE, Rocky Mountain spotted fever, tuberculosis, brucellosis	Corticosteroids, acute stress, acute infection, aplastic anemia, myelotoxic therapies	
Eosinophils	SLE, polyarteritis nodosa, Churg-Strauss angiitis, RA, Sjögren syndrome, eosinophilic fasciitis, Wegener's granulomatosis, eosinophil myalgia syndrome, pemphigus, allergic disorders, asthma, Hodgkin disease, polycythemia vera, hypereosinophilic syndrome, parasitic infection, inflammatory bowel disease	Corticosteroids, acute stress, bacterial infection	
Basophils	CML, polycythemia, myelodysplasia, Hodgkin's disease		
Platelets	Inflammation (i.e., RA), infection, malignancy, sarcoidosis, essential thrombocytosis, polycythemia vera, CML, postsplenectomy, iron deficiency anemia, oral contraceptives	Hyperthyroidism, pregnancy, acute infection, chemotherapy, radiation Drugs (gold salts, penicillamine, chloroquine, sulfasalazine, penicillin, heparin, quinidine, estrogen, cyclophosphamide, chlorambucil), infection (EBV, herpes), SLE, hypersplenism, aplastic anemia, ITP, TTP, DIC, radiation, toxemia of pregnancy Wiskott-Aldrich syndrome, autoimmune thrombocytopenia, leukemia, hypersplenism	May be falsely elevated with cryoglobulins, malaria, or fragmented RBCs; platelet clumping may decrease counts and be caused by EDTA collection tubes, cold agglutinins
MPV	ITP, recovery from thrombocytopenia, myeloproliferative disorders, hyperthyroidism, massive hemorrhage, splenectomy, preeclampsia, smokers, vasculitis		Increased with effective thrombopoiesis.

Hgb, hemoglobin; Hct, hematocrit; WBC, white blood cell; MCV, mean corpuscular volume; MTX, methotrexate; SSZ, sulfasalazine; RBC, red blood cell; RDW, red cell distribution width; IDA, iron deficiency anemia; ACD, anemia chronic disease; SLE, systemic lupus erythematosus; BM, bone marrow; PAN, polyarteritis nodosa; NSAID, nonsteroidal antiinflammatory drug; MCTD, mixed connective tissue disease; RA, rheumatoid arthritis; CLL, chronic leukocytic leukemia; EBV, Epstein-Barr virus; CMV, cytomegalovirus; TTP, thrombotic thrombocytopenic purpura; DIC, disseminated intravascular coagulation; MPV, mean platelet volume; ITP, idiopathic thrombocytopenic purpura.

els are seen with inflammatory states because ferritin behaves as an acute-phase reactant. There is usually an elevated total iron-binding capacity.

—*Hemolytic anemia:* May be owing to hemoglobinopathies (i.e., sickle cell, thalassemia, hemoglobin C), hereditary spherocytosis or elliptocytosis, paroxysmal nocturnal hemoglobinuria, transfusion reaction, autoimmune hemolytic anemia (i.e., Coombs positive, SLE, viral infection, lymphoma, drugs, idiopathic), prosthetic heart valves, disseminated intravascular coagulation, thrombotic thrombocytopenic purpura, scleroderma renal crisis, hemolytic-uremic syndrome, malaria, snakebite, or glucose-6-phosphate or pyruvate kinase deficiency.

—*Aplastic anemia:* May be seen with NSAIDs (e.g., phenylbutazone, diclofenac), gold, penicillamine, azathioprine, cyclophosphamide, chlorambucil, methotrexate, viral infections, and hepatitis.

WBC Abnormalities

—*LE cells:* Phagocytic cells that have ingested an opsonized nucleus. Although rarely done or available, they may be incidentally found in joint, pleural, or pericardial fluid. They are found in 75% of patients with SLE but are also seen in mixed connective tissue disease, RA, Sjögren syndrome, chronic active hepatitis, PBC, and drug-induced lupus or with ANA-inducing drugs.

—*Hypersegmented neutrophils:* With macrocytic anemia.

—*Toxic granulation:* Seen with severe bacterial or viral infections and sepsis.

—*Atypical lymphocytes:* Seen in viral infections (e.g., mononucleosis, mumps, cytomegalovirus, hepatitis), drug reactions, serum sickness, pertussis, and brucellosis.

Platelet Abnormalities

—*Platelet clumping:* May falsely lower platelets but increase leukocyte counts; may be induced by EDTA and large platelets associated with thrombocytopenia.

—*Giant/large platelets:* Recovery of thrombocytopenic states, myeloproliferative syndromes, hyperthyroidism, Bernard-Soulier syndrome.

—*Mean platelet volume:* Mean platelet volume is increased with large (young/immature) platelets and with increased platelet turnover and is inversely proportional to platelet count.

Confounding Factors: CBC is rendered inaccurate by hemolysis, hemodilution with intravenous fluids, and hypercalcemia (causes coagulation). Accuracy is lowered when numbers approach critical values (i.e., platelets $<10,000/mm^3$).

Indications: CBC is useful in the evaluation or diagnosis of anemia, infection, connective tissue disorders, or neoplasia and in monitoring the effects of medication.

Cost: $20–30.

Comment: A peripheral smear should be requested and examined when evaluating anemia, suspected hemolysis, leukemia, or thrombocytopenia.

BIBLIOGRAPHY

ARA Glossary Committee. Miscellaneous tests in the rheumatic diseases: A. Blood studies. In: *ARA Glossary Committee, JL Decker, chairman. Dictionary of the rheumatic diseases, vol II: diagnostic testing. American Rheumatism Association.* Atlanta: Contact Associates International Ltd., 1985:2–6.
Wallach J. *Interpretation of diagnostic tests,* 6th ed. Boston: Little, Brown, 1996.

CEREBROSPINAL FLUID STUDIES

Description: CSF tests may be used in diagnosing or distinguishing between benign, infectious, autoimmune, inflammatory, hemorrhagic, obstructive, and neoplastic disorders.

Method: The clinician should look for signs of increased intracranial pressure (i.e., papilledema) or perform cranial imaging [computed tomography or magnetic resonance imaging (MRI)] before doing lumbar puncture. CSF should be aseptically obtained, with the opening pressure and appearance of fluid recorded. Routine CSF studies include cell and differential counts, glucose and protein determinations, and serologic tests for syphilis. When infection is considered, microbiologic assays may include Gram staining; culture for bacteria, fungi, or mycobacteria; or detection of microbial antigens (e.g., cryptococcal, pneumococcal, meningococcal, or *Haemophilus influenzae*) by latex agglutination. With suspected inflammatory or autoimmune causes, oligoclonal bands or quantitation of IgG and albumin may be useful.

—*Q albumin:* Estimates the state of the blood-brain barrier (BBB) integrity (or the rate of albumin transfer between compartments); requires a paired sample of serum and CSF for analysis.

$$Q \text{ albumin} = \frac{\text{CSF Albumin} \times 10^3}{\text{Serum Albumin}} \quad nl < 9$$

—*IgG index:* Calculates the amount of *in situ* IgG production within the CSF (intrathecal synthesis of IgG); requires a paired sample of serum and CSF for analysis; tends to be increased in a variety of conditions including multiple sclerosis, neuropsychiatric lupus, and neurosyphilis.

$$\text{IgG Index} = \frac{\text{CSF IgG} \times \text{Serum albumin}}{\text{CSF albumin} \times \text{Serum IgG}} \quad nl < 0.7$$

Another measure of *in situ* IgG production is the IgG synthetic rate. IgG synthetic rate measures in situ IgG, corrects for transfer of IgG and albumin across BBB and considers the molecular weight of albumin and IgG. Many advocate this calculation as the more reliable indicator of IgG synthesis.

$$\text{IgG synthetic rate} = [(\text{IgG}_{csf} - \text{IgG}_{ser}/369) - (\text{Alb}_{csf}\,\text{Alb}/230)(\text{IgG}_{ser}/\text{Alb}_{ser})(0.43)] \times 5 \quad nl < 3.3$$

—*Oligoclonal bands:* Indicate the presence of clonally restricted immunoglobulins identified by high-resolution electrophoresis or isoelectric focusing. Test requires a paired sample of serum and CSF for analysis. Oligoclonal bands are seen in nearly 90% of patients with multiple sclerosis. They are also found in a minority of patients with SLE, neuro-Behçet's syndrome, neurosyphilis, cerebral vasculitis, Guillain-Barré syndrome, and encephalitis.

Normal Values: See Table 6. CSF is normally clear, colorless, and without cells. Blood or RBCs may indicate a traumatic tap or subarachnoid or intracerebral hemorrhage. Xanthochromia indicates hemorrhage.

Abnormal in: See Table 6. Tests should be used selectively to establish/confirm clinical suspicions. Ordering all CSF tests is likely to be expensive and provide misleading rather than diagnostic information.

Confounding Factors: A traumatic tap alters the reliability of cell counts, glucose and protein determinations, IgG index, and Q albumin.

Indications: In patients with suspected meningitis, encephalitis, subarachnoid or intracerebral hemorrhage, neurosyphilis, multiple sclerosis, neuropsychiatric lupus, primary CNS vasculitis, or inflammatory conditions with suspected CNS involvement (i.e., Behçet syndrome, sarcoidosis).

Cost: Cell count, $20–30; CSF protein, $30–50; IgG index, $130–190; antineuronal antibody, $180.

BIBLIOGRAPHY

Andersson M, Alvarez-Cermeno J, Bernardi G, et al. Cerebrospinal fluid in the diagnosis of multiple sclerosis: a consensus report. *J Neurol Neurosurg Psychiatry* 1994;57:897–902.

CHLAMYDIA TESTS

Description: A variety of tests are useful in diagnosing infection or past exposure to chlamydial species (*Chlamydia trachomatis, Chlamydia psittaci,* and *Chlamydia pneumoniae*).

Method: Chlamydial infection is best detected by analysis of specimens taken from urethral, cervical, conjunctival, nasopharyngeal, or rectal swabs. Genitourinary specimens are most reliable when not contaminated with urine. In males, urethral swabs should be inserted >2 cm into the urethra. In females, swabs of the cervix/endocervix should be sufficient to collect infected epithelial cells. Serum antibody assays are also available but are less reliable. Available tests include
—*Enzyme immunoassay or direct fluorescent antibody testing of urethral or cervical swabs:* Useful and >80% sensitive in diagnosing active infection.
—*Polymerase chain reaction (PCR) (using DNA probe for chlamydial RNA):* Very sensitive and reliable; recommended if available. Specimens are collected in a special medium provided by laboratory.

Table 6
CSF Findings in Selected Neurologic Conditions

Disorder	Opening Pressure (mm Hg)	WBC (cells/mm³)	Cell Type	Predominant Glucose	Protein (mg/dL)	IgG Index	Q albumin	Oligoclonal Bands (% Positive)
Normal results[a]	60–180	0–5	Lymphocytes, monocytes	>60% of serum value	15–45	<0.7	<9.0	Negative
Bacterial meningitis	High	100–10,000	PMNs	Low or normal	100–500	<0.7	>15.0	Negative
Cryptococcal or tuberculous meningitis	High	50–500	Lymphocytes	Low or normal	100–500	Normal or high	15–100	Negative
Lupus cerebritis	Normal or high	0–50	Lymphocytes	Normal or low	Normal	65% >0.7	67% <9.0 33% 9–15	0–40%
Multiple sclerosis	Normal	0–20	Lymphs	Normal	Normal	80% >0.7	75% <9.0	>90%
Neuro-Behçet syndrome	Normal	>100	Lymphocytes, monocytes	Normal	Increased	20%–50% >0.7	40% >9.0	<10%
Neurosarcoid	Normal or high	100–500	Lymphocytes, monocytes	Normal or low	40–100	25%–80% >0.7	12%– 80% >9.0	0–50%
Neurosyphilis	Normal or high	<100	Lymphocytes, monocytes	Normal or low	40–200	>80%	>80%	50%

[a] Normal reference values may vary according to laboratory.
CSF, cerebrospinal fluid; WBC, white blood cell.

—*Culture:* Definitive, difficult, unreliable, 2- to 7-day turnaround time.

—*Serologic tests for IgG or IgA anti*-Chlamydia *antibodies:* Most useful in the diagnosis of systemic infection (i.e., infantile pneumonia, lymphogranuloma venereum, or psittacosis).

—*Infrequently used:* Microimmunofluorescence or complement fixation assays.

Positive in: More than 50% of patients with reactive arthritis (Reiter's syndrome) have positive results, as do those with nongonococcal urethritis, ocular infections, psittacosis, or lymphogranuloma venereum. Acute and convalescent serum titers may be necessary to prove infection. Titers of $\geq$1:640 suggest active infection.

Confounding Factors: Recent antibiotic therapy may alter culture but not serologic or PCR results.

Indications: Tests may be useful in patients with suspected reactive arthritis, ocular and urogenital infections, or psittacosis. Serologic or culture evidence of infection may be an indication for antibiotic therapy.

Cost: Enzyme immunoassay, $100–120; DNA probe, $60–80; culture, $100–120.

CHOLESTEROL CRYSTALS

Description: Crystals of cholesterol are occasionally found in joints, bursae, tendons, pericardial and pleural fluid, and skin. Two morphologic forms occur: highly birefringent, large, flat, rectangular plates with notched corners (80–100 μm) and needle-shaped, strongly birefringent crystals (2–20 μm). The former are more common and appear as "stacked panes of glass."

Method: Crystals are best identified by polarized light microscopy but may be seen with ordinary light microscopy.

Found in: Cholesterol crystals are often found in the synovial fluid of patients with RA, SLE, osteoarthritis, hyperlipidemia, and chronic tophaceous gout. They are also found in xanthomas, cholesterol tophi, calcinosis cutis, rheumatoid nodules, and pleural and pericardial effusions owing to RA, tuberculosis, or malignancy. Their significance and contribution to inflammation are unclear.

Indications: Crystals are usually an incidental finding, and testing is rarely requested.

COMPLEMENT

Synonyms: C3, C4, total hemolytic complement activity (CH50).

Description: Complement is an organized system of >20 serum proteins (mostly made in the liver) that help protect the host from invading organisms.

Historically, the name complement is derived from the notion that factors present in the serum complemented the ability of immunoglobulin to destroy bacteria. Activation of complement depends on sequential cleavage of individual components. This amplifies the ultimate response and generates many complement split products, a number of which serve important biologic functions. The complement system is organized into classical and alternate pathways, both of which merge and activate C3 and lead to the formation of the membrane attack complex. The cascade is regulated by a variety of inhibitory factors and cell surface receptors.

In the classic pathway, complement is normally inactive in the serum until it becomes activated by immune complexes or antibody-coated surfaces. C1 recognizes either of these and activates the classical pathway components C4, C2, and C3. C1 esterase inhibitor regulates the classic pathway and is dysfunctional in hereditary angioedema.

The alternate pathway is activated by endotoxin, bacterial cell wall polysaccharides, and proteolytic enzymes.

Complement is an important part of the antigen-nonspecific part of the immune response and helps control infections by several mechanisms: (a) complement components and complement split products bound to the surface of bacteria function as opsonins, enhancing phagocytosis of bacteria; (b) complement split products C3a and C5a (anaphylotoxins) activate mast cells, leading to recruitment and activation of neutrophils and other cells; (c) the membrane attack complex (C5b-9) can punch a hole in the membrane of pathogens; and (d) immune complexes with complement fragments attached are more easily cleared by the reticuloendothelial system.

Method: Individual complement components (C3, C4) may be directly quantified by such specific immunologic methods as rate nephelometry or radial immunodiffusion. Complement consumption, which is probably the most common clinical indication for complement testing, is best assessed by measuring serum C3 and C4.

The overall complement cascade can be functionally assessed by the CH50, which measures the ability of a patient's serum to lyse foreign blood cells. Although this test has the advantage of assessing the function all the components, it is labor intensive and performed infrequently in many laboratories. Thus, it is best used to indicate deficiency of one of the terminal complement proteins (e.g., in a patient with recurrent neisserial infections and a C5-9 deficiency, C3 and C4 determinations will be normal, but CH50 will be very low). In the future, complement consumption will likely be assessed by direct measurements of complement split products (e.g., C3a), which are more specific and sensitive for this purpose.

Normal in: Complement is normal in Henoch-Schönlein purpura, Goodpasture syndrome, polyarteritis nodosa, and Wegener granulomatosis.

Abnormal in: Although complement is important in host defense, activation of the complement system is detrimental to the host in a variety of diseases. Conditions associated with specific serum complement profiles are shown in Table 7.

Table 7
Complement Profiles in Various Disease States

Condition	C3	C4	C1	C1-Inh (Antigenic)	C1-Inh (Functional)
Immunologic activation of the classical pathway (e.g., by immune complexes in SLE)	↓	↓	↓	N	N
Alternate pathway activation (e.g., by bacterial cell walls)	↓	N	N	N	N
Tissue injury (proteolytic cleavage of C3, e.g., in DIC)	↓	N	N	N	N
Hereditary angioedema type I (85% of cases)	N	↓	N	↓	↓
Hereditary angioedema type II (15% of cases)	N	↓	N	N	↓
Acquired angioedema type I (paraprotein related)	N or ↓	↓	↓	↓	↓
Angioedema type II (anti-C1 inhibitor antibody related)	N or ↓	↓	↓	N or ↓	↓

SLE, systemic lupus erythematosus; DIC, disseminated intravascular coagulation.

—*SLE:* Serial determinations of C3 and C4 are often performed in patients with SLE. Depressed C3 and C4 levels may indicate disease activity and tissue damage (e.g., glomerulonephritis). Patients with SLE whose complement proteins are within the normal range may fare better than those with persistent complement consumption. Among patients with SLE, however, there is a higher than normal prevalence of null alleles for C4; therefore, C3 may be a better measure. Immune complex formation further activates the complement cascade and contributes to tissue damage.

—*Other diseases:* Associated with immune complex formation, complement consumption, and low serum complement levels are serum sickness, active viral hepatitis, mixed cryoglobulinemia, rapidly progressive and poststreptococcal glomerulonephritis, and infective endocarditis. Low levels may be seen with advanced liver disease. In addition, direct enzymatic activation of the alternate pathway and low serum complement levels may be seen in conditions such as disseminated intravascular coagulation and myocardial infarction. Low complement levels may be seen in IgA nephropathy and hypersensitivity vasculitis.

—*Complement deficiencies:* Deficiencies of the early components of the classical pathway (C1, C4, C2) interfere with the ability to handle immune complexes, which results clinically in an SLE-like condition. Deficiencies of the terminal components (C5, C6, C7, C8) lead to increased susceptibility to infection, particularly with neisserial organisms. Deficiencies or abnormal function of the inhibitor of C1 lead to unrestrained activation of the classical pathway and the clinical syndrome of angioedema.

—*Inflammation:* Many complement components function as acute-phase reactants (e.g., ESR, CRP) and may be elevated in inflammatory conditions (e.g., RA, ulcerative colitis, rheumatic fever, thyroiditis).

Indications: Tests of individual complement proteins such as C3 and C4 are used to assess the activity of diseases characterized by immune complex formation and consumption of these components. Complement assays are useful in diagnosing and monitoring SLE and diagnosing hereditary angioedema.

Cost: C3, $43–85; C4, $43–80; CH50, $90–150; inhibitor of C1, $90–130.

BIBLIOGRAPHY

Frank MM. Complement in the pathophysiology of human disease. *N Engl J Med* 1987;316:1625–1630.
Glovsky MM. Applications of complement determinations in human disease. *Ann Allergy* 1994;72:477–486.

CREATINE PHOSPHOKINASE (CPK)

Synonyms: Creatine kinase, CK.

Description: CPK is an intracellular enzyme found in high concentrations in skeletal muscle, myocardium, and brain. Damage to these tissues results in elevated serum levels of CK. Three isoforms are used to determine the tissue origin of serum CK: skeletal muscle (MM), myocardium (MB), and brain (BB).

Method: Analysis may be part of a selected automated chemistry profile or may be ordered separately. Serum should be collected in a plain red-top tube. Avoid hemolysis. All determinations of CK levels should be done before invasive diagnostic procedures such as electromyography or muscle biopsy. Ultraviolet spectrophotometry is most common.

Normal Values: Values depend on the method used but generally range from 50 to 200 U/L for males; values for females are 25% lower. Black individuals (males more so than females) may have CK levels above normal values. Such values do not correlate with muscle mass and are not associated with an occult myopathic process. Normal values are seen in renal or pulmonary infarction, pericarditis, thyrotoxicosis, and steroid myopathy.

Increased in: Most patients with dermatomyositis or polymyositis have elevated serum levels of CK. Unless the clinical picture is unclear (e.g., in a patient with chest pain as well as limb weakness), determination of the isoenzyme pattern is not necessary. Although skeletal muscle (MM) is the usual isoenzyme pattern in patients with myositis, elevated MB fractions may occur because of inflammatory damage to, or regeneration of, skeletal muscle, which can express the MB isoform. If CK levels are elevated at the outset of myositis, serial measurements may provide a useful index of therapeutic response.

A significant minority (35%) of patients with active dermatomyositis or polymyositis do not show CK elevations, and in these cases, measurement of other muscle enzymes such as aldolase may be useful. Low levels of CK, sometimes below the normal range, may predict a poor prognosis, especially in patients with malignancy-associated dermatomyositis. Reasons for the lack of CK elevation in some patients with polymyositis/dermatomyositis are not clear but may include the loss of muscle mass or the presence of circulating inhibitors of this enzyme.

Other causes of CK elevation include alcoholic myopathy, myxedema (hypothyroidism), malignant hyperthermia syndrome, Duchenne muscular dystrophy, seizure, eosinophil-myalgia syndrome, late pregnancy (parturition), moderate to severe hemolysis, cocaine use, rhabdomyolysis, cerebrovascular accident, myocardial injury, cardioversion, or muscle trauma. Intramuscular injections and vigorous exercise can also cause CK elevations and should be avoided before phlebotomy.

Decreased in: Those with low muscle mass, severe dermatomyositis or polymyositis, alcoholic liver disease, early pregnancy (20 weeks), and RA may show low CK values.

Indication: CK may be useful in the diagnosis and treatment of inflammatory myositis, muscular dystrophy, myocardial disease, and rhabdomyolysis.

Cost: $30–100.

BIBLIOGRAPHY

Wei N, Pavlidis N, Tsokos G, et al. Clinical significance of low creatine phosphokinase values in patients with connective tissue diseases. *JAMA* 1981;246:1921–1923.
Worrall JG, Phongsathorn V, Hoope RJL, et al. Racial variation in serum creatine kinase unrelated to lean body mass. *Br J Rheumatol* 1990;29:371–373.

CRYOGLOBULINS

Definition: Cryoglobulins are immunoglobulins that reversibly precipitate in the cold (4°C). The reversibility of precipitation by warming the sample to body temperature (37°C) distinguishes cryoglobulins from other cold-precipitable proteins such as cryofibrinogen.

Classification: Cryoglobulins are usually classified into one of three categories, depending on the characteristics of their component immunoglobulins (Table 8).

Type I includes monoclonal antibodies, which can be of any of the major immunoglobulin classes (IgA, IgG, IgM). Such monoclonal proteins may be produced by malignant clonal expansion of B lymphocytes. Monoclonal cryoglobulins are commonly seen in multiple myeloma and Waldenström's macroglobulinemia (see p. 152).

Type II cryoglobulins are referred to as mixed, indicating that both monoclonal and polyclonal antibodies are present. The most common mixed cryoglobulin consists of a monoclonal IgM with RF activity that binds polyclonal IgG. Such complexes are associated with idiopathic mixed cryoglobulinemia, hepatitis C, Sjögren's syndrome, and lymphoproliferative disorders.

Table 8
Classification of Cryoglobulins

Type	Immunoglobulin Components	Other Features
I	Monoclonal only	High levels may be seen
II	Mixed (monoclonal-polyclonal)	IgM-RF often present
III	Mixed polyclonal	Levels usually below 1%

RF, rheumatoid factor.

Type III cryoglobulins do not contain any monoclonal components and are most commonly associated with connective tissue diseases such as RA and SLE. Type III cryoglobulins are usually present in low concentrations, often with cryocrits <1%.

Method (Collection of Sample): Serum samples to be processed for detection of cryoglobulins must be collected carefully to ensure accurate quantitation. Samples cannot be collected during routine scheduled phlebotomy. The laboratory that is to receive the sample must be notified in advance to prepare for processing. Because some cryoprecipitation may occur even at room temperature (22°C), collection must be in a Vacutainer tube prewarmed to 37°C in a portable water bath. The bath can be fashioned from a small covered Styrofoam box or jug with an indwelling thermometer. Blood is drawn into the prewarmed tube, which is then placed in the warm water bath for immediate transport to the laboratory. Samples may be rejected if the specimen has cooled to <36°C. Once received, the blood is allowed to clot completely at 37°C. This procedure is designed to keep all cryoprecipitable proteins in the serum rather than in the blood clot. The clotted sample is spun in a warm centrifuge, and serum is removed and stored at 4°C. Samples are usually kept in the cold for 72 hours to allow precise quantitation, although cryoprecipitate accumulation can often be detected visually after 24 hours. The volume of cryoprecipitate is quantitated in a tube similar to a hematocrit tube, and results are expressed as a percentage of the serum volume. High levels may reach values of ≥10%; levels <1% are difficult to quantitate accurately. Alternatively, the precipitate can be centrifuged out of the cold serum, washed, and resuspended in warm buffer. The amount of protein is then determined spectrophotometrically, and values are expressed as milligrams per total volume of serum.

Typing: After quantitation, cryoprecipitate components may be characterized by counterimmunoelectrophoresis. Specific antibodies are used to detect heavy chains identifying the major immunoglobulin classes as well as the accompanying light chains. Expression of exclusively λ or κ light chains by an immunoglobulin in the precipitate indicates monoclonality. Detection of RF positivity within the cryoprecipitate (tested under warmed conditions) is often useful in characterization.

Normal Values: Values are usually negative (cryocrit, <1%; serum, <80 μg/mL).

Clinical Associations: Cryoglobulins are found in a wide variety of disorders, including infection (e.g., infective endocarditis, hepatitis, Epstein-Barr virus, syphilis), autoimmune disorders (e.g., SLE, RA, polyarteritis nodosa, Sjögren's syndrome, scleroderma, Kawasaki disease), lymphoproliferative disorders (e.g., multiple myeloma, lymphoma, Waldenström's macroglobulinemia), and hyperviscosity syndrome, or it may be idiopathic (essential mixed cryoglobulinemia).

The most clinically important syndromes associated with cryoglobulins are nephritis and cutaneous vasculitis (see p. 152). Essential mixed cryoglobulinemia may demonstrate an acute glomerulonephritis, and patients with this syndrome should be screened for the presence of cryoglobulins in serum. Cryoproteins present a unique appearance in renal biopsies and are usually recognized without special staining. Cutaneous vasculitis with palpable purpura, especially in the lower extremities, should suggest cryoglobulinemia. Biopsy of the rash commonly demonstrates leukocytoclastic vasculitis. Recently, associations of hepatitis C virus infection with type II mixed cryoglobulins have been reported, and this viral infection may represent a significant number of cases previously considered to be idiopathic or essential.

Indications: Cryoglobulin testing should be considered in patients suspected of cryoglobulinemia (i.e., palpable purpura, systemic illness) or those with no known cause for acute glomerulonephritis, severe Raynaud phenomenon, cutaneous vasculitis, or hyperviscosity syndrome.

Cost: $30–65.

CYTOKINES

Synonyms: Other names, such as interleukin (IL), reflect the importance of cytokines in intercellular interactions between white blood cells. Other names reflect the predominant cell type from which they derive (e.g., monokines, lymphokines) or the functions with which they were first associated (e.g., B-cell growth factor, endogenous pyrogen, or chemokine).

Definition: To perform their functions optimally, cells of the immune system must communicate with each other. Such communication can be accomplished in two ways. Cells may physically touch each other, relaying information via specific cell-surface receptors (e.g., adhesion molecules). Alternatively, cells may secrete molecules (cytokines) that interact with receptors on other cells. Many cytokines are small glycoproteins with varying cellular origins (Table 9) that bind with high affinity to specific receptors.

Role: Cytokines serve critical roles in (a) immune reactions (they modulate antigen presentation, activation of immunocompetent cells, and the determination of whether immune reactions are predominantly humoral or cellular); (b) inflammatory reactions (cytokines cause recruitment and activation of cells and also initiate the acute-phase response); and (c) hematopoiesis (several cytokines promote the growth and maturation of various cell lineages).

Table 9
Major Cytokines, Cellular Sources, and Biologic Functions

Cytokine	Major Sources	Functions
IL-1	Macrophages, many other cell lines	Activates lymphocytes, stimulates acute-phase response, CNS effects (fever, increased sleep, anorexia), bone and cartilage destruction, stimulates various inflammatory mediators (leukotrienes, prostaglandins), increases IL-6, activates endothelium
IL-2	T cells, NK cells	Critical autocrine growth factor for T cells; increases killing of tumors by NK cells (creating LAK cells)
IL-3	T cells	Stimulates growth of multiple cell lineages
IL-4	T cells, mast cells	Increases antibody synthesis (e.g., IgE), may inhibit cell-mediated T-cell responses
IL-5	T cells, mast cells	Promotes maturation, activation, and survival of eosinophils
Il-6	Macrophages, lymphocytes	Promotes terminal B-cell maturation, synthesis of acute-phase reactants
IL-8	Macrophages	A "chemokine," promotes endothelial cells chemotaxis of neutrophils to inflammatory sites
IL-10	Macrophages, T cells	Inhibits synthesis of other cytokines (e.g., IL-2, IFN-γ)
TNF	Macrophages, lymphocytes	Stimulates acute-phase response, endothelial cells CNS effects (fever, increased sleep, cachexia), bone and cartilage destruction, increases IL-1, IL-6, IL-8, activates endothelium
IFN-γ	T cells	Critical cytokine for macrophage activation, activates endothelium, inhibits humoral response
GM-CSF	T cells	Stimulates growth of macrophage, endothelial cells granulocyte precursors

IL, Interleukin; CNS, central nervous system; NK, natural killer; LAK, lymphocyte-activated killer cell; TNF, tumor necrosis factor; IFN, interferon; GM-CSF, granulocyte-macrophage colony-stimulating factor.

More than 50 cytokines and their receptors have been identified, and the range of functions of these molecules expands continuously. Cytokines may exert their varied effects in an autocrine (acting on the cell from which they were secreted), paracrine (acting on cells in the same area), or endocrine (acting on distal cells) manner. Cytokines are typically pleiotropic, i.e., a single cytokine typically has numerous functions and acts on various cell types. In addition, there is significant redundancy; several cytokines may have overlapping functions. Rather than acting in isolation, cytokines act in an organized network. Some cytokines have antagonistic functions; others are synergistic.

Disease Associations: The role of cytokines in various diseases has been illustrated by demonstrating increased concentrations of some cytokines in specific conditions. For example, the synovial fluid of patients with inflammatory arthritides such as RA contains elevated amounts of the proinflammatory cytokines IL-1 and tumor necrosis factor-α. In addition, the efficacy of various immunosuppressive therapies depends in large part on their ability to inhibit cytokines (e.g., corticosteroids inhibit IL-1, IL-6, and other cytokines; cyclosporine inhibits IL-2). Moreover, specific therapies directed against cytokines, such as anti-cytokine monoclonal antibodies or receptors, are currently being used for various inflammatory diseases.

Method: Several of the cytokines listed in Table 9 are available from special clinical laboratories. Most assays for secreted circulating cytokines are enzyme immunoassays performed on serum or plasma.

Indications: Cytokine levels are not clinically indicated in the diagnosis or monitoring of patients with rheumatic or autoimmune disease. They are primarily used in some research situations to evaluate a patient's immunologic status or response to biologically specific therapies.

Cost: These tests are expensive. IL-1, $320; IL-6, $230; IL-8, $520; IL-2, $220; IL-2R, $30–205; interferon gamma, $185.

DENSITOMETRY

Synonyms: Single-photon absorptiometry, dual-energy x-ray absorptiometry (DEXA).

Description: Densitometry is a noninvasive procedure that uses a radiation source to quantitate bone mineral density. This imaging technique is widely used in the evaluation of osteoporosis and other metabolic bone disorders. Densitometry is far superior to radiography in estimating bone mass. Newer techniques for measuring bone density that do not use radiation [ultrasonography (US), MRI] are under evaluation.

Method: Bone is exposed to a radiation source (photons or gamma rays), and as the rays pass through the bone, the amount of attenuation is quantitated. Observed results are compared with gender- and age-specific normal values. The differences between observed and expected values may be used to assess the risk of fracture. The most common method currently in use is DEXA, which allows a shorter scanning time and is more precise than single-photon absorptiometry. Single-photon absorptiometry produces a radiation dose of 15 mrem and DEXA produces <5 mrem. Unlike some other methods, DEXA can be used to assess both trabecular and cortical bone.

Commonly, two sites (lumbar spine and hip) are evaluated. These are common sites of fracture, and each represents a different bone-type trabecular bone in the spine and cortical bone in the hip. The patient is positioned with the hips flexed to reduce the normal lumbar lordotic curvature and a posteroanterior view is obtained. Vertebral bodies with compression fractures should be avoided. The procedure usually takes 10 to 20 minutes. Intravenous contrast is not used.

Normal Values: Most equipment reports standards for normal individuals of both genders in age-specific categories. Results are expressed relative to both the age-matched, gender-matched group and to normal young controls of the same gender. The T score is most important amongst these and refers to the number of standard deviations the bone mineral density differs from gender-matched normal young individuals. Normal T scores are greater than -1.0.

Increased in: T scores may be increased in fractures and in rare bone disorders such as osteopetrosis or with heterotopic bone formation and ankylosis (e.g., ankylosing spondylitis).

Decreased in: T scores between -1.0 and -2.5 indicate osteopenia (low bone mass). Values equal to or less than -2.5 indicate osteoporosis and a significant risk for fracture. Bone mineral density may be low in postmenopausal women, hypogonadal men, patients with excess endogenous or exogenous glucocorticoids, immobilized patients (or limbs), hyperthyroidism, and primary hyperparathyroidism.

Confounding Factors: Fractures, even in very thin bones, can cause false elevations in calculated bone density. Heavy calcification in the abdominal aorta can confound readings for the lumbar spine. Residual barium may produce significant artifact.

Indications: With the advent of numerous therapies to treat osteoporosis, diagnosis of this condition has become more important, but there is no universal agreement on when to perform densitometry. New guidelines for DEXA testing have been developed by the National Osteoporosis Foundation and include (a) all women aged 65 and older; (b) younger postmenopausal women with one or more risk factors; (c) postmenopausal women who present with fracture; (d) estrogen-deficient women at clinical risk of osteoporosis; (e) individuals with vertebral abnormalities; (f) individuals starting or receiving long-term glucocorticoid therapy; (g) individuals with primary hyperparathyroidism; (h) individuals while being monitored on osteoporosis drug therapy.

An initial two-site DEXA is reasonable for high-risk patients or individuals who have already sustained a fracture. After initiation of treatment, it is also reasonable to repeat the examination yearly to determine whether the chosen therapy has been effective.

Cost: The usual cost is $150–$350 for one or more sites. Medicare allots $126 for the entire examination, regardless of the number of sites. Medicare allows DEXA once every 2 years (or every 12 months if the patient is on steroids).

BIBLIOGRAPHY

American College of Rheumatology Task Force on Osteoporosis Guidelines. Recommendations for the prevention and treatment of glucocorticoid-induced osteoporosis. *Arthritis Rheum* 1996;39:1791–1801.

National Osteoporosis Foundation. Physician's guide to prevention and treatment of osteoporosis. Available at http://www.nof.org/physguide/index.htm.

DNA ANTIBODIES

Synonyms: Anti-DNA, dsDNA, native DNA, nuclear DNA (nDNA) Farr assay, *Crithidia luciliae* assay, DNA-binding assay.

Description: Autoantibodies that react with dsDNA (anti-DNA or anti-dsDNA) are important in both the diagnosis and pathogenesis of SLE. Diagnostically, anti-dsDNA antibodies are relatively specific for SLE and are part of the American College of Rheumatology classification criteria for SLE (see p. 364). The presence of anti-dsDNA antibodies defines a subset of patients with SLE who are expected to have more severe disease. In particular, these antibodies are associated with the development of lupus nephritis. The concentration (or titer) of DNA antibodies may give some indication of disease activity when followed serially. Some patients with lupus demonstrate higher titers of dsDNA antibodies and lower serum complement levels during disease flares, and, conversely, these indices normalize with appropriate medication and clinical improvement. Pathogenically, immune complexes containing anti-dsDNA antibodies can be found in the circulation and deposited in the tissues of patients with SLE. Specific characteristics of anti-DNA antibodies (e.g., their isotype and overall electrical charge) predispose to renal disease. Single-stranded DNA antibodies are commonly found in SLE but are distinctly different from dsDNA antibodies and are not specific for SLE or associated with nephritis.

Method: Several methods can assess the presence of anti-dsDNA antibodies. The *Crithidia luciliae* assay uses immunofluorescence to detect antibodies binding to a structure called the kinetoplast (which is rich in dsDNA) near the tail of this organism. It has been used for many years and is relatively specific for anti-dsDNA antibodies (antibodies to denatured or single-stranded DNA do not give positive results in this assay). Results are reported as titers (i.e., the highest dilution of serum that still gives positive staining). Other tests for DNA antibodies include radioimmunoassay (the Farr assay) and ELISA. Results from these various tests are reported in different units, and one must be familiar with the laboratory performing these tests.

Increased in: Anti-DNA antibodies are relatively specific for SLE. On rare occasion, low titers are found in healthy older persons or in patients with Sjögren's syndrome, and autoimmune or infectious hepatic disease.

Indications: Anti-DNA antibodies may be of value in establishing the diagnosis of SLE in difficult cases, determining the prognosis of patients known to have SLE, and indicating disease activity in SLE. These are not absolutes; patients with SLE without anti-DNA antibodies may have severe lupus nephritis and vice versa. Also, anti-DNA titers do not correspond to disease activity in every patient with SLE.

Relative Cost: The *Crithidia luciliae* assay, Farr assay, and ELISA all cost approximately $50.

ELECTROMYOGRAPHY (EMG)

Synonyms: EMG, electrodiagnostic studies.

Description: EMG is a diagnostic test used to evaluate patients with suspected muscle disease. EMG is often performed in conjunction with nerve conduction testing (see p. 90).

Method: This test assesses the electrical activity and physiologic function of muscle by placing needle electrodes into selected muscle groups. The procedure does not use external electrical stimulation. Muscle action potentials are produced as waveforms (recorded on an oscilloscope), with specific patterns corresponding to various types of pathologic processes in muscle tissues. EMG is generally performed by specially trained individuals (i.e., neurologist or physiatrist). Because the test is relatively nonspecific, it is important that the clinician provide as much clinical information as possible along with the EMG request to aid in interpretation of the findings.

Normal in: EMG is not useful or diagnostic in fibromyalgia, polymyalgia rheumatica, restless legs, and muscle cramps.

Abnormal in: For patients with inflammatory muscle disorders such as polymyositis or dermatomyositis, characteristic EMG findings include (a) generally increased insertional activity and spontaneous discharges (indicating muscle irritability); (b) decreased amplitude and duration of motor unit action potentials; and (c) an increased number of polyphasic potentials. Although none of these findings is necessarily specific for a given myopathic diagnosis, other potential causes of muscle weakness, such as neuropathies, can often be excluded from further consideration.

Indications: EMG is primarily used to distinguish between weakness caused by disorders of muscle (e.g., muscular dystrophy, inflammatory myositis), peripheral motor neuron (e.g., peripheral neuropathy, radiculopathy), or neuromuscular junction (e.g., myasthenia gravis, Eaton-Lambert syndrome).

Contraindications: EMG is contraindicated with thrombocytopenia, severe coagulopathy, and anticoagulant use.

Confounding Factors: If a muscle biopsy is contemplated, the EMG needles should be placed on the side opposite the biopsy site because low-grade inflammatory infiltrates may result from needle insertion. EMG itself may also result in minor elevations of the CPK.

Relative Cost: EMG with nerve conduction testing is $600–800 per limb.

Comments: Although EMG testing is generally considered noninvasive, patients should be told that mild to moderate discomfort may be noted. If possible, aspirin/NSAIDs should be stopped (five half-lives) before the procedure.

FUNCTIONAL ASSESSMENT

Synonyms: American College of Rheumatology functional classification, Arthritis Impact Measurement Scale, Health Assessment Questionnaire, Modified Health Assessment Questionnaire, Bath Ankylosing Spondylitis Activity Index.

Description: A variety of validated scales have been developed to assess the functional status of patients with arthritis. There are three main types: (a) assessment of functional capacity by either patient self-report or physician; (b) quantitative joint examinations; (c) measurement of performance. Although these assessment tools have been applied primarily in clinical trials of new drugs and evaluation of disability status, they are now being used in clinical practice where functional and clinical outcomes may be easily measured, recorded, and studied longitudinally.

Assessment of Capacity: The American College of Rheumatology has devised a four-class scale to determine the global functional status, primarily in patients with RA. This physician-determined scale is based on the patient's ability to perform activities of daily living including self-care and vocational and avocational activities (Table 10).

Global scales measuring pain or overall functional status may be determined using a 10-cm visual analog scale ranging from no problems (score = 0 cm) to very severe limitations (score = 10 cm). These are often used in clinical trials but can be applied to numerous diseases and situations and can be independently completed by the patient or physician or both.

The most established self-report scale is the Health Assessment Questionnaire (HAQ). A total of 20 items regarding activities of daily living are scored by the patient on a scale of 0 (no problem), 1 (some difficulty), 2 (much difficulty), or 3 (extreme difficulty or unable to do). A shorter modified version of the HAQ, the Modified Health Assessment Questionnaire (mHAQ) (Table 11), with eight questions also scored from 0 through 3, has been advocated as eas-

Table 10
American College of Rheumatology Functional Classification in Rheumatoid Arthritis

Class	Description
I	Able to perform all activities of daily living
II	Able to perform activities of daily living and vocational activities; limited in avocational activities
III	Able to perform activities of daily living but not vocational or avocational activities
IV	Limited in all activities, including self-care

ier to perform in usual clinical situations. The mHAQ score is the mean value of these eight questions. This scale has been very useful in following patients with RA in both clinical trials and practice settings.

The Arthritis Impact Measurement Scales (AIMS) involves a longer questionnaire and has been validated in both RA and psoriatic arthritis. Patients with relatively low educational levels may have difficulty completing this scale without assistance.

A more generalized assessment of overall health is the Short-Form 36 Health Status Questionnaire (or SF-36), which can be administered in person or by telephone and covers general aspects of function in life activities, including social interactions. It has been used in large studies assessing health care delivery as well as in evaluating responses to new treatments in clinical trials.

Various disease-specific questionnaires have been developed. For instance in lupus, the SLE Disease Activity Index and Systemic Lupus Activity

Table 11
Modified Health Assessment Questionnaire

Please check the column that is the best answer for your abilities at this time:

At this moment, are you able to:	Without any difficulty (0)	With some difficulty (1)	With much difficulty (2)	Unable to do (3)
Dress yourself, including tying shoelaces and doing buttons?	_____	_____	_____	_____
Get in and out of bed?	_____	_____	_____	_____
Lift a full cup or glass to your mouth?	_____	_____	_____	_____
Walk outdoors on flat ground?	_____	_____	_____	_____
Wash and dry your entire body?	_____	_____	_____	_____
Bend down to pick up clothing from the floor?	_____	_____	_____	_____
Get in and out of a car?	_____	_____	_____	_____
Turn regular faucets on and off?	_____	_____	_____	_____

Measure are two indices of activity and severity that have also been used in clinical trials. A questionnaire for patients with fibromyalgia, the Fibromyalgia Impact Questionnaire, has been validated and tested in small studies. In those with osteoarthritis of the knee, the Western Ontario and McMaster Universities Osteoarthritis Index (WOMAC) is a commonly used, validated functional assessment tool. For ankylosing spondylitis trials, the Bath Ankylosing Spondylitis Activity Index (BASDAI) also uses patient-derived questionnaires to assess activity.

Quantitative Joint Examination: Counts of tender and swollen joints are a standard means for measuring disease activity and response to therapy in patients with RA. These indices can also be applied to other forms of arthritis, including osteoarthritis and lupus arthritis. Generally, 66 and 68 joints are scored for swelling and tenderness, respectively. A joint is assigned a value of 1 if abnormal (tender or swollen) and 0 if normal. The sum of these is called the (tender or swollen) joint count. A tender or swollen joint score is the sum of the individual joints scored on a scale of 1 to 3. Joint pain is scored as 0 (no pain), 1 (tenderness), 2 (tenderness with wincing), or 3 (wince and withdrawal). Joint swelling is scored as 0 (none), 1 (swelling, just appreciable), 2 (swelling within normal joint contours), or 3 (swelling outside of normal joint contours). Studies suggest that evaluation of fewer accessible joints (e.g., the 28 joint count that examines only the upper extremities and knees) provides as much information as examining all joints.

Assessment of Performance: In RA, the walking time (for 25 or 50 ft) and grip strength (measured using a modified sphygmomanometer) are commonly used functional measures that show correlations with other measures of disease status and are reliable and reproducible.

Confounding Factors: Most validation studies of questionnaires have been done in white, English-speaking populations. Their applicability to those who are non-English speaking or of low educational levels cannot be assumed. However, some forms have been validated in Spanish and French.

Indications: These assessments have been used in trials of new therapeutic agents, especially in patients with RA. Applications in other diseases such as SLE or fibromyalgia are less well established. Insurance companies, other third-party payers, and disability assessment organizations have begun to use these outcome measures. Thus, their use in evaluating patient outcomes in clinical practice is likely to become more common.

Cost: Time is the major cost involved, but even the longer questionnaires such as the Arthritis Impact Measurement Scale or Health Assessment Questionnaire can be completed in <20 minutes. Some questionnaires can be completed by telephone or through the mail. A computerized data entry system may facilitate longitudinal and comparative analyses.

BIBLIOGRAPHY

Bellamy N, Buchanan WW. Clinical evaluation in the rheumatic disease. In: Koopman WJ, ed. *Arthritis and allied conditions: a textbook of rheumatology.* Baltimore: Williams & Wilkins, 1996:47–79.

Hochberg MC, Chane RW, Dwosh I, et al. The American College of Rheumatology 1991 revised criteria for the classification of global functional status in rheumatoid arthritis. *Arthritis Rheum* 1992;25:498–502.

Pincus T, Brooks RH, Callahan LF. Prediction of long-term mortality in patients with rheumatoid arthritis according to simple questionnaire and joint count measures. *Ann Intern Med* 1994;120:26–34.

HEPATITIS: SEROLOGIC TESTS

Description: Serologic tests are used in the diagnosis and management of viral hepatitis A, B, and C. Serologic tests are also available for viral hepatitis D, E, and G, but they have limited clinical application in rheumatology.

Method: Methods include immunodiffusion, ELISA, recombinant immunoblot assays, PCRs, and branched DNA (bDNA) assays.

Normal Value. Tests are normally negative in healthy persons.

Abnormal in: Serologic pattern varies with hepatitis type and duration.
   —*Hepatitis A virus*
   • Antihepatitis A virus IgM is detected in acute hepatitis A. It appears with the onset of symptoms, is detectable for as long as 24 weeks, and confirms the diagnosis.
   • Antihepatitis A virus IgG is detected after the acute period and persists for life. It indicates previous exposure, recovery, and immunity to hepatitis A.
   —*Hepatitis B virus*
   • Hepatitis B surface antigen (HBsAg) is the earliest indicator of HBV infection; it appears in 27 to 41 days, persists during acute illness, and disappears within 6 months with recovery. Persistence after 6 months implies chronic carrier state.
   • Antibody to HBsAg indicates clinical recovery and immunity to hepatitis B virus; it appears after immunization against hepatitis B virus.
   • Hepatitis B "e" antigen (HBeAg) is associated with infectivity. It appears shortly after HBsAg and disappears before HBsAg disappears, being present for 3 to 6 weeks. Persistence beyond 10 weeks suggests progression to chronic carrier state, chronic hepatitis. Presence correlates with neonatal transmission of hepatitis B virus.
   • Antibody to hepatitis B e antigen correlates with decreasing infectivity and good prognosis.
   • Antibody to core antigen includes antihepatitis B core total, antihepatitis B core IgM, and antihepatitis B core IgG. Antihepatitis B core to-

tal appears early in infection and persists lifelong. The IgM component is found for a short time during acute viral infection and persists during the "window" period (after disappearance of HBsAg and before appearance of anti-HBs) and is thus a marker of recent infection. The IgG component persists lifelong and indicates prior exposure to HBV.

—*Hepatitis C virus:* Four assays are available for the diagnosis of hepatitis C virus: ELISA, recombinant immunoblot assays, PCR, and a bDNA assay:

- Antibody to hepatitis C virus (ELISA) reflects actual viral replication and infectivity rather than immunity. Its sensitivity is approximately 80% in chronic carriers and only approximately 15% in the first 6 months after acute infection. It is present in several high-risk groups: posttransfusion hepatitis (70%–85%), intravenous drug users (70%), patients on hemodialysis (20%), homosexual men positive for human immunodeficiency virus-1 (8%). Its prevalence in normal blood donors is between 0.5% and 2%.
- Recombinant immunoblot assay is used as a supplemental test if the ELISA is borderline positive (differentiates false-positive from true-positive results).
- PCR and bDNA assays both measure the amount of HCV. PCR efficiently detects very low levels of the virus.

Table 12
Diagnostic Approach in Suspected Acute Viral Hepatitis

Screening	Result	Secondary Test	Diagnosis[a]
Anti-HAV IgM HBsAg Anti-HBc IgM	Positive Negative Negative		Acute HAV infection
Anti-HAV IgM HBsAg Anti-HBc IgM	Negative Positive Positive		Acute HBV
Anti-HAV IgM HBsAg Anti-HBc IgM	Negative Positive Negative	Anti-HBc IgG positive Anti-HBc IgG negative	Chronic carrier Acute HBV
Anti-HAV IgM HBsAg Anti-HBc IgM	Negative Negative Positive	Anti-HBs positive Anti-HBs negative	Convalescence "Window" period
Anti-HAV IgM HBsAg	Negative Negative	Anti-HBs positive	Convalescence, immune, passive transfer
Anti-HBc IgM	Negative	Anti-HBs Negative	Possible HCV infection

[a]Diagnosis based on screening and secondary test results.
HAV, hepatitis A virus; IgM, immunoglobulin M; HBsAg, hepatitis B surface antigen; HBc, hepatitis B core.

Confounding Factors: False positives are common with anti-hepatitis C virus antibodies and are seen in many autoimmune diseases, with passive antibody transfer and prolonged blood storage. False negatives may occur in early infection and immunosuppression.

Indications: Serologic tests are used for diagnosis of acute hepatitis (Table 12), screening potential blood donors, gauging the response to therapy in chronic hepatitis, monitoring for immunization, investigation of polyarteritis nodosa (25% of cases, usually intravenous substance abusers, are HBsAg, anti-hepatitis B surface, or hepatitis C virus positive), suspected cryoglobulinemia (anti-hepatitis C virus or hepatitis C virus RNA occurs in more than 80% of patients with essential mixed cryoglobulinemia).

Cost: Hepatitis A virus antibody, $40–90; HBsAg, $55; hepatitis C virus antibody, $85; hepatitis C virus recombinant immunoblot assay, $160–260.

Comments: Hepatitis C virus testing continues to improve with newer generations of ELISA and recombinant immunoblot assays, with decreasing numbers of false positives. A logical stepwise approach is preferred to indiscriminate testing.

BIBLIOGRAPHY

Wallach J. Hepatobiliary diseases and diseases of the pancreas. In: *Interpretation of diagnostic tests,* 6th ed. Boston: Little, Brown, 1996:187–205.

HLA-B27

Description: HLA-B27, one of the HLA-B alleles, is expressed on all human cells and is involved in presentation of antigen to CD8$^+$ T cells. HLA-B27 is often associated with spondyloarthropathies such as ankylosing spondylitis, Reiter's syndrome, psoriatic arthritis, and enteropathic arthritis.

Method: Collect 15 mL of blood into tubes containing acid-citrate-dextrose solution B and mix to avoid coagulation. Do not refrigerate or freeze. HLA-B27 may be detected by a microcytotoxicity assay in which mononuclear cells are exposed to test antiserum and complement. HLA-B27 also can be detected by flow cytometry using HLA-B27–specific antibodies.

Normal Values: HLA-27 is a normal gene found in as many as 8% of normal individuals (6%–8% of whites, 3%–4% of African Americans, and 1% of Asians).

Increased in: HLA-B27 is associated with a variety of spondyloarthropathies. The frequency of this allele is shown in Table 13. HLA-B27 positivity is associated with a propensity for axial disease (spondylitis) and uveitis. The actual risk of an HLA-B27–positive person developing ankylosing spondylitis is esti-

Table 13
Population Frequency of HLA-B27

Population	Frequency of HLA-B27 (%)
Ankylosing spondylitis	90
Ankylosing spondylitis with uveitis/aortitis	>95
Reiter syndrome	75–80
Juvenile spondylitis	80
Psoriatic arthritis	
Peripheral arthritis	<10
Spondylitis	50
Enteropathic arthritis	
Peripheral arthritis	<10
Spondylitis	50
General population	
Whites	6–8
African Americans	3–4
Asians	1

mated to be 1% to 2%. Only 20% of HLA-B27-positive individuals infected with arthritogenic bacteria (*Salmonella, Shigella*) develop a reactive arthropathy. Also, only 20% of HLA-B27–positive first-degree relatives of HLA-B27–positive patients with spondylitis develop ankylosing spondylitis. HLA-B27 positivity may correlate with more aggressive disease in reactive arthritis but not in ankylosing spondylitis.

Indications: HLA-B27 assay is used infrequently as a diagnostic test in suspected cases of spondyloarthropathy. It should not be routinely ordered for evaluation or screening of patients with low back pain because the prevalence of HLA-B27 may be as high as 8%, yet the prevalence of spondyloarthropathy is perhaps one per 1,000 individuals. Ordering this test is more likely to yield more false-positive than true-positive results. It is diagnostically valuable when the incomplete syndrome is present or when the pretest probability lies between 30% and 70%. It has no value for screening (low pretest probability) or in patients with classic disease presentations (high pretest probability).

Cost: $80–110.

BIBLIOGRAPHY

Gardner GC, Kadel NJ. Ordering and interpreting rheumatologic laboratory tests. *J Am Acad Orthop Surg* 2003;11:60–67.

HLA-DR4

Definition: The major histocompatibility complex locus designated HLA-DR4 was first associated with RA in studies reported by Stastny in 1978. Using the technique of mixed lymphocyte culture, patients with RA were found to be more alike than were normal individuals, suggesting the presence of a shared cell-associated antigen. This shared antigen was later identified on chromosome 6 as a member of the major histocompatability complex D locus, designated HLA-DR4. The DR molecule consists of two transmembrane chains, designated α and β. The β chain shows extensive polymorphisms and is used to identify subtypes of DR4.

Normal Values: The prevalence of HLA-DR4 is highest in northern European whites and lowest in those of Mediterranean ancestry.

Increased in: Studies in diverse ethnic groups show that the incidence of HLA-DR4 is significantly higher in patients with RA than in the matched normal control population. In white populations of North America, most published series indicate that 60% to 65% of patients with RA are positive for HLA-DR4, which is more than twice the incidence of this allele in the normal population. Moreover, the presence of this allele seems to define a more aggressive variant of RA, with a greater incidence of articular erosions, rheumatoid nodules, secondary Sjögren syndrome, and other extraarticular features of RA. Molecular techniques have been used to identify subtypes of the serologically identified HLA-DR4 molecule that are associated with a significantly elevated risk of RA. These include the HLA-DR4 alleles designated DRB1*0401 and DRB1*0404 as well as the closely related alleles of HLA-DR1 designated DRB1*0101.

- Sequence analyses have further demonstrated that these alleles known to be associated with increased susceptibility and severity of RA also share a common amino acid sequence at positions 67, 70, 71, and 74 in the β chain of the DR4 molecule. This common sequence has been called the "shared epitope". Identification of the antigen recognized by the shared motif carries the potential to reveal the causative antigen in RA. Furthermore, interference with the pathogenetic binding site through production of blocking antibodies or peptides may offer therapeutic benefit. Studies examining the feasibility of this approach are currently in progress.
- The association of HLA-DR with other arthropathies is weaker but, when present, seems to define individuals with a greater risk of chronic, severe polyarthritis (e.g., Lyme disease, psoriatic arthritis).

Clinical Applications: At present, HLA typing is not useful in the clinical management of patients with RA. It appears that patients with DR4, especially those with two copies of the disease-related shared epitope, have more severe disease than patients with RA without any shared epitope alleles. Nonetheless, patients show significant variability in clinical course, and no predictive or prognostic value has been demonstrated. Therefore, therapeutic decisions should be made based on the clinical disease features, not the HLA type.

Cost: HLA-DR4 (DRβ1), $170—230.

BIBLIOGRAPHY

Olsen NJ, Callahan LF, Brooks RH, et al. Associations of HLA-DR4 with rheumatoid factor and radiographic severity in rheumatoid arthritis. *Am J Med* 1988;84:257–264.

Weyand CM, Hicok KC, Conn DL, et al. The influence of HLA-DRB1 genes on disease severity in rheumatoid arthritis. *Ann Intern Med* 1992;117:801–806.

Winchester R. Genetic determination of susceptibility and severity in rheumatoid arthritis. *Ann Intern Med* 1992;117:869–871.

IMMUNE COMPLEXES

Description: Immune complexes composed of antibody and antigen are responsible for pathophysiologic findings in various autoimmune and infectious diseases. The ability of immune complexes to cause injury depends on their deposition in some tissues and subsequent activation of the complement system, phagocytic leukocytes, and other inflammatory mediators.

Deposition of immune complexes in specific tissues depends on a number of factors related to the immune complex itself as well as local factors. For example, the size of immune complexes is critical. Very small immune complexes (typically seen early in an immune response, in states of antigen excess) are readily eliminated and seldom cause tissue injury. Very large immune complexes (usually seen late in the immune response, in states of antibody excess) are efficiently removed by phagocytic cells of the reticuloendothelial system and seldom cause tissue injury. Immune complexes that are prone to deposit and cause injury are often those formed when circulating antigen and antibody are present in roughly equal amounts. Thus, in a immune reaction to a foreign protein, the clinical picture of immune complex deposition may be seen transiently as the immune response switches from a state of antigen excess to one of antibody excess. Other factors that affect tissue deposition of immune complexes include the electric charge of the complex, local blood pressure, and flow patterns (e.g., turbulence).

Methods: Circulating immune complexes may be detected by several methods. Physical methods, such as precipitation with high molecular weight polymers, such as polyethylene glycol, take advantage of the large size of immune complexes and allow direct quantification of the protein concentration in the complex. Other physical methods include gel filtration, cryoprecipitation, and nephelometry. Immune complexes activate the complement cascade via interaction with the C1q component of complement. Thus, C1q can be used in various assays such as a solid-phase radioassay to estimate the concentration of immune complexes in samples. As they activate the complement cascade, complement fragments such as C3d become bound to immune complexes. Assays such as the Raji cell assay take advantage of this by quantifying the amount of immune complex that binds to cell surface complement receptors. Samples should be sent to the laboratory immediately or refrigerated because complement and immune complexes deteriorate at room temperature.

Normal Value: Immune complexes are normally not present or not detected.

Clinical Associations: Clinical expression of immune complex disease varies with the tissues involved. For example, deposition of immune complexes in the kidney (e.g., in bacterial endocarditis) causes glomerulonephritis. Serum sickness, a constellation of symptoms that includes arthralgias, arthritis, lymphadenopathy, fever, and urticarial, petechial, or macular skin lesions, results from widespread deposition of immune complexes in various organs.

Immune complex formation and deposition play a part in a number of diseases. The relevant antigens include exogenous antigens (e.g., drugs, foreign proteins, vaccines); infectious agents (e.g., bacteria such as staphylococci, streptococci, mycoplasma, treponemes; parasites such as plasmodia, *Toxoplasma, Schistosoma;* viruses such as hepatitis B, Epstein-Barr, cytomegalovirus); endogenous or self-antigens (as in SLE, RA, cryoglobulinemia, tumor antigens). In some cases, specific antigens may be typically associated with particular end-organ manifestations, such as arthritis associated with hepatitis B or the glomerulonephritis associated with staphylococcal endocarditis. In other cases, many antigens may produce a similar constellation of symptoms, such as serum sickness related to various endogenous or infectious agents.

Confounding Factors: Some RFs, cryoglobulins, cold agglutinins, and paraproteins may cause false-positive results.

Cost: Raji, $140–165; C1q, $95–130.

Comment: Immune complex assays are seldom used in clinical practice because they are expensive, etiologically nonspecific, poorly correlated with each other, and slow because many are performed primarily in reference laboratories. Some investigators and researchers still use these assays as sequential indicators of disease activity in diseases characterized by immune complex formation (e.g., SLE) or to aid in the diagnosis of patients with multisystem disease. Because circulating immune complexes are very efficient at activating the complement system, some investigators use direct measurements of complement proteins or their split products (see Complement, p. 58) to provide indirect evidence of immune complex involvement in disease processes.

IMMUNOGLOBULINS (IgG, IgA, IgM, IgE)

Description: Immunoglobulins are serum antibodies produced by plasma cells and are the major component of the humoral immune response. Measurement of serum immunoglobulins of different isotypes (i.e., IgG, IgA, IgM, IgE) may be useful in a variety of immunodeficiency, infectious, allergic, and lymphoproliferative diseases.

Method: Serum immunoglobulins are currently measured by specific immunologic methods such as ELISA.

Normal Values: Concentrations may vary slightly depending on the laboratory and the particular methods used, but, in general, normal values for serum immunoglobulins in healthy adults are as follows: IgG, 550 to 1,900 mg/dL; IgM, 50 to 150 mg/dL; and IgA, 60 to 350 mg/dL. IgE is usually present in far smaller amounts.

Serum immunoglobulin concentrations depend on a number of developmental, genetic, and environmental factors, among which the most important is age. IgG synthesized by the mother crosses the placenta in increasing amounts beginning at approximately 3 months of fetal development. At birth, this maternal contribution to the newborn's IgG stops, and total IgG levels slowly decrease until the contribution from the newborn increases at approximately 4 to 6 months of age. Levels of immunoglobulins increase throughout childhood, generally reaching adult concentrations by age 12.

Abnormal Values: Values vary according to clinical situation, therapy, and isotype.

—*IgE:* Most methods currently used do not ascribe any significance to very low concentrations of IgE (i.e., normal persons may have undetectable serum concentrations of IgE). Elevated serum IgE concentrations correlate with a proclivity to allergic conditions such as allergic rhinitis, asthma, atopic skin disease, anaphylactic shock, and some parasitic infections. However, determination of IgE specific for particular antigens is of greater significance in evaluating patients with allergic diseases than measurements of total IgE. Antigen-specific IgE may be determined by *in vivo* tests such as the cutaneous scratch tests using particular allergens or by *in vitro* methods such as the radioallergosorbent test.

—*IgM:* IgM usually circulates in a large molecular weight pentamer and remains almost entirely within the vasculature and does not cross the placenta. It is the earliest immunoglobulin synthesized in response to antigenic challenge. Decreased IgM levels may be seen in humoral immunodeficiencies such as common variable immunodeficiency or in conditions of excess protein loss such as nephrotic syndrome. Polyclonal increases in IgM may be seen during the course of various infections or autoimmune disorders in which there is polyclonal stimulation of the immune response. Monoclonal elevations in IgM are seen in neoplastic proliferations of B cells, e.g., Waldenström macroglobulinemia. Because of their large size, IgM aggregates are more likely to affect plasma viscosity and cause clinical symptoms than are other immunoglobulin isotypes. Clinically important IgM antibodies are directed against RF and the ABO blood groups.

—*IgA:* Serum concentrations of IgA reflect the amounts of two isotypes, IgA1 and IgA2. Although these are present in approximately equal amounts in serum, IgA1 is the predominant IgA isotype secreted onto mucosal surfaces.

This secreted form is an important part of the immune response to pathogens present on mucosal surfaces. Serum IgA levels, therefore, may not reflect the functional status of IgA-mediated responses. Indeed, serum concentrations of IgA below the lower limits of normal, the most commonly observed humoral immunodeficiency, are found in one in 700 persons. Although the vast majority of these patients are asymptomatic, decreased serum levels of IgA may also be seen in immunodeficient patients, e.g., those with common variable immunodeficiency.

—*IgG:* IgG is present in approximately equal amounts in the intravascular and extravascular compartments and comprises nearly 80% of the circulating immunoglobulin. It is the most important immunoglobulin isotype in secondary (anamnestic) immune responses. Total serum IgG represents the sum of the four IgG subclasses (IgG1, IgG2, IgG3, and IgG4), which are numbered in descending order of their concentration in normal serum. Thus, isolated deficiencies of IgG1 typically are evidenced as a decrease in total IgG [as well as decreased gamma fraction of serum protein electrophoresis (SPEP)]. By contrast, deficiencies of IgG3 or IgG4 may be masked within a normal total IgG concentration.

Confounding Factors: Leaving samples at room temperature for hours may result in lower immunoglobulin levels. Radiation therapy, chemotherapy, and high-dose corticosteroids may also lower serum immunoglobulin levels.

Indications: Quantitative serum immunoglobulin (IgG, IgA, IgM) determinations are appropriate for initial evaluation of a patient with suspected humoral (antibody) immunodeficiency (see p. 217). If these are normal but there is a very high clinical suspicion of humoral immunodeficiency, it may be appropriate to obtain IgG subclasses or antigen-specific antibody titers (e.g., serum titers of antipneumococcal antibody in patients who have been appropriately vaccinated). Testing is also indicated in the diagnosis of some paraproteinemias such as multiple myeloma and Waldenström macroglobulinemia.

Cost: $150–200.

ISCHEMIC FOREARM EXERCISE TEST

Definition: A common test used to diagnosis metabolic diseases of muscle.

Description: This test was first used by McArdle to describe the absence of elevated blood lactate levels during exercise in patients with a myophosphorylase deficiency (McArdle disease) and has subsequently been useful in detecting other storage disorders. In McArdle disease, the enzyme deficiency impairs the metabolism of glycogen (a source of energy) to lactate in muscle. Because this test is often poorly tolerated and may have hazardous consequences in patients with McArdle disease, some have advocated the use of nonischemic test methods (see Alternatives section).

Method: Ischemic forearm exercise testing requires that the patient's non-dominant, exercised arm have the antecubital vein cannulated and then a blood pressure cuff on the same arm is inflated (>20 mm Hg above systolic pressure) to occlude venous return. The arm is then maximally exercised to exhaustion using intermittent anisometric maximal forearm contractions (i.e., squeezing a ball or inflated blood pressure cuff) to the point of ischemia or exhaustion. The blood pressure cuff is released. Blood samples are taken at baseline and then serially (1, 3, 5, and 10 minutes) after exercise.

Normal Values: Normal individuals will show at least a threefold increase in serum lactate and ammonia levels without an increase in CPK or potassium.

Abnormal Values: Patients with McArdle disease (myophosphorylase deficiency) show an increase in ammonia levels but not in serum lactate. Patients with a myoadenylate deaminase deficiency will show an increase in lactate but not ammonia levels. Although forearm ischemic testing is >90% sensitive with glycogen storage disorders, only 50% of patients with mitochondrial myopathies will show abnormalities with elevated baseline lactate levels that will normalize in response to exercise.

Confounding Factors: Results may be altered by catheter placement but not by preexercise dietary intake.

Adverse Effects: Cramping, myalgia, contractures, and, rarely, myoglobinuria or rhabdomyolysis are seen (usually in patients with glycogenolytic disorders such as McArdle disease). Compartment syndrome is rarely reported.

Indications: Useful in the evaluation of patients suspected of having McArdle disease and other like disorders of muscle metabolism.

Alternatives: A standardized nonischemic forearm exercise test has been proposed and shows promise. This uses a nonischemic grip test that can be used in patients with exercise intolerance. In this test, an isometric 70% maximum voluntary contraction of 30 seconds is followed by serial blood samples at 1, 2, 3, 4, 6, and 10 minutes post-contraction to measure lactate and ammonia levels. This alternative test takes nearly 30 minutes and was not associated without significant toxicity. Patients with McArdle disease failed to increase their blood lactate levels but did increase serum ammonia and, in some, CPK levels in response to isometric exercise.

Cost: Approximately $1400 (includes procedure, labs, interpretation)

BIBLIOGRAPHY

Hogrel JY, Laforet P, Yaou RB, et al. A non-ischemic forearm exercise test for the screening of patients with exercise intolerance. *Neurology* 2001;56:1733–1738.
Wortmann RL, Vladutiu GD. The clinical laboratory evaluation of the patient with noninflammatory myopathy. *Curr Rheumatol Rep* 2001;3:310–316.

LABIAL SALIVARY GLAND BIOPSY

Synonyms: Labial or lip biopsy, minor salivary gland biopsy.

Description: Incisional biopsy of minor salivary glands in the lower lip is useful in the evaluation of xerostomia and the diagnosis of Sjögren's syndrome.

Method: Patients should suspend aspirin or NSAIDs intake 3 to 7 days before the procedure. This outpatient procedure is usually done by a surgeon using local anesthesia. The lower lip is everted, and normal mucosa is incised with a 2-cm horizontal incision. At least five minor salivary glands are removed and sent for histopathologic examination.

Complications: Complications include numbness in the lower lip (<1%), local bleeding, infection, and pain.

Abnormal Pathology: A diagnosis of Sjögren's syndrome can be entertained if there is more than one focus of lymphocyte clusters ($\geq$50 round cells in $\geq$4 mm^2 of glandular tissue), with acinar atrophy and hypertrophy of ductal epithelial and myoepithelial cells. The reliability of the biopsy is improved if normal-appearing acini are also seen adjacent to foci of inflammation. Myoepithelial islands may not be seen with minor salivary gland biopsies. Focal lymphocytic sialoadenitis is graded as a focus score, indicating the number of inflammatory foci seen. A focus score of >1 has a 95% specificity and 63% sensitivity for Sjögren's syndrome. A focus score of $\geq$10 implies near confluent inflammation.

Confounding Factors: False-positive results may be seen with lichen planus or mucosal trauma.

Indications: The procedure is indicated when Sjögren's syndrome is suspected, especially when the clinical presentation is incomplete or other tests are inconclusive or negative.

Contraindications: Coagulopathy, anticoagulant therapy, local infection, mouth ulcers, and sensitivity to lidocaine or epinephrine are contraindications.

Alternative Procedures: Noninvasive procedures include salivary flow rate, sialography, or salivary scintigraphy.

Cost: $80–200 (does not include hospital charges or consultation).

Comment: Positive labial salivary gland biopsy does not imply coexistent ocular inflammation. In patients with parotid swelling, biopsy of the parotid may be considered, especially if other diagnoses (e.g., parotid tumors) are suspected.

BIBLIOGRAPHY

Daniels TE. Labial salivary gland biopsy in Sjögren's syndrome. *Arthritis Rheum* 1984;27: 147–156.

LYME DISEASE ANTIBODY

Description: A serologic test that may be used to confirm the diagnosis of Lyme disease.

Method: Screening for serum antibodies against *Borrelia burgdorferi* is done using ELISA or, less commonly, an indirect immunofluorescent assay. Additional specificity is provided by Western immunoblot confirmation (more than three bands is considered confirmatory). PCR has been used to confirm *B. burgdorferi* DNA in ticks but is not yet standardized for routine clinical use in humans.

Normal Values: This test is normally negative.

Increased in: Specific IgM antibody peaks within 3 to 6 weeks after Lyme disease onset. IgG titers increase more slowly and are often present when arthritis begins. CSF antibody levels help confirm neuroborreliosis.

Confounding Factors: Serology may be normal in early disease or with an attenuated immune response to a partially treated infection. Cross-reactivity with other spirochetes such as *Treponema pallidum* can lead to false-positive results. False positives also occur in <20% of patients with high-titer RF. High serum lipid levels and hemolysis may interfere with results.

Indications: Serologic testing should only be done when individuals are strongly suspected of having Lyme disease because of (a) the low prevalence of Lyme disease in nonendemic areas; (b) significant false-positive and false-negative rates; and (c) considerable intra- and interlaboratory variation in results.

Cost: Enzyme immunoassay, $75–110; Western blot, $120–160; PCR, $130–180.

Comments: Lyme disease remains a clinical diagnosis with laboratory studies helpful for confirmation. Half of patients with early Lyme disease (erythema chronicum migrans, constitutional features), and nearly all those with late Lyme disease (carditis, neuritis, arthritis) or in remission have positive serologic test results.

MAGNETIC RESONANCE IMAGING

Synonyms: Nuclear magnetic resonance.

Description: MRI is an imaging method that uses a magnetic field to detect changes in the spin orientation of hydrogen nuclei, or protons, located in living tissues. Patients are placed within a magnetic coil and then exposed to pulsed radiofrequency waves that cause the protons in tissues to change spin orientation. After the pulse, the magnet measures the time required for protons to return to baseline, which is translated into a signal used to characterize tissue composition.

Methods: Most studies involve acquisition of two or more types of images, the most common of which are designated T1- and T2-weighted. These images use different repetition times and sample after different echo times. The T1-weighted image usually provides greater anatomic detail, but the T2-weighted image is more likely to show common tissue pathology such as inflammation, which is associated with increased free water content.

Confounding Factors: Patients with indwelling magnetic metal cannot be evaluated; this includes those with pacemakers, insulin pumps, sutures or artificial components in the eye, wire sutures in brain tissues, and rods or screws in bones. Most joint replacement components in current use are made of non-magnetic materials, so these patients can be safely scanned. Wire sutures in areas such as the abdomen also do not present problems.

Adverse Effects: No radiation exposure is involved, and, at present, there are no known health risks associated with exposure to the magnetic field. A minority of patients may experience claustrophobia or other discomfort. At times, these reactions require stopping the examination; in other cases, use of sedative agents is required to complete the scan.

Indications: Unlike standard radiographs, MRI can define soft tissues in great detail, so joint structures such as ligaments, tendons, synovium, and articular cartilage can be evaluated. Examples of joint abnormalities that can be delineated with MRI include meniscal tears, ligamentous damage, tendon rupture, Baker cysts, pigmented villonodular synovitis, and simple effusions. MRI has largely replaced invasive radiologic procedures (e.g., arthrography) in evaluation of rotator cuff and shoulder disorders. Inflammation in muscles can be detected in patients with myositis and related syndromes. MRI may be useful in evaluating the integrity of bone and nerve tissues in the spine.

Cost: $1,000–2,000. Expense is significantly greater than per site other techniques. MRI should therefore be used selectively.

BIBLIOGRAPHY

Ghozlan R, Vacher H. Where is imaging going in rheumatology? *Baillieres Best Pract Res Clin Rheumatol* 2000;14:617–633.
Santiago Restrepo C, Gimenez CR, McCarthy K. Imaging of osteomyelitis and musculoskeletal soft tissue infections: current concepts. *Rheum Dis Clin North Am* 2003;29:89–109.

MYOGLOBIN

Description: Myoglobin is an oxygen-binding intracellular muscle protein that stores and delivers oxygen to mitochondria. It is found in skeletal and cardiac muscle and may be released into the circulation after damage to muscle cells.

Method: Myoglobin is measured by radioimmunoassay in serum and by dipstick in urine. Myoglobin is chemically similar to hemoglobin and is detected by the usual dipsticks used for urinalysis. A strongly positive hemoglobin indicator on the dipstick in the absence of erythrocytes may signal myoglobinuria and should prompt measurement of urine myoglobin.

Normal Values: Concentration in serum is normally ≤ 90 ng/mL and 0 to 2 mg/mL in urine.

Increased in: Myoglobin is released into the circulation after muscle damage, most commonly caused by injuries such as blunt trauma, heat stroke, ischemia, or inflammation. Release may occur during the course of inflammatory muscle disorders such as polymyositis. In some but not all cases, muscle swelling or tenderness occurs.

Elevated serum levels are also seen in patients with overlap disease with myositis, alcoholic myopathy, hypothermia, shock, severe renal failure, myocardial infarction, or recent cardioversion.

Myoglobinuria may be detected in any instance of excessive serum myoglobin and may also be found in those with familial myoglobinuria, transient "march" myoglobinuria, diabetic ketoacidosis, marked hypokalemia, and severe infections.

Indications: Myoglobin is determined to assess the magnitude of muscle damage or the risks to renal function after muscle damage.

Comment: Myoglobin is cleared by the kidney and excreted in the urine. For reasons that are not well understood, myoglobin is toxic to renal tubular cells, and excess myoglobin (myoglobinuria) may cause acute tubular necrosis and renal failure.

Cost: Urine dipstick is inexpensive; serum radioimmunoassay, $90–130; urine radioimmunoassay, $95–130.

MYOSITIS-SPECIFIC AUTOANTIBODIES

Synonym: Anti-synthetase antibodies

Description: Approximately 60% to 80% of patients with inflammatory myopathies have autoantibodies. Some of these, such as ANAs, are seen in other syndromes and are not specifically associated with muscle disorders. However, approximately half of patients with autoantibodies show antibody specificities that are exclusively seen in association with inflammatory muscle disease. Most myositis-specific autoantibodies (MSAs) are directed against intracellular (usually cytoplasmic) ribonucleoproteins that are involved in protein translation. The most common are a family of antibodies directed against aminoacyl-tRNA synthetases. Antibodies to histidyl-tRNA, also called Jo-1 antibodies, are the most common and most clinically assayed of these antisynthetase antibodies. Other MSAs include anti–Mi-2 and anti–signal-recognition particle antibodies.

Method: MSAs are detected by indirect fluorescent antibody assay.

Normal Values: MSAs are normally not present.

Clinical Associations: Some researchers suggest that MSAs may be more useful in defining clinical subsets of inflammatory muscle disorders than currently used clinical categories, such as polymyositis and dermatomyositis. This proposal is based on observations indicating that the clinical disease course, including mortality rates, is correlated with the pattern of autoantibody expression. Some of these clinical associations are summarized in Table 14.

—*Jo-1:* Jo-1 is seen in patients with polymyositis, interstitial lung disease, and arthritis; 20% of all patients with inflammatory myositis are Jo-1 positive. Patients with antibodies to synthetases have a higher incidence of interstitial lung disease than patients in the other groups; responses to treatment interventions are intermediate. The "antisynthetase syndrome" is characterized by the occurrence of inflammatory myositis, arthritis, interstitial lung disease, Raynaud phenomenon, photosensitive facial rashes, "mechanics (or machinists) hands" (cracked, fissured, hypertrophic changes over the distal fingers), and fever.

—*Mi-2:* Antibodies to Mi-2 are seen almost exclusively in patients with the clinical syndrome of dermatomyositis. These patients tend to respond best to treatment.

—*Signal-Recognition Particle (SRP):* Patients with antibodies to SRP tend to have the clinical syndrome of acute onset polymyositis without a rash, have variable cardiac involvement, and generally respond poorly to treatment. Limited studies in children suggest a similar clinical pattern in juvenile myositis syndromes.

Table 14
Syndromes Associated with Myositis-Specific Autoantibodies

Autoantibody	Characteristic Clinical Features	Response to Treatment
Anti-Jo-1 and other antisynthetases	Relatively acute onset; frequent interstitial lung disease, fever, arthritis, Raynaud phenomenon	Moderate response to therapy but persistent disease
Anti-Signal recognition particle	Very acute onset, severe weakness, palpitations (no rash)	Poor response to therapy
Anti-Mi-2	Relatively acute onset, classic dermatomyositis rash, cuticular overgrowth	Good response to therapy

Indications: MSA assays are primarily used in research to characterize subsets of inflammatory myositis. The utility of antisynthetase antibodies has largely been investigated at tertiary academic sites, and it is unknown whether the same associations will be seen in a primary care practice setting. Because MSAs are relatively expensive, not readily available, and of uncertain prognostic value, their routine in patients with myositis is not recommended.

Cost: Jo-1, $120–150; Mi-2, $170–220.

BIBLIOGRAPHY

Hengstman GJ, van Engelen BG, Vree Egberts WT, et al. Myositis-specific autoantibodies: overview and recent developments. *Curr Opin Rheumatol* 2001;13:476–482.
Targoff IN. Laboratory testing in the diagnosis and management of idiopathic inflammatory myopathies. *Rheum Dis Clin North Am* 2002;28:859–890.

NAILFOLD CAPILLAROSCOPY

Synonym: Wide-field nailfold capillaroscopy.

Description: Easily performed, this test examines nailfold capillary architecture by microscopy. Although not truly specific, the test is useful in distinguishing primary and secondary Raynaud phenomenon. Secondary Raynaud disease refers to Raynaud phenomenon in the setting of another connective tissue disorder (e.g., systemic sclerosis, CREST syndrome, RA, or SLE).

Method: A clean nailbed from the third and fourth (preferred) fingers should be examined at room temperature using low-power magnification from either an ophthalmoscope (+40 diopters), hand-held illuminating microscope (10–40×, available from Radio Shack), or a wide-field stereomicroscope (12–14×) using a low-voltage lamp that does not heat the skin. Videomicroscopy has also been used. Place a drop of grade B immersion oil, mineral oil, or lubricant gel (e.g., K-Y Jelly) proximal to the cuticle. Look for evenly arranged capillary loops arising from the nailbed with a hairpin appearance. There may be finger to finger variation.

Normal: Normal vessels are thin, uniform, evenly spaced, and symmetric in distribution (Fig. 1). Normal capillary loops have a hairpin appearance. Normal vessels are seen in most rheumatic disorders, including fibromyalgia, osteoarthritis, gout, primary Raynaud phenomenon, and eosinophilic fasciitis. Minor vessel abnormalities and a few avascular areas are uncommonly seen in normal individuals. However, extensive hemorrhage and avascular dropout and bizarre or giant vessels are rarely seen in normal controls.

Abnormal: Commonly seen abnormalities may include absent ("dropout" areas) or dilated capillary loops. Vessel architecture may be described as irregu-

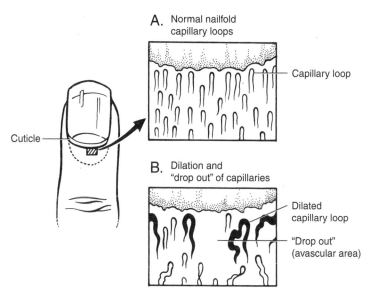

A. Normal nailfold capillary loops

Capillary loop

Cuticle

B. Dilation and "drop out" of capillaries

Dilated capillary loop

"Drop out" (avascular area)

Figure 1. Nailfold capillaroscopy.

lar, tortuous, elongated, bizarre, bushy, engorged, or corkscrew in appearance. Spacing between loops may be uneven or irregular (Fig. 1).

—*Primary Raynaud phenomenon:* Normal capillaries are most common and suggest a good prognosis and low risk of future development of scleroderma and related disorders.

—*Scleroderma:* The scleroderma pattern (also seen with CREST and mixed connective tissue disease) is one of enlarged or dilated capillary loops with areas of intervening vessel dropout. Dropout is specific for scleroderma. Tortuous vessels, distortion, or "budding" of capillaries may be seen. Capillary hemorrhages and bizarre vessel architecture are common. The extent of capillary lesions may correlate with the severity of end-organ damage and survival rates.

—*Dermatomyositis:* Patients with dermatomyositis are frequently abnormal, with vessel changes similar to scleroderma. Giant, engorged vessels with hemorrhage may be seen macroscopically. Patients with SLE may be abnormal with corkscrew-appearing capillaries.

—*Others:* Nailfold capillary abnormalities have also been described in patients with diabetes mellitus, RA, psoriasis, and Behçet syndrome.

Indications: Nailfold capillaroscopy is useful as a bedside aid to the differential diagnosis of Raynaud phenomenon or an undifferentiated connective tissue disease. Many undifferentiated patients with abnormal capillary findings progress to a fully manifest syndrome. Capillaroscopy may be of some value in documenting the extent of microvascular disease in patients with scleroderma, CREST, mixed connective tissue disease, and dermatomyositis.

Cost: Inexpensive; procedure takes 3–5 minutes to perform using an ophthalmoscope, hand-held microscope, or dermatoscope (Fig. 1).

NERVE CONDUCTION TESTING

Synonyms: Nerve conduction velocity, latency studies.

Definition: Evaluation of peripheral nerves by nerve conduction testing involves measurement of the velocity of an electrical stimulus in a target nerve.

Method: The test is done by percutaneous stimulation of a nerve at two separate points along its course and recording the electrical response (evoked action potentials) on the skin (for sensory nerves) or an associated muscle (for motor nerves). This test helps to evaluate both generalized and localized neuropathies that might affect peripheral nerves or muscle function. Nerve conduction testing is usually performed by a specially trained physiatrist or neurologist, often at the same time as electromyography (see p. 69). Referrals should include a clinical history and the reason for the procedure.

Normal in: Nerve conduction is normal in primary muscle disorders, myasthenia gravis radiculopathies, and amyotrophic lateral sclerosis.

Abnormal in: Detection of abnormalities in all extremities suggests generalized disorders such as polyneuropathy, mononeuritis multiplex, or Guillain-Barré syndrome. If only localized abnormalities are found, then mechanical problems with nerve entrapment (e.g., carpal tunnel syndrome) or localized inflammatory problems such as mononeuritis multiplex should be considered. Measurements to confirm a diagnosis of carpal or tarsal tunnel syndrome can be limited to the involved extremity, whereas a more generalized problem requires evaluation of all limbs.

Confounding Factors: A cardiac pacemaker (or implanted defibrillator) may influence evoked potentials. Results are unreliable or unobtainable in agitated or uncooperative patients. Results are not affected by medications.

Indications: Nerve conduction velocity testing is a noninvasive procedure appropriate for evaluating peripheral neuropathies. Specifically, nerve conduction velocity is useful in determining the extent of nerve involvement (i.e., polyneuropathy versus mononeuritis multiplex) and whether a demyelinating or axonal process is present. It is often useful in distinguishing neuropathic from myopathic causes of muscle weakness. Diagnostic findings may occur in patients with entrapment syndromes (e.g., carpal tunnel syndrome), Guillain-Barré syndrome, Eaton-Lambert syndrome, and myasthenia gravis.

Cost: $200–500 per limb (cost includes evaluation by the neurologist or physiatrist).

PROTEIN: URINE

Description: Quantitative tests for proteinuria are commonly performed. Normal persons may secrete approximately 150 mg of protein into the urine in a 24-hour period. Albumin constitutes only a fraction of this (15–40 mg); the remainder is composed of many different proteins derived predominantly from the renal cells. The most prevalent of these is the Tamm-Horsfall mucoprotein derived from the loop of Henle, which is made in amounts of as much as 50 mg/day. Increased amounts of protein in the urine result most commonly from glomerular damage that allows plasma proteins to enter the urine.

Method: Proteinuria is initially screened for by dipstick testing. This colorimetric chemical reaction depends on urine protein concentration rather than absolute amount. Thus, results may vary considerably depending on how concentrated the urine is. The test is semiquantitative, with results typically reported as 0, trace, + (or 30 mg/dL), ++ (or 100 mg/dL), and +++ (or >300 mg/dL). Proteinuria can be better quantified with a 24-hour urine collection. A close estimate of 24-hour protein excretion may also be obtained from a single ("spot") urine sample if the amount of protein is correlated with the concentration of creatinine in the same sample. This gives an estimate of the amount that would be excreted in 24 hours.

Individual proteins in a urine sample may be determined by protein electrophoresis (similar to SPEP, see Serum Protein Electrophoresis section). This distinguishes proteinuria reflecting glomerular injury (largely albumin) from tubular proteinuria (diverse proteins that migrate in the α, β, and γ regions) from proteinuria related to myeloma (proteins that typically migrate in the γ region). The specific type of immunoglobulin in the urine may be identified by immunoelectrophoresis. Patients with diabetes mellitus often secrete increasing amounts of albumin in their urine as the disease progresses. Albumin present in the urine in the early stages of diabetes is often missed by dipstick. Microalbuminuria can be detected by several test reagents now available that allow detection of concentrations as low as 5 mg/dL.

Normal Values: Normally, approximately 150 mg of protein is excreted into the urine in a 24-hour period. Amounts >500 mg/day are often considered clinically significant. Excretion of >3.5 g of protein is considered massive proteinuria. Massive proteinuria associated with hypoalbuminemia, edema, and hyperlipidemia is known as the nephrotic syndrome.

Increased in: Proteinuria may be seen in a variety of conditions (Table 15).

Confounding Factors: Dipstick analysis of urine for protein is most sensitive to albumin, so substantial amounts of other proteins may be missed. Because

Table 15
Causes of Proteinuria

Glomerular disease
  Minimal change disease
  Mesangial proliferative glomerulonephritis (e.g., IgA nephropathy)
  Focal segmental glomerulonephritis/glomerulosclerosis
  Membranous glomerulonephritis
  Crescentic glomerulonephritis
Glomerular disease associated with systemic conditions
  Autoimmune
    Systemic lupus erythematosus (lupus nephritis)
    Wegener granulomatosis
    Henoch-Schönlein purpura
    Goodpasture syndrome
    Amyloidosis
    Sjögren syndrome
    Microscopic polyarteritis
    Rheumatoid arthritis
  Infectious/postinfectious
    Poststreptococcal
    Subacute bacterial endocarditis
    Human immunodeficiency virus
  Neoplastic
    Leukemia/lymphoma
    Wilms tumor
Hereditary proteinuria
Proteinuria associated with drugs
  Intramuscular gold salts
  D-Penicillamine
  Impure heroin
  Amphotericin B
  Aminoglycosides
Benign proteinuria (typically <2.0 g/d)
  Orthostatic

---

dipstick urinalysis is so dependent on protein concentration, significant amounts of excreted protein may be missed in a dilute urine sample. Analysis of a concentrated early morning urine specimen is one way to address this problem. The common assumption that microhematuria itself causes proteinuria is usually false; 1 mL of blood contains 5 million red blood cells but only 70 mg of protein. When diluted in urine, this usually falls below the level of detection for proteinuria. Thus, proteinuria in the setting of microhematuria (as opposed to massive hematuria) usually reflects glomerular damage. Last, some drugs may cause false-positive dipstick results (e.g., tolbutamide, chlorpromazine, high-dose penicillin, sulfonamide, cephalosporin, iodine contrast).

Indications: Determination of proteinuria is useful in a number of diseases. In rheumatology, it is most commonly used to determine the extent of glomerular injury from diseases such as SLE or drugs such as gold (Table 15).

Cost: Urinalysis, $14–26; 24-hour urine protein quantification, $60–80.

RADIOGRAPHY

Synonyms: X-ray, conventional radiography, roentgenograms.

Description: Radiography is an imaging method used in assessment of osseous and soft tissue structures. Conventional radiography is useful in the diagnosis and staging of articular and osseous disorders.

Method: Symptomatic structures should be imaged from several views to allow a circumferential view of articular structures. Both the imaging equipment and film used in conventional radiography vary, as do the clarity and resolution of films obtained. The quality of radiographs can be enhanced by using faster machines and single-emulsion film cassettes without an intensifying screen. Ensuring patient comfort during the imaging procedure results in more reliable images. Those in pain or with severe deformities that limit proper positioning may have difficulty complying with the imaging process.

Recommended Views: The use of proper technique, patient positioning, and selected views may eliminate the need for further diagnostic studies. The following is a list of commonly requested views during routine radiography. These may be modified in accord with the clinical picture or after consultation with an experienced musculoskeletal radiologist.
—*Hand/wrist:* Posteroanterior and oblique ("pincer" or "ball catchers") views.
—*Elbows:* Anteroposterior (AP) and lateral views.
—*Shoulders:* AP (with internal and external rotation) views; consider axillary view.
—*Cervical spine:* AP, obliques, lateral (extension and flexion), and open-mouthed views.
—*Lumbar spine:* AP, obliques, lateral, and L5–S1 views.
—*Hips:* AP of the pelvis and "frog leg" (external rotation) views.
—*Sacroiliac joints:* AP pelvis and AP with 30-degree cephalad angle.
—*Knees:* Standing AP and lateral views; axial ("sunrise") view is best for the patella.
—*Ankles:* AP and lateral views.
—*Feet:* AP, oblique, and lateral views.

Abnormal Findings: A limited number of abnormalities can be identified by standard radiography. Such reports often comment on soft tissue alterations (e.g., effusions, calcification), articular malalignment (e.g., swan-neck deformity), bone stock (e.g., osteopenia, osteoporosis), joint space (implying cartilage thickness), changes in cortical bone (e.g., fracture, erosions, osteophytes, periosteal reaction), or subcortical bone (e.g., cysts). A poor correlation exists between clinical symptoms and radiographic changes in many disorders, but this is especially true in osteoarthritis. Findings of osteopenia are nonspecific because it is seen in a variety of inflammatory and metabolic disorders.

Indications: Plain x-rays are most appropriate when there is a history of trauma, suspected chronic infection, progressive disability, or monarticular involvement; when therapeutic alterations are considered; or as a baseline assessment for what appears to be a chronic process. Diagnostic patterns of radiographic change may be seen in conditions such as gout, pseudogout, RA, psoriatic arthritis, spondyloarthropathy, reflex sympathetic dystrophy, osteonecrosis, osteoarthritis, and diffuse idiopathic skeletal hyperostosis. Generalized bone surveys are not routinely recommended, unless evidence of skeletal metastases or Paget disease of bone is sought. In most inflammatory disorders, early radiographs rarely help to establish a diagnosis and may only reveal soft tissue swelling or juxtaarticular demineralization.

Alternatives: Bone scans (see p. 49), computed tomography, and MRI (see p. 84) are other modalities often used in evaluation of rheumatic complaints. Such modalities are far more costly and also have limited indications.

Cost: $100–300 per site (depends on locale and extent).

RAPID PLASMA REAGIN

Synonyms: VDRL (venereal disease research laboratory) test, Wassermann test, reaginic antibody test.

Description: The RPR test detects antibodies that bind cardiolipin (so named because they were initially derived from cow heart). Historically, this test was of substantial importance because results were positive in patients with syphilis. Subsequently, a variety of tests and techniques were developed to check for reactivity to this antigen.

Method: The RPR test is a flocculation test (results may be determined macroscopically or microscopically).

Normal Values: RPR is not normally detected. (Negative results may be seen in early primary and late syphilis.)

Abnormal in: The RPR is sensitive but nonspecific.

—*Syphilis:* The sensitivity of RPR depends on the stage: 75% in primary syphilis, >99% in secondary syphilis, and 70% in late latent or tertiary syphilis. The diagnosis of syphilis is suggested by high or rising titers in the correct clinical setting. Alternatively, patients suspected of having syphilis may be assessed using a more specific test for treponemal infection, such as the FTA-ABS (fluorescent treponemal antibody absorption test) and MHA-TP. Patients positive for the RPR but negative for these treponema-specific tests are said to have a biologic false-positive RPR. Although not specific for syphilis, the RPR may be a prognostic aid in following the response to therapy because successful treatment of syphilis should be accompanied by reversion of the RPR to negative after a period of time (e.g., 1 year for primary syphilis).

—*Other:* Positive RPR results may be found in patients with a variety of other diseases, including mononucleosis, leprosy, hepatitis, SLE, and the APL syndrome.

Confounding Factors: False-positive results are seen in ≤2% of pregnant women.

Indications: The RPR test may be used to screen for primary or secondary syphilis in asymptomatic individuals with multiple sexual partners, to confirm the diagnosis of secondary syphilis in the presence of syphilitic lesions, to gauge efficacy of therapy, or to identify a biologic false-positive RPR.

Cost: $20–38.

RHEUMATOID FACTOR

Description: RFs are autoantibodies that react with the Fc portion of IgG. The major immunoglobulin classes are capable of demonstrating RF activity, but the usual routine laboratory assays detect primarily IgM RF.

Methods: Classically, IgM RF in serum is detected by agglutination of IgG-coated particles. The source of IgG may be human or rabbit because human IgM RF reacts with IgG molecules from various species. The particles may be latex beads or tanned erythrocytes. Addition of test serum in graded amounts (dilutions) may lead to agglutination of the coated particles and a positive result. The most dilute serum concentration that causes agglutination is the titer reported. The Rose-Waler test or sensitized sheep cell agglutination test was used previously. Although less sensitive, it was more specific than current assays. The specificity of the sheep cell agglutination test has been replaced by anti-CCP antibodies that are more specific than RF (for RA) but have comparable sensitivity (see p. 36).

Other, more quantitative techniques include measurement of complexes that form between IgM RF and IgG by rate nephelometry or by capture of IgM RF on IgG-coated plastic wells, detected using enzyme-linked reagents (e.g., enzyme immunoassay, ELISA). Results from these assays may be reported in international units using standardized reagents. Normal ranges should be supplied for each assay.

Normal Values: RF is normally not detected.

Clinical Associations: RF is found in a variety of conditions (Table 16).

Table 16
Conditions Associated with Rheumatoid Factor Positivity

Immune system disorders
  Rheumatoid arthritis
  Sjögren syndrome
  Systemic lupus erythematosus
  Sarcoidosis
  Waldenström macroglobulinemia
Infectious diseases
  Subacute bacterial endocarditis
  Tuberculosis
  Leprosy
  Syphilis
  Lyme disease
  Viral infections
  Parasitic diseases (e.g., leishmaniasis)
Malignancies
  Leukemias
  Lymphomas
Miscellaneous conditions
  Elderly individuals
  Interstitial pulmonary fibrosis
  Chronic liver disease
  Chronic renal disease

—*RA:* Approximately 80% of patients with RA are seropositive for RF. The remaining 20% are said to be seronegative. Distinction between seropositive and seronegative RA has been considered of some importance because patients without RF are thought to have milder disease and a less severe disease course. Nonetheless, some of the more severe extraarticular manifestations of RA, such as vasculitis and nodules, occur almost exclusively in high-titer seropositive patients. Treatment with some second-line drugs, notably gold salts and penicillamine, can lower or abolish RF positivity, whereas others (e.g., cyclosporine) do not affect RF titers.

—*Other conditions:* RF can be detected in patients with diseases other than RA (Table 16). These disorders can be grouped into four major categories: immune system disorders, infections, malignancies, and other miscellaneous conditions. These processes suggest that long-term stimulation of the immune system may lead to production of RF.

—*Normals:* RF positivity is seen in 5% of healthy, young individuals and as many as 15% of elderly individuals. These "normal" individuals are not more likely to develop RA or arthritis. More sensitive techniques (radioimmunoassay, ELISA) can demonstrate RF production by mitogen-stimulated blood mononuclear cells from normal individuals, indicating that this autoantibody is part of the normal immune repertoire. Furthermore, sequences encoding immunoglobulins with RF activity exist in the normal human genome. These findings suggest that RF has an important role in the normal immune response, perhaps enhancing clearance of infectious agents or senescent cells from the circulation.

Confounding Factors: Prevalence of RF positivity increases with age. Some patients with cryoglobulinemia, monoclonal paraproteinemias, or very high lipid levels may demonstrate RF activity.

Indications: RF is not specific for RA but can be seen in a wide variety of other conditions. Therefore, RF measurement should be ordered intelligently and reserved for individuals with possible RA based on the history and physical examination. Even in these situations, RF positivity should not be overinterpreted. RF should only be used as a confirmatory rather than screening test. For example, in patients with arthralgia only and a low pretest probability (i.e., 1%) of having RA, a positive RF result has a positive predictive value of 7% (only seven patients in 100 with a positive result are likely to have RA). Conversely, in patients with recent-onset symmetric polyarthritis of the knees and wrists and a moderate likelihood (pretest probability = 50%) of having RA, a positive test result has a positive predictive value of 89% (89 in 100 patients are likely to have RA).

Cost: $35–50.

Comment: High levels of RF somewhat increase the specificity of the RA test but do not correlate with more severe disease or with fluctuations of disease activity in an individual patient. Therefore, measurement of serial RF levels is rarely, if ever, indicated. Exceptions are during the first year of disease, when conversion from seronegativity to seropositivity may occur or with long-term use of some second-line drugs (as noted above), when conversion to seronegativity may correlate with a good therapeutic response. Some of the very highest RF titers are seen not in patients with RA but in those with other disorders such as Sjögren syndrome, macroglobulinemias, or leishmaniasis. In these patients, titers may exceed 1:10,000 using the latex-agglutination test.

BIBLIOGRAPHY

Carson DA, Chen PP, Kipps TJ. New roles for rheumatoid factor. *J Clin Invest* 1991;87:379–383.
Jansen AL, van der Horst-Bruinsma I, van Schaardenburg D, et al. Rheumatoid factor and antibodies to cyclic citrullinated peptide differentiate rheumatoid arthritis from undifferentiated polyarthritis in patients with early arthritis. *J Rheumatol* 2002;29:2074–2076.

ROSE-BENGAL STAIN

Description: Rose bengal, a vital stain that detects dead or dying cells, is used to evaluate corneal abnormalities in patients with symptomatic or suspected keratoconjunctivitis sicca.

Method: This test is performed by an ophthalmologist. After instillation of a topical anesthetic, the dye is introduced using sterile paper strips, and corneal staining is observed with a slit lamp.

Normal Results: A normal cornea does not take up the stain.

Abnormal Results: A punctate pattern of staining in the interpalpebral area is characteristic of sicca syndrome.

Indications: Patients appropriate for referral include those with symptomatic dry eyes, usually manifested by a foreign body sensation, redness, or pain; the patient may also note decreased tear formation. However, it is also likely that symptoms do not correlate with the ocular findings in some patients. Loss of the normal tear film can result in ocular problems such as infections, and thus, establishing a diagnosis allows institution of appropriate treatment and preventive measures. Keratoconjunctivitis sicca has multiple causes including inflammatory conditions such as Sjögren syndrome (primary or secondary). Diminished tear secretion also occurs with normal aging.

Cost: $200–350 (cost includes procedure and ophthalmology consultation).

SCHIRMER TEST

Description: The Schirmer test is a simple, crude measure of ocular tear formation and is useful in evaluating patients with dry eye symptoms.

Method: Standardized, commercially available strips of filter paper are folded 5 mm from the end (usually indicated by a notch), and the short end of the fold is placed inside the lower palpebral-conjunctival sac. Normal tear formation spontaneously wets this strip, which will extend downward (at least 15 mm from the eyelid) over a 5-minute period. For most normal individuals, this amount of wetting actually occurs in far less than the suggested time. Less than 15 mm of wetting suggests deficient tear formation. This test is most commonly carried out by an ophthalmologist, although other physicians may perform it at the bedside or in the clinic if the calibrated Schirmer strips are available.

Abnormal in: Moistening <5 mm of filter paper is consistent with Sjögren syndrome and keratoconjunctivitis sicca. A positive Schirmer test result suggests, but is not diagnostic of, keratoconjunctivitis sicca and should be confirmed with a rose bengal dye test. Moistening of 5 to 10 mm is equivocal and may require further testing.

Indications: The Schirmer test is used for evaluation of suspected Sjögren syndrome or dry eye syndrome (owing to, e.g., medications, blepharitis, allergies, autoimmune disorders).

Cost: Schirmer strips can be purchased for less than $20.

Comment: Patients should discontinue artificial tear use before the procedure. Although topical anesthetic is not required for this test, some patients may find the strip uncomfortable in the eye unless an anesthetic is used. More sensitive measures of tear formation include fluorescein dye staining and rose bengal staining.

SERUM PROTEIN ELECTROPHORESIS

Definition: SPEP measures the major blood proteins, albumin, and globulins.

Method: Because proteins are heterogeneous in surface charge and size, they can be separated electrochemically. In zone electrophoresis, serum is placed on an inert surface such as cellulose acetate and exposed to an electrical current. Different proteins in the serum will move at different rates, thus migrating to different locations where they can be quantified. When proteins are present in normal concentrations, this yields the familiar pattern of SPEP that includes albumin and the globulins (α_1, α_2, β, and γ). α-Globulins include the acute-phase proteins. Immunoglobulins (IgG, IgA, and IgM) migrate predominantly in the γ-globulin fraction and to a lesser extent in the β fraction (particularly IgM).

Normal Values: Variation may occur between laboratories. Total protein ranges from 6.6 to 7.9 g/dL; albumin, 3.3 to 4.5 g/dL; α_1, 0.1 to 0.4 g/dL; α_2, 0.5 to 1.0 g/dL; β, 0.7 to 1.2 g/dL; and γ, 0.5 to 1.6 g/dL.

Abnormal Findings: Analysis of the individual subfractions on the SPEP may yield important information about several disease states.

Total Protein: A decrease in all protein fractions (which would also be seen as a decrease in total protein on chemistry profile) occurs during massive protein loss, typically from the kidney or gastrointestinal tract. An increase in total protein may result from increases in individual fractions, especially the γ-globulins. Increased protein levels are seen in chronic inflammatory diseases, infections, liver disease, and dehydration.

—*Albumin.* Decreases in albumin may be seen with renal diseases, particularly those associated with membranous glomerular lesions and resultant proteinuria. In such cases, there may be a compensatory increase in proteins in other fractions. Hypoalbuminemia may also be seen in severe liver disease, reflecting impaired synthetic capacity, and as a result of major dermatologic burns. α_1-Antitrypsin constitutes a substantial portion of the α_1-globulin fraction of the SPEP; thus, decreases in this fraction may signal α_1-antitrypsin deficiency.

—α-*Globulins.* Various proteins synthesized during the acute-phase response migrate in the α_1-globulin fraction; therefore, this fraction increases in patients with inflammatory diseases, infections, or malignancies. Increases in the α_2-globulin fraction, which encompasses proteins such as haptoglobin, are commonly seen in patients with hypoalbuminemia, for example, secondary to nephrotic syndrome.

—γ-*Globulins.* Decreases in γ-globulins reflect decreases in IgG, the immunoglobulin present in largest quantity. Decreases in IgG, or hypogammaglobulinemia, may indicate immunodeficiency of the antibody-mediated component of the immune response. Likewise, increases in the γ-globulin fraction largely reflect increases in serum IgG. When this increase is polyclonal (indicated by a diffuse "hump" on the SPEP), it often reflects a response to infection or an autoimmune disease. When a single clone of B cells produces excess amounts of IgG, as in multiple myeloma, the IgG molecules are identical and thus yield a sharp "spike" on SPEP. The immunoglobulin molecules can be specifically identified by immunoelectrophoresis.

—*Other uses:* Urine protein electrophoresis is particularly useful in detecting light chains (Bence-Jones proteins) secreted by some myelomas. Electrophoretic analysis of CSF for oligoclonal protein bands is used to support the diagnosis of multiple sclerosis.

Indications: SPEP is frequently used in the evaluation of weight loss, fever of unknown origin, hypoalbuminemia, elevated serum protein, or suspected multiple myeloma malignancy, autoimmune disease, or malnutrition.

Cost: $50–75.

SIALOGRAPHY

Description: Sialography is an imaging modality used to identify salivary gland disorders and salivary duct architecture. Interest in sialography has waned with the advent of less invasive imaging modalities, including ultrasonography, scintigraphy, and MRI.

Anatomy: Parotid glands drain via the Stensen duct opposite the upper second molar. The submandibular glands drain via the Wharton duct lateral to the lingual frenulum. Sublingual glands drain via smaller ducts in to the oral cavity.

Method: A water-soluble contrast agent is instilled after cannulation of the parotid duct or submandibular ducts. Visualization of ductal architecture may be achieved with fluoroscopy or multiple view radiographs, although digital subtraction and computed tomography techniques may also be used. Secretory sialography is primarily used to assess glandular function The use of an oral sialogogue (such as citric acid) allows a subjective indication of delayed emptying from functional or obstructive causes. Interventional sialographic methods allow dilation of ductal strictures or removal of calculi.

Complications: The procedure has a very low complication rate. Allergic reactions, worsening of local inflammation, or infection has rarely been reported.

Abnormal in: Abnormal function or structure can be seen in Sjögren syndrome, sialectasis, sialadenitis, sarcoidosis, human immunodeficiency virus–related salivary disease, benign lymphoepithelial proliferation, trauma, or laceration. It may be helpful in distinguishing benign from malignant tumors. As many as 15% of autoimmune patients (e.g., RA, SLE, scleroderma) will have abnormal sialographic studies, even in the absence of xerostomia or secondary Sjögren syndrome. The results of sialography, MRI sialography, and labial biopsies often overlap. Chronic sialadenitis shows decreased secretion and increased stasis.

Indications: Sialography is used to evaluate strictures, calculi, inflammatory lesions, or trauma. It may be indicated when symptoms (xerostomia) are not otherwise explained by age, medications, or illness. It is also indicated with chronic parotitis or recurrent sialoadenitis to exclude stricture or calculus. It is not indicated for the evaluation of mass lesions, for which US and MRI are more effective tools.

Contraindication: Allergy to iodine or acute sialadenitis.

Alternatives: Although sialography, scintigraphy, and/or minor labial gland biopsy may be used in the diagnosis and assessment of Sjögren syndrome, this clinical and serologic diagnosis seldom requires such extensive investigation. Xerostomia may be evaluated with ^{99m}Tc-sodium pertechnetate scintigraphy. Ultrasound, using power Doppler technology, is being increasingly used to identify ductal strictures, calculi, and mass lesions. Computed tomography sialography has been replaced by MRI.

Cost: Approximately $300.

BIBLIOGRAPHY

Gritzmann N, Rettenbacher T, Hollerweger A, et al. Sonography of the salivary glands. *Eur Radiol* 2003;13:964–975.

Kalk WW, Vissink A, Spijkervet FK, et al. Parotid sialography for diagnosing Sjogren syndrome. *Oral Surg Oral Med Oral Pathol Oral Radiol Endod* 2002;94:131–137.

ULTRASONOGRAPHY

Description: US uses reflections of sound waves to define tissue anatomy. There has been increasing interest in the musculoskeletal applications of US.

Method: Conventional gray scale (B-mode) US can define articular and periarticular structures. It is particularly useful for tendons and disruption in the bony cortex (i.e., erosions). Also, synovial hypertrophy, as seen in inflammatory arthritides, can be detected. Typically, transducers in the range of 7.5 to 10 MHz frequency have been used for US of musculoskeletal structures. Higher frequencies provide greater resolution and finer tissue detail. However, tissue penetration and hence field of vision decrease with increasing frequency. Other developments in US include Doppler and power Doppler techniques. Doppler US assesses the mean frequency shift of sound waves echoing from moving objects and is particularly suited for defining large-vessel, high-velocity blood flow. Power Doppler US encodes the amplitude of the Doppler signal and is useful for assessing blood flow in smaller vessels, such as those in the inflamed synovium.

Indications: Many joints are amenable to US examination. Joint fluid, synovium, and periarticular structures are readily visualized. US is very useful in the delineation of abnormalities in the periarticular structures of the shoulder, such as the rotator cuff apparatus, and is therefore very useful in the evaluation of a painful shoulder. US of the knee allows identification of popliteal (Baker) cysts versus deep vein thrombosis in patients with acute, painful swelling of the calf. For many joints, US can facilitate the accurate placement of needles and hence injected medications within the joint space. In the small joints of the hands and feet, US has a sensitivity that is comparable with MRI in detecting periarticular erosions; both of these modalities are superior to conventional radiography in that regard. Power Doppler imaging has been shown to correlate with measures of inflammation and thus may be a useful tool for the longitudinal assessment of disease activity within joints in conditions such as RA.

Advantages/Limitations: Relatively low cost, lack of exposure to ionizing radiation, lack of adverse effects, ease of performance, and ready access make US attractive. Limitations of US include the dependence of imaging techniques on the skill of the examiner and a limited ability to view some joints (e.g., the fourth metacarpophalangeal joint).

Cost: Typical charges for musculoskeletal US examination are $150–260.

BIBLIOGRAPHY

Ostergaard M, Szkudlarek M. Imaging in rheumatoid arthritis: why MRI and ultrasonography can no longer be ignored. *Scand J Rheumatol* 2003;32:63–73.
Taylor P. The value of sensitive imaging modalities in rheumatoid arthritis. *Arthritis Res Ther* 2003;5:210–213.

URIC ACID

Synonyms: Urate, monosodium urate.

Description: Uric acid is the end product of purine metabolism and is excreted in the urine. It is primarily used in the diagnosis of gout. Uric acid is not soluble at a pH <7.4.

Method: Uric acid may be measured singly or as part of an automated chemistry panel. These automated enzymatic methods depend on the generation of peroxide during oxidation of urate by uricase.

Normal Values: In men, serum uric acid levels increase during childhood and reach adult levels after puberty. In women, urate levels remain constant until after menopause, when they increase (as does the incidence of gout). Gender differences are owing to estrogen, which exerts a uricosuric effect. Although normal values vary between laboratories, serum values in men range from 4.0 to 8.6 mg/dL and in women from 3.0 to 5.9 mg/dL. Urinary uric acid levels are normally <750 mg/24 hours. Urinary levels >750 mg/24 hours in gout (or >1,100 mg/24 hours in asymptomatic hyperuricemia) indicate that the patient is a urate overproducer and may need allopurinol therapy.

Abnormal in: Serum uric acid values may be abnormally high or low (Table 17). Although hyperuricemia may indicate gout, levels do not correlate with

Table 17
Abnormalities of Serum Uric Acid

Increased Values	Decreased Values
Renal failure	Drugs
Gout	Adrenocorticotropic hormone
Asymptomatic hyperuricemia	Uricosuric drugs (sulfinpyrazone,
Increased purine turnover	probenecid, high-dose salicylates)
Lymphoproliferative disorders	Allopurinol
Myeloproliferative disorders	Wilson disease
Chemotherapy or radiotherapy	Fanconi syndrome
Hemolytic anemia	
Toxemia of pregnancy	
Psoriasis	
Drugs	
Diuretics (except p-spironolactone)	
Low-dose salicylates	
Ethanol	
Diet: purine-rich foods (meat, legumes)	
Metabolic acidosis	
Lead poisoning	
Hypoparathyroidism	
Primary hyperparathyroidism	
Hypothyroidism	
Sarcoidosis	

the severity of disease. Hyperuricemia levels >9 mg/dL are associated with increased risk of gout and nephrolithiasis. Nonetheless, treatment of asymptomatic hyperuricemia may not be necessary until values are >13 mg/dL in men or 10 mg/dL in women. Although nearly all patients with gout demonstrate hyperuricemia at some time during their illness, as many as 40% of patients having an acute gouty attack have normal serum uric acid levels.

Indications: Serum uric acid assays are most useful in monitoring the response to treatment in gout, renal failure, and neoplasia or during chemotherapy; 24-hour urinary uric acid determinations may be valuable in assessing the risk of nephrolithiasis or in making therapeutic decisions in gout (e.g., whether to treat with probenecid or allopurinol).

Cost: $10–25.

Comments: Urinary uric acid determinations are most reliable when the patient is on a low-purine diet and not taking uricosuric drugs. Serum uric acid levels are labile and vary from day to day.

BIBLIOGRAPHY

Wallach J. Core blood analytes: alterations by diseases. In: *Interpretation of diagnostic tests*, 6th ed. Boston: Little, Brown, 1996:37–38.

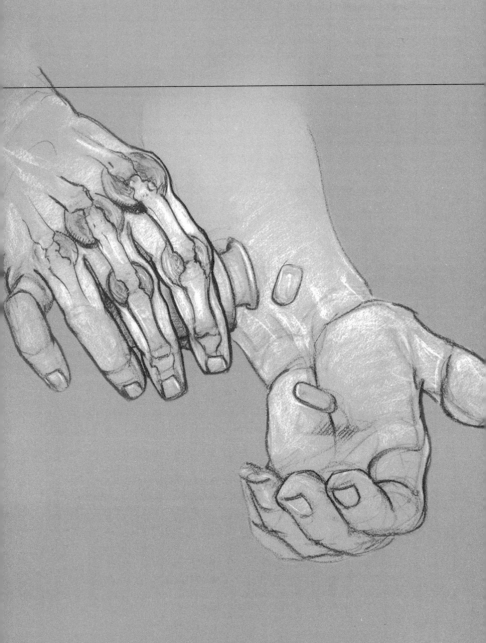

RHEUMATIC DISEASES

This section is devoted to specific musculoskeletal disorders or complaints. Diseases and topics are listed alphabetically for easy retrieval using the most commonly used or accepted diagnostic label. Disorders may also be found by searching the index for alternative terms or synonyms. The depth of information presented is roughly proportional to the prevalence and complexity of the disorder. Where appropriate, abbreviations are used and reflect the most commonly used abbreviations or acronyms in clinical practice. Abbreviations used throughout this text are listed at the beginning of the book.

Useful clinical, diagnostic, and therapeutic information is presented under template headings that may include Synonyms, ICD-9 Codes, Definition, Etiology, Genetics, Pathology, Uncommon Findings, Complications, Diagnostic Tests, Imaging, Biopsy Findings, Keys to Diagnosis, Diagnostic Criteria, Differential Diagnosis, Therapy, Surgery, Prognosis, Monitoring, Comments, and Bibliography. When necessary, the reader is referred to other sections or appendices for supplemental information on related topics, diagnostic tests, or medications. Guidance on the dosing and use of pharmacologic agents is available in Section III of this text.

CHAPTER 2

RHEUMATIC DISEASES

ACROMEGALY

Synonyms: Gigantism, acromegalia.

ICD-9 Code: 253.0.

Definition: Overproduction of growth hormone by a pituitary tumor causes acromegaly. This syndrome is accompanied by distinct findings in the musculoskeletal system that may contribute to early detection and diagnosis.

Cardinal Findings: Excess growth hormone causes acromegaly in adults and, if the onset is before epiphyseal closure, gigantism in children. Clinically, patients develop distinctive coarse facial features; thickening of the skin; enlarged mandible, hands, and feet; prominent forehead and supraorbital ridge; enlarged tongue and viscera; hirsutism; oily skin; and excessive sweating. The musculoskeletal complaints result from premature osteoarthritis (OA), kyphosis, pseudogout, entrapment neuropathies [e.g., carpal tunnel syndrome (CTS)], or a mild proximal myopathy. Many patients complain of nonspecific arthralgias affecting the shoulder, knees, hips, and spine.

Complications: Increased cardiovascular morbidity and mortality from hypertension, cardiomyopathy, heart failure, or valvular regurgitation. Patients may also develop diabetes (25%), galactorrhea (5%), parathyroid and islet cell adenomas, or sleep apnea.

Diagnostic Tests: Serum somatomedin C (insulin-like growth factor-I) is more sensitive and cost-effective than serum growth hormone levels. Increased prolactin levels (seen in 40% of patients) should be sought; 80% of patients have evidence of insulin resistance, but only 20% develop clinical diabetes mellitus.

Imaging: Radiographic findings may be diagnostic and include generalized widening of the joint spaces because of overgrowth of cartilage. Bone remodeling and spur formation are common. Look for widening/prominence of phalangeal tufts or vertebral "scalloping" (exaggerated posterior vertebral concavity), especially in the lumbar spine. In later stages of the disease, OA is obvious. In some cases, deposition of calcium pyrophosphate within joint tissues can lead to the clinical syndrome of pseudogout. Radiography or MRI may disclose an abnormal sella turcica and pituitary tumor.

Therapy: Treatment goals include (1) normalization of growth hormone/insulin-like growth factor-I levels, (2) tumor mass reduction, and (3) preservation of pituitary function. Surgical (transsphenoidal) resection of the pituitary tumor may be followed by radiation therapy or pharmacotherapy with pegvisomant (growth hormone receptor antagonist), octreotide (somatostatin analogue), or bromocriptine. Pegvisomant is highly effective in normalizing insulinlike growth factor-I levels and clinical symptoms but does not reduce tumor size. It has fewer side effects and is indicated when there is resistance or intolerance to somatostatin analogues.

Prognosis: In most cases, the joint findings of acromegaly are not reversed with correction of growth hormone overproduction. One exception is the commonly observed CTS, which may improve after surgical or medical ablation of the pituitary tumor.

BIBLIOGRAPHY

Clemmons DR. Optimizing control of acromegaly: integrating a growth hormone receptor antagonist into the treatment algorithm. *J Clin Endocrinol Metab* 2003;88:4759–3767.
Melmed S. Acromegaly. *N Engl J Med* 1990;322:966.

ACUTE RHEUMATIC FEVER (ARF)

Definition: ARF is a febrile illness occurring as a delayed sequela of infection with group A streptococci and is characterized by inflammatory lesions of connective tissue.

ICD-9 Codes: With arthritis, 390.0; with carditis, 391.9.

Etiology: ARF occurs 2 to 3 weeks after untreated severe group A β-hemolytic streptococcal pharyngitis (in as many as 3% of untreated cases). It may be more common with some streptococcal M serotypes. Cutaneous infections (impetigo) never cause ARF.

Pathology: The exact mechanisms are unclear. Humoral response leads to immune-complex deposition. Cell-mediated immune damage to the heart is potentially owing to molecular mimicry secondary between streptococcal cell wall antigens (M proteins or group A carbohydrate) and myocardial tissue. Streptococcal extracellular toxins, which can act as superantigens, may also be pathogenic. Host factors, including some HLA and non-HLA antigens, may increase susceptibility to rheumatogenic strains.

Demographics: The peak age of incidence is 5 to 15 years. ARF remains endemic and is the major cause of valvular heart disease in the developing world. Risk factors include poverty, crowded living conditions, and youth. Nonetheless, outbreaks of ARF have recently appeared in some regions and populations in the United States.

Cardinal Findings: Only two-thirds of patients recall an antecedent pharyngitis. The onset is heralded by a migratory or additive polyarthritis (knees, ankles, wrists) that may last 2 to 4 weeks. Abdominal pains occur early and may be severe. Jones Criteria serve as a guideline for diagnosis. Carditis occurs early in <15% and is less common in adults. Post-streptococcal reactive arthritis (see p. 360) may be a form fruste of ARF, without carditis and with different extraarticular manifestations (i.e., tenosynovitis).

Uncommon Findings: Erythema marginatum (an evanescent, erythematous eruption of the torso with a serpiginous border and central clearing) and nodules are rare in adults. Most cases of Sydenham chorea occur in women. Arthritis of the small joints of the hands or feet alone occurs in <1% of cases. Jaccoud arthropathy, a nonerosive, reducible, deforming arthritis of the hands, occurs rarely when there are repeated episodes. Epistaxis and pneumonia are other uncommon findings.

Diagnostic Testing: Elevated levels of anti-streptolysin O, anti-DNase B, anti-NADase, antistreptokinase, and antihyaluronidase all provide presumptive evidence of recent streptococcal infection. Although none of these tests is specific for ARF, at least one titer is elevated in 90% of streptococcal infections. Elevated levels of acute-phase reactants [erythrocyte sedimentation rate (ESR) and/or C-reactive protein (CRP)] and anemia of chronic inflammation are often present. Throat culture for streptococcal infection is usually negative at the time of ARF; if positive, it may only indicate noninfectious carriage. An electrocardiogram, chest radiograph, or echocardiogram may also be necessary to diagnose first-degree atrioventricular block or carditis.

Diagnostic Criteria: Jones Criteria define classic features of ARF. Major manifestations include polyarthritis, carditis, chorea, subcutaneous skin nodules, and erythema marginatum. Minor manifestations include previous ARF or rheumatic heart disease, arthralgias, fever, elevated acute-phase reactants, and a prolonged PR interval on the electrocardiogram. The presence of two major or one major and two minor criteria indicates a high probability of ARF, if supported by evidence of recent streptococcal infection.

Keys to Diagnosis: A young patient with fever and painful migratory polyarthritis after pharyngitis may be suggestive of ARF.

Therapy: Treatment with antibiotics (penicillin or alternative) is necessary to eradicate group A streptococci. Although the arthritis is sensitive to high-dose salicylates (4–8 g/day in divided doses or a serum salicylate level of 20–30 mg/dL), other NSAIDs may be used with success. A prompt and prominent response to salicylates/NSAIDs supports the diagnosis. Refractory arthritis and severe carditis may require corticosteroids. Prevention and prompt management of recurrent pharyngitis is essential. Long-term prophylactic penicillin (or erythromycin if penicillin allergic) is often recommended. Post-streptococcal reactive arthritis is less responsive to nonsteroidal antiinflammatory drugs (NSAIDs) than ARF.

Prognosis: Acute mortality secondary to carditis is very uncommon. The most serious chronic sequela is rheumatic heart disease, which most commonly involves the mitral valve. Rheumatic heart disease develops within 10 to 20 years of the initial attack. Joint disease in ARF is generally self-limiting, lasting less than 6 weeks on average, and chronic arthropathy is rare. Poststreptococcal reactive arthritis has a generally benign prognosis.

BIBLIOGRAPHY

Amigo MC, Martinex-Lavin M, Reyes P. Acute rheumatic fever. *Rheum Dis Clin North Am* 1993;19;333–350.
Rullan E, Sigal LH. Rheumatic fever. *Curr Rheumatol Rep* 2001;3:445–452.
Tani LY, Veasy LG, Minich LL, et al. Rheumatic fever in children younger than 5 years: is the presentation different? *Pediatrics* 2003;112:1065–1068.

ADULT-ONSET STILL'S DISEASE (AOSD)

Synonyms: Still disease, systemic juvenile arthritis, Wissler-Fanconi syndrome, subsepsis hyperallergica.

ICD-9 Code: 714.3.

Definition: AOSD is a systemic inflammatory disease that typically afflicts young adults. It is characterized by quotidian fevers, evanescent rashes, and chronic polyarthritis.

Etiology: Unknown. AOSD is the adult continuum of systemic juvenile arthritis. Both exhibit the same manifestations and clinical course. However, a prodromal sore throat is more common in adults and occurs without evidence of infection. Hence, AOSD has infrequently been associated with a variety of viral infections, including rubella, Epstein-Barr virus, Coxsackie B4, and mumps, although no single agent has been proven to be the cause. Although periodic fevers have been linked to tumor necrosis factor (TNF) receptor gene mutations, AOSD has not. Excess production of interleukin (IL)-6, IL-1, and IL-18 has been reported in AOSD.

Incidence: AOSD is uncommon. Fever of unknown origin in 5% to 9% of patients is caused by AOSD. Most major medical centers may see one to two cases per year.

Demographics: Usual onset age is between 16 and 35 years (~75% of cases), with 10% presenting after age 50 years. Males and females are equally affected. AOSD has been reported worldwide, affecting all races and ethnic groups.

Cardinal Findings: Onset is often heralded by a prodromal sore throat (70%). Symptoms progress within 1 to 3 weeks. Nearly 90% of patients have the triad of quotidian fevers, evanescent rash, and arthritis. Quotidian (spiking, daily) fevers may be as high as 102° to 105°F and usually recur at the same time each day, either late afternoon (3–6 PM) or late night (11 PM–2 AM). The evanescent rash is faintly erythematous or salmon pink, maculopapular, and most evident with febrile episodes. It commonly appears on the trunk, neck, or extremities and may be associated with dermatographism, Koebner phenomenon (lesions arising at sites of trauma/pressure), pruritus, or urticaria. Fixed dermal plaques have been rarely described. Arthritis tends to predominate with time and behaves like rheumatoid arthritis (RA), involving the wrist, knee, ankle, and small joints of the fingers. As many as 25% of patients develop a destructive polyarthritis. Other prominent manifestations (seen in 50% of patients) include myalgias, carpal ankylosis, weight loss, lymphadenopathy, hepatomegaly, splenomegaly, pleuritis, or pericarditis.

Diagnostic Tests: No test is diagnostic. Patients with AOSD should be seronegative for rheumatoid factor (RF) and antinuclear antibody (ANA). Neutrophilic leukocytosis, thrombocytosis, markedly elevated ESR or serum ferritin (acute-phase reactants), hypoalbuminemia, and elevated hepatic enzymes are common during active inflammatory diseases. Ferritin levels >1,000 ng/mL are seen in 50% of patients, and very high levels (as high as 30,000 ng/mL) are occasionally seen. Radiographs are nondiagnostic. Nearly half of patients develop carpal ankylosis with chronic arthritis.

Diagnostic Keys: This is a clinical diagnosis of exclusion. The evanescent rash and circadian fever (102°F) may be the most distinctive features of AOSD.

Diagnostic Criteria: Major criteria (2 points each) include: quotidian fevers ≥102°; evanescent Still's rash; seronegative tests for ANA and RF; elevated ESR >40 mm/h and white blood cell (WBC) count; and carpal ankylosis. Minor criteria (1 point) include: onset age before 35 years; arthritis; prodromal sore throat; serositis; hepato- or splenomegaly (or lymphadenopathy or elevated hepatic enzymes); or cervical or tarsal ankylosis. Probable AOSD requires ≥10 points and 12-week disease duration. Definite AOSD requires ≥10 points and 6-month disease duration.

Differential Diagnosis: Acute viral infection (e.g., Epstein-Barr virus, rubella), dermatomyositis (DM), Reiter's syndrome, inflammatory bowel disease, acute leukemias, and lymphoma are often mistaken for AOSD. Less common possibilities include bacterial endocarditis, sarcoidosis, Sweet's syndrome, tuberculosis, and granulomatous hepatitis. Periodic fevers, Familial Mediterranean fever (FMF), TNF receptor–associated periodic syndrome (TRAPS), and hyper-IgD syndrome may also mimic AOSD or systemic juvenile rheumatoid arthritis.

Therapy: Initially, NSAID therapy at antiinflammatory doses can be used. Sustained-release indomethacin (75–150 mg/day) is effective in 40% to 60% of patients. Aspirin is seldom effective. Corticosteroids should be reserved for patients with markedly elevated hepatic enzymes, pericardial tamponade, severe serositis, or pneumonitis and those resistant to NSAIDs. High-dose prednisone (40–80 mg/day) is necessary to control the systemic manifestations. Weekly oral methotrexate (MTX) (7.5–20 mg/wk) has been used successfully to limit steroid exposure. Systemic features are infrequently controlled with hydroxychloroquine, azathioprine, or cyclosporine. Chronic polyarthritis can be managed in the same manner as RA. TNF inhibitors are more effective in treating the arthritis than the systemic features of AOSD. Difficult cases may respond to colchicine, anakinra, or anti–IL-6 receptor antibody therapy.

Prognosis: Flares of systemic disease may last from 6 to 24 months. In most, the clinical course displays either intermittent bouts of systemic disease or chronic arthritis. Death is uncommon (9% of cases) and results from complications of therapy, pericardial tamponade, hepatic failure, or disseminated intravascular coagulation.

BIBLIOGRAPHY

Cush JJ. Adult onset Still's disease. *Bull Rheum Dis* 2000;49:1–4.
Cush JJ, Medsger TA, Christy WA, et al. Adult-onset Still's disease: clinical course and outcome. *Arthritis Rheum* 1987;30:186–194.

ALCAPTONURIA

Synonyms: Ochronosis.

ICD-9 Code: 270.2.

Definition: This rare metabolic disorder is caused by a deficiency of the enzyme homogentisic acid oxidase and the accumulation of homogentisic acid that binds to collagen, resulting in darkened pigment deposition in cartilage, intervertebral discs, and skin.

Demographics: The disorder is transmitted as an autosomal recessive gene; heterozygotes do not have ochronosis. The incidence of homozygotes is estimated to be one in 200,000.

Cardinal Findings: Skin changes are usually first noted after age 20 years. The delayed onset of skin and cartilaginous changes leaves many undiagnosed until they are elderly, when the clinical findings are striking. The dark pigmentation may be seen in the pinna and external canal of the ear or in skin overlying the nasal and malar areas of the face. Pigmentation is often described as slate blue, gray, or coal colored. This pigment may even appear in axillary sweat and stain clothing. Articular manifestations usually begin in the spine. Peripheral joint pain and subsequent OA may affect the knees, shoulders, and hips. Hands, feet, elbows, and ankles are usually spared.

Diagnostic Tests: The diagnosis is confirmed by demonstrating homogentisic aciduria. Urine samples may be dark colored or become dark if left to stand. Nearly 50% of patients develop a noninflammatory, yellow- or amber-colored synovial effusion.

Imaging: Spinal radiographs show a characteristic pattern of densely calcified intervertebral discs with intervening osteoporotic vertebral bodies, giving the appearance of a "rugger jersey" spine. Degenerative changes or chondrocalcinosis may occur in peripheral joints.

Therapy: Definitive medical therapies are not available; although a low protein diet and ascorbic acid have been advocated. Treatment of the arthritis is symptomatic.

BIBLIOGRAPHY

Schumacher HR, Holdsworth DE. Ochronotic arthropathy. I. Clinicopathologic studies. *Semin Arthritis Rheum* 1977;6:207–246.

AMYLOIDOSIS

ICD-9 Code: 277.3.

Definition: Amyloidosis is a multisystem disorder caused by deposition of fibrillar protein aggregates that interfere with structural integrity and function of targeted organs or tissues. Four major forms are distinguished by the deposited protein and the clinical associations (Table 1).

Etiology: Primary amyloidosis is commonly associated with plasma cell dyscrasias such as multiple myeloma or may be seen with other malignancies such as medullary carcinoma of the thyroid. Secondary amyloidosis occurs most commonly in association with inflammatory syndromes such as FMF or RA. β_2-Microglobulin amyloidosis occurs in association with hemodialysis.

Pathology: The various proteins associated with amyloidosis all show a characteristic fibrillary array, most clearly seen by electron microscopy. Under the light microscope, amyloid deposits are visualized by staining with Congo red. When viewed under polarized light, the stained fibers show a characteristic apple-green birefringence.

Table 1
Syndromes of Systemic Amyloidosis

Type	Clinical Syndromes	Protein
Immunoglobulin (AL)	Primary, myeloma-associated amyloidosis	Ig light chains
Reactive (AA)	Secondary to inflammatory disease	Amyloid A [also called serum amyloid A (SAA)]
Hereditary	Familial	Various non-Ig proteins
β_2-Microglobulin	Hemodialysis associated	β_2-Microglobulin

Demographics: Patients can be of almost any age, from childhood to elderly, depending on the underlying cause. Primary amyloidosis shows a male predominance.

Cardinal Findings: In primary amyloidosis, the most commonly involved organs are the kidney, heart, liver, and skin; skeletal muscle and the tongue may also be affected. Peripheral neuropathies are seen, but the central nervous system (CNS) is generally not involved. Secondary amyloidosis most commonly presents with nephrotic syndrome or gastrointestinal (GI) bleeding. Macroglossia is not seen with secondary amyloidosis. The initial finding in hemodialysis-associated amyloid is often CTS.

Uncommon Manifestations: In primary amyloidosis, amyloid deposits may be seen in the synovium and occasionally in the synovial fluid.

Diagnostic Tests: Biopsies of affected tissues are usually required. The tissues are stained with Congo red and viewed under polarized light. Kidney and peripheral nerve biopsy specimens can be useful if there are known abnormalities in these tissues; otherwise, a blind abdominal fat pad aspirate should be attempted.

Keys to Diagnosis: Suspect amyloid in a patient with multisystem disease, especially those with new-onset cardiomyopathy, peripheral neuropathy, renal insufficiency, or nephrotic syndrome. Biopsy demonstration of amyloid deposits is diagnostic.

Therapy: In primary amyloidosis, chemotherapy with melphalan and prednisone is usually recommended, although it is not clear that this treatment prolongs survival. Cardiomyopathy is especially resistant to medical therapy. In secondary amyloidosis, treatment should be directed at controlling the underlying inflammatory process. Colchicine has some utility in patients with amyloid secondary to FMF. Recent uncontrolled studies have shown the benefit of TNF inhibitors in patients with amyloidosis and in those with primary and secondary amyloidosis.

Surgery: Surgery is not generally indicated. Organ transplantation (heart, kidney) may be attempted in some cases.

Prognosis: In primary amyloidosis, only 20% of patients are alive 5 years after diagnosis. Disease progression is generally slower in secondary forms, with some patients surviving 10 years after diagnosis.

BIBLIOGRAPHY

Hussein MA, Juturi JV, Rybicki L, et al. Etanercept therapy in patients with advanced primary amyloidosis. *Med Oncol* 2003;20:283–290.
Westmark P. Diagnosing amyloidosis. *Scand J Rheumatol* 1995;24:327–329.

ANKYLOSING SPONDYLITIS (AS)

Synonyms: AS, Marie-Strumpell disease, Bechterew's syndrome

ICD-9 Code: 279.8.

Definition: AS is a common inflammatory enthesopathy and arthropathy that preferentially affects the axial skeleton, often beginning in the sacroiliac joints and ascending to involve the remaining spine.

Etiology: AS has a strong genetic component because >90% of white patients are HLA-B27 positive (see p. 75), and a significant minority have a positive family history for AS. AS develops in 1% to 2% of HLA-B27–positive individuals. There is a 20% risk of AS in HLA-B27–positive first-degree relatives of patients with AS. Others have postulated that AS may result from exposure to some arthritogenic bacteria that resemble HLA-B27, resulting in molecular mimicry. There are 25 subtypes of B27, with B*2705 as the most common.

Pathology: The spondyloarthropathies (SpA) typically demonstrate enthesitis early, followed by erosive changes, osteitis, and, ultimately, fibrous ankylosis. Synovial biopsy changes are similar to those seen in RA, with synoviocyte proliferation, inflammatory cell infiltration into the sublining layer, and juxtaarticular erosive changes. AS and the other SpA share a propensity for inflammation at the entheses (sites of tendon or ligament attachment to bone), with resultant reactive bone formation.

Demographics: Epidemiologic studies suggest that the prevalence of AS in a white population is between 0.5 and five cases per 1,000 persons. The age- and gender-adjusted incidence rate in Rochester, MN, is 7.3 per 100,000 person-years. HLA-B27 and AS are less prevalent in African Americans. AS commonly affects young men more frequently than women, with an estimated male:female ratio ranging from 2.5:1 to 5:1. AS in women is often underdiagnosed, primarily because of milder axial disease and occult extraarticular manifestations. Women with AS may have a delayed disease onset, less hip involvement, less aggressive axial disease, more peripheral arthritis, severe osteitis pubis, and a higher incidence of isolated cervical spine disease. Peak age at onset is between 15 and 30 years. Onset is rare after age 50. Juvenile spondylitis, a minority subset of juvenile arthritis, includes those with onset of AS between the ages of 9 and 16 years.

Cardinal Findings: Symptoms often begin in young adulthood. The insidious onset of inflammatory low back pain or stiffness is often the initial symptom of AS. Bilateral symmetric sacroiliitis is highly suggestive of AS. Although sacroiliitis begins at an early age, it may take as long as 10 years to become evident by conventional radiography. Sacroiliac pain is localized over the sacroiliac joints and less commonly down the posterior thigh. Patients usually complain of prolonged morning stiffness that is only relieved by increased activity or antiinflammatory medications. Often these young patients actively pursue sports and physical activity as a means of alleviating their symptoms. Constitutional complaints of fever, anorexia, and weight loss may also be seen. With progressive axial involvement, pain and stiffness result in difficulty with ambulation and activities of daily living. Fusion of the axial spine occurs in an ascending fashion, with early lumbar and late cervical spine involvement.

An asymmetric oligoarticular, inflammatory, peripheral arthritis is seen in 30% of patients with AS. Synovitis of the hip can be destructive and may lead to concentric loss of joint space, especially in men. Involved joints also typically include the ankles, wrists, shoulders, elbows, and small joints of the hands or feet. Radiographically, peripheral articular changes may be erosive and similar to RA.

Extraarticular disease in AS primarily affects the eye. Ocular involvement is seen in as many as 40% of patients and is more frequently observed in HLA-B27–positive individuals. Uveitis (see p. 386) presents as acute, unilateral, orbital pain with photophobia and progressive loss of vision if untreated.

Examination reveals restricted spinal movement from axial stiffness, fusion, and paraspinal muscular spasm. Often the earliest finding is a loss of normal lumbar lordosis and resultant "flattening" of the lumbar spine. Left untreated, progressive axial inflammation may lead to a fixed forward flexion posture, most evident in the hip and neck. Chest expansion, as measured by the inspiratory minus expiratory chest circumference, normally exceeds 5 cm. Patients with AS demonstrate diminished expansion (<4 cm). Cervical spine mobility can be serially assessed by measuring the occiput (or tragus) to wall distance.

Lumbar spine mobility is assessed by the Schober test (see p. 116). Although the patient stands upright with heels together, a 10-cm span is marked from the fifth lumbar vertebra cephalad. Upon maximal forward flexion, the distance between marks is remeasured. Normal spinal flexion expands the surface area over the flexed spine to >15 cm. Flexion in patients with spondylitis and limitation of spinal motion usually measures ≤14 cm.

Uncommon Findings: Thoracocervical kyphoscoliosis, aortitis, aortic insufficiency, aortic root dilation, and conduction defects (heart block) are uncommon. Others include mitral valve disease, myocardial dysfunction, pericarditis, pulmonary fibrosis, and amyloidosis.

Complications: Minor or incidental trauma may result in serious spinal fractures in those with ankylosis of the spine. Such fractures may result in spinal cord damage and carry a high mortality rate. Fractures may be identified on plain radiographs, bone scans, or MRI. Other rare complications of AS include cauda equina syndrome, osteoporotic compression fractures, spondylodiscitis, restrictive lung disease, apical fibrosis, cardiac conduction defects, aortic insufficiency, and uveitis.

Diagnostic Tests: Elevated ESR or CRP levels and anemia of chronic disease are commonly seen. Mild elevations of alkaline phosphatase and IgA levels may be seen. Serologies for autoantibodies are unnecessary because of their absence. HLA-B27 determination is seldom necessary to establish the diagnosis but may be diagnostic in questionable cases without distinctive radiographic changes. HLA-B27 is found in ~90% of white but only 50% of African-American patients with AS.

Imaging: Radiographs are often normal early in the disease and demonstrate normal mineralization before the onset of ankylosis. Once present, ankylosis results in marked immobility and subsequent generalized osteoporosis. Sacroiliitis is indicated by early erosions and pseudo-widening and, later, by ileal sclerosis or fusion of the inferior, synovium-lined portion of the sacroiliac joint. These findings are easily observed on plain radiographs of the pelvis and seldom require computed tomography (CT) or MRI, although these may detect diagnostic changes earlier. Axial radiographic findings also include vertebral enthesitis (manifest as "shiny corners"), marginal bridging syndesmophytes, fusion of the posterior facet joints, and "squaring" of lumbar and thoracic vertebrae. Collectively, these findings may produce the classic appearance of a "bamboo spine." Axial damage or fibrosis tends to have a bilateral symmetric distribution.

Diagnostic Criteria: Two different sets of diagnostic criteria have been developed (Table 2).

Keys to Diagnosis: AS must be distinguished from other causes of mechanical or degenerative low back pain. AS is suggested by (1) young age at onset, (2) strong family history of low back pain, (3) presence of inflammatory low

Table 2
Diagnostic Criteria for Ankylosing Spondylitis

Rome Criteria, 1961
  Clinical criteria
  1. Low back pain and stiffness for >3 mo, not relieved by rest
  2. Pain and stiffness of the thoracic region
  3. Limited motion in the lumbar spine
  4. Limited chest expansion
  5. History or evidence of iritis or its sequelae
  Radiologic criterion
  6. Radiographs showing characteristic bilateral sacroiliac changes
  Definite AS = grade 3–4 bilateral sacroiliitis and 1 clinical criterion or at least 4 clinical criteria
Modified New York, 1984
  1. Low back pain for at least 3 months; duration improved by exercise and not relieved by rest
  2. Limitation of the lumbar spine in sagittal and frontal planes
  3. Chest expansion decreased relative to normal values for age and sex
  4. Bilateral sacroiliitis grades 2–4
  5. Unilateral sacroiliitis grades 3–4
  Definite AS = unilateral grade 3–4 sacroiliitis or bilateral sacroiliitis grades 2–4 and 1 clinical criterion

back pain (lasting >3 months, with prolonged morning stiffness and improved by activity or exercise), (4) limited spinal mobility on examination, (5) elevated ESR or CRP, and, if needed, (6) HLA-B27 positivity.

Differential Diagnosis: The differential diagnosis includes other SpA (enteropathic arthritis, Reiter's syndrome, psoriatic spondylitis), osteitis condensans ilii, diffuse idiopathic skeletal hyperostosis (DISH), and other causes of hyperostosis (e.g., fluorosis, hypervitaminosis A).

Therapy: The goal of treatment is to reduce pain and stiffness and maintain posture and mobility. Both nonpharmacologic and pharmacologic measures should be used in all.

—*Nonpharmacologic:* Patients should be educated about the disorder and the importance of joint protection, appropriate exercise, intermittent rest, physical therapy, and dietary and vocational counseling. Patients with axial disease should engage in lifelong physical therapy to maintain posture and prevent slow deformity. Patient support can be found through the Spondylitis Association of America (www.spondylitis.org).

—*NSAIDs:* NSAIDs are effective in controlling inflammatory back pain/ stiffness, peripheral arthritis, and enthesitis. These agents modify symptoms but do not suppress disease progression. NSAIDs are the mainstay of therapy for most patients. A few NSAIDs are approved by the U.S. Food and Drug Administration for use in AS and/or Reiter's syndrome. These include indomethacin, diclofenac, naproxen, sulindac, aspirin, and phenylbutazone. Of these, indomethacin, especially the sustained-release formula (1–2 mg/kg per day), is recommended because of its prolonged duration of effect and antiinflammatory potency. Other NSAIDs are used according to individual tolerability and efficacy. Phenylbutazone is very effective but is rarely used, primarily because of the unacceptable risk of aplastic anemia. Phenylbutazone is no longer commercially available and may only be acquired through a few select compounding pharmacies.

—*Corticosteroids:* Systemic corticosteroids are seldom used in the SpA. They are most effective in controlling localized disease. They are used primarily as local therapy by intraarticular injection (i.e., mono- or oligoarthritis), topical management of ocular complications (conjunctivitis or uveitis), and, on occasion, intralesionally to control enthesitis. Uncontrolled reports suggest beneficial effects of intraarticular corticosteroids administered by guided arthrocentesis into the sacroiliac joints.

—*Disease-modifying antirheumatic drugs (DMARDs):* When the condition is chronic, progressive, NSAID unresponsive, or associated with uncontrolled peripheral inflammatory arthritis, the addition of a DMARD (e.g., sulfasalazine, MTX) should be considered for patients with peripheral arthritis. These agents have a delayed onset of action (2–4 months). Randomized, placebo-controlled trials of sulfasalazine (or MTX) indicate efficacy in patients with peripheral arthropathy and enthesopathy. Unfortunately, these agents have not been shown to be effective in controlling the axial symptoms or ankylosis of AS. Other DMARDs (azathioprine, gold salts, antimalarials, cyclosporine) have not been well studied in AS. Limited studies suggest the benefit of pamidronate in controlling axial symptoms. TNF inhibitors have revolutionized the treatment of axial AS. Multiple studies with etanercept and infliximab have shown dramatic improvement in symptoms and spinal mobility measures. It is currently unclear whether TNF inhibitors will alter the radiographic progression of axial disease in AS, although this is under investigation.

Surgery: Surgical intervention in AS is primarily reserved for those with advanced peripheral arthritis, usually affecting the hip or knee. Total joint replacement may be indicated when pain and immobility markedly interfere with the patient's lifestyle. The success of arthroplasty may be limited by post-surgical heterotopic bone formation. Surgical stabilization of spinal fractures should be undertaken with extreme caution. Correction of spinal deformities caused by advanced, aggressive ankylosis is not advised.

Prognosis: The clinical course and disease severity are highly variable. Inflammatory back pain and stiffness are prominent early in the disease, whereas chronic, aggressive disease may produce pain and marked axial immobility or deformity. Early-onset age and diagnosis portend a more severe outcome.

BIBLIOGRAPHY

Braun J, Pham T, Sieper J, et al., and the ASAS Working Group. International ASAS consensus statement for the use of anti-tumour necrosis factor agents in patients with ankylosing spondylitis. *Ann Rheum Dis.* 2003;62:817–824.

Clegg DO, Reda DJ, Weisman MH, et al. Comparison of sulfasalazine and placebo in the treatment of ankylosing spondylitis. A Department of Veterans Affairs cooperative study. *Arthritis Rheum* 1996;39:2004–2012.

Davis JC, van der Heijde D, Braun J, et al., and the Etanercept Study Group. Recombinant human tumor necrosis factor (etanercept) for treating ankylosing spondylitis: a randomized controlled trial. *Arthritis Rheum* 2003;48:3230–3236.

Hammer RE, Malka SD, Richardson JA, et al. Spontaneous inflammatory disease in transgenic rats expressing HLA-B27 and human β2m: an animal model of HLA-B27-associated human disorders. *Cell* 1990;63:1099–1112.

Khan MA. Update on spondyloarthropathies. *Ann Intern Med* 2002;136:896–907.

ANTIPHOSPHOLIPID ANTIBODY (APL) SYNDROME

Synonyms: Anticardiolipin (ACL) syndrome, Hughes syndrome.

ICD-9 Code: 289.81.

Definition: APL syndrome refers to a constellation of clinical findings, including vascular thrombosis, fetal wastage, and thrombocytopenia, that are seen in association with the lupus anticoagulant and ACL or APL antibodies.

Etiology: The etiology of APL syndrome is unknown. Patients with a variety of infections, cancers, and other conditions may develop ACL antibodies, but fewer develop clinical APL syndrome. ACL antibodies may be found in as many as half of patients with systemic lupus erythematosus (SLE). Clinical APL syndrome occurs only in a minority of those with the antibody. The precise pathogenesis of the APL syndrome is unknown. It is hypothesized that antibodies to negatively-charged phospholipids, such as cardiolipin, alter the normal anticoagulant function of the vascular endothelium. Alternatively, ACL and other APL antibodies may potentiate platelet activation, resulting in thrombosis.

Demographics: APL syndrome occurs most commonly among young women, but all ages and both sexes may become involved. The prevalence of APL antibodies (without clinical symptoms) is far more common than APL syndrome (with an abnormal test).

Cardinal Findings: Clinical characteristics of APL syndrome are shown in Table 3. Recurrent venous or arterial thromboses are the most prominent feature. A history of thrombosis in a patient thought to be otherwise at low risk of such an event often prompts the search for APL syndrome. Other common presentations include recurrent spontaneous abortions and refractory thrombocytopenia.

Complications: Catastrophic APL syndrome refers to fulminant organ failure from widespread thromboses. Precipitating events often include infection, surgery, trauma, anticoagulant cessation, pregnancy, or the use of estrogen-containing compounds. A thrombotic microangiopathy usually affects the kidney, gut, heart, lungs, and brain but may also affect the skin, adrenals, and pancreas. This may result in renal, pulmonary or adrenal failure, alveolar hemorrhage, and bowel infarction, among others complications. This may be confused with thrombotic thrombocytopenic purpura (TTP) or disseminated intravascular coagulation (DIC) because these patients may also have thrombocytopenia, DIC, schistocytes, and severe anemia. Mortality is high,

Table 3
Characteristics of the Antiphospholipid Antibody Syndrome

Common
  Venous thrombosis (e.g., pulmonary embolus, deep venous thrombosis, retinal vein
    thrombosis, Budd-Chiari syndrome)
  Arterial thrombosis (e.g., cerebrovascular accident, myocardial infarction)
  Thrombocytopenia
  Recurrent fetal loss
Less common
  Livedo reticularis
  Cutaneous ulceration
  Hemolytic anemia
  Endocardial/cardiac valvular vegetations (Libman-Sacks endocarditis)
  Chorea, myelopathy

and treatment may require multiple modalities, including high-dose corticosteroids, cyclophosphamide, heparin, gamma-globulin, and plasmapheresis.

Diagnostic Tests: Diagnosis of APL syndrome depends on two distinct types of laboratory tests: functional hematologic tests (the lupus anticoagulant test) or assays for specific antibodies (e.g., ACL antibody test) (see p. 121). Although many patients with APL syndrome may have abnormal results in both types of test, others may manifest only one abnormal test result. Although they are not exactly the same, the terms APL and ACL are often used interchangeably.

There are several laboratory tests that define the presence of a lupus anticoagulant. A prolonged partial thromboplastin time (PTT) with a normal prothrombin time is suggestive. If the PTT does not correct with a 1:1 dilution with normal serum, as would be expected if the prolonged PTT were owing to a deficiency of clotting factors, the presence of an inhibitor such as the lupus anticoagulant is suggested. The dilute Russell viper venom time and the kaolin clot time are clotting tests that depend on phospholipids and are thus interfered with when APL antibodies are present. Finally, correction of a prolonged PTT by addition of excess phospholipids, as is done in the platelet neutralization test and the hexagonal phospholipid test, suggests that a lupus anticoagulant is present.

Enzyme-linked immunosorbent assay (ELISA) is used to identify antibodies that bind to negatively charged phospholipids, including cardiolipin, phosphatidylcholine, and others. Although several antibody isotypes (e.g., IgG, IgA, IgM) may have ACL activity, high-titer IgG ACL correlates most strongly with the clinical syndrome of APL syndrome. Recently, it has been demonstrated that most pathogenic ACL antibodies have binding activity only in the presence of another serum protein, β_2-glycoprotein-I (see p. 121).

Differential Diagnosis: Other considerations for recurrent thrombotic events might include protein C, protein S, antithrombin III or factor V Leiden deficiency, dysfibrinogenemias, hyperhomocystinemia, nephrotic syndrome, malignancies, Behçet's syndrome, paroxysmal nocturnal hemoglobinuria, TTP, Buerger diseases, sickle cell anemia, hyperlipidemia, severe diabetes, or hypertension. Recurrent fetal loss may also be associated with anti-Ro antibodies, coexistent infection or inflammatory diseases, or anatomic abnormalities of the female reproductive tract.

Keys to Diagnosis: An international consensus conference concluded that APL syndrome is defined by at least one clinical criterion (vascular thrombosis, pregnancy complications) and one laboratory testing criterion (lupus anticoagulant, ACL antibodies).

Therapy: Treatment of APL syndrome depends to some extent on the occurrence and severity of the clinical manifestations. Acutely, patients with severe thromboembolic events (e.g., pulmonary embolism) are treated with anticoagulation in the same manner as those without APL syndrome. Because patients with APL syndrome are prone to recurrent thromboses, many physicians recommend that patients with a single serious clotting event be treated with long-term oral anti-coagulation, typically with warfarin. Patients with recurrent events should re-ceive anticoagulation unless there are compelling reasons not to do so. Treatment that achieves an international normalized ratio >2 appears to be more efficacious than less intense anticoagulation. When anticoagulation is not feasible, low doses of aspirin are commonly used as adjunctive therapy, although data supporting the efficacy of this approach are lacking. In some circumstances (e.g., pregnancy), warfarin is contraindicated because it crosses the placenta. Daily treatment with heparin is an alternative. Low molecular weight heparin therapy has also been successfully used in patients with APL syndrome. The role of clopidogrel remains to be defined. Because APL syndrome relates to antibody production, corticos-teroids and other immunomodulatory agents have been tried for some patients. However, good data supporting this approach are lacking.

BIBLIOGRAPHY

Alarcon-Segovia D, Deleze M, Oria CV, et al. Antiphospholipid antibodies and the antiphos-pholipid syndrome in SLE: a prospective analysis of 500 consecutive patients. *Medicine* 1989;68:353–365.
Asherson RA, Cervera R. Catastrophic antiphospholipid syndrome. *Curr Rheumatol Rep* 2003;5:395–400.
Gezer S. Antiphospholipid syndrome. *Dis Mon* 2003;49:696–741.
Luzzana C, Gerosa M, Riboldi P, et al. Up-date on the antiphospholipid syndrome. *J Nephrol* 2002;15:342–348.

ARTHRALGIA/MYALGIA

Synonyms: "Hurts all over," widespread pain.

ICD-9 Code: Arthralgia, 719.4; Myalgia, 729.1.

Definition: The evaluation of patients with widespread arthralgias and/or myalgias can be a challenge because many disorders may manifest these pro-tean symptoms. Widespread pain can be defined as pain that extends beyond joint margins to involve large areas or whole limbs. Alternatively, it is de-scribed as pain on both sides of the body, above and below the waist, and in-cludes axial pain as well. The examiner should search for revealing historical features or evidence of articular or periarticular pathology (i.e., swelling, ery-thema, warmth) before considering the disorders mentioned herein.

ICD-9 Codes: Arthralgia, site unspecified, 719.40; myalgia/myositis, 729.1

Etiology: The most common cause of widespread arthralgias and myalgias is fi-bromyalgia (see p. 177) and myofascial pain syndrome. It is also possible that widespread pains may be drug induced, infectious, endocrinologic/metabolic, autoimmune, neoplastic, or psychiatric in origin (Table 4).

Cardinal Findings: Many patients manifest moderate to severe fatigue and morning stiffness (lasting minutes to hours); thus, these features have little dis-

Table 4
Differential Diagnosis of Arthralgias and Myalgias ("Hurts All Over")

Drug-induced
    Antiinfectives: quinolones, amphotericin, acyclovir
    Biologic agents: interferon, IL-2, IL-6, immunotoxins
    Supplements: excessive vitamin A, fluoride
    Lipid-lowering agents: clofibrate, statins (e.g. lovastatin)
    Cardiac: quinidine, propranolol, nicardipine
Infectious
    Viral syndromes
    Dengue fever
    Vaccines
Endocrine/metabolic
    Hypothyroidism/myxedema
    Hyperparathyroidism
    Hypercortisolism
    Corticosteroid withdrawal
    Adrenal insufficiency
    Hypophosphatemia
Autoimmune
    Systemic lupus erythematosus
    Polymyalgia rheumatica
    Inflammatory myositis
Neoplastic/hematologic
    Leukemia
    Lymphoma
    Multiple myeloma
    Metastases to bone
    Sickle cell crisis
Psychiatric
    Depression
    Psychogenic rheumatism
    Malingering
    Somatization disorder
Other
    Fibromyalgia
    Chronic fatigue syndrome
    Hypermobility syndrome
    Silicone implant syndrome (most have fibromyalgia)

IL, interleukin.

criminant value. The patient should be questioned about fever (i.e., ≥100°F) or weight loss because these may suggest conditions with significant morbidity. Symptoms suggesting endocrinopathies should be sought (i.e., heat or cold intolerance). Symptomatic rashes, muscle weakness, myalgias, muscle cramping, depression, or sleep disturbance may also provide important clues. It is equally important to review the patient's medication history, medical and surgical history, health maintenance, and social history when evaluating diffuse musculoskeletal complaints.

Efforts should be directed toward identifying the source and extent of joint or muscle pain; many patients in this group will have periarticular rather than articular pain. The clinician should carefully examine for the trigger point tender areas of fibromyalgia. Signs of ligamentous laxity may indicate hypermobility syndrome. Lymphadenopathy, masses, organomegaly, and stigmata of thyroid, adrenal, or muscle disease (see p. 248) should be sought.

Diagnostic Testing: Routine laboratory testing should include a complete blood count (CBC), chemistries, and an ESR. Extreme elevation of the ESR (>60 mm Hg) seldom occurs without evidence of serious illness. Conversely, normal or low-level elevations of the ESR are less diagnostic and should not be overinterpreted. Serologic testing for ANA or RF (or batteries of rheumatic screening tests) are unlikely to yield useful information. Similarly, thyroid function studies or CPK should only be done if symptoms and signs (beyond arthralgias) warrant.

Differential Diagnosis: Table 4 lists the many disorders that may manifest widespread arthralgias/myalgias. Although fibromyalgia is most common among these, the clinician should be careful to not confuse fibromyalgia with influenza and other viral infections, thyroid or adrenal disease, metabolic bone disease (e.g., osteomalacia/rickets, hyperparathyroidism), polymyalgia rheumatica, Still disease, the early onset of a connective tissue disease (lupus, RA, myositis), multiple myeloma, bony metastases, or depression with somatization.

Imaging: Imaging will seldom reveal diagnostic information not gleaned from the physical examination. Rarely, bony metastases are found by plain radiographs or scintigraphy. The predictive value of whole body scintigraphy has been advocated for the evaluation of widespread pain without supportive physical findings.

Therapy: Patients should be treated symptomatically, and narcotic analgesics should be avoided until a confident diagnosis is made. Thereafter, therapeutic choices are defined by the diagnostic entity rather than the general complaint. If the complaint is drug induced, then drug withdrawal usually results in rapid improvement. Treatment of the underlying condition may also improve the musculoskeletal complaint.

BIBLIOGRAPHY

McBeth J, Macfarlane GJ, Hunt IM, et al. Risk factors for persistent chronic widespread pain: a community-based study. *Rheumatology* 2001;40:95–101.
Puttick MPE, Esdaile JM. Evaluation of the patient with pain all over. *CMAJ* 2001;164:223–227.

ATRIAL MYXOMA

Synonyms: Cardiac myxoma.

ICD-9 Code: 212.7.

Definition: Atrial myxoma is a benign cardiac tumor that may lead to valvular obstruction or emboli. Embolic manifestations may be confused with a systemic necrotizing vasculitis.

Pathology: Tumors are typically found in the left atrium (75%), right atrium (20%), or ventricles (5%), usually as a single pedunculated tumor attached to the septum, valve, or chordae tendineae. Large myxomas may produce valve obstruction and emboli. Increased amounts of IL-6, produced by myxoma cells, are responsible for many of the systemic and constitutional manifestations. Asymptomatic tumors may be found at autopsy.

Demographics: Atrial myxomas usually affect adults between 30 and 60 years of age. They are uncommon in blacks and rarely familial (autosomal dominant). No gender preference exists.

Cardinal Findings: Atrial myxomas produce systemic, obstructive, and embolic symptoms. Fever, weight loss, arthralgia, myalgia, Raynaud phenomenon, rash, and clubbing may occur. Cardiac findings include new-onset congestive heart failure, chest pain, and dyspnea that improves when supine. Arterial emboli may cause central neurologic deficits, mononeuritis multiplex, or skin lesions.

Complications: Congestive heart failure pulmonary emboli, and pulmonary hypertension may occur.

Diagnostic Tests: Anemia, leukocytosis, increased ESR, thrombocytosis or thrombocytopenia, hypergammaglobulinemia, and hypocomplementemia are common.

Imaging: Diagnosis is usually made by echocardiography, but CT or MRI can also be used. Occasionally, vasculitic findings may be seen on angiogram or in biopsy specimens.

Therapy: Tumors are surgically excised and may recur.

BIBLIOGRAPHY

Burke AP, Virmani R. Cardiac myxoma. A clinicopathologic study. *Am J Clin Pathol* 1993;100:671–680.
Sack KE. Mimickers of vasculitis: cardiac myxoma. In: Koopman WJ, ed. *Arthritis and allied conditions,* 13th ed. Baltimore: Williams & Wilkins, 1997:1529–1530.

BACTERIAL ARTHRITIS

Synonyms: Septic arthritis, infectious arthritis, gonococcal arthritis.

ICD-9 Codes: Pyogenic arthritis, 711.0; gonococcal arthritis, 098.5; bacterial arthritis unspecified, 711.4.

Definition: Bacterial arthritis is a bacterial infection of the joint space that may affect any type of joint.

Etiology: Most cases of bacterial arthritis are hematogenously disseminated. Others may occur by direct invasion (e.g., trauma) or contiguous spread (e.g., osteomyelitis). Reasons for invasion of the joint space by bacteria are not known, but preexisting articular abnormalities (e.g., RA, OA) or previous surgery may contribute to entry of the infectious agent. Comorbid conditions such as diabetes mellitus or drugs (corticosteroids) that impair immune function may be contributing factors.

At-Risk Populations: Those at risk include the very young, elderly, or immunosuppressed (e.g., by cytotoxics or corticosteroids); those with chronic arthropathies (e.g., RA, OA), prosthetic joints, repeated joint aspiration or injection, or systemic illness (e.g., chronic liver disease, neoplasia, sickle cell); intravenous substance abusers; and those engaged in high-risk sexual activity or who have had recent trauma or surgery.

Pathology: Joint cultures are usually positive for the causative agent unless antibiotics have been previously given. An important exception is gonococcal arthritis, in which >90% of synovial fluid cultures are often negative, even with appropriate culture techniques. Common pathogens in septic arthritis include staphylococci (*Staphylococcus aureus, Staphylococcus epidermidis*), streptococci (*Streptococcus pyogenes, Streptococcus pneumoniae*), neisseriae (*Neisseria gonorrhoeae, Neisseria meningitidis*), *Haemophilus influenzae, Salmonella, Proteus mirabilis*, and *Bacteroides fragilis*.

Demographics: All age groups are susceptible. An increasing percentage of patients have a chronic underlying disease (e.g., RA, diabetes), but healthy individuals can also be affected. Septic arthritis in children is usually caused by *S. aureus*, group B streptococci, or *H. influenzae*. Young adults are likely to have gonococcal or staphylococcal infection. The elderly are commonly affected by bacterial arthritis owing to staphylococcal, streptococcal, gram-negative, and polymicrobic infections.

Cardinal Findings: The classic presentation is an acute monarticular arthritis with effusion, warmth, and erythema, often accompanied by fever. Polyarticular onset occurs in a minority of cases and carries a poorer prognosis.
—*Gonococcal arthritis:* Typically seen in young, sexually active (often menstruating) females. Gonococcal arthritis often affects the knees, ankles, wrists, or elbows as monarthritis or oligoarthritis. Tenosynovitis and migratory arthralgias are common, and characteristic pustular (often painful) lesions are found on the skin. Fever may be absent, and a minority will have genitourinary, pharyngeal, or rectal symptoms on presentation. If suspected, every orifice should be swabbed and cultured for gonococcus on Thayer-Martin culture medium. A small minority of patients have a positive synovial fluid culture.

—*Staphylococcal arthritis:* Usually monarticular (seldom polyarticular), staphylococcal arthritis affects the knee, hip, shoulder, elbow, wrist, or ankle, and >90% of patients exhibit high fevers. Involvement of the sternoclavicular joint, shoulder, or sacroiliac joint should raise suspicion of a staphylococcal infection and, possibly, intravenous substance abuse. Patients with preexisting arthritis (e.g., RA) are prone to infection with *S. aureus.*

—*Prosthetic joints:* Fewer than 2% of those with joint replacements develop a septic joint. Those at greatest risk are patients with RA, with distant infections, or who use corticosteroid or are undergoing revision arthroplasty. When septic arthritis immediately follows the procedure, *S. epidermidis, S. aureus,* or skin anaerobes are the most common pathogens. High fevers and purulent effusions develop. Late prosthetic infection (>1 year postoperatively) is usually less symptomatic and is most likely to be caused by *S. aureus,* non–group A streptococci, and gram-negative organisms.

—*Intravenous substance abuse:* Common sites of infection include the shoulder, sternoclavicular, and sacroiliac joints. Infections in the sacroiliac joint may present as low back or buttock pain with only subtle suggestions of infection. These patients are commonly infected by *S. aureus* and gram-negative organisms (e.g., *Pseudomonas aeruginosa*).

Diagnostic Tests: Joint aspiration and culture of synovial fluid is usually diagnostic in those with nongonococcal septic arthritis (Table 5). Blood should also be cultured and is frequently positive in nongonococcal arthritis. Other measures, such as the synovial fluid WBC count and ESR or CRP elevations, are only suggestive. Joint aspiration and the interpretation of synovial fluid results are discussed on p. 17. Aspiration should be performed with a large-bore

Table 5
Suspected Bacterial Arthritis: Important Tasks in the First 48 Hours

1. Aspirate fluid from the joint *unless*
   a. Overlying skin/soft tissues appear infected
   b. The joint has been surgically replaced
2. Send the fluid to the laboratory for
   a. Leukocyte count and differential
   b. Culture and sensitivity
   c. Crystal identification
3. Initiate presumptive antibiotic treatment
   a. Intravenous therapy
   b. Include coverage for *Staphylococcus aureus*
4. Repeat joint aspiration in 24 h and then daily for
   a. SF leukocyte count; repeat until declining
   b. Culture; repeat until sterile
5. Obtain orthopedic consultation for
   a. Suspected septic hips (adults or children)
   b. Suspected infections of prosthetic joints
   c. Consideration of open drainage if repeat SF WBC not declining

SF, synovial fluid; WBC, white blood cell.

needle to remove as much purulent material as possible. Synovial fluid WBC counts should be >30,000 cells/mm³ with gonococcal arthritis and >50,000 cells/mm³ with nongonococcal septic arthritis. The percentage of neutrophils is as important as cell counts and usually exceeds 85% in septic arthritis. The presence of crystals in synovial fluid does not exclude a coexistent infection. Gram stains are useful in making initial antibiotic choices, but culture confirmation is required. Needle aspiration should not be performed through skin or soft tissues that show signs of infection. If the joint in question has been surgically replaced, orthopaedic consultation should be considered before any joint aspiration or injection.

Imaging: Radiographs are seldom revealing and may only show soft tissue swelling with acute septic arthritis. Radiographic changes may take 2 to 3 weeks to become apparent. Thus, an early diagnosis must be established on clinical grounds and synovial fluid culture. The presence of gas formation should suggest infection with *Escherichia coli* or anaerobes. Radiography and other modalities may be necessary to diagnose an infected prosthetic joint. Radiographs may show bone resorption and radiolucency at the implant-bone interface, with or without evidence of overlying periosteal reaction. Technetium bone scanning may suggest an infected prosthesis before changes on plain radiography. MRI and gallium- and indium-labeled WBC scanning have not been shown to be of value in such patients.

Keys to Diagnosis: Acute monarticular arthritis with fever is the most common presentation, but polyarticular and subacute afebrile presentations also occur. In patients with inflammatory types of arthritis (e.g., RA), activity in one joint that seems out of proportion to that in others should raise suspicion of septic arthritis. Acute inflammatory monarthritis in the setting of positive blood cultures should strongly suggest septic arthritis.

Differential Diagnosis: Bacterial arthritis may often be confused with other forms of infectious arthritis (viral, fungal, mycobacterial). The infectious arthropathies are compared in Table 6. Bacterial arthritis should also be distinguished from acute crystal-induced arthritis (e.g., gout, pseudogout), Reiter's syndrome, Lyme disease, septic bursitis, overlying cellulitis, osteomyelitis, foreign body reaction, fracture, or mechanical joint derangement.

Therapy: Parenteral antibiotics must be given as soon as possible after the initial joint aspiration. Although culture results are pending (usually 24–48 hours), the initial antibiotic should include coverage for *S. aureus* (Table 6). Parenteral therapy is recommended for at least 3 weeks for *S. aureus* and gram-negative organisms, 7 days for gonococcal infection, and 2 weeks for most other organisms (e.g., *S. pyogenes*, *H. influenzae*). Follow-up therapy with oral antibiotics is of unproven benefit. With the availability of long-lasting intravenous access lines and home care teams, prolonged hospitalization is not required. Before hospital discharge, serial joint taps must show a steady and

Table 6
Comparison of Infectious Arthropathies

Bacterial Arthritis

	Staphylococcal	Gonococcal	Gram-negative
Pattern	Acute monarticular	Acute monarticular or migratory polyarticular with tenosynovitis	Acute monarticular
Demographics	All ages	Sexually active young adults	IV drug abuse; very young or very old
Synovial fluid	WBCs >50,000	WBCs >30,000	WBCs >50,000
Cultures	Usually positive	Usually negative	Usually positive
Treatment	Nafcillin (± rifampin) or vancomycin	Ceftriaxone	Aminoglycoside + semisynthetic penicillin or third-generation cephalosporin
Outcome	Guarded, inversely correlated with age	Generally good	Generally good, poor in elderly

Nonbacterial Arthritis

	Viral	Fungal	Mycobacterial
Pattern	Acute polyarticular	Chronic monarticular	Chronic monarticular
Demographics	All ages	Immunocompromised host	All ages
Synovial fluid	WBCs <20,000	Variable WBCs	WBCs 10,000–20,000
Cultures	Usually negative	Usually negative	Usually negative; requires biopsy
Treatment	Symptomatic	Amphotericin B (± 5-fluorocytosine)	INH, rifampin, and pyrazinamide
Outcome	Self-limited with preserved joint bone	Mixed; deformity possible	Mixed; destructive changes are possible

IV, intravenous; WBC, white blood cells; INH, isoniazid.

marked decrease in synovial fluid WBCs and sterile synovial fluid culture. There is no role for intraarticular antibiotics.

Surgery: The role of surgical drainage is controversial except in inaccessible sites such as the hip, where a surgical approach (open drainage or fluoroscopically-guided needle aspiration) is often required. In children, all septic hips require arthrotomy to reduce intraarticular pressure and allow adequate drainage. Most other joints can be treated by serial needle aspirations and do not require surgical drainage unless the leukocyte count does not drop as expected or cultures do not rapidly become sterile.

Prognosis: In general, mortality rates are below 5%. Prognosis is poorest in the elderly and those with gram-negative infections, polyarticular involvement, prosthetic joints, or delayed diagnosis. If less than 1 week elapses before initiation of therapy, the prospect for maintaining normal joint function is very good; if the time before treatment is 1 month or more, the outcome is usually poor. Infections of prosthetic joints present major surgical problems, usually requiring removal of the components, prolonged antibiotic treatment, and then revised reconstruction. Such cases should be referred to an orthopedist at the outset.

BIBLIOGRAPHY

Bernard L, Hoffmeyer P, Assal M, et al. Trends in the treatment of orthopaedic prosthetic infections. *J Antimicrob Chemother* 2004;53:127–129.
Gupta MN, Sturrock RD, Field M. A prospective study of 75 patients with adult-onset septic arthritis. *Rheumatology* 2001;40:24–30.
Ho G Jr. Septic arthritis update. *Bull Rheum Dis* 2002;51:1–4.
Piro MH. Septic arthritis. *Rheum Dis Clin North Am* 1997;23: 239–258.
Shirtliff ME, Mader JT. Acute septic arthritis. *Clin Microbiol Rev* 2002;15:527–544.

BACTERIAL ENDOCARDITIS

Synonyms: Infective endocarditis, subacute bacterial endocarditis (SBE).

ICD-9 Code: Infective endocarditis, 421.0; prosthetic valve endocarditis, 996.61.

Definition: Infective endocarditis implies infection of valvular or mural endocardium. Endocarditis is an uncommon cause of fever, arthralgia, and low back pain.

Etiology: Most infections occur over abnormal valves or damaged endocardial surfaces, where abnormal blood flow patterns lead to development of platelet-thrombin clots that serve as foci for infections. Some cases occur in intravenous drug abusers and are caused by more highly virulent staphylococcal and streptococcal organisms. Subacute endocarditis may be caused by β-hemolytic streptococci, *Streptococcus bovis,* and enterococci. Endocarditis with intravenous drug abuse may be caused by *S. aureus, Pseudomonas* spp, gram-negative species, and *Candida* spp.

Pathology: Infections are usually formed over areas of sterile vegetations consisting of platelets and fibrin. Most occur in high-pressure areas, usually on the left side of the heart. Underlying valves may show thickening from previous damage.

Demographics: Those at risk include older individuals; those with rheumatic valvular disease or prosthetic valves; intravenous drug abusers; those with indwelling catheters; and those with bacteremia.

Cardinal Findings: Most patients have fever (with or without night sweats) and a cardiac murmur. Tender nodules on the fingertips (Osler's nodes) and splinter hemorrhages under the fingernails may be seen. Anorexia, weight loss, arthralgias, frank arthritis, low back pain, and splenomegaly are common. Back pain may be caused by bacteremia or septic emboli resulting in septic discitis. A small number of patients develop septic arthritis owing to seeding with the causative organism. Multiple joints may be involved.

Complications: Congestive heart failure, ruptured valve cusp or chordae tendineae, abscesses (myocardial, aortic root, brain), or infarction (lung, spleen, bowel, or myocardium) from emboli may be seen. Renal failure from glomerulonephritis has been described.

Diagnostic Tests: Positive blood cultures are diagnostic, but a significant minority of patients remain culture negative. Previous treatment with antibiotics may alter culture results. Elevated levels of acute-phase reactants (ESR, CRP) are expected. In subacute endocarditis, an anemia of chronic disease, low complement levels, and positive RF may be seen.

Imaging: Echocardiography, including transesophageal approaches, is recommended.

Differential Diagnosis: Patients may present with fever of unknown origin. Splinter hemorrhages and Osler nodes may suggest a systemic vasculitis (e.g., Churg-Strauss, cryoglobulinemia). Multiple swollen joints and inflamed joints might suggest gout or Reiter's syndrome. Some patients are transiently positive for RF, so polyarthritis might be mistaken for RA. Other possibilities include osteomyelitis, rheumatic fever, and tuberculosis.

Therapy: Definitive therapy requires an extended course of appropriate antibiotics. Subsequent antibiotic prophylaxis is recommended for all invasive procedures.

Surgery: Heart valve replacement may be required.

Prognosis: Long-term outcome is dictated by the severity of the underlying heart disease or drug addiction or development of complications.

BIBLIOGRAPHY

Roberts-Thomson PJ, Rischmueller M, Kwiatek RA, et al. Rheumatic manifestations of infective endocarditis. *Rheumatol Int* 1992;12:61–63.

BEHÇET'S SYNDROME

Definition: Behçet's syndrome is a syndrome of recurrent, painful oral and genital lesions associated with uveitis and other forms of systemic inflammation.

ICD-9 Codes: 136.1; with arthropathy, 711.2.

Etiology: Behçet's syndrome is a relapsing small vessel vasculitis of uncertain etiology. There is evidence suggesting immune-complex deposition, hyperfunctioning neutrophils, increased levels of circulating IL-6, and a decreased CD4:CD8 T cell ratio. HLA-B5 and subtype HLA-B51 may be risk factors in afflicted Japanese patients.

Pathology: Histology of skin lesions may show perivascular inflammation or vasculitis, with both neutrophilic and monocytic infiltrates.

Demographics: Behçet's syndrome is most common in the eastern Mediterranean (Turkey) and Japanese (prevalence approximately one in 1,000) populations. In the United States, the prevalence is 0.3 to 6.6 cases per 100,000. The male:female ratio is 2:1 to 5:1, and the mean age of onset is approximately 40 years. Behçet's syndrome is one of the leading causes of acquired blindness in Japan.

Cardinal Findings: The prevalence of findings ranges widely betwen nonendemic (i.e. North American) and endemic (i.e. Turkish) populations. Aphthous stomatitis (100% prevalence) is usually the first manifestation. Very painful lesions occur in crops and may last 1 to 2 weeks and often heal with scarring. Oral ulcers are most commonly found on the buccal or gingival mucosa or tongue. Painful genital ulcers (70%–100%) occur on the vulva or vagina in women (often during menses) and penis or scrotum in men. Genital ulcers resemble oral aphthae but tend to recur less frequently. Ocular findings (50%–90%) are usually bilateral and occur 2 to 3 years after initial symptoms. Anterior uveitis, with hypopyon (pus in anterior chamber of the eye), and posterior uveitis may result in visual loss and be caused by retinal, macular, or choroidal vessel vasculitis. Arthritis (40%–50%) is usually episodic, monarticular, or oligoarticular. Large joints are more commonly affected than small joints. Arthralgias are more common than frank arthritis. Cutaneous lesions (30%–65%) include pustules, erythema nodosum, papules/pseudofolliculitis, and severe acneform lesions. Nodules are also seen secondary to superficial phlebitis. Pathergy, nearly unique to Behçet syndrome, occurs when pricking the skin with a needle leads to development of a sterile pustule. Central nervous system (5%–30%) manifestations of headaches, meningoencephalitis, ocular and other cranial nerve palsies, seizures, cerebrovascular insufficiency, brainstem syndrome leading to cerebellar ataxia, and pseudobulbar palsy have all been reported. Phlebitis/arteritis (25%) with thromboses of large veins/arteries and aneurysms (of the aorta and pulmonary arterial tree) may occur. Chiari syndrome, dural sinus thrombosis, limb ischemia, stroke, and renovascular hypertension have been reported.

Uncommon Findings: Colitis and epididymitis are seen in a minority of patients. Nephritis and amyloidosis have rarely been noted. The rarely seen MAGIC syndrome (*m*outh *a*nd *g*enital ulceration with *i*nflamed *c*artilage) has overlapping features of Behçet's syndrome and relapsing polychondritis.

Complications: The most feared common complication is blindness from eye manifestations. Neurologic and vascular complications (thrombotic events) are responsible for most of the severe morbidity and potential mortality.

Diagnostic Testing: Nonspecific measures of systemic inflammation include elevated acute-phase reactants (ESR and CRP), leukocytosis, anemia of chronic inflammation, and thrombocytosis. With significant CNS involvement, the cerebrospinal fluid (CSF) typically shows a mononuclear cell pleocytosis and elevated protein levels. Patients with thromboses may have APL antibodies.

Differential Diagnosis: Other forms of systemic vasculitis [polyarteritis nodosa (PAN)] and SLE should be considered. Oral and genital lesions may be confused with inflammatory bowel disease or Reiter's syndrome. The oral ulcers of SLE or Reiter's syndrome are usually painless and palatal. Uveitis should raise the possibility of other inflammatory disease (i.e., the SpA) as well as infectious causes. Skin manifestations resemble those of Sweet's syndrome, disseminated gonococcus or Stevens-Johnson syndrome. Large vessel vasculitis may mimic Takayasu's arteritis.

Keys to Diagnosis: Look for the triad of oral ulcers, genital lesions, and uveitis. Although pathergy is nearly pathognomonic, it is infrequently seen among North American whites.

Diagnostic Criteria: Criteria of the International Study Group are
   A. Recurrent oral ulceration (at least three times in 1 year), plus
   B. Two of the following four criteria:
      1. Recurrent genital ulcerations
      2. Eye lesions-uveitis or retinal vasculitis
      3. Skin lesions-erythema nodosum, pseudofolliculitis, papulopustular lesions, or unexplained acne
      4. Pathergy

Therapy: Intermittent prednisone (10–40 mg/day) is effective in the control of recurrent ulcerations, but long-term use should be discouraged because of the risk of steroid toxicity. Colchicine, dapsone, and levamisole may also be used to treat skin/mucocutaneous manifestations. Active uveitis or CNS disease merits aggressive therapy with high-dose corticosteroids, cytotoxic agents (e.g., azathioprine, chlorambucil, cyclophosphamide), or cyclosporine. Thalidomide and TNF inhibitors have been used successfully for refractory oral and genital ulcers and sight-threatening eye disease. Colchicine, NSAIDs, or sulfasalazine may be effective for Behçet's syndrome–associated arthritis. Chronic anticoagulation may be required for thrombotic complications.

Prognosis: Oral and genital lesions frequently predate vascular and neurologic manifestations by months or years. Relapses are common over a 5- to 7-year period before a reduction in disease activity may occur.

BIBLIOGRAPHY

International Study Group for Behçet's Disease. Criteria for diagnosis of Behçet's disease. *Lancet* 1990;335:1078–1080.

Yazici H. Behçet's syndrome: an update. *Curr Rheumatol Rep* 2003;5:195–199.

BRUCELLOSIS

Synonyms: Undulant fever, Malta fever.

ICD-9 Code: 023.9.

Definition: Systemic infection with *Brucella* is uncommon and may cause fever, peripheral arthritis, sacroiliitis, or spondylitis.

Etiopathogenesis: Humans may acquire *Brucella* by ingesting infected unpasteurized dairy products (e.g., cheese), exposure to aerosolized bacteria, or contact with broken skin or conjunctiva. *Brucella* is a gram-negative coccobacillus. *Brucella* arthritis is usually caused by direct seeding of the synovium. Some cases appear to be "reactive" (i.e., not caused by direct infection). *Brucella* septic arthritis is usually monarticular or axial, is persistent, and requires antibiotic therapy. The reactive arthritis is usually intermittent, self-limited, sterile, nondestructive, and polyarticular.

Demographics: *Brucella* has a worldwide distribution. Most cases are reported from South America. *Brucella* spp include *Brucella abortus* (zoonotic source, cow), *Brucella melitensis* (goat), and *Brucella suis* (pig). Although *B. abortus* is most common in the United States, *B. melitensis* is most common worldwide. Infection occurs at all ages and in both genders. Those at risk include veterinarians, farm and slaughterhouse workers, and persons ingesting unpasteurized milk or cheese.

Cardinal Findings: Acute infection is associated with bacteremia and may show fever (101°–104°F), arthralgias, headache, or malaise. Fever, diaphoresis, and weight loss may be undulant. Hepatosplenomegaly and uveitis are common. In the subacute form, fever is less common. Acute peripheral arthritis of the lower extremities (e.g., hip or knee) is common. Arthralgias and myalgias are seen in more than half of patients. Sacroiliitis is usually unilateral and nondestructive. Spondylitis commonly affects the lumbar spine.

Uncommon Findings: Lymphadenopathy, pulmonary symptoms, orchitis, tendinitis, bursitis, and epicondylitis.

Complications: Local microabscesses (i.e., paraspinal abscess often manifesting as antibiotic resistance), endocarditis, thrombophlebitis, hepatitis, and CNS infection may occur.

Diagnostic Tests: Routine laboratory testing may show leukopenia, relative lymphocytosis, thrombocytopenia, or abnormal hepatic enzymes. Culture of organism from joint fluid is slow (3–4 weeks) and is positive in <50% of samples. Bone marrow culture may improve culture yield or show granulomas. Serologic tests (ELISA or agglutination reaction) for IgM or IgG (chronic) anti-*Brucella* antibody are usually positive.

Imaging: Sacroiliitis appears as blurring of articular margins of the sacroiliac joints, seldom with erosions. Spondylitis appears as intervertebral erosions, disc narrowing, and reactive osteophytes with a "parrot-beak" appearance. Scintigraphy may be useful in identifying spondylitis or sacroiliitis.

Keys to Diagnosis: Bacteriologic or serologic evidence of infection signals the diagnosis, which requires a high index of suspicion, especially in the at-risk population.

Differential Diagnosis: Spondyloarthropathies, septic arthritis, psittacosis, tuberculosis, human immunodeficiency virus (HIV), and rickettsial infections must be considered.

Therapy: At least 4 to 6 weeks of combination antibiotic therapy with tetracycline (doxycycline) plus a second agent (rifampin, streptomycin, or trimethoprim) is effective in most.

Monitoring: Clinical response and serum antibody levels should be monitored for a year after treatment.

Prognosis: Most patients do very well. The relapse rate is 5%. Mortality is rare and usually owing to endocarditis.

BIBLIOGRAPHY

Colmenero J, Reguera JM, Fernandez-Nebro A, et al. Osteoarticular complications of brucellosis. *Ann Rheum Dis* 1991;50:23–26.

Zaks N, Sukenik S, Alkan M, et al. Musculoskeletal manifestations of brucellosis: a study of 90 cases in Israel. *Semin Arthritis Rheum* 1995;25:97–102.

CALCINOSIS AND CALCIPHYLAXIS

Synonyms: Calcinosis cutis, dystrophic calcification.

ICD-9 code: Calcinosis cutis, 709.3; tumoral calcinosis, 275.49; calciphylaxis, 440.23.

Definition: Cutaneous and subcutaneous deposition of calcium is often referred to as calcinosis cutis or tumoral calcinosis. Calciphylaxis is a rare disorder that affects patients with long-standing end-stage renal disease, many of whom have secondary hyperparathyroidism. This condition primarily manifests painful nodular lesions.

Etiology: There are five types of calcinosis cutis: metastatic calcinosis, dystrophic calcinosis, iatrogenic calcinosis, idiopathic calcinosis and calciphylaxis. Metastatic calcinosis results from hypercalcemia or hyperphosphatemia and affects the kidneys, lungs, stomach, and, less commonly, the finger tips and periarticular structures. Dystrophic calcification occurs as a result of previously damaged skin and tissues, spares internal organs, and has normal serum calcium and phosphate levels. Dystrophic calcification in the skin seems to correlate with MRI evidence of cutaneous edema or vasculitis, suggesting calcific change is a response to injury. Iatrogenic forms result from extravasation of intravenous agents containing calcium or phosphate. Idiopathic calcification occurs without apparent cause or tissue degeneration. Calciphylaxis is a life-threatening condition caused by progressive cutaneous necrosis caused by small vessel calcification. Calciphylaxis is rare, and typically occurs in patients with end-stage renal disease.

Pathology: Calcinosis may affect the skin, subcutaneous layers including the fascia and muscle. Calcific lesions are rich in hydroxyapatite but may also contain calcium oxalate and uric acid in crystalline form. Lesions are also rich in macrophages, IL-1, IL-6, and TNF.

Risk Factors: Dystrophic calcification commonly occurs in children (more so than adults) with dermatomyositis (DM) and in scleroderma (diffuse and limited) and is rare in mixed connective tissue disease (MCTD). Calcinosis cutis may also occur as a consequence of subcutaneous injections with heparin or other parenteral agents or as a response to trauma.

Cardinal Features: Calcinosis often manifests as painful new lesions in the skin. They appear insidiously such that calcinosis is often a late finding in juvenile DM, CREST syndrome, and diffuse scleroderma. Calcific deposits commonly are found over the fingers, forearms, elbows, knees, and buttocks. Calciphylaxis presents as plaque-like, nodular, or bullous lesions progress to necrotic, ulcerative, painful, nodular lesions on the digits, extremities, and trunk. Patients may develop gangrene of the digits, extremities, buttocks, or abdomen. Uncommonly, it manifests as painful myopathy or severe livedo reticularis that progresses to cutaneous gangrene.

Uncommon Findings: Tumoral calcinosis is an uncommon condition with large calcific masses affecting the soft tissues, bursae, and joints (knees, wrist, fingers, feet, temporomandibular joint). These need not be painful. Tumoral calcinosis is seen in patients with renal failure, hyperparathyroidism, myelitis, calcium pyrophosphate dihydrate (CPPD) crystal deposition disease, sarcoidosis, trauma, or microtrauma. Also rare are "milk of calcium" effusions are nonseptic collections of noncrystalline calcium seldom found in joints and tissues.

Complications: Cutaneous calcific lesions may cause skin breakdown, with the release of a chalky exudate. Such open lesions are subject to secondary bacterial infection. Tumoral collections of calcium may cause local compressive effects leading to pain, nerve impingement, or even myelopathy. Complications of calciphylaxis include cutaneous gangrene and sepsis. Unfortunately, there is a very high mortality rate owing to secondary sepsis. Calcification of the lungs or ischemic infarction of major organs is rare. It may be associated with functional protein C or S deficiency.

Diagnostic Tests: Serum calcium, phosphate, and alkaline phosphatase levels are normal for most with calcinosis cutis. With calciphylaxis, parathyroid hormone levels are elevated in 90% of patients. Look for hypercalcemia and hyperphosphatemia. The calcium-phosphate product ($Ca^{2+} \times PO_4$) exceeds 70 in 80% of patients. Deep incisional biopsies are preferred over punch biopsies.

Imaging: Subcutaneous, fascial, and muscular calcification is usually identified by soft tissue radiographs but may also be found on a CT scan. Vascular calcifications are seen in calciphylaxis.

Keys to Diagnosis: The presence of tender, hard, bead-like or gravel-like lesions beneath the skin that may ulcerate. Diagnosis is confirmed by either soft tissue radiography or calcium exudates from eroded skin lesions. Vascular calcifications or painful nodules in patients with end-stage renal disease indicates the presence of calciphylaxis.

Differential Diagnosis: Calcific deposits are seldom confused with tophi, rheumatoid nodules, or xanthoma. Vasculitis, panniculitis, and type 1 primary hyperoxaluria must be distinguished from calciphylaxis.

Therapy: There is no proven effective therapy for cutaneous calcification. Anecdotal reports suggest that oral aluminum hydroxide; calcium channel blockers (e.g., diltiazem); and bisphosphonate (e.g., alendronate, pamidronate, risedronate) therapy may be effective in some. The use of colchicine and warfarin appears to be even less successful. There is no specific therapy for calciphylaxis other than proper wound care and antibiotics. Corticosteroids are not helpful.

Prognosis: Lesions tend to be chronic and less commonly are relapsing or remittent. Calciphylaxis has a significant mortality rate of 60% to 80%.

BIBLIOGRAPHY

Khafif RA, DeLima C, Silverberg A, et al. Calciphylaxis and systemic calcinosis. Collective review. *Arch Intern Med* 1990;150:956–959.
Martinez S. Tumoral calcinosis: 12 years later. *Semin Musculoskel Radiol* 2002;6:331–339.
Touart DM, Sau P. Cutaneous deposition diseases. Part II. *J Am Acad Dermatol* 1998;39:527–544.

CALCIUM PYROPHOSPHATE DIHYDRATE CRYSTAL DEPOSITION DISEASE (CPPD)

Synonyms: Pseudogout, chondrocalcinosis, pyrophosphate arthropathy.

ICD-9 Codes: Pseudogout, 712.2; CPPD crystal deposition disease, 712.2; chondrocalcinosis, 712.3.

Definition: CPPD crystal deposition disease includes arthritic syndromes associated with CPPD crystal deposition disease in articular tissues. The following definitions are used here:

—*Chondrocalcinosis:* Calcification of articular cartilage (identified by x-ray).

—*Chronic CPPD crystal deposition disease:* Structural bone and cartilage abnormalities associated with intraarticular deposition of CPPD crystals.

—*Pseudogout:* Clinical syndrome of acute synovitis caused by intraarticular CPPD crystal deposition, the most common form of CPPD crystal deposition disease.

Etiology: The cause of CPPD crystal deposition disease is unknown. Formation of CPPD crystals in cartilage may be related to matrix changes or result from elevated levels of calcium or inorganic pyrophosphate. Some cases appear to be hereditary, whereas others are idiopathic.

Pathology: CPPD crystals are found in joint capsules and fibrocartilaginous structures. The earliest deposition is seen at the lacunar margin of chondrocytes. Neutrophils can be seen invading matrix structures, with erosion of cartilage and degradation of collagen fibrils. Synovial proliferation can resemble rheumatoid pannus.

Demographics: Data on CPPD crystal deposition disease are largely derived from radiographic surveys of chondrocalcinosis of the knee. Predominantly a condition of the elderly, it has a peak age of 65 to 75 years and female predominance (F:M ratio, 2–7:1). The prevalence of chondrocalcinosis in the general population is 5% to 8% and increases to >15% by the ninth decade. It is ubiquitous in geographic distribution. Familial predisposition has been reported in several groups, some of whom have early-onset, severe, polyarticular disease (third to fourth decades).

Disease Associations: Several conditions are associated with CPPD crystal deposition disease: hyperparathyroidism, hypocalciuria, hypercalcemia, hemochromatosis, hemosiderosis, hypophosphatasia, hypomagnesemia, hypothyroidism, gout, neuropathic joints, amyloidosis, trauma, OA, and aging.

Cardinal Findings: Findings vary according to the type of disease.

—*Pseudogout:* Pseudogout often begins as self-limited acute arthritic attacks lasting from 1 day to 4 weeks and may be as severe as and resemble acute gout. Attacks are often provoked by concurrent medical illnesses or surgery. The knee joint is involved in 50% of cases, followed by the wrist, shoulder, ankle, and elbow. Podagra (first metatarsophalangeal arthritis) has been reported. Patients are asymptomatic between attacks. Men are predominantly affected. As many 20% have concurrent hyperuricemia, and 5% have monosodium urate crystals in synovial fluid as well. The diagnosis is suggested by the clinical presentation and confirmed by synovial fluid analysis (CPPD crystals) or radiography (chondrocalcinosis).

—*Chronic CPPD crystal deposition disease:* Chronic CPPD crystal deposition disease predominantly affects women as a chronic, progressive, often symmetric polyarthritis affecting the knees (most common) but also the wrists, metacarpophalangeal (especially second and third) joints, hips, spine, shoulder, elbows, and ankles. Some patients have episodic pseudogout. Patients typically have chronic pain, morning and inactivity stiffness, limitation of movement, and functional impairment. Symptoms may be restricted to a few joints. Affected joints reveal signs of OA with varying degrees of synovitis. Variations in compartmental knee involvement may cause valgus or varus deformities. Chronic CPPD crystal deposition disease differs from pseudogout in its chronicity, tendency to affect the metacarpophalangeal joints and spine, and the pattern of progressive OA with intermittent inflammation/synovitis.

—*Chondrocalcinosis:* Generally an incidental radiographic finding, chondrocalcinosis is usually seen in asymptomatic individuals, typically in the elderly.

Uncommon Findings: Severe synovitis in chronic CPPD crystal deposition disease may produce a pseudorheumatoid pattern. Charcot-like arthropathy of the knee has been ascribed to CPPD crystal deposition disease in some patients. Rarely, a predominantly axial pattern is seen, simulating AS. Tendinitis, tenosynovitis, bursitis, and tophaceous CPPD crystal deposition may occur.

Diagnostic Tests: Synovial fluid usually shows a mean leukocyte count of $20,000/mm^3$ with >90% neutrophils, and blood-tinged effusions may be seen. Compensated polarized light microscopy reveals rhomboidal or rod-like intracellular crystals with weakly positive birefringence. In pseudogout, joint fluid should always be sent for Gram and culture to exclude a septic process.

An increase in acute-phase reactants (ESR or CRP) can be seen along with an elevated leukocyte count, but these are not diagnostic. In chronic arthropathy, an elevated serum ferritin level and a mild anemia are not uncommon. Routine screening for metabolic causes of CPPD crystal deposition disease should be reserved for those with early-onset arthritis (age ≤55 years), florid polyarticular disease, or recurrent acute attacks out of proportion to the degree of chronic arthropathy. In such patients, the following screening tests are suggested: serum calcium, serum alkaline phosphatase, serum magnesium, and serum ferritin levels and tests of liver function.

Imaging: Calcification of articular fibrocartilage may be visible as punctate and linear densities, most frequently seen in the fibrocartilaginous menisci of the knee. Other sites of calcification include the articular discs of the distal radioulnar joint (triangular fibrocartilage), the symphysis pubis, the glenoid and acetabular labra, and the annulus fibrosus of the intervertebral discs. Calcification of hyaline cartilage occurs in the midzonal layer, appearing as a radiopaque line that runs parallel to the cortex of the underlying bone. Typically, the larger joints are involved. Degenerative arthropathy is similar to that observed in OA, with visible subchondral cysts, sclerosis, osteophytes, and joint space narrowing, all of which are often pronounced.

DISEASES

Keys to Diagnosis

—*Pseudogout:* The presence of an acute synovitis in one or a few joints, with radiographic chondrocalcinosis and/or synovial CPPD crystals strongly suggests pseudogout. Synovial fluid may be purulent, mandating exclusion of sepsis (which may coexist).

—*Chronic CPPD crystal deposition disease:* In most cases, a characteristic joint pattern, radiographic findings, and CPPD crystals in joint fluid easily establish a diagnosis. Polyarticular involvement with modestly elevated ESR and RF may cause confusion with RA. The infrequency of systemic features, lack of radiographic erosions, and periarticular osteopenia often permit differentiation from RA. Differentiation from OA is possible by involvement of metacarpophalangeal joints, radiographic findings, and the presence of superimposed acute attacks.

Diagnostic Criteria: See Table 7.

Differential Diagnosis: Pseudogout and CPPD crystal deposition disease may be misdiagnosed as gout, pseudogout, OA, septic arthritis, inflammatory OA, neuropathic arthritis, or hypertrophic osteoarthropathy.

Therapy

—*Pseudogout:* General principles of management include relief of symptoms, identification and treatment of triggering illnesses, and rapid mobilization. Although aspiration alone can relieve symptoms, intraarticular steroid in-

---

Table 7
Diagnostic Criteria for CPPD

  I. Demonstration of CPPD crystals by definitive means (x-ray diffraction, chemical analysis)
 II. A. Identification of CPPD crystals by compensated polarized light microscopy
    B. Presence of typical calcifications on roentgenograms
III. A. Acute arthritis, especially of the knees
    B. Chronic arthritis, especially of the knee, hip, wrist, carpus, MCPs, elbow, or shoulder; differentiated from OA by demonstrating the following features:
     1. Uncommon site for primary OA (MCP joints, wrist, elbow, shoulder)
     2. Radiographic appearance (isolated compartment narrowing in wrist, knee)
     3. Subchondral cyst formation
     4. Severe progressive degeneration (subchondral bony collapse, intraarticular radiodense bodies)
     5. Variable and inconstant osteophyte formation
     6. Tendon calcifications
     7. Involvement of the axial skeleton
Diagnosis
    Definite CPPD crystal deposition disease: criteria I or II.A and II.B
    Probable CPPD crystal deposition disease: criterion II.A or II.B
    Possible CPPD crystal deposition disease: criterion III.A or III.B

CPPD, calcium pyrophosphate crystal deposition disease; MCP, metacarpophalangeal; OA, osteoarthritis.

jection is appropriate, either concurrently with the first aspiration or after Gram staining and culture results are negative. Acetaminophen or NSAIDs can be of additional benefit. Colchicine (see p. 437) may be used as acute therapy for pseudogout but is rarely necessary. Colchicine may also be useful as prophylaxis in those with recurrent attacks of pseudogout. Systemic corticosteroids can be used if other treatments are contraindicated, although their efficacy remains untested in controlled trials.

—*Chronic CPPD crystal deposition disease:* No specific therapy exists for chronic CPPD crystal deposition disease, and treatment of any underlying metabolic abnormalities usually does not reverse joint damage. The aims of management are to relieve symptoms and improve function. Chronic NSAID or colchicine therapy may be effective. Troublesome individual joints can be managed with injection of intraarticular steroids. Joint arthroplasty may eventually be needed.

Prognosis: Although pseudogout usually responds well to therapy, chronic CPPD crystal deposition disease is often progressive and in some may lead to significant disability and deformity.

BIBLIOGRAPHY

Agudelo CA, Wise CM. Crystal-associated arthritis in the elderly. *Rheum Dis Clin North Am* 2000;26:527–546.

Doherty M. Calcium pyrophosphate dihydrate crystal-associated arthropathy. In: Hochberg MC, Silman AJ, Smolen JS, et al., eds. *Rheumatology*, 3rd ed. Edinburgh: Mosby, 2003:1937–1050.

CARCINOMA POLYARTHRITIS

Synonyms: Cancer polyarthritis.

ICD-9 Code: 716.59.

Definition: RA-like polyarthritis in the setting of underlying malignancy.

Etiology: Carcinoma polyarthritis may be secondary to antigenic cross-reactivity between synovium and tumor or be caused by altered cellular and humoral immune mechanisms.

Demographics: Carcinoma polyarthritis occurs most commonly with solid tumors; breast cancer accounts for approximately 80% of cases.

Cardinal Findings: Characteristic features include (1) close temporal relationship of explosive-onset arthritis with malignancy diagnosis (joint symptoms seldom precede malignancy by more than 10 months); (2) late age at onset for inflammatory arthritis; (3) asymmetric joint involvement, often affecting lower extremity joints, with relative sparing of wrists and small joint of hands; (4) absence of rheumatoid nodules and absent or low titer of serum RF. Carcinoma polyarthritis is occasionally mistaken for hypertrophic osteoarthropathy or AOSD (when associated with high fever).

Diagnostic Testing: ESR is often nonspecifically elevated, reflecting the tumor burden. As many as 20% of patients may have low-titer RF or ANA. Synovial biopsy specimens show only nonspecific synovitis. As in RA, bone erosions may develop.

Therapy: Therapy is aimed at alleviating the underlying cancer (tumor resection may improve arthritis). NSAIDs or corticosteroids may be necessary to control arthritis inflammation.

BIBLIOGRAPHY

Bennet RM, Ginsberg MH, Thomsen S. Carcinoma polyarthritis. The presenting symptom of an ovarian tumor and association with a platelet activating factor. *Arthritis Rheum* 1976;19:953–958.

CARPAL TUNNEL SYNDROME

Synonyms: CTS, median nerve entrapment syndrome.

ICD-9 Code: 354.0.

Definition: Entering the hand, the median nerve and the flexor tendons pass through the carpal tunnel within the wrist. The carpal tunnel is formed on the bottom by the volar surface of the carpal bones of the wrist and on top by the transverse carpal ligament (flexor retinaculum), which encloses the tunnel (Fig. 1). CTS is a constellation of symptoms that result from the compression of structures within this restricted space. In most cases, symptoms result from compression of the median nerve, which innervates the thenar muscles, the lumbricales on the radial side of the hand, and the skin overlying the radial side of the palm and the first, second, third, and radial side of the fourth digits.

Risk Factors: A number of conditions may be associated with development of this condition (Table 8). Among the most important may be overuse or repetitive stress injury, although this is somewhat controversial. Nevertheless, in some series, more than half of the patients evaluated were considered to have CTS of occupational origin. It has been estimated that one in 10 office workers may develop CTS (presumably from computer overuse).

Demographics: CTS is the most common entrapment neuropathy, with a prevalence of approximately 250 to 500 cases per 100,000 population. It may affect as many as two million Americans every year.

Cardinal Findings: Early in CTS, patients may complain only of paresthesia or numbness of the fingers or hand rather than frank pain. These symptoms may be

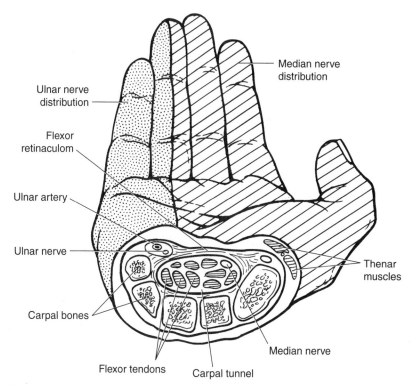

Figure 1. Anatomic cross section of the carpal tunnel. Median nerve (*hatched area*) and ulnar nerve *(stippled area)* innervation is shown.

Table 8
Causes of Carpal Tunnel Syndrome

Repetitive motion injury[a]
Pregnancy[b]
Rheumatoid arthritis[b]
Hypothyroidism[b]
Diabetes mellitus[b]
Amyloidosis (e.g., with multiple myeloma)
Acromegaly
Infectious diseases (e.g., mycobacteria, fungi)
Ganglion cysts
Carpal bone osteophytes
Trauma
Idiopathic

[a]Accounts for >50% of cases.
[b]These conditions, in combination, account for nearly 25% of cases.

accentuated at night and may be relieved by shaking the hand. Symptoms are more common in the dominant hand but may be bilateral. As the condition progresses, patients may report more severe pain in the distribution of the median nerve that may be exacerbated by particular movements. Some patients may relate sensations of pain or numbness in areas that anatomically should not be affected (e.g., proximal to the wrist). As CTS becomes more chronic, frank muscle weakness, muscle atrophy (e.g., thenar muscle atrophy), and hypesthesia may develop. Tinel's sign or Phalen's sign is sometimes used to aid in the diagnosis of CTS (see p. 13). Tinel's sign is positive if repetitive tapping over the flexor retinaculum and medial nerve at the wrist (with the hand in slight dorsiflexion) elicits numbness, dysesthesia, or electric-like sensations in the first 3-1/2 fingers. The Phalen test is positive if symptoms are elicited when the patient holds the dorsal surfaces (or backs) of the hands against each other with the wrists in forced flexion. Unfortunately, in several large research series, the sensitivity and specificity of these tests for diagnosing CTS were nearly 50%. Thus, a positive or negative result must be interpreted within the context of the clinical suspicion.

Diagnostic Tests: Because the pathophysiology relates to entrapment and impaired function of the median nerve, electrodiagnostic tests may be considered the gold standard for diagnosis of this disorder. Thus, nerve conduction velocity testing would be expected to reveal findings such as prolonged distal nerve latency conduction times. In experienced hands, these tests may have a sensitivity of 90% and a specificity of 60%. The findings present on nerve conduction velocity vary with the extent of involvement and may progress over time. Laboratory studies may aid in the diagnosis of associated conditions (Table 8), and tests should be chosen based on clinical presentation. Imaging studies are of little value in evaluating CTS.

Keys to Diagnosis: CTS should be strongly considered in any individual who presents with numbness or pain in the hand. Because it is so prevalent, many patients may be expected to have atypical presentations. A clinical history of pain or numbness affecting the hand in the distribution of the median nerve and pain or weakness of the thenar muscles (e.g., in flexing or opposing the thumb) should arouse clinical suspicion of CTS. Patients demonstrating classic symptoms and signs need not undergo further electrodiagnostic testing.

Differential Diagnosis: A variety of less common conditions may present with wrist or hand pain and be confused with CTS. Early, mild synovitis of the wrist, for example, with RA or crystalline arthritis, may mimic CTS. Likewise, ganglion cysts of the volar aspect of the wrist or bony osteophytes of the carpal bones may cause wrist pain. As noted above, all these conditions may also be associated with true CTS, which may make a determination of the exact cause of pain more difficult. Entrapment of the median nerve at another location or cervical radiculopathy may mimic CTS, but these are uncommon. Patients with ulnar or radial nerve entrapment may also report similar complaints. Ulnar nerve entrapment may produce pain, numbness, or clumsiness of the fourth and fifth fingers, hypothenar atrophy, or "clawing" of fourth and fifth digits. Radial nerve palsy may result in wrist drop, with flexion of the metacarpophalangeal joints and numbness of the thumb, index, and middle fingers.

Therapy: Treatment of CTS begins with avoiding overuse and splinting the wrist and hand in a neutral position (in slight extension). Nighttime splinting of the affected wrist(s) may suffice. Most physicians add an NSAID if there are no contraindications and wrist inflammation or arthritis exists. For those unresponsive to conservative maneuvers, local injection with a corticosteroid may be used. Although steroid injections are often successful in the short term, many patients have recurrent symptoms.

A large number of cases arise from repetitive overuse at the workplace. Thus, correct ergonomics may be important in preventing CTS. For example, it is recommended that those who type at computer terminals for long periods of time sit with the back straight, feet flat on the floor, forearms parallel to the floor, and wrists "floating" (i.e., not resting continually on anything). In addition, it is important to take breaks every so often to stretch and rest the arms and hands.

Surgery: Surgical decompression of the carpal tunnel may be indicated when conservative measures fail or when there is evidence of persistent sensory loss or thenar atrophy. Surgical release of the transverse carpal ligament may relieve the compression on the nerve. Symptoms may recur after surgery. Although carpal tunnel release is usually an outpatient, open surgical procedure, newer techniques are being evaluated (e.g., arthroscopic decompression, balloon dilatation of the carpal tunnel, and laser stimulation of the affected nerve). The comparative efficacy and risks of these newer techniques remain to be determined.

BIBLIOGRAPHY

Dawson DM. Entrapment neuropathies of the upper extremities. *N Engl J Med* 1993;329:2013–2018.

Golding RN, Rose DM, Selvarajah L. Clinical tests for carpal tunnel syndrome—an evaluation. *Br J Rheumatol* 1986;25:388–390.

Slater RR, Bynum DK. Diagnosis and treatment of carpal tunnel syndrome. *Orthop Rev* 1993;22:1095–1105.

CENTRAL NERVOUS SYSTEM ANGIITIS

Synonyms: Primary CNS angiitis, isolated CNS angiitis, granulomatous angiitis of CNS.

ICD-9 Code: 437.4 (vasculitis).

Definition: The term *CNS angiitis* encompasses a variety of inflammatory conditions that result in decreased blood flow in cerebral vessels (Table 9). Neuro-

Table 9
Conditions Associated With or Resembling CNS Angiitis

Primary CNS angiitis
  Biopsy proven
  Angiographically proven
Secondary CNS angiitis
  Systemic vasculitides: giant cell arteritis, Takayasu's arteritis, Wegener's granulomato-
    sis, polyarteritis nodosa, Churg-Strauss angiitis, Behçet's syndrome
  Inflammatory disorders: rheumatoid arthritis, SLE, Sjögren syndrome, sarcoidosis
  Infections: tuberculosis, fungi (coccidioidomycoses, actinomycoses, cryptococcus),
    spirochetal disease (syphilis, Lyme disease), viruses (HIV, CMV, herpes)
  Drug induced: cocaine, amphetamines, sympathomimetics (ephedrine, phenyl-
    propanolamine), thiazides
Vasculopathic conditions
  Antiphospholipid syndrome
  Atherosclerotic disease
  Hypertension
  Thrombotic thrombocytopenia purpura
  Persistent or recurrent vasospasm
  CNS lymphoma
  Moyamoya disease

CNS, central nervous system; SLE, systemic lupus erythematosus; HIV, human immunodeficiency virus;
CMV, cytomegalovirus.

logic defects may be focal or diffuse, depending on the location and extent of the lesions. Primary CNS angiitis is an idiopathic inflammatory disorder with characteristic clinical, angiographic, or histologic findings of vasculitis limited to the CNS.

Pathology: Primary CNS angiitis may demonstrate granulomatous or non-granulomatous vasculitis affecting the leptomeningeal and cortical small- and medium-sized vessels.

Demographics: This rare disorder is commonly seen in adults aged 20 to 60 years.

Cardinal Findings: Symptoms of primary CNS angiitis may include headache, confusion, neurocognitive dysfunction, cranial neuropathy, seizures, and focal motor or sensory defects. Physical examination may reveal fever, hypertension, focal neurologic deficits, papilledema, and funduscopic abnormalities. Other systemic features, such as arthralgias or myalgias, are uncommon. Nearly 10% of patients exhibit a myelopathy.

Diagnostic Testing: In patients suspected of having CNS angiitis, routine laboratory test results are frequently normal. Nonspecific findings may include an elevated ESR or leukocytosis. Serologies (ANA, RF, ANCA) should be normal. CSF analysis may reveal several abnormalities, including increased CSF protein, lymphocytic pleocytosis, and increased CSF immunoglobulins (see CSF studies, p. 55). The CSF results may also be normal and be of greatest value in excluding other causes.

The role of leptomeningeal biopsy is controversial. Although pathognomonic, granulomatous or nongranulomatous vasculitis with mononuclear infiltrates is found in <50% of patients. Sensitivity is increased by using biopsy specimens from both brain tissue and leptomeninges or by taking tissue samples from areas abnormal on MRI. However, the procedure may yield false-negative results in >25% of cases. Biopsy is particularly helpful in establishing or excluding other diagnoses such as lymphoma and sarcoidosis.

Imaging: CNS imaging results are often abnormal. However, they may not allow precise determination of the cause. CT scans may show infarcts or be entirely normal. It may be most useful in helping to rule out other conditions, such as subarachnoid hemorrhage or tumor. As many as 15% of patients have mass lesions on CT scans or MRI. MRI frequently reveals abnormal signals in the areas of affected vessels. MRI is most effective in identifying myelopathy owing to vasculitis.

Angiography characteristically shows diffuse vascular "beading" with areas of alternating stenosis and dilatation. Although these changes are consistent with vasculitis, they are not diagnostic; they may also be seen in noninflammatory vasculopathies.

Keys to Diagnosis: Primary CNS angiitis should be suspected in young to middle-aged individuals presenting with headache, focal neurologic findings, normal or slightly abnormal CSF results, and angiographic evidence of intracerebral vasculitis. Medications, infections, or associated inflammatory and noninflammatory vascular disorders must be considered and excluded.

Differential Diagnosis: See Table 9.

Therapy: Aggressive immunomodulatory therapy is indicated for proven primary CNS angiitis. Usual recommendations include high-dose prednisone in conjunction with cytotoxic drugs such as cyclophosphamide for a period of 6 to 12 months.

Prognosis: The prognosis of CNS angiitis can be variable. Primary CNS angiitis may be fatal if untreated. However, early diagnosis and aggressive treatment have led to more favorable outcomes, although some may be left with fixed neurologic deficits.

BIBLIOGRAPHY

Calabrese LH, Duna GF, Lie JT. Vasculitis in the central nervous system. *Arthritis Rheum* 1997;40:1189–1201.

Cohen SB, Hurd ER. Neurological complications of connective tissue and other "collagen-vascular" diseases. *Semin Arthritis Rheum* 1981;11:190–212.

West SG. Central nervous system vasculitis. *Curr Rheumatol Rep* 2003;5:116–127.

DISEASES

CHOLESTEROL EMBOLI SYNDROME

Synonyms: Multiple cholesterol emboli syndrome, pseudovasculitis.

ICD-9 Code: 445.0; affecting the kidney, 593.83.

Definition: Cholesterol emboli syndrome is an uncommon complication of atherosclerosis with obstruction of small arteries and arterioles by cholesterol crystals. Symptoms are caused by embolization from ulcerated or denuded large vessel plaques and may mimic systemic necrotizing vasculitis.

Demographics: Cholesterol emboli syndrome occurs in adults (>50 years of age) with advanced atherosclerotic vascular disease, frequently after angiographic or other invasive vascular procedures. It may also follow anticoagulation or thrombolytic therapy. The lower aorta is the most common source of emboli.

Cardinal Findings: Skin and renal manifestations predominate. Skin manifestations include livedo reticularis, "blue toes," splinter hemorrhages, ulcerations, purpura/petechiae of the lower extremities, or gangrene. Renal impairment may initially be subacute but can progress over weeks to months to severe renal insufficiency. As many as 40% of patients may require dialysis. Less common clinical features include ischemia of the gut leading to perforation or hemorrhage and CNS involvement manifest as amaurosis fugax or stroke. Constitutional symptoms such as fever, weight loss, myalgias, and fatigue are occasionally seen and add to the difficulty in differentiating this entity from systemic necrotizing vasculitis.

Diagnostic Testing: Laboratory test findings are nonspecific and include elevated acute-phase reactants (ESR and CRP) and eosinophilia. Urine may reveal granular or hyaline casts, proteinuria, and eosinophiluria. Skin, muscle, or, less commonly, renal biopsy specimens show pathognomonic findings of cholesterol clefts in the lumina of small vessels. Arteritis varies from a mild inflammatory response to obliterative endarteritis. Diagnosis is made premortem in only 30% to 40% of cases.

Therapy: Anticoagulation is contraindicated and, if already initiated, should likely be discontinued. It may be helpful to locate and resect the source of emboli. A role of steroid therapy has not been established. Treatment is largely supportive. Mortality may be as high as 60% to 90% because of renal involvement and frequent comorbidities.

BIBLIOGRAPHY

Hauben M, Norwich J, Shapiro E, et al. Multiple cholesterol emboli syndrome—six cases identified through the spontaneous reporting system. *Angiology* 1995;46:779–784.
Scolari F, Tardanico R, Zani R, et al. Cholesterol crystal embolism: a recognizable cause of renal disease. *Am J Kidney Dis* 2000;36:1089–1109.

CHURG-STRAUSS ANGIITIS

Synonyms: Allergic angiitis and granulomatosis

ICD9 Code: 446.2.

Definition: Churg-Strauss angiitis is granulomatous vasculitis of small and medium-sized vessels associated with pulmonary disease and hypereosinophilia.

Etiology: This systemic vasculitis is of uncertain etiology.

Pathology: Churg-Strauss angiitis is necrotizing vasculitis with prominent eosinophilic tissue infiltrates and granulomas involving both medium and small arteries, capillaries, and venules.

Demographics: This very rare disorder is more prevalent in middle-aged men with antecedent asthma and rhinitis.

Cardinal Findings: Asthmatic manifestations with fluctuating pulmonary infiltrates (resembling Loeffler's syndrome), chronic eosinophilic pneumonia, and eosinophilic gastroenteritis may antedate frank vasculitis. Vasculitis may present with worsening respiratory status accompanied by systemic manifestations similar to those of polyarteritis nodosa (PAN). These include severe constitutional symptoms, arthralgias, mononeuritis multiplex, and occasional cardiac or gastrointestinal symptoms. Lung and skin findings are more common in Churg-Strauss angiitis than in PAN.

Uncommon Findings: In contrast to PAN, glomerulonephritis is not usually seen, and renal disease is present in only 40% of patients. In contrast to Wegener's granulomatosis, in Churg-Strauss angiitis the pulmonary lesions seldom cavitate, and the upper airway disease is less destructive.

Diagnostic Testing: Nonspecific measures of systemic inflammation include elevated acute-phase reactants (ESR and/or CRP), leukocytosis, anemia of chronic inflammation, and thrombocytosis. Peripheral blood eosinophilia and elevated IgE levels are often present. Circulating immune complexes, hypocomplementemia, and hyperglobulinemia have been observed but do not aid in the differential diagnosis. P-ANCA is occasionally present. A diagnosis is strongly supported by histopathologic evidence of small and medium vessel angiitis with eosinophils.

Keys to Diagnosis: The presentation is similar to that of PAN but with concomitant pulmonary involvement and a strong allergic component.

Diagnostic Criteria: 1990 ACR criteria include (a) asthma; (b) eosinophilia (>10% on WBC differential); (c) mononeuropathy or polyneuropathy; (d) migratory or transient pulmonary infiltrates; (e) paranasal sinus abnormalities; and (f) extravascular eosinophils on biopsy of a blood vessel. The presence of 4 or more of these 6 criteria constitutes a diagnosis for the purposes of classification (85% sensitivity; 99.7% specificity). A history of allergy is a criterion in other classification systems.

Therapy: High-dose corticosteroids are used ($\geq$1 mg/kg prednisone, occasionally started using a 1-g bolus of methylprednisolone). Cytotoxic therapy with cyclophosphamide or less commonly azathioprine is often used initially or added later as a steroid-sparing agent.

Prognosis: Survival is slightly better than in polyarteritis nodosa, with up to 90% of patients alive 1 year after the diagnosis.

BIBLIOGRAPHY

Gay RM, Ball GV. Vasculitis. In: Koopman WJ, ed. *Arthritis and allied conditions: a textbook of rheumatology.* 13th ed. Baltimore: Williams & Wilkins, 1997:1500–1501.
Lhote F, Guillevin L. Polyarteritis nodosa, microscopic polyangiitis and Churg Strauss syndrome: clinical aspects and treatment. *Rheum Dis Clin North Am* 1995;21:911–948.
Masi AT, Hunder GG, Lie JT, et al. The American College of Rheumatology 1990 criteria for the classification of Churg-Strauss syndrome (allergic granulomatosis and angiitis). *Arthritis Rheum* 1990;33:1094–1100.

CREST SYNDROME

Synonyms: Limited scleroderma (diffuse scleroderma is discussed on p. 344).

ICD9 Code: 710.1

Definition: "CREST syndrome" is more appropriately referred to as "limited scleroderma." In this variant of systemic sclerosis, skin thickening (sclerodactyly) is found distal to the elbow or knee and rarely affects the face or neck. The CREST constellation of findings includes: *C*alcinosis, *R*aynaud's phenomenon, *E*sophageal dysmotility, *S*clerodactyly, and *T*elangiectasias. Calcinosis is the least common of these findings. Table 10 compares features of limited and diffuse scleroderma.

Etiology: Unknown (see etiology of scleroderma p. 344)

Demographics: Both diffuse and limited forms of scleroderma affect females more than males, with a female:male ratio of 3:1. The limited variant of scleroderma is more prevalent than the diffuse form, which is quite rare. Although Raynaud's phenomenon is quite common and affects up to 10% of female nonsmokers, only a small minority of Raynaud's patients develop limited or diffuse scleroderma.

Cardinal Findings: Virtually all patients manifest sclerodactyly and Raynaud's phenomenon (see p. 312). This should prompt a search for esophageal

Table 10
Comparison of Limited and Diffuse Systemic Sclerosis

Feature	Limited[a]	Diffuse[a]
Sclerodactyly	+++++	+++++
Raynaud's phenomenon	+++++	+++++
Telangiectasias	++++	+++
Dysphagia	++++	++++
Calcinosis	++	+
Arthralgia/arthritis	++	++++
Pulmonary fibrosis	+	++
Pulmonary hypertension	+	0
Tendon friction rubs	0	+++
Renal crisis	0	+
Anticentromere Ab[b]	+++	+/0
Anti-Scl-70 Ab	+	++

[a]Relative percentages: +++++ 81–100%; ++++ 61–80%; +++ 41–60%; ++ 21–40%; + 1–20%.
[b]Ab, antibody.

dysmotility or cutaneous telangiectasias, often found over the lips, tongue, hands, and face. Tight skin is usually most prominent in the fingers and toes and is less common over the hand or wrist. If severe, skin thickening may lead to problematic ischemic/traumatic ulcerations over the distal fingertips or DIP or PIP joints. Tendon friction rubs are rarely seen in limited scleroderma. Esophageal dysmotility manifests as food "sticking" substernally at the lower esophageal sphincter. Subcutaneous calcinosis is found in 30% to 40% of patients. Calcific deposits are usually "hard"; are located over the fingers, forearms, or lower extremities; and may be painful, intermittently inflamed, or ulcerate.

Uncommon Findings: Small bowel disease is infrequently encountered in those with longstanding CREST syndrome and may manifest as bloating, cramping, diarrhea, or malabsorption. Interstitial lung fibrosis is much more common in diffuse scleroderma but has been described in the limited form. Those with longstanding CREST syndrome are at greatest risk for developing progressive pulmonary hypertension, usually late in the disease.

Diagnostic Testing: The vast majority of patients are ANA positive. Anticentromere antibodies are found in more than 50% of patients with limited scleroderma but only 10% of those with diffuse disease. Anticentromere antibodies may also be found in patients with primary biliary cirrhosis. A minority of CREST patients have anti-RNP antibodies. Pulmonary function test (PFT) results are abnormal in two-thirds of patients, with a reduced forced vital capacity or DLCO. Nailfold capillaroscopy (see p. 88) is usually abnormal.

Imaging: Chest radiography (CXR) is indicated in those with pulmonary symptoms. Up to one-third of patients may show evidence of pulmonary fibrosis. High-resolution computerized tomography may be used to resolve discrepancies between symptoms and PFTs or CXR.

Differential Diagnosis: CREST should be distinguished from diffuse scleroderma, eosinophilic fasciitis, overlap syndrome, drug-induced sclerodactyly, PBC, and other causes of pseudosclerodactyly (e.g., diabetes, hypothyroidism).

Therapy: Treatment of limited scleroderma is primarily directed at symptomatic relief of joint pain, Raynaud's phenomenon, and esophageal reflux and dysmotility (see "Scleroderma, Therapy," p. 347). Smoking cessation, hand warming (mittens, hand warmers, etc.), and care of the distal extremities should be emphasized. There is no proven role for penicillamine or other disease-modifying therapies in limited scleroderma. Cutaneous ulcerations may pose a therapeutic challenge. Treatment should hinge on warm soaks, vasodilator and antiplatelet agents, and treatment of superinfection.

BIBLIOGRAPHY

Furst DE, Clements PJ, Saab M, et al. Clinical and serological comparison of 17 chronic progressive systemic sclerosis (PSS) and 17 CREST syndrome patients matched for sex, age, and disease duration. *Ann Rheum Dis* 1984;43:794–801.
Mitchell H, Bolster MB, LeRoy EC. Scleroderma and related conditions. *Med Clin North Am.* 1997;81:129–149.

CRYOGLOBULINEMIA

ICD9 Code: 273.2

Definition: These clinical syndromes are associated with the presence of cold-precipitable immunoglobulins (i.e., cryoglobulins).

Etiology: Cryoglobulins are produced by activated B cells, which may be oligoclonal or monoclonal. Some cases are associated with lymphoid malignancies, chronic immune-system disorders (e.g., RA or Sjögren's syndrome), or infection (e.g., hepatitis, infective endocarditis). Cryoglobulins are classified as type I (monoclonal), type II (mixed monoclonal and polyclonal), or type III (mixed polyclonal). Disease association with each type is discussed under "Cryoglobulins" (p. 62).

Pathology: Skin lesions often show leukocytoclastic vasculitis. Renal involvement is usually associated with a proliferative glomerulonephritis. Characteristic protein deposits in subendothelial regions are seen on electron microscopy. Serum samples contain reversibly precipitable immunoglobulins which may be monoclonal, polyclonal, or mixed. Hepatitis C or B antigenemia may be present.

Demographics: Most patients are in the fifth decade or older. Associations with an underlying disease, such as RA, follow the gender distribution characteristic of that disorder.

Cardinal Findings: Palpable purpura may be present on the lower extremities and rarely extends above the waist. Proteinuria may be present and in some cases can be accompanied by significant edema. Peripheral neuropathy with symptoms of pain, dysesthesia, or motor abnormalities may be the predominant finding in some patients. Cryoglobulinemia may present as a multisystem disorder with fever, cutaneous vasculitis, arthralgia, hepatosplenomegaly, lymphadenopathy, and glomerulonephritis.

Uncommon Manifestations: Raynaud's phenomenon and hyperviscosity syndrome are uncommon manifestations of cryoglobulinemia.

Diagnostic Tests: Serum collection, processing, and characterization of cryoglobulins must be carried out using proper procedure (see p. 62). Complement levels should be measured. Some cryoglobulins may demonstrate rheumatoid factor activity and should be tested for it. Hepatic enzyme elevations may be related to liver involvement or underlying hepatitis C or B infection, which should be assayed. Peripheral neuropathy or mononeuritis can be confirmed by nerve conduction tests. In some cases, biopsy of a nerve that is abnormal on EMG testing is useful. Skin biopsy evidence of leukocytoclastic vasculitis supports the diagnosis of cryoglobulinemia.

Keys to Diagnosis: Palpable purpura in a dependent distribution is most suggestive of cryoglobulinemia. A systemic disorder with involvement of the skin, kidney, peripheral nerves, and liver should suggest the possibility of cryoglobulinemia.

Differential Diagnosis: Conditions that may mimic cryoglobulinemia include vasculitis (e.g., polyarteritis nodosa, Henoch-Schönlein purpura), SLE, and lymphoma. Henoch-Schönlein purpura is more likely to be seen in young adults or children. Isolated renal involvement may occur with cryoglobulinemia and often requires renal biopsy for definitive diagnosis and exclusion of other forms of glomerulonephritis.

Therapy: If an underlying disorder is identified, therapy should be aimed at that process. Hepatitis C may be treated with IFN-α/ribavirin. Acute complications of the cryoglobulins themselves, such as rapidly progressive renal failure or symptoms associated with hyperviscosity, should be treated with a course of intensive plasmapheresis. Cyclophosphamide and steroids are used to treat patients with renal or nervous system involvement.

Surgery: Surgery is only used for diagnostic biopsy such as kidney or nerve.

Prognosis: In the absence of renal or neurologic involvement, many patients remain stable for years. Rapidly progressive glomerulonephritis is associated

DISEASES

with a poorer prognosis. All patients should be monitored for transformation to neoplastic disease.

BIBLIOGRAPHY

Abel G, Zhang QX, Agnello V. Hepatitis C virus infection in type II mixed cryoglobulinemia. *Arthritis Rheum* 1993;36:1341–1349.
Anaya JM, Talal N. Sjogren's syndrome and connective tissue diseases associated with other immunologic disorders. In: Koopman WJ, ed. *Arthritis and allied conditions: a textbook of rheumatology.* 13th ed. Baltimore: Williams & Wilkins, 1997:1561–1580.
Brouet JC, Clauvel JP, Danon F, et al. Biologic and clinical significance of cryoglobulins: a report of 86 cases. *Am J Med* 1974;57:775–788.

DEQUERVAIN'S TENOSYNOVITIS

Synonyms: deQuervain's disease, stenosing tenosynovitis

ICD9 Codes: 727.04

Definition: deQuervain's tenosynovitis represents inflammation of the tendon sheath surrounding the abductor pollicis longus and extensor pollicis brevis muscles (see p. 195). It generally develops after overuse of the involved muscles (e.g., repetitive grasping with the thumb against resistance).

Demographics: Commonly affects women more than men. It is one of the most common forms of occupational overuse syndrome. It is also common during pregnancy, postpartum, and in other instances where no history of overuse can be elicited.

Cardinal Findings: Patients typically present with pain and tenderness in the area about the radial styloid that is worsened with movement. Uncommonly, local swelling of the involved tendons is seen. The diagnosis may be confirmed with the Finkelstein test (see p. 13), in which pain is elicited by stretching the involved tendons. To perform this test, the patient places the thumb inside a clenched fist and then moves or deviates the fist downward toward the ulnar side. Pain elicited with this maneuver suggests deQuervain's tenosynovitis.

Therapy: Treatment is guided by severity and may include splinting (to protect against further overuse), administration of topical analgesia (e.g., ice), NSAIDs, or local injection of corticosteroids (see p. 438). Surgery is rarely indicated.

BIBLIOGRAPHY

Moore JS. deQuervain's tenosynovitis. Stenosing tenosynovitis of the first dorsal compartment. *J Occup Environ Med* 1997;39:990–1002.
Schumacher HR Jr, Dorwart BB, Korzeniavski OM. Occurrence of deQuervain's tendinitis during pregnancy. *Arch Intern Med* 1985;145:2083–2084.

DIABETES MELLITUS: MUSCULOSKELETAL MANIFESTATIONS

Synonyms: Cheiroarthropathy, neuropathic joints, Charcot joints, diabetic amyotrophy, syndrome of limited joint mobility.

ICD-9 Codes: Diabetic neuropathic arthropathy, 250.6; diabetic complication NEC, 250.9; diabetic amyotrophy, 250.6 (358.1); arthropathy associated with endocrine disorder, 713.0.

Definition: These are symptomatic abnormalities of skin, bones, joints, and tendons that may be associated with, or result from, type 1 or 2 diabetes mellitus.

Etiology: Some abnormalities result from diabetes-induced nerve and blood vessel damage; others are caused by excess collagen accumulation in periarticular structures and skin, which occurs with aging but is accelerated in diabetics. Others have hypothesized that nonenzymatic glycosylation of proteins leads to accumulation of advanced glycosylation end products that may contribute to the pathology.

Pathology: Skin and tendons show excessive fibrosis owing to collagen accumulation. Muscle biopsy specimens may show type 2 fiber atrophy without significant inflammatory infiltrate.

Demographics: Musculoskeletal manifestations are most common in patients with longstanding type 1 diabetes but may also occur in some patients with type 2 diabetes.

Disease Associations: Associations between diabetes mellitus and gout, CTS, osteoporosis, or hyperostosis (DISH) have been suggested but are not well established.

Clinical Findings: The most common musculoskeletal conditions seen in diabetics include
—*Pseudosclerodactyly:* Thickened, waxy skin changes are most apparent in the fingers.
—*Syndrome of limited joint mobility* (cheiroarthropathy or diabetic contractures): The fingers are commonly affected, with stiffness, limited movement and contractures. Flexion contractures of the proximal and distal interphalangeal joints results in the "prayer sign," an inability to close the gap between opposed palms and fingers. It is associated with advanced disease and diabetic microvascular disease elsewhere.
—*Periarthritis:* Adhesive capsulitis of the shoulder is commonly seen in patients with type 1 older than 40 years of age. Patients complain of shoulder pain (especially at night) and difficulty raising their arms. Joint examination reveals limited range of motion (especially abduction).

—*Dupuytren contractures* (see p. 163) and trigger fingers are relatively common.

—*Neuropathic (Charcot) arthropathy* (see p. 255) commonly affects the tarsal and metatarsal joints with painless bony hypertrophy. Diagnosis is made by radiography.

—*Diabetic neuropathy* may cause pain and dysfunction in the extremities and may also lead to symptomatic muscle weakness.

—*Diabetic amyotrophy* is an asymmetric ischemic myopathy that results in weakness and pain. Diabetic amyotrophy is typically seen in adults over 50 years of age and should be considered with pain, limb girdle muscle atrophy, and fasciculation. Prominent involvement of the iliopsoas, quadriceps, and adductor thigh muscles causes difficulty standing, rising from a seated position, or climbing stairs. The diagnosis may be made by MRI or muscle biopsy.

Uncommon Findings: There are reports of acanthosis nigricans and severe insulin resistance owing to circulating antireceptor antibodies in patients with SLE and scleroderma.

Diagnostic Tests: Muscle biopsy or EMG may be required to confirm tissue involvement. Diagnosis of these manifestations does not depend upon the presence of hyperglycemia or an elevated hemoglobin-A1c.

Keys to Diagnosis: The onset of musculoskeletal symptoms in patients with established type 1 or 2 diabetes mellitus should lead to consideration of one of the above entities.

Differential Diagnosis: Skin changes (pseudosclerodactyly) in diabetics resemble those seen in scleroderma, but abnormalities on nailfold capillaroscopy are absent. Muscle weakness may suggest inflammatory myopathy, but the diabetic form is more likely to be asymmetric. The presence of neuropathic joints and neurologic changes in the extremities may resemble changes seen with syphilis.

Therapy: Some musculoskeletal manifestations may be slowed by improved glycemic control. Physical therapy may be helpful in managing or improving the range of motion in affected shoulders or fingers. Tendinitis is managed symptomatically with NSAIDs and physical therapy, but local application of heat is relatively contraindicated because of safety concerns. Neuropathic joints are treated primarily with rest and local measures to prevent infections.

Prognosis: Some manifestations show improvement or stabilization with improved glycemic control, and radiculopathy or weakness may spontaneously remit. Other problems, notably skin or tendon thickening and neuropathic joint abnormalities, are not likely to improve with glycemic control and may cause permanent dysfunction.

BIBLIOGRAPHY

Crispin JC, Alcocer-Varela J. Rheumatologic manifestations of diabetes mellitus. *Am J Med* 2003;114:753–757.

Pastan RS, Cohen AS. The rheumatologic manifestations of diabetes mellitus. *Med Clin North Am* 1978;62:829–839.

Tsokos GC, Gordon P, Antonovych T, et al. Lupus nephritis and other autoimmune features in patients with diabetes mellitus due to autoantibody to insulin receptors. *Ann Intern Med* 1985;102:176–181.

DIALYSIS: MUSCULOSKELETAL MANIFESTATIONS

Synonym: Hemodialysis-related arthropathy.

ICD-9 Code: Amyloid arthropathy, 713.7.

Definition: These are syndromes related to muscles and joint structures seen in patients undergoing long-term renal dialysis.

Etiology: The cause of most hemodialysis-associated syndromes is unknown. Secondary hyperparathyroidism can lead to development of bone abnormalities. β_2-Microglobulin amyloidosis and crystal deposition arthritis result from abnormalities of renal clearance.

Pathology: Arthritic syndromes associated with dialysis show erosive bone changes in <25%. Most synovial fluids are noninflammatory, except those associated with crystals. β_2-Microglobulin deposits are observed in bone cysts and soft tissues such as those within the carpal tunnel.

Cardinal Findings: Arthralgias are common. A minority of patients show erosive changes in small joints of the hands. Amyloid deposition most commonly presents as CTS or characteristic bone cysts seen on radiographs.

Uncommon Findings: Myelopathy with paresis caused by amyloid deposition has been reported.

Diagnostic Tests: Biopsies of affected tissues are required to establish a diagnosis of amyloidosis. Radiographs of affected joints show bone cysts, erosions, or subperiosteal resorption of bone. Synovial fluid analyses are required to evaluate crystal deposition diseases.

Keys to Diagnosis: Persistent symptoms referable to joints or periarticular tissues in the setting of hemodialysis should prompt further investigation.

Differential Diagnosis: Hyperparathyroidism, idiopathic CTS (not related to amyloid deposition), and other metabolic disorders should be considered.

Therapy: Amyloid deposition in some patients may be slowed by changing the membrane used for dialysis. Symptomatic CTS may require surgical intervention. Nonspecific arthralgias and other joint complaints may be treated symptomatically, with use of analgesics dictated by the underlying medical condition and the drugs mode of clearance or half-life. Treatment of crystal arthritis may also be limited by the underlying condition.

Prognosis: Patients with amyloid are difficult to treat and have a more limited prognosis than those with other dialysis-related syndromes, which probably do not significantly alter the patient's course.

BIBLIOGRAPHY

Menerey K, Braunstein E, Brown M, et al. Musculoskeletal symptoms related to arthropathy in patients receiving dialysis. *J Rheumatol* 1988;15:1848–1854.

DIFFUSE IDIOPATHIC SKELETAL HYPEROSTOSIS (DISH)

Synonyms: Forestier disease, ankylosing hyperostosis.

ICD-9 Code: 721.6.

Definition: DISH is not an arthropathy, but rather a bone-forming diathesis primarily affecting the spine, with ossification of tendons and ligaments. Diagnosis is often incidentally found on chest radiography.

Etiology: The etiology of DISH is unknown.

Demographics: This common disorder occurs in 12% of those older than age 65 years. Men are more commonly affected than women by a ratio of 2:1.

Associated Disorders: DISH is associated with CPPD crystal deposition disease, gout, RA, and OA, but not AS. DISH may be associated with diabetes mellitus, obesity, hyperlipidemia, or hyperuricemia.

Cardinal Findings: Patients are usually asymptomatic but may complain of thoracolumbar or neck stiffness. Large osteophytes of the cervical spine may cause dysphagia in as many as 25% of patients. Enthesopathy is common. Large osteophytes elsewhere may cause recurrent Achilles tendinitis or tennis elbow.

Complications: Excessive heterotopic bone formation may complicate hip surgery. Relatively minor trauma may result in fractures through ankylosed segments with subsequent neurologic impairment. Rarely, ossification of the posterior longitudinal ligament may result in myelopathy.

Diagnostic Tests: Test results are normal for age (e.g., ESR). No association with HLA-B27 is seen in most studies.

Diagnostic Criteria: Resnick has proposed the following. All three criteria are required.
1. Flowing spinal calcification involving ≥4 contiguous vertebrae
2. Preservation of disc height and lack of degenerative disc disease
3. Absence of apophyseal and sacroiliac joint ankylosis or erosions

Imaging: Radiographic findings are diagnostic in DISH and include spinal and extraspinal findings.

—*Spinal findings:* There is normal bone mineralization. Anterolateral ossification of the anterior longitudinal ligament (and surrounding soft tissues) of the spine results in flowing, bridging, often bulky osteophytes that involve at least four contiguous vertebrae. Disc spaces are preserved. Involvement of the thoracic (nearly 100%), lumbar (>90%), and cervical spine (75%) is common.

—*Extraspinal findings:* Pelvic films are frequently abnormal with "whiskering" of the iliac crests, ossification of the symphysis pubis, or large bony osteophytes at the acetabular margin of the hip. The lower third (synovium-lined portion) of the sacroiliac joint should not be involved in DISH. Other sites of extensive ossification (or spurring) may include the calcaneus, patella, tibial tuberosity, and olecranon. Calcification of the sacrotuberous and iliolumbar ligaments may be seen.

Differential Diagnosis: AS, other spondylorthropathies, OA, intervertebral osteochondrosis, hypoparathyroidism, retinoid therapy, fluorosis, and hypervitaminosis A must be distinguished.

Therapy: No specific therapy retards development of new bone. Analgesic agents and NSAIDs may be used for pain or stiffness. Rarely is surgical removal of calcific masses indicated. The use of low-dose radiation after hip surgery to minimize heterotopic bone formation has not been tested.

BIBLIOGRAPHY

Belanger TA, Rowe DE. Diffuse idiopathic skeletal hyperostosis: musculoskeletal manifestations. *J Am Acad Orthop Surg* 2001;9:258–267.
Mader R. Diffuse idiopathic skeletal hyperostosis: a distinct clinical entity. *Isr Med Assoc J* 2003;5:506–508.

DRUG-INDUCED LUPUS

ICD-9 Code: 995.2.

Definition: Drug-induced lupus is an uncommon complication of several commonly used medications. It is characterized by development of lupus-like symptoms, ANA positivity, and symptom resolution upon withdrawal of the offending drug. Drug-induced lupus differs from SLE by affecting an older population with milder symptoms and by having a different autoantibody profile (i.e., fewer autoantibodies) and a more favorable outcome.

Etiology: Numerous drugs have been implicated in causing drug-induced lupus (Table 11). Mechanisms underlying this disorder remain unclear but may involve either (a) similarities between drug and self antigens, resulting in immunologic cross-reactivity; (b) drug-induced alteration in immunogenicity of autoantigens (i.e., drugs may react with histones or deoxyribonucleoprotein); or (c) altered immunoregulation by drug or its metabolites.

Risk Factors: Other factors may contribute to the onset of drug-induced lupus. The slow acetylator phenotype clearly increases the risk of hydralazine-induced ANA positivity and drug-induced lupus but is less important in procainamide- and isoniazid-associated drug-induced lupus and does not appear to influence the risk of drug-induced lupus owing to other drugs or idiopathic SLE. There are few genetic associations with drug-induced lupus. Only HLA-DR4 has been suggested to be linked with hydralazine-induced lupus.

Pathology: CNS and renal findings are rare in drug-induced lupus. However, other lupus manifestations and pathology may occur in drug-induced lupus and be pathologically indistinguishable from SLE, including ANA positivity, LE cells, inflammatory pleuritis, pericarditis, and synovitis.

Demographics: Drug-induced lupus affects a greater percentage of males, whites, and the elderly than does idiopathic SLE (Table 12). For all implicated drugs, the incidence of drug-induced ANA positivity alone is far greater (often two- to fivefold more common) than the actual drug-induced lupus syndrome. Prevalence varies for each drug, and reliable rates have only been reported for

Table 11
Agents Implicated in Causing Drug-Induced Lupus[a]

Definite/Common	Probable/Uncommon	Possible/Rare
Procainamide	Phenytoin	Gold salts
Hydralazine	Carbamazepine	Oral contraceptives
Isoniazid	Primidone	Nitrofurantoin
Quinidine	Ethosuximide	Griseofulvin
Sulfasalazine	Propylthiouracil	Interferon (alpha, gamma)
Chlorpromazine	Methylthiouracil	Methyldopa
	Penicillamine	TNF inhibitors
	Lithium carbonate	(etanercept, infliximab,
	Acebutolol	adalimumab)
	Practolol	
	Minocycline	

[a]Drugs are listed according to strength of association and frequency of antinuclear antibodies or drug-induced lupus.
TNF, tumor necrosis factor.

hydralazine and procainamide, the most commonly associated drugs. The rates of drug-induced lupus are dose related for hydralazine and time dependent for procainamide. Between 60% and 90% of patients taking procainamide for >12 months develop ANA positivity, and roughly one-third of these develop drug-induced lupus. Approximately 60% or more of patients treated with TNF inhibitors will be found to have a positive ANA, and approximately 10% to 15% will have a positive anti–double-stranded DNA if these are checked on multiple occasions during the course of therapy; however, cases of drug-induced lupus related to these agents are uncommon. Rates of ANA positivity approach 50% for those taking 400 mg/day of hydralazine or more, but only 10% develop drug-induced lupus. With lower doses of hydralazine, lower percentages are seen. The incidence of ANA positivity in those treated with isoniazid, methyldopa, chlorpromazine, or quinidine ranges from 10% to 30%, yet very few develop clinical features of drug-induced lupus syndrome. Drug-induced lupus caused by minocycline has only been seen after prolonged exposure (>12 months) to the antibiotic.

Cardinal Findings: Most patients present with insidious onset of constitutional features (e.g., low-grade fever, fatigue, anorexia, weight loss, arthralgias, or myalgias). However, the pattern of organ involvement differs from that of idiopathic SLE (Table 11).
—*Renal:* Kidney involvement is rare in drug-induced lupus and has only been sporadically described with hydralazine-induced lupus. Such findings include sporadic proteinuria, abnormal urinary sediments, impaired creatinine clearance, or biopsy-proven nephritis. Most of these findings tend to resolve with drug withdrawal.
—*CNS:* CNS involvement is very rare in drug-induced lupus. There are few reports of neuropathy.
—*Skin:* Lupus skin findings (e.g., malar rash, oral ulcers, photosensitivity, vasculitic skin lesions) are uncommon in most patients with drug-induced lu-

Table 12
Comparison of Drug-Induced Lupus and SLE

Feature	Hydralazine Lupus	Procainamide Lupus	SLE
Demographics			
Female:male	1.6:1	0.9:1	9:1
Black:white	0.2:1	0.5:1	2.7:1
Mean onset age (y)	50	62	29
Clinical features			
Renal	13%	0	44%
Neurologic	7%	1%	45%
Skin	27%	11%	71%
Articular	86%	82%	92%
Pulmonary	3%	41%	1%
Serosal (pleuropericardial)	18%	46%	46%

SLE, systemic lupus erythematosus.

pus, with the notable exception of drug-induced lupus related to TNF inhibitors.

—*Musculoskeletal:* As in SLE, articular findings are common. Myalgias, arthralgias, and synovitis tend to be symmetric and polyarticular and involve the knees and fingers. Polymyalgia rheumatica has also been described. Because most patients receiving TNF inhibitors have inflammatory arthritis, it is difficult to ascribe musculoskeletal symptoms to drug-induced lupus in such patients.

—*Pulmonary:* Alveolar infiltrates are common in procainamide-induced lupus but are rarely seen with other implicated drugs (Table 11). Chronic interstitial lung disease has been described, but pulmonary hemorrhage has not.

—*Serositis:* Symptomatic pleural or pericardial effusions are common in drug-induced lupus, especially in procainamide-induced lupus. LE cells and ANA may be found in serosal fluids.

Uncommon Findings: CNS, renal, and lupus skin disease are uncommon. There have been uncommon reports of pericardial tamponade and constrictive pericarditis.

Diagnostic Tests: Requisite findings in drug-induced lupus include lupus clinical features in association with ANA positivity (or a positive LE cell preparation). Patients with drug-induced lupus have very high titers (e.g., >1:1,280) of ANA, often in a diffuse or speckled pattern. Such ANAs are directed toward deoxyribonucleoproteins (i.e., histones). Antihistone antibodies are commonly found in drug-induced lupus but are also seen in SLE and, therefore, cannot distinguish between the two. Nonetheless, antibodies against specific histone complexes have been identified for procainamide and sulfasalazine (against H2A-H2B), hydralazine (H3-H2A), and quinidine (H1-H2B). Antibodies against double-stranded DNA and complement levels should be negative or normal with the exception of drug-induced lupus related to TNF inhibitors. Leukopenia, lymphopenia, and Coombs-positive hemolytic anemia have all been well described in drug-induced lupus. Elevated ESR may been seen during active drug-induced lupus. Lupus anticoagulants and APL antibodies have frequently been reported, but thromboses and APL syndrome are rare.

Keys to Diagnosis: This diagnosis can be suspected in older adults taking an implicated drug who develop lupus-like features described above. Development of ANA alone does not suffice for the diagnosis or for withdrawal of the drug.

Diagnostic Criteria: Most patients meet the American College of Rheumatology (ACR) criteria for the diagnosis of SLE (see p. 372), although this is not necessary. The diagnosis of drug-induced lupus can be established if there are (a) no history of SLE before drug exposure, (b) one or more clinical features of SLE in addition to ANA positivity, and (c) resolution of symptoms and ultimately the ANA with drug withdrawal. Rechallenge with the offending agent is not necessary.

Therapy: Most patients respond promptly to drug withdrawal and symptomatic therapy. Commonly, patients benefit from rest, analgesics, and possible NSAIDs when treating constitutional, articular, or serosal manifestations. Infrequently, corticosteroids are necessary to treat refractory pleural/pericardial effusions, pericardial tamponade, moderate to severe pneumonitis, or symptomatic hemolytic anemia. Pericardiocentesis or surgery is rarely necessary for pericardial tamponade.

Course: The vast majority experience rapid resolution of their symptoms on drug withdrawal. ANA positivity may persist for 6 to 12 months after cessation.

Comment: Drugs implicated in causing drug-induced lupus (Table 11) can be safely used in patients with idiopathic SLE without risk. Identification of ANA positivity alone (without clinical features of lupus) is not a sufficient reason to withdraw potentially beneficial therapy.

BIBLIOGRAPHY

Brogan BL, Olsen NJ. Drug-induced rheumatic syndromes. *Curr Opin Rheumatol* 2003;15:76–80.
Cush JJ. Safety overview of new disease-modifying anti-rheumatic drugs. *Rheum Dis Clin North Am* 2004;30:237–255.
Louis M, Rauch J, Armstrong M, et al.. Induction of autoantibodies during prolonged treatment with infliximab. *J Rheumatol* 2003;30:2557–2562.
Rich MW. Drug-induced lupus. The list of culprits grows. *Postgrad Med* 1996;100:299–302.
Schlienger RG, Bircher AJ, Meier CR. Minocycline-induced lupus. A systematic review. *Dermatology* 2000;200:223–231.

DUPUYTREN'S CONTRACTURE

ICD-9 Code: 728.6.

Definition: Dupuytren's contracture results from thickening and shortening of the palmar fascia of the hand. Flexion deformities of involved fingers may cause considerable morbidity.

Etiology: The etiology is unknown; it may be familial (autosomal dominant) in as many as 10% of patients.

Demographics: Dupuytren's contracture may be seen in 3% to 5% of adults. Men are affected approximately five times more frequently than women, and the incidence increases with age. It occurs most commonly in whites, particularly northern Europeans.

Associated Conditions: Dupuytren's contracture is often seen in those with alcoholism, diabetes, epilepsy, hypercholesterolemia, RA, or reflex sympathetic dystrophy.

Cardinal Findings: Findings may be unilateral or bilateral. In early disease, painless nodularity of the fascia may be mistaken for local tenosynovial swelling. As the disease progresses, classic, thick, cord-like swelling of the fascia that is easily palpable below the thickened and puckered dermis. The fibrotic process can extend to involve the digital fascia. Shortening of the fascia results in flexion contracture of the fingers, particularly the fourth finger, although digits two through five may also be involved.

Therapy: Physical therapy and local therapies, such as heat, are often recommended for patients with mild contracture. Intralesional corticosteroids injections have varied success. More severe cases may require surgical release of the contracture.

BIBLIOGRAPHY

Thurston AJ. Dupuytren's disease. *J Bone Joint Surg Br* 2003;85:469–477.

ENTEROPATHIC ARTHRITIS

Synonyms: Inflammatory bowel disease–associated arthritis, Crohn's arthritis (also see Whipple's disease [p. 312] or intestinal-bypass syndrome [p. 221]).

ICD-9 Code: Arthritis associated with inflammatory bowel disease, 713.1; Crohn's enteritis, 555.9; Ulcerative colitis, 556.9.

Definition: Enteropathic arthritis refers to the inflammatory arthritis seen with Crohn's disease or ulcerative colitis. It is the most common extraintestinal finding and occurs in 5% to 20% of patients. In both, clinical and histologic gut inflammation, altered intestinal permeability, and the onset of an inflammatory peripheral or axial arthritis may be seen.

Etiology: There is no association between HLA-B27 and colitic peripheral arthritis. However, HLA-B27 is found in 50% of patients with spondylitic colitis. Thus, in the presence of HLA-B27-negative AS, enteropathic arthritis should be considered.

Pathology: GI manifestations and pathology may be insidious or subclinical. In ulcerative colitis, mucosal lesions appear in the colon as ulceration, edema, friability, or microabscesses. In Crohn's disease, lesions may be present anywhere in the GI tract, although the terminal ileum and colon are most common. Lesions may be ulcerative (aphthoid), patchy, or transmural, with evidence of granulomas. Synovial biopsy reveals chronic, nonspecific inflammatory changes.

Demographics: Peripheral arthritis affects men and women equally. All age groups are affected. Although the onset of arthritis follows established intestinal inflammation in adults, the converse may be seen in children. In contrast with peripheral arthritis, axial disease is more common in men and may precede the onset of colitis.

Cardinal Findings: Triad features of Crohn's disease includes abdominal pain, weight loss, and diarrhea. Ulcerative colitis is characterized by diarrhea and intestinal blood loss. Disease onset is sometimes heralded by low-grade fever, painful oral (aphthous) ulcers, or ocular (conjunctivitis, anterior uveitis) or cutaneous manifestations (erythema nodosum, pyoderma gangrenosum). In most, GI manifestations antedate or coincide with the onset of arthritis.

Axial arthritis occurs in 10% to 15% of patients with inflammatory bowel disease and is clinically and radiographically indistinguishable from AS. Chronic low back pain/stiffness and limited range of motion are common. The activity of axial disease does not parallel gut involvement.

Peripheral arthritis is seen in nearly 20% of patients. Peripheral arthritis manifests as an inflammatory, nonerosive, asymmetric oligoarthritis or monarthritis affecting large joints (knees, ankles, elbows), especially of the lower extremities. It is usually chronic but may be migratory and resolve in weeks or months. Enthesitis (i.e., heel pain) and "sausage digits" (toes or fingers) may occur. The activity of peripheral arthritis parallels gut inflammation. Peripheral arthropathy more frequently occurs in those with extraintestinal manifestations (e.g., erythema nodosum, uveitis).

Uncommon Findings: Clubbing, erosive arthritis, pericarditis, amyloidosis, thrombophlebitis, and pyoderma gangrenosum are rarely seen.

Diagnostic Tests: Abnormalities may include increased ESR or CRP, thrombocytosis, and hypochromic anemia. Synovial fluid WBC counts ranges from 2,000 to 50,000 cells/mm^3.

Imaging: Axial disease is radiographically indistinguishable from AS. Periostitis and radiographic enthesitis may be present.

Keys to Diagnosis: The presence of spondylitis or a seronegative oligoarthritis along with GI symptom evidence of inflammatory bowel disease may suggest this diagnosis.

Differential Diagnosis: Articular disease may be confused with seronegative RA, other spondyloarthropathies, or Behçet's syndrome. Arthritis and GI manifestations may be seen in the vasculitides, Whipple's disease, celiac sprue, intestinal-bypass syndrome, scleroderma, amyloidosis, Henoch-Schönlein purpura, FMF, postdysenteric reactive arthritis, and lymphoma and in those with GI toxicity related to antirheumatic therapies.

Therapy: Control of colitis may improve the peripheral arthritis but not axial disease. Treatment options are similar to those used in AS. NSAIDs tend to be helpful. Rarely will NSAIDs exacerbate the enteritis. Corticosteroids are not advised in spondylitis but may be useful in low doses for peripheral arthritis or when injected intraarticularly for uncontrolled mono- or oligoarthritis. Sulfasalazine, MTX, and azathioprine should be reserved for those with uncontrolled peripheral arthritis, with or without active colitis. TNF inhibitors may be indicated with refractory axial disease.

Surgery: Joint surgery is seldom indicated. Bowel surgery may be indicated but not for arthritis alone.

BIBLIOGRAPHY

Holden W, Orchard T, Wordsworth P. Enteropathic arthritis. *Rheum Dis Clin North Am* 2003;29:513–530.

ENTHESOPATHY

Synonyms: Enthesitis, Achilles tendonitis, plantar fasciitis, heel spur syndrome, or calcaneal periostitis.

ICD-9 Code: Enthesopathy, unspecified site, 726.90; spinal enthesopathy 720.1.

Definition: A periarticular condition that affects the entheses: sites of tendinous or ligamentous attachments to bone. These may be inflammatory or degenerative and are seldom owing to endocrinopathy, trauma, or drugs.

Etiology: In spondyloarthropathy (SpA), local inflammation is responsible for the onset or perpetuation of enthesitis. Factors underlying metabolic or degenerative causes are unknown but may be anatomic or mechanical.

Pathogenesis: There are two types of entheses: fibrous and fibrocartilaginous. The fibrous type is a dense connective tissue that attaches tendon or ligament to membranous bone. The fibrocartilage entheses have a transitional zone of fibrocartilage that attaches to endochondral bone at the epiphyses or apophyses. At these sites, fibrocartilage functions to resist shear and compressive forces. Fibrocartilage entheses are primarily affected in enthesopathy. There are innumerable entheses affected by disease. They often lie adjacent to bursal, synovial, and spinal structures that may also become involved. Inflammation of the entheses is the primary pathology in SpA.

Demographics: Enthesitis is seen in 25% to 60% of patients with SpA and thus may occur at any age or affect either gender. With advancing age, degenerative changes affect the entheses as well.

Disease Associations: Enthesopathy has been reported in AS, reactive arthritis, psoriatic arthritis, enteropathic arthritis, SpA, juvenile spondylitis, RA, leprosy, trauma, OA, DISH, acromegaly, fluorosis, retinoid therapy, hypoparathyroidism, hyperparathyroidism, POEMS syndrome, and X-linked hypophosphatemia.

Cardinal Findings: Enthesitis most often manifests as pain, seldom with swelling. The most common site of involvement is the heel with tenderness at either the distal insertion of the Achilles tendon posteriorly or the proximal insertion of the plantar fascia on the inferior os calcis. Other common sites include the toes and fingers (resulting in sausage digits), elbow epicondyles, pes anserinus, symphysis pubis, ischium, anterior superior iliac crest, greater trochanter, spinous processes, and costochondral junctions. Enthesitis involving the muscle insertions on the anterolateral ribs may be mistaken for chest pain or pleurisy.

Uncommon Findings: May manifest as low back pain or may be asymptomatic and incidentally found on imaging. Uncommonly enthesitis will result in avulsion or rupture of a tendon.

Diagnostic Tests: Laboratory tests reflect the nature of the underlying pathology and cause. HLA-B27 may be indicated in young patients with an equivocal presentation to suggest a SpA.

Imaging: Radiographs have traditionally been most often used to assess enthesopathy. The hallmarks of enthesopathy include bony erosions and reactive new bone formation. This may be accompanied by periostitis, periarticular sclerosis, or cysts. Such findings will only be evident with advanced or established disease because such findings take years to be evident. Scintigraphy may be used because of its greater sensitivity in early disease often when radiographic abnormalities are absent. Scintigraphic skeletal surveys may be used to quantitate or define enthesitis not apparent by physical examination. MRI is helpful in the early identification of perientheseal soft tissue edema, thickening of the entheses, early erosion of bone, or adjacent bone marrow edema. MRI is particularly useful in identifying sites of polyenthesopathy. The "shiny corners" or vertebral osteitis associated with SpA are manifest examples of enthesitis on MR imaging. Ultrasonography has also been investigated in patients with SpA and enthesopathy and is effective in delineating enthesopathic abnormalities and improvement with therapy.

Diagnostic Criteria: Enthesitis is one of several criteria included by the European Spondyloarthropathy Study Group for the diagnosis of SpA. Several clinical trials tools have been developed to quantify the degree of enthesitis. These include enthesopathy indices developed by Mander et al. (66 sites), Mastricht et al., and the assessment in ankylosing spondylitis (ASAS) enthesitis index (13 regions).

Differential Diagnosis: Other causes of periarticular pain, including fracture, should be considered (see p. 259).

Therapy: Nonpharmacologic measures (e.g., weight loss, activity modification, stretching, orthotics, splints) may prove useful in some. First-line drug therapy often includes the use of antiinflammatory doses of NSAIDs, if not otherwise contraindicated. Although there are no studies to show the superiority of cyclooxygenase (COX)-1 versus COX-2 inhibitors, there are anecdotal claims that enthesitis may respond better to indomethacin or diclofenac. Although systemic corticosteroids are ineffective and should be discouraged, some patients will benefit from intralesional injections of corticosteroids. Disease-modifying therapy with sulfasalazine or MTX appears to be effective. For patients not responding to NSAIDs or DMARDs, the use of TNF inhibitor therapy has proven to be highly effective in many resistant cases. There is no role for surgery in most.

BIBLIOGRAPHY

Kohler L, Kuipers JG, Zeidler HK. Enthesopathy. In: Hochberg MC, Silman AJ, Smolen JS, et al., eds. *Rheumatology*, 3rd ed. Edinburgh: Mosby, 2003:1275–1281.
McGonagle D. Diagnosis and treatment of enthesitis. *Rheum Dis Clin North Am* 2003;29:549–560.

EOSINOPHILIA MYALGIA SYNDROME

ICD-9 Code: 710.5. Eosinophilia myalgia syndrome is considered a variant form of scleroderma. Most cases have been associated with ingestion of L-tryptophan.

Etiology: Ingestion of specific lots of L-tryptophan in 1989–1990 resulted in new cases of eosinophilia myalgia syndrome because of a trace contaminant (1,1'-ethylidene-bis-L-tryptophan) arising from a manufacturing change. Sporadic cases reported since then may be owing to similar trace contaminants in other supplements or to inborn errors of tryptophan metabolism.

Pathology: Full-thickness skin biopsy specimens show thickened fascia with accumulation of collagen in the dermis. Inflammatory infiltrates, which may contain eosinophils, are found in subcutaneous fat (panniculitis) and surrounding small blood vessels or muscle spindles.

Demographics: An epidemic of cases appeared after 1989 and quickly subsided after the suspect preparation was recalled. Most of the epidemic-associated patients were female.

Cardinal Findings: Myalgias are severe and may be debilitating. A minority of patients show muscle enzyme elevations. Skin induration is most commonly seen on the trunk, generally sparing the extremities and face. CNS involvement, manifested by difficulty with memory or other cognitive problems and peripheral neuropathy, occurs in most patients. Uncommonly it results in interstitial lung disease or cardiac involvement with conduction changes and possibly sudden death.

Diagnostic Tests: Peripheral eosinophilia is seen in most patients.

Keys to Diagnosis: Skin thickening and myalgias suggests the diagnosis; rare cases may not be associated with ingestion of L-tryptophan. A full-thickness skin biopsy is needed.

Differential Diagnosis: The skin changes of eosinophilia myalgia syndrome resemble eosinophilic fasciitis. However, eosinophilic fasciitis does not usually exhibit cognitive dysfunction and myalgias. Localized forms of scleroderma and underlying malignancies should be also considered.

Diagnostic Criteria: (a) Eosinophil count $>1 \times 10^9/L$, (b) generalized myalgias that limit activity, and (c) absence of underlying malignancy.

Therapy: Acute symptoms respond to treatment with glucocorticoids, but late symptoms, including cognitive dysfunction, are relatively resistant to therapy.

Surgery: Surgery is not generally indicated except diagnostic skin biopsy.

Prognosis: A chronic phase develops in more than half of patients, with muscle cramps and CNS abnormalities that may impair normal daily activity.

BIBLIOGRAPHY

Pincus T. Eosinophilia-myalgia syndrome: patient status 2–4 years after onset. *J Rheumatol* 1996;23:19–25.
Winkelmann RK, Connolly SM, Quimby SR, et al. Histopathologic features of the L-tryptophan-related eosinophilia-myalgia syndrome. *Mayo Clinic Proc* 1991;66:457–463.

EOSINOPHILIC FASCIITIS

Synonyms: Schulman syndrome, diffuse fasciitis with eosinophilia.

ICD-9 Code: 728.89.

Definition: Eosinophilic fasciitis is a rare disorder of unknown cause characterized by inflammation in the skin that leads to skin tightening limited to the extremities and spares the face. Onset is often abrupt and may be preceded by vigorous exercise.

Etiology: Most cases are sporadic and of unknown cause. Few cases are associated with exposure to organic solvents, drugs (i.e., simvastatin), *Borrelia* infection, or hematologic disorders (myelodysplasia, leukemia, lymphoma, aplastic anemia).

Pathology: Full-thickness skin biopsy must include the fascia. Specimens show collagen accumulation in the dermis, with panniculitis and a cellular infiltrate, often containing significant numbers of eosinophils.

Demographics: Onset is usually in middle age. Males and females are equally affected.

Cardinal Findings: Pitting edema may be an early finding. Symmetric skin thickening, with a corrugated (*peau d'orange*) appearance, frequently affects (in decreasing frequency) the forearms, legs, hands, trunk, and neck. If periarticular areas are involved, joint contractures may develop. In contrast to scleroderma, Raynaud phenomenon is absent and nailfold capillaroscopy is normal.

Uncommon Findings: Pulmonary hypertension, thromboembolic disease, and liver abnormalities have been reported.

Keys to Diagnosis: Peripheral eosinophilia and hypergammaglobulinemia are usually present. Serologic tests for ANA and RF are negative. Skin biopsy specimens may show skin thickening accompanied by tissue eosinophilia.

Differential Diagnosis: Rare cases of this syndrome develop in association with underlying malignancies. Eosinophilia myalgia syndrome associated with ingestion of L-tryptophan more commonly shows muscle, CNS, and visceral involvement. Other localized forms of scleroderma should be considered.

Therapy: Treatment with prednisone benefits most patients. Hydroxychloroquine, penicillamine, and MTX may also be beneficial.

Prognosis: Most patients respond to medical therapy and show significant improvement. Spontaneous remissions have been reported.

BIBLIOGRAPHY

Claw DW, Crofford LJ. Eosinophilic rheumatic disorders. *Rheum Dis Clin North Am* 1995;21: 231–246.
Mori Y, Kahari VM, Varga J. Scleroderma-like cutaneous syndromes. *Curr Rheumatol Rep* 2002;4:113–122.

ERYTHEMA NODOSUM

Synonym: Panniculitis (see p. 284).

ICD-9 Code: 695.2.

Definition: Erythema nodosum is an acute, usually self-limited septal panniculitis characterized by tender subcutaneous nodules, typically on the anterior tibial surface.

Etiology: Half of cases have an underlying associated condition (see below). Pathogenesis is unknown but may be related to circulating immune complexes. There is an association with HLA-B8.

Pathology: Acute (neutrophilic) and chronic (granulomatous) septal inflammation is seen in subcutaneous adipose tissue and around blood vessels.

Demographics: Women are predominantly affected, with an M:F ratio of 1:3. It is most common in those between the ages of 25 and 40 years. Incidence has been reported to be two to three cases per 100,000 population.

Disease Associations: It may be idiopathic or seen with some infections (streptococcus, tuberculosis, leprosy, fungal or enteric infections), systemic disorders (Behçet's syndrome, sarcoidosis, inflammatory bowel disease, pregnancy) or with some drugs (penicillin, sulfonamides, oral contraceptives).

Cardinal Findings: There is sudden onset of one or more tender, erythematous or violaceous nodules on the anterior tibial surface, rarely over the thighs or forearms. Lesions are deep nodules, 1 to 10 cm in diameter, that evolve into softer, ecchymotic lesions and usually heal in 6 to 8 weeks without scar formation. In dark-skinned individuals, lesions are usually hyperpigmented. Symptoms such as fever and arthralgia usually relate to the associated condition. Synovitis typically involves the ankles or knees. Loefgren's syndrome, a specific variant of sarcoidosis, describes the triad of bilateral hilar adenopathy, erythema nodosum, and polyarthralgia or polyarthritis.

Uncommon Findings: Cutaneous ulceration is extremely rare. Migratory and chronic forms have been described.

Diagnostic Tests: A careful clinical search to identify associated conditions should be undertaken. The ESR is usually elevated.

Keys to Diagnosis: Look for tender, erythematous, subcutaneous nodules on anterior tibial surface.

Differential Diagnosis: Erythema nodosum may be confused with vasculitis with nodular lesions, Weber-Christian disease, or panniculitis associated with pancreatitis.

Therapy: Treat any underlying condition. Symptomatic management includes bed rest, cold compresses, and NSAIDs. A short course of systemic corticosteroids or potassium iodide can be very helpful.

Prognosis: Erythema nodosum is usually self-limited, with resolution in 6 to 8 weeks. Prognosis may be determined by the associated disorder, if any.

BIBLIOGRAPHY

Requena L, Sanchez-Yus E. Panniculitis. Part I. Mostly septal panniculitis. *Am Acad Dermatol* 2001;45:163–183.

FAMILIAL MEDITERRANEAN FEVER (FMF)

Synonyms: Periodic fever, familial recurrent polyserositis.

ICD-9 Code: 277.3.

Definition: FMF is an intermittent febrile disorder with inflammatory serositis, arthritis, and rash.

Etiology: FMF is an autosomal recessive disorder associated. The genetic defect is in the gene MEFV, which encodes pyrin, a 781-amino-acid protein that associates with the cytoskeleton in neutrophils and activated monocytes.

Twenty-eight mutations in this gene have been described, most in exon 10. Different mutations may be associated with variable prognoses and complications, such as amyloidosis. Heterozygous carriers of this gene are asymptomatic.

Pathology: Synovial biopsy shows nonspecific inflammation. Skin lesions show dense dermal infiltration with neutrophils and no evidence of vasculitis.

Demographics: Eastern Mediterranean persons (especially Armenians, Arabs, Turks, and Sephardic Jews) are most frequently affected. It is uncommon in other Mediterranean populations. In Iraqis and Sephardic Jews, the prevalence of FMF is between 1:250 and 1:1,000. The prevalence in Ashkenazi Jews is 1:73,000. The male:female ratio is 3:2. Less than half have a family history of FMF.

Cardinal Findings: Acute, recurrent, unpredictable attacks of fever, serositis (e.g., peritonitis, pleuritis), arthritis, and an erysipelas-like rash are seen. More than 80% of attacks begin before age 20, and initial attacks are very rare after age 40. Although fever and serosal attacks usually last 12 to 72 hours, arthritis may last for several weeks. Disease-free intervals may last days or months. Attacks may be precipitated by menses, stress, or physical exercise.

—*Fever:* The magnitude of fever varies.
—*Serositis:* Nearly all patients (>95%) have abdominal attacks at some time. Peritoneal attacks manifest as localized or generalized pain, abdominal distention, or signs of peritoneal inflammation. Constipation or diarrhea may accompany the attack. Pleural attacks occur in 25% to 50% of patients and tend to be unilateral and associated with a pleural rub and effusion on chest x-ray.
—*Arthritis:* Seen in as many as 75% of patients, arthritis tends to be acute, very painful, and monarticular and typically affects the knee, ankle, and hip. Synovial effusion is usually detectable. Persistent synovitis is uncommon but may last for weeks or months. Such patients may have radiographic evidence of osteopenia or joint damage. Febrile myalgias may also be intense and last for weeks.
—*Erysipelas-like rash:* Seen in 20% to 46% of patients, rash may occur with fever, is usually on the anterior lower extremity, and may be uni- or bilateral. Lesions are sharply demarcated, erythematous, tender, and sometimes swollen. Purpura is less common.

Uncommon Findings: Pericarditis is rare. Scrotal edema and pain have been described.

Complications: Amyloidosis develops in 10% to 40% and is unrelated to severity or frequency of FMF. Such patients may exhibit proteinuria, renal failure, or intestinal malabsorption. Less than 5% of children manifest Henoch-Schönlein purpura. FMF may coexist with PAN.

Diagnostic Tests: Genetic testing for MEFV mutations is possible; however, the diagnosis can still be made on clinical grounds, particularly in high-risk populations. Leukocytosis, elevated ESR, and inflammatory synovial fluid are usually seen. A normochromic, normocytic anemia may be found. Transient albuminuria and microscopic hematuria may be seen during the febrile attacks. Sterile exudative peritoneal or pleural fluid, with a neutrophil predominance, is common. C5a-inhibitor and IL-8 may be decreased in serosal or joint fluid (these tests are not routinely available).

Differential Diagnosis: Acute appendicitis, porphyria, hereditary angioedema, systemic juvenile arthritis (Still disease), rheumatic fever, septic arthritis, and endometriosis or pelvic inflammatory disease in women should be considered. Other febrile syndromes should be considered (see below).

Therapy: Symptomatic relief is the goal of therapy. Corticosteroids are ineffective. Colchicine prophylaxis (0.6 mg b.i.d. or t.i.d.) reduces the frequency of attacks, protects against amyloidosis, and stabilizes or lessens the proteinuria. Intravenous colchicine should be avoided.

BIBLIOGRAPHY

Kastner DL. The hereditary periodic fevers. In: Hochberg MC, Silman AJ, Smolen JS, et al., eds. *Rheumatology,* 3rd ed. Edinburgh: Mosby, 2003:1717–1734.

FEBRILE SYNDROMES

Synonyms: Periodic fever, hereditary periodic fever.

ICD-9 Code: Periodic Fever, 277.3; cyclic neutropenia, 288.0.

Definition: Several distinct diseases all associated with joint pain and fever, among other symptoms, have been shown to relate to defects in single genes. These include FMF (see p. 171); TNF receptor–associated periodic syndrome (TRAPS); hyperimmunoglobulinemia D (Hyper IgD) with periodic fever syndrome; familial cold autoinflammatory syndrome; Muckle-Wells syndrome; neonatal-onset multisystem inflammatory disease (NOMID); periodic fever with aphthous stomatitis, pharyngitis, and adenitis (or Marshall syndrome); and Blau syndrome. These disorders are characterized by recurrent febrile episodes with systemic inflammation commonly affecting the joints.

Etiology: FMF (autosomal recessive) relates to defects in a 10-exon gene on the short arm of chromosome 16, MEFV, that encodes pyrin, a 781-amino-acid protein that associates with the cytoskeleton of neutrophils and activated monocytes. TRAPS (autosomal dominant), which had been known as familial Hibernian fever before the discovery of the genetic defect, related to defects in the gene encoding p55 TNF receptor type I (CD120a). Hyperimmunoglobulinemia D with periodic fever syndrome (autosomal recessive) relates to defects in the gene encoding mevalonate kinase, an enzyme central to cholesterol synthesis. Blau syndrome (autosomal dominant) relates to mutations in NOD2, a gene also associated with susceptibility to Crohn's disease. Familial cold autoinflammatory syndrome, Muckle-Wells syndrome, and NOMID (autosomal dominant) all relate to mutations in a single gene, CIAS1, that encodes cryopyrin, a protein similar to pyrin that is also expressed primarily in neutrophils and monocytes.

Incidence: These disorders are rare but are more common with some ages and ethnicities.

Cardinal Findings: FMF is a prototype for these disorders and is characterized by several-day episodes of fever, monarticular arthritis, rash, and abdominal pain. Many of these disorders also manifest rash, mucosal inflammation, adenopathy, and serositis, and thus the diagnosis may rest with age, demographic features, or genetic testing. These disorders are characterized below.

—*TNF receptor–associated periodic syndrome (Hibernian fever):* Characterized by fever, arthralgia, myalgia, migratory rash, and abdominal pain lasting a week or longer (as long as 6 weeks). Primarily described in those of Irish, Scottish, and Australian ancestry.

—*Hyperimmunoglobulinemia D with periodic fever syndrome:* The usual onset is before 1 year of age. Symptoms last 3 to 7 days and may include recurrent fever, abdominal pains, arthralgia or arthritis, rash, diarrhea, headaches, and elevated ESR/CRP. Hyper IgD syndrome primarily affects those of Dutch, French, or Western European ancestry.

—*Familial cold autoinflammatory syndrome:* Characterized by the infantile onset of 1- to 3-day episodes of urticaria with fever, arthralgia, or conjunctivitis and may be induced by cold.

—*Muckle-Wells syndrome:* This syndrome has its onset by adolescence and is associated with fever arthralgia, urticaria, conjunctivitis, sensorineural hearing loss, hypergammaglobulinemia, and an intense acute-phase response. Amyloidosis may complicate Muckle-Wells syndrome.

—*Neonatal-onset multisystem inflammatory disease:* It is also known as chronic infantile cutaneous and articular disorder and has symptoms similar to those of Muckle-Wells syndrome on a more chronic basis.

—*Periodic fever with aphthous stomatitis, pharyngitis, and adenitis (PFAPA or Marshall syndrome):* Usually has its onset before age 5 years and remits spontaneously within 4 to 8 years. Symptoms include periodic fevers >40°C at fixed intervals every 2 to 8 weeks and usually resolve within 4 days. Aphthous ulcers, pharyngitis, and adenitis are seen in 70% to 90%. Periodic fever with aphthous stomatitis, pharyngitis, and adenitis is not familial and without diagnostic tests. Short doses of corticosteroids are recommended.

—*Cyclic neutropenia:* This is a disorder of recurrent fever (every 15–35 days) lasting as long as 14 days and coincides with episodic neutropenia (polymorphonuclear leukocytes >500/mm^3). Patients complain of malaise, pharyngitis, mouth ulcers, and lymphadenopathy. This is an autosomal dominant disorder wherein a stem cell regulatory defect results from a mutation of neutrophil elastase gene and apoptosis of polymorphonucleocyte precursors. Treatment options include steroids, cyclosporine, and granulocyte colony-stimulating factor.

—*Relapsing fever* is not a genetic defect but rather to a tick-borne infection with the spirochete *Borrelia recurrentis*. It manifests as headache, fever, myalgia, arthralgia, photophobia, and abdominal pains. Episodes occur every 10 to 14 days. Diagnosis is by serology. It may give false-positive results for tests for Lyme disease.

Keys to Diagnosis: The diagnosis of these conditions is still largely made on clinical grounds. FMF testing for mutations in the MEFV gene are available. TRAPS may be screen for by MEFV gene testing (to exclude FMF) and serum p55 TNF receptor levels (low). Genomic DNA sequencing for mutations of p55 TNF-R1 testing are not routinely available but may be necessary to confirm the diagnosis.

Differential Diagnosis: Other causes of fever of unknown origin should be considered including lymphoma, thromboembolic disease, endocarditis, polymyalgia rheumatica, temporal arteritis, Still's disease, occult abscess, drug fever, and factitious fever (e.g., thermometer manipulation, self-injection of pyrogenic material). Also, there are numerous febrile arthritis-dermatitis syndromes, including lupus, DM, psoriatic arthritis, sarcoidosis, Behçet's syndrome, erythema nodosum, leukocytoclastic vasculitis, PAN, cryoglobulinemia, hepatitis B or C, inflammatory bowel disease, intestinal bypass arthritis, Lyme disease, rheumatic fever, reactive arthritis, gonococcal or meningococcal arthritis, Parvovirus B19, rubella, SAPHO syndrome, and Sweet's syndrome.

Therapy: Colchicine has been the mainstay of treatment for FMF for many years and hence has been tried in Muckle-Wells and other syndromes as well. NSAIDs are commonly tried, and corticosteroids may be used intermittently for severe cases. Recently, there has been success using cytokine directed biologic agents, particularly soluble forms of the TNF receptor (etanercept) for TNF receptor–associated periodic syndrome or neonatal-onset multisystem inflammatory disease and IL-1 inhibitor (anakinra) for familial cold autoinflammatory syndrome and Muckle-Wells syndrome.

BIBLIOGRAPHY

Hoffman H, Patel D. Genomic-based therapy: targeting interleukin-1 for autoinflammatory diseases. *Arthritis Rheum* 2004;50:345–349.
Kastner DL. The hereditary periodic fevers. In: Hochberg MC, Silman AJ, Smolen JS, et al., eds. *Rheumatology*, 3rd ed. Edinburgh: Mosby, 2003:1717–1734.

FELTY'S SYNDROME

ICD-9 Code: 714.1.

Definition: Felty's syndrome is defined as the triad of erosive deforming arthritis, splenomegaly, and leukopenia.

Risk Factors: Felty's syndrome occurs almost exclusively among patients with severe, erosive, deforming RA who have high titers of RF in their serum. Furthermore, patients with Felty's syndrome commonly have the HLA-DR4 and other alleles associated with disease severity in RA.

Etiology: The cause of Felty's syndrome is unknown. Neutropenia may result from splenic sequestration of granulocytes. Defective granulocytic phagocytosis and chemotaxis may contribute to the susceptibility to infection.

Demographics: Felty's syndrome is rare and primarily affects whites.

Cardinal Findings: Although patients with Felty's syndrome have evidence of deforming erosive RA, active synovitis may not be present at the time of diagnosis. Patients often display other extraarticular manifestations (e.g., rheumatoid nodules, Sjögren's syndrome, rheumatoid vasculitis, episcleritis, pericarditis, or neuropathy) and may have evidence of weight loss, leg ulcers, recurrent infections, and splenomegaly. Splenomegaly may not be detected in all patients with extraarticular manifestations of RA and leukopenia. However, splenomegaly in Felty's syndrome may be massive.

Diagnostic Tests: The leukopenia of Felty's syndrome is typically a neutropenia (<2,000/mm^3). Although lymphocyte numbers may be depressed in some patients, a number of patients with Felty's syndrome have an increased number of large granular lymphocytes (LGL) in the circulation. Platelet counts are usually normal and thrombocytopenia is rare. As expected with severe RA, most patients are anemic. Despite the splenomegaly, leukopenia, and neutropenia, most patients with Felty's syndrome do not develop serious infections. RF is uniformly present and may be accompanied by other autoantibodies (e.g., ANA, perinuclear ANCA [P-ANCA]).

Differential Diagnosis: Splenomegaly is uncommon in RA without evidence of Felty's syndrome or neutropenia. Other causes of splenomegaly in patients with RA should be considered, including drug reactions, myeloproliferative diseases, lymphoma, amyloidosis, tuberculosis, and other chronic infections.

Therapy: Treatment of Felty's syndrome parallels the treatment of severe RA. Many patients are treated with low-dose corticosteroids or receive a second-line agent or DMARD. Splenectomy may be considered in those with massive splenomegaly or recurrent infections. Patients with significant neutropenia and fever or documented infection may benefit from parenteral growth factor therapy (e.g., granulocyte colony-stimulating factor), although such agents may exacerbate the synovitis of RA.

BIBLIOGRAPHY

Bowman SJ. Hematological manifestations of rheumatoid arthritis. *Scand J Rheumatol* 2002;31:251–259.

FIBROMYALGIA

Synonyms: Fibrositis, myofascial pain syndrome, neurasthenic pain syndrome.

ICD-9 Codes: 729.1.

Definition: Fibromyalgia is a very common syndrome. Widespread soft tissue pains, fatigue, and poor sleep are characteristic.

Etiology: The cause is unknown. Numerous studies have speculated on contributory role(s) for trauma, stress, depression, poor cardiovascular fitness, abnormalities of thalamic pain processing, and loss of non–rapid eye movement (stage IV) sleep.

Pathogenesis: Although most of the pain arises from nociceptors in muscle, numerous muscle studies (e.g., histopathology, electromyography (EMG), exercise testing, nuclear magnetic resonance spectroscopy) have failed to identify consistent abnormalities. Central mechanisms may underlie these heightened pain responses. Sleep electroencephalographic studies have documented alpha wave intrusion during delta (stage IV) sleep and a reduction in rapid eye movement sleep. Recent studies using single-photon emission computed tomography demonstrate lower cerebral blood flow in the thalamus and caudate nucleus of patients with fibromyalgia than in normal controls. Such studies suggest that central mechanisms may play a key role.

Demographics: Fibromyalgia is estimated to affect between three and six million or as many as 2% of Americans. Population studies suggest that the prevalence of widespread pain ranges from 10% to 23% and increases with age. Most reported series show that ≥80% of patients with fibromyalgia are female. The average age at presentation is between 30 and 50 years, although fibromyalgia has been uncommonly described in children and is probably underreported in the elderly. Racial and ethnic variances have not been described. Fibromyalgia often accompanies other rheumatic disorders, where it is referred to as secondary fibromyalgia. Twenty to 30% of patients with RA and SLE and as many as 50% of patients with Sjögren's syndrome have secondary fibromyalgia.

Cardinal Findings: All patients exhibit widespread pain affecting the upper and lower torso and both sides of the body. Asymmetric or focal areas of soft tissue pain and spasm may be referred to as myofascial pain syndrome. Patients typically complain of axial pain affecting the neck, interscapular area, and low back. Others may initially present with focal joint pains (e.g., shoulder, elbow, hip), only to demonstrate other evidence of widespread pain on examination. In addition to arthralgias and myalgias, patients complain of prominent fatigue, malaise, and morning stiffness, often lasting hours. Gel phenomenon and activity-induced articular pains are common. Articular symptoms often wax and wane and may be related to exacerbating factors. Many patients com-

D
I
S
E
A
S
E
S

plain of joint swelling, although objective evidence of effusion or synovial proliferation is lacking.

Sleep disturbance occurs in the vast majority of patients, with difficulty falling asleep, staying asleep, frequent awakening, restlessness, or early morning awakening. Most patients admit to only sleeping for short intervals throughout the night and feeling worse or tired on awakening. This results in the loss of the normal progression of sleep stages, and it is thought that loss of slow or delta wave (stage IV) sleep is especially disturbed. Obese males (more so than females) with fibromyalgia should be evaluated for an underlying sleep apnea syndrome.

Tender trigger points, some of which may not be apparent to the patient, are required for the diagnosis. Trigger points are defined as a focal painful response elicited by 4 kg of digital pressure (enough to blanch a thumbnail) over specific locations (Fig. 2). The physical examination should test all 18 trigger points. For purposes of disease classification, the ACR requires that at least 11 of these points be tender to have the diagnosis and be included in clinical trials.

Patients with fibromyalgia are often plagued by associated disorders that include migraine headache, irritable bowel syndrome, premenstrual syndrome, chronic fatigue syndrome, depression, allergic rhinitis, multiple drug allergies, or temporomandibular joint pain.

Numerous psychiatric disorders have been associated with fibromyalgia, yet less than 20% of patients exhibit major depression. Anxiety, panic attacks, and inadequate coping mechanisms have all been found in a minority of patients.

Uncommon Findings: Atypical chest pains (often with chest wall tenderness), Raynaud phenomenon, restless leg syndrome, numbness, memory loss, and cognitive dysfunction have been reported. The latter are more likely the result of poor sleep than sleep medications.

Diagnostic Tests: Extensive laboratory testing is rarely indicated, and wide batteries of rheumatic screening tests should be avoided. Although there are patients with secondary fibromyalgia, the diagnosis of fibromyalgia should not prompt additional testing to identify an associated or underlying disorder. Use of the ANA or thyroid function tests should be predicated on symptoms that suggest SLE or hypothyroidism, respectively.

Imaging: MRI and CT scans are normal and should not be performed unless otherwise indicated.

Keys to Diagnosis: Several clues should strongly suggest the diagnosis of fibromyalgia. Most common is the presentation of a patient who claims widespread and impressive musculoskeletal symptoms whose history is not substantiated by physical findings or abnormalities (e.g., no joint swelling). This should prompt a search for soft tissue trigger points and supportive features such as a sleep disturbance. Patients who present with musculoskeletal symptoms and a history of psychiatric disorders (e.g., depression) should be evaluated for fibromyalgia.

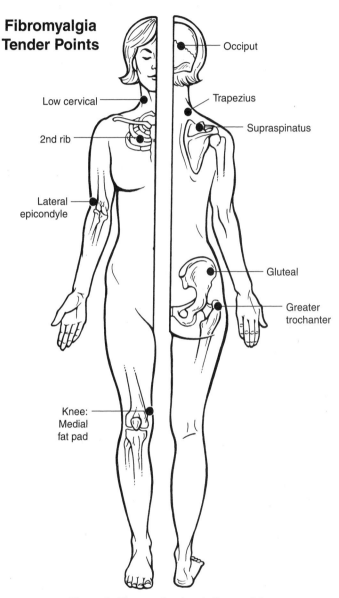

Fibromyalgia Tender Points

Occiput

Low cervical

Trapezius

2nd rib

Supraspinatus

Lateral epicondyle

Gluteal

Greater trochanter

Knee: Medial fat pad

Figure 2. Trigger point sites in fibromyalgia.

Diagnostic Criteria: Diagnostic criteria based entirely on these clinical features have been developed primarily for use in clinical studies (Table 13). These criteria may be instructive in establishing a diagnosis of fibromyalgia, but in practice, it is not necessary that ≥11 trigger points be present. The diagnosis

Table 13

American College of Rheumatology 1990 Criteria for the Classification of Fibromyalgia*[a]*

---

1. History of widespread pain
   Definition: Pain is considered widespread when all the following are present: pain in the left side of the body, pain in the right side of the body, pain above the waist, and pain below the waist. In addition, axial skeletal pain (cervical spine or anterior chest or thoracic spine or low back) must be present. In this definition, shoulder and buttock pain is considered as pain for each involved side. "Low back" pain is considered lower segment pain.
2. Pain in 11 of 18 tender point sites on digital palpation
   Definition: Pain, on digital palpation, must be present in at least 11 of the following 18 tender point sites:
   Occiput: bilateral, at the suboccipital muscle insertions
   Low cervical: bilateral, at the anterior aspects of the intertransverse spaces at C5-7
   Trapezius: bilateral, at the midpoint of the upper border
   Supraspinatus: bilateral, at origins, above the scapula spine near the medial border
   Second rib: bilateral, at the second costochondral junctions, just lateral to the junctions on upper surfaces
   Lateral epicondyle: bilateral, 2 cm distal to the epicondyles
   Gluteal: bilateral, in upper outer quadrants of buttocks in anterior fold of muscle
   Greater trochanter: bilateral, posterior to the trochanteric prominence
   Knee: bilateral, at the medial fat pad proximal to the joint line
   Digital palpation should be performed with an approximate force of 4 kg
   For a tender point to be considered positive, the subject must state that the palpation was painful; tender is not to be considered painful.

---

[a]For classification purposes, patients will be said to have fibromyalgia if both criteria are satisfied. Widespread pain must have been present for at least 3 months. The presence of a second clinical disorder does not exclude the diagnosis of fibromyalgia.

---

should be considered for someone with multiple tender trigger points, evidence of widespread pain, and a sleep disturbance.

Differential Diagnosis: Many rheumatic disorders manifest prominent soft tissue pain during the onset period or during disease flares. Disorders that may masquerade as fibromyalgia include hypothyroidism, psychogenic rheumatism, hypochondriasis, somatoform pain disorder, chronic fatigue syndrome, drug-induced myopathy, hypermobility syndrome, polymyalgia rheumatica, or the onset/flare of a connective tissue disease (e.g., SLE, polymyositis (PM), vasculitis, SpA).

Therapy: Patients with fibromyalgia differ from each other in the scope and severity of symptoms. Treatment approaches should be tailored to the individual patient and are best coordinated by a single physician who knows the patient well. Single agent or solitary measures are seldom effective. Successful management relies on the combined use of pharmacologic agents, physical modalities, and psychological measures to ensure an effective, multifaceted approach.

—*Pharmacologic agents:* No single drug will alleviate the patient's pain. Hence, pharmacologic pain relief is but one component of a comprehensive treatment plan. The four goals of therapy are to improve pain, optimize restorative sleep, promote stretching exercise, and, if present, treat depression. Pain relief can be achieved using drugs that target pain, muscle tension, or abnormal patterns of sleep. Analgesic medications may be used to decrease pain. Commonly used agents include acetaminophen (3–4 g/day), NSAIDs, or nonnarcotic analgesics, such as tramadol (50–100 mg b.i.d.) or propoxyphene (50–100 mg b.i.d.) when NSAIDs cannot be used. The clinician should avoid the temptation to escalate NSAID use (with resultant GI risks) or to resort to chronic narcotic analgesic use to control recalcitrant pain. Tricyclic antidepressants are useful analgesic adjuncts and should also be considered as first-line therapy. These drugs tend to normalize sleep patterns while providing muscle relaxing and analgesic effects. Bedtime trazodone (50–150 mg) or amitriptyline (10–75 mg) are commonly used agents for pain and sleep control. Doses should be escalated to optimize nighttime sleep without causing attendant daytime drowsiness. Trazodone may be less sedating than amitriptyline (see Appendix D, p. 533). Other sleep aids may include the use of bedtime zolpidem (5–10 mg) or zaleplon (5–20 mg). Patients should be counseled on sleep hygeine. Muscle relaxants such as cyclobenzaprine, carisoprodol, and orphenadrine may benefit patients with muscle spasm as a predominant symptom and may also promote better sleep. Drowsiness during daytime hours may be undesirable, so these agents may be given at bedtime only, either alone or with other sleep aids. The use of newer antidepressant agents, such as sertraline, fluoxetine, and venlafaxine (see Appendix D, p. 533). may also augment patient pain control. However, there is less experience with these drugs in fibromyalgia than with the tricyclic antidepressants, and their expense is generally greater. Gabapentin, dextromethorphan, and guaifenesin are uncommonly used adjuncts to control pain but have not been tested in clinical trials. Pain can be reduced further through appropriate stretching and exercise and with control of depression or anxiety.

—*Physical modalities:* Supervised therapy or instructional exercise programs are important in the overall therapeutic plan in fibromyalgia. Physical therapists who perform the technique of myofascial release are helpful in treating patients with significant muscle spasm or muscle tension. Some patients benefit from conventional massage therapy, but this is usually temporary unless combined with a more sustained program. Supervised therapy in a heated pool (aquatherapy) may allow patients with pain or weakness to exercise with less discomfort. Exercises that emphasize stretching, such as yoga and Tai Chi may be useful and should be done at least initially under supervision. In some studies, a program of conditioning aerobic exercise has improved symptoms in some patients. A supervised program of exercise starting at a low level thus may be of benefit as part of the treatment plan.

—*Psychologic approaches:* Many patients with fibromyalgia exhibit symptoms of psychological distress, including anxiety and depression. A minority will have symptoms that will require psychiatric evaluation and treatment. Others may benefit from cognitive-behavioral therapy. Such a program can include training in relaxation and coping skills as well as guidance in reinforcing positive behaviors.

Monitoring: The frequency of monitoring is determined by the medications used and response to therapy. At each follow-up visit, the clinician should assess the magnitude of the patient's pain, the quality and quantity of sleep, limitations on activities of daily living, the number of tender trigger points, and the impact of outside stressors or new sources of pain on current status.

Prognosis: Longitudinal studies suggest that the duration of disease is often many years and that only a minority of patients (10%–20%) improve over time and the number of patients requesting disability benefits is increasing. Fibromyalgia is a significant cause of long-term disability and, given the high prevalence of this condition and relatively young age of most patients, the economic and social impact of this disorder is profound. In many, disability can be avoided by vocational counseling, modification of work schedule and activities, and avoidance of exacerbating factors (e.g., trauma, stress, poor sleep, depression, arthritis).

BIBLIOGRAPHY

Clauw DJ, Crofford LJ. Chronic widespread pain and fibromyalgia: what we know, and what we need to know. *Best Pract Res Clin Rheumatol* 2003;17:685–701.
Forseth KO, Gran JT. The prevalence of fibromyalgia among women aged 20–49 years in Arendal, Norway. *Scand J Rheumatol* 1991;21:74–78.
Moldofsky H, Scarisbrick P. Induction of neurasthenic musculoskeletal pain syndrome by selective sleep stage deprivation. *Psychosom Med* 1976;38:35–44.
Silver DS, Wallace DJ. The management of fibromyalgia-associated syndromes. *Rheum Dis Clin North Am* 2002;28:405–417.
Wolfe F, Ross K, Anderson J, et al. The prevalence and characteristics of fibromyalgia in the general population. *Arthritis Rheum* 1995;38:19–28.

FROSTBITE

ICD-9 Code: Multiple sites, 991.3; hand, 991.1; foot, 991.2.

Definition: Frostbite injury to the extremities can result in vascular damage and thrombi with associated chondrocyte damage. As a result, patients with frostbite may develop osteoarthritis (OA) months or even years after exposure.

Cardinal Findings: Frostbite injury tends to occur in the distal extremities, particularly in the hands and feet. Findings of OA related to frostbite may resemble primary (e.g., Heberden and Bouchard nodes) or erosive OA. In children, frostbite exposure may result in premature closure of the epiphyses and impaired growth, usually of the fingers.

Imaging: Typical radiographic findings include demineralization, periostitis, subchondral (juxtaarticular) cysts, joint space narrowing, and formation of osteophytes.

Therapy: Because the signs and symptoms of frostbite arthritis develop some time after exposure, there is no specific therapy for this condition. Therapy is comparable with that for idiopathic OA (see p. 268).

BIBLIOGRAPHY

Glick R, Parhami N. Frostbite arthritis. *J Rheumatol* 1979;6:456–460.

FUNGAL ARTHRITIS

ICD-9 Codes: Arthropathy associated with mycoses, 711.8 (code underlying disease first: sporotrichosis, 117.1; *Candida* arthritis, 112.9; coccidioidomycosis, 114.9; blastomycosis, 116.0; cryptococcosis, 117.5; histoplasmosis, 115.9).

Demographics: With the exception of those with sporotrichosis and histoplasmosis, most with serious fungal bone or joint infection are immunocompromised from systemic illnesses (e.g., HIV), malignancy, chronic disease (diabetes), chronic inflammatory disorders, or drugs (e.g., corticosteroids, TNF inhibitors).

Specific Infections

Sporotrichosis: Osteoarticular infections may be caused by *Sporothrix schenckii,* which has worldwide distribution. Exposure is through the skin, often secondary to plant thorn injury in gardeners and agricultural or other outdoor workers. Infection begins in the skin as a painful skin nodule. Indolent unifocal arthritis most commonly involves the knee but also can affect the wrist, hand, ankle, and elbow. Tenosynovitis is also possible. Polyarticular arthritis is rarely seen in disseminated skin and bone infection occurring in immunocompromised hosts. Diagnosis is made by culture from skin, synovial fluid, or bone. Amphotericin B is being superseded by oral itraconazole for lymphocutaneous, articular, and osseous disease, with 70% to 100% cure rates. Surgical resection is sometime necessary.

***Candida* Arthritis:** Commonly caused by *Candida albicans,* infection is owing to direct seeding of a joint or by hematogenous spread, often from an indwelling transcutaneous catheter. It manifests as a monarthritis in 60% to 75% of patients, most commonly affecting the knee. Diagnosis is established by culture of synovial fluid and/or blood. The preferred treatment is systemic am-

D
I
S
E
A
S
E

photericin B. Prognosis is poor, and mortality rates are high because of comorbidities and frequent, concurrent candidemia.

Coccidioidomycosis: Infection with *Coccidioides immitis* is commonly seen in the western and southwestern United States, with a higher incidence in summer months. Primary respiratory infection occurs after inhalation of spores and may be associated with constitutional and systemic manifestations, including erythema nodosum and migratory arthritis. Disseminated infection is rare (except in immunocompromised hosts) and is associated with frequent bone involvement and monarthritis, particularly of the knee. It can progress to an indolent arthritis with pannus. Histologic examination reveals noncaseating granulomas with fungal spores. Diagnosis is suggested by a positive skin test result that is seen in 80% of patients within 1 to 3 weeks of infection. Synovial fluid culture is difficult but occasionally positive. Serologies are positive in diffuse disease. Chest radiographs may also be abnormal. Treatment options include itraconazole or fluconazole for limited to moderate disease. Amphotericin B is recommended for disseminated infection.

Blastomycosis: *Blastomyces dermatitidis* causes an uncommon infection in the Mississippi and Ohio River valleys and Middle Atlantic states of the United States. Primary respiratory infection occurs after inhalation of spores. Acutely, arthralgias and myalgias are common. Uncommonly, there is lymphatic or hematogenous dissemination to bone, joints, and skin. Joints are less commonly involved than bone and may be owing to direct extension from adjacent osteomyelitis. Skeletal involvement is occasionally asymptomatic. Long bones, ribs, and vertebrae are most commonly affected and appear osteolytic on radiographs. Soft tissue or vertebral abscesses may occur. Fungi may be detected in synovial fluid after KOH preparation. Culture on Sabouraud medium is confirmatory. Serologic tests are available, sensitive, but nonspecific and are not routinely recommended. Itraconazole may be effective with mild to moderate disease. Amphotericin B is reserved for severe infection in immunocompromised hosts.

Cryptococcosis: Infection with *Cryptococcus neoformans* is seen worldwide, especially in the immunocompromised host. Primary respiratory infection occurs after inhalation of spores (ubiquitous, found in pigeon droppings). Bone involvement is uncommon (<10% of cases), and infectious arthritis is rare. The latex agglutination test for cryptococcal antigen is generally positive. Limited disease may be treated with fluconazole alone. Amphotericin B with 5-fluorocytosine is recommended for severe cases.

Histoplasmosis: Infection with *Histoplasma capsulatum* is most commonly seen in the Mississippi and Ohio River valleys of United States but is also found worldwide. Primary respiratory infection is usually asymptomatic. Spores tend to grow and persist in soil contaminated with avian or bat excreta. Histoplasmosis is usually a benign, self-limited, respiratory illness. Acute infections may be heralded by erythema nodosum, arthralgia, or acute oligo- or polyarthritis. Chronic infection is very rare. The diagnosis is confirmed by histopathology (caseating granulomas) or by culture. Itraconazole is indicated for mild to moderate disease. Amphotericin B, with or without surgical debridement, may be necessary with severe disease or if the host is severely immunocompromised.

BIBLIOGRAPHY

Hansen BL, Andersen K. Fungal arthritis. A review. *Scand J Rheumatol* 1995;24:248–250.

GANGLION CYSTS

ICD-9 Code: 727.40.

Definition: Ganglions are cystic masses that arise in proximity to joint capsules or tendon sheaths but do not communicate with the joint cavity. They are most common with repetitive strain or overuse, trauma, or inflammatory arthritis.

Pathology: Ganglia are formed by a dense capsule of mesenchymal connective tissue that encloses one or more cavities. These cavities are thin walled and contain a viscous, mucinous fluid.

Cardinal Findings: Ganglia arise most commonly on the dorsal aspect of the wrist; however, they also occur on the volar aspect of the wrist, the medial and lateral aspects of the knee, the dorsum of the foot, and the anterior aspect of the lower leg. Although most ganglia are asymptomatic, symptoms may relate to their location and impingement on adjacent structures (e.g., restriction of motion, paresthesias). They may become painful if traumatized. Recently formed ganglia are easily compressible; with chronicity, they may become more indurated and nodule-like.

Therapy: Patients with ganglia may seek medical therapy for symptoms related to tendinous, neural, or vascular impingement or for cosmetic reasons. Ganglia may resolve spontaneously and recur over time. Treatment varies according to duration and symptoms. Ganglia of only a few months' duration may be treated by firm compression. This can be accomplished with a firm object such as a padded coin secured by an elastic bandage for several weeks. Alternatively, the mucinous fluid can be removed with a large-bore needle. Corticosteroid injection may also be used. Chronic or recurrent ganglionic cysts may require excision.

BIBLIOGRAPHY

Soren A. Clinical and pathologic characteristics and treatment of ganglia. *Contemp Orthop* 1995;31:34–38.

DISEASES

GOODPASTURE'S SYNDROME

Synonyms: Antiglomerular basement membrane antibody disease.

ICD-9 Code: 446.21.

Definition: Goodpasture syndrome is an autoimmune disorder characterized by pulmonary hemorrhage and rapidly progressive glomerulonephritis in association with antibodies to alveolar and glomerular basement membrane (GBM).

Etiology: The cause of Goodpasture's syndrome is unknown. Most cases are without cause, but some are preceded by respiratory infections (e.g., influenza), toxic lung injury or drug exposure (D-penicillamine). The pathogenesis of Goodpasture's syndrome is related to anti-GBM antibodies.

Pathology: Immunofluorescent staining of biopsy specimens from the lungs and kidneys of patients with Goodpasture's syndrome reveals a characteristic linear pattern of anti-GBM antibody deposition. Crescentic glomerulonephritis is seen in 80% of patients. The specific antigenic epitopes recognized by anti-GBM antibodies were recently shown to be present on the α_3 chain of type IV collagen. Type IV collagen is the major component of basement membranes and provides structural support. Although other chains of type IV collagen occur widely throughout the body, the α_3 chain has more limited expression. This provides an explanation for why end-organ involvement of Goodpasture's syndrome is typically limited to the lungs and kidneys.

Demographics: Goodpasture's is rare and mostly affects white men in their third decade, although all races and ages may be affected.

Cardinal Findings: Approximately 75% of those with Goodpasture's syndrome have both pulmonary and renal involvement; the remainder have only rapidly progressive glomerulonephritis. Isolated pulmonary disease is rare. Hemoptysis is the initial complaint in most patients, and alveolar infiltrates may be seen on chest radiographs. Other symptoms include cough and dyspnea. Smoking history may be associated with pulmonary hemorrhage. Renal manifestations generally lag behind pulmonary signs and symptoms.

Diagnostic Tests: Laboratory studies often reveal an anemia that may be related to both anemia of chronic disease and iron deficiency, depending on the severity and chronicity of the pulmonary hemorrhage. Patients may also be hypoxic. Less than half of patients demonstrate renal insufficiency at initial evaluation, but more than 80% eventually display azotemia or proteinuria. Hematuria is very common. Anti-GBM assays are performed by ELISA in a number of reference laboratories, and anti-GBM is present in >95% of patients with Goodpasture's syndrome (see p. 37).

Imaging: Chest radiographs usually reveal diffuse, extensive alveolar infiltrates.

Differential Diagnosis: Various other pulmonary/renal syndromes (see p. 310, such as SLE, cryoglobulinemia, and several types of vasculitis, must be distinguished.

Keys to Diagnosis: The diagnosis of Goodpasture syndrome may be secured by demonstrating linear antibody staining of the basement membrane of renal or pulmonary biopsy specimens. However, patients are often quite ill during the initial course of the disease, making biopsy more difficult. Tests for serum anti-GBM antibodies are most commonly used to diagnose Goodpasture syndrome because of their widespread availability and high sensitivity and specificity.

Therapy: Goodpasture syndrome used to be associated with a poor prognosis and high associated mortality. Recently, the prognosis has improved, in part because of the availability of diagnostic tests and advances in immunomodulatory interventions, although improvements in the intensive care of critically ill persons have no doubt contributed. Because most patients present in extreme distress (e.g., hemoptysis, hypoxia), large boluses of corticosteroids (e.g., 1 g methylprednisolone intravenously for 3–4 days) are commonly used. Plasmapheresis appears to benefit many patients and is also commonly used. Many patients are treated with cytotoxic drugs, such as daily oral cyclophosphamide, in conjunction with plasmapheresis. In contrast to some other pulmonary renal syndromes, such as SLE, production of anti-GBM antibodies is usually self-limited. Thus, these aggressive immunomodulatory therapies may often be stopped when the patient has demonstrated significant clinical improvement.

BIBLIOGRAPHY

Gravelyn TR, Lynch JP. Alveolar hemorrhage syndromes. *IM Intern Med Special* 1987;8:63–83.

Hudson BG, Tryggvason K, Sundaramoorthy M, et al. Alport's syndrome, Goodpasture's syndrome, and type IV collagen. *N Engl J Med* 2003;348:2543–2556.

Levy JB, Turner AN, Rees AJ, et al. Long-term outcome of anti-glomerular basement membrane antibody disease treated with plasma exchange and immunosuppression. *Ann Intern Med* 2001;134:1033–1042.

Shah MK, Hugghins SY. Characteristics and outcomes of patients with Goodpasture's syndrome. *South Med J* 2002;95:1411–1418.

GOUT

ICD-9 Codes: Gouty arthritis, 274.0; gouty nephropathy, 274.1; uric acid nephrolithiasis, 274.11.

Definition: Gout is an inflammatory disorder caused by tissue deposition of monosodium urate (MSU) crystals. Several descriptive terms are often used in association with gout:

—*Acute gout:* Single or recurrent attacks of inflammatory mono- or oligoarthritis.

—*Tophaceous gout:* Accumulation of crystalline MSU aggregates in soft tissues; nodular aggregates are referred to as tophi. Usually associated with chronic arthropathy.

—*Hyperuricemia:* Serum level of uric acid above which supersaturation of MSU in extracellular fluids theoretically occurs ($\geq$6.8 mg/dL).

—*Asymptomatic hyperuricemia:* The state in which the serum uric acid level is abnormally high (>7.0 mg/dL in men, >6.0 mg/dL in postmenopausal women), but no symptoms of gout or nephrolithiasis have occurred.

—*Primary gout:* Gout resulting from abnormalities in purine metabolism or from idiopathic decreased renal excretion of urate.

—*Secondary gout:* Gout resulting from increased serum uric acid levels resulting from an associated disorder (e.g., neoplasms, lymphoproliferative disease, chronic renal failure) or drug therapy (e.g., diuretics, ethanol, cytotoxics).

—*Saturnine gout:* Gout caused by chronic lead intoxication, from either occult or occupational exposure or the ingestion of moonshine. This accounts for <5% of cases. Hyperuricemia results from lead-induced tubulointerstitial renal damage. Saturnine gout should be expected when the magnitude of hyperuricemia exceeds the reduction in glomerular filtration.

Etiology: The common denominator of gout is hyperuricemia. Uric acid, the product of purine degradation, is synthesized mainly in the liver. Two-thirds of the uric acid pool is excreted by the kidney, with the remainder secreted into the intestine. The causes of hyperuricemia can be divided into disorders of overproduction and disorders of decreased renal clearance of urate (Table 14). Most cases of gout (90%) are owing to underexcretion of uric acid; overproduction because of inherited enzyme defects [hypoxanthine-guanine adenine phosphoribosyltransferase deficiency (also known as Lesch-Nyhan syndrome) or overactivity of 5-phosphoribosyl 1-pyrophosphate synthetase] accounts for <1% of cases.

The pathogenesis of acute gout involves the response of polymorphonuclear leukocytes to formation of MSU crystals. Acute gout is thought to result from formation of new crystals rather than from release of crystals from preformed MSU synovial deposits or tophi. Crystals are coated with IgG, which reacts with Fc receptors on polymorphonuclear cells that phagocytose the crystals. Intracellularly, the crystals are stripped of their protein coats and disrupt the cell, releasing a variety of inflammatory mediators.

Pathology: The most frequent sites of MSU deposition are cartilage, epiphyseal bone, periarticular structures, and the kidney. Deposition in other sites is rare. Crystal aggregates cause a foreign body reaction. A tophus is composed of MSU crystals, a proteoglycan-rich intercrystalline matrix, and surrounding fibrous tissue. Affected joints may develop cartilage degeneration, erosion of marginal bone, and synovial proliferation. In the kidney, crystal deposition causes arteriosclerosis and interstitial fibrosis.

Table 14
Causes of Hyperuricemia

Overproducers: increased purine synthesis or urate production
  Idiopathic
  Inherited enzyme defects
    Hypoxanthine-guanine phosphoribosyltransferase deficiency
      Complete (Lesch-Nyhan syndrome)
      Incomplete
    Phosphoribosylpyrophosphate synthetase overactivity
  Diseases with purine overproduction
    Lympho- and myeloproliferative disorders
    Hemolytic disorders
    Malignant diseases
    Obesity
    Drugs and diet
      Ethanol
      Cytotoxic drugs
      Warfarin
      Purine-rich diets
Underexcreters: decreased renal clearance of urate
  Primary idiopathic uric acid underexcretion
  Secondary uric acid underexcretion
    Chronic renal failure
    Hypertension
    Dehydration
    Obesity
    Hyperparathyroidism
    Hypothyroidism
    Drugs
      Ethanol
      Diuretics
      Low-dose salicylate
      Cyclosporine
      Ethambutol
      Pyrazinamide
      Levodopa

Demographics: The prevalence of asymptomatic hyperuricemia in adult Americans is 5% to 8%. The prevalence of gout is estimated to be 13 cases per 1,000 men and 6.4 cases per 1,000 women in North America. The risk of developing gout increases with higher uric acid levels: The annual incidence in relation to serum uric acid concentration is 0.1% for those with a serum uric acid level <7.0 mg/dL, 0.5% for levels between 7.0 and 8.9 mg/dL, and 4.9% for levels >9.0 mg/dL.

    More than 90% of patients with primary gout are men. Women rarely develop the disorder before menopause because estrogen is thought to enhance uric acid excretion. The peak incidence for men is in the fifth decade.

Risk Factors: Factors provoking episodes of acute gouty arthritis include trauma, surgery, immobility, alcohol ingestion, starvation, overindulgence in purine-rich foods, and drugs that raise urate concentrations (Table 14). Alcohol (ethanol) increases serum lactate levels, which blocks renal excretion of urate. Primary gout is often associated with obesity, hyperlipidemia, diabetes mellitus, hypertension, and atherosclerosis. Secondary gout may be associated with alcoholism and myeloproliferative and lymphoproliferative disorders. Gout is more prevalent among patients of African descent, largely because of the prevalence of hypertension.

Cardinal Findings

—*Acute gout:* Acute gouty arthritis is the most common early clinical manifestation of gout. The metatarsophalangeal joint of the first toe is the most common site (often referred to as podagra) of involvement, affecting 75% to 90% of patients at some time in the course of their disease, with 50% experiencing their first attack of acute gout in this joint. Approximately 80% of initial attacks are monarticular, typically involving joints of the distal lower extremity: the metatarsophalangeal joints, ankle, or knee. Wrist, finger, or elbow involvement is rare early but may occur with tophaceous gout or in the elderly with nodal OA, renal insufficiency, and diuretic use. Onset is usually abrupt, often waking the patient at night. The affected joints may be warm, swollen, and tender, with diffuse periarticular erythema that is often confused with cellulitis or thrombophlebitis. Fever may occur. Attacks may be associated with impressive soft tissue pitting edema. Early attacks generally subside spontaneously over 3 to 10 days, even in the absence of treatment. Postinflammatory desquamation of the skin overlying the joint may occur. Patients are typically symptom free after an acute attack. Subsequent episodes may occur more frequently, involve more joints, and persist longer. Trivial episodes of pain lasting a few hours may precede the first dramatic attack of acute gout. Although affected joints usually recover completely, erosions may develop in those with repeated attacks. Polyarticular attacks may also occur in those with established, poorly controlled disease. Such attacks may display a migratory or additive pattern or involve periarticular structures such as tendons and bursae.

—*Intercritical gout:* The interval between acute gouty attacks is termed the intercritical period. If necessary, MSU crystals can be recovered from previously affected joints in this symptom-free period. The duration of this period varies; most untreated patients experience a second episode within 2 years. A minority evolve into chronic polyarticular gout without pain-free intercritical periods. At this stage, the clinical picture can be confused with RA, especially if tophi are mistaken for rheumatoid nodules. However the two (RA, gout) rarely coexist because there is a negative association between the two.

—*Chronic tophaceous gout:* This form of gout is characterized by the deposition of solid urate (tophi) in connective tissues, including articular structures, with an eventual destructive arthropathy. Tophaceous gout may be associated with early age at onset, long duration of active untreated disease, frequent attacks, high serum urate levels, upper extremity involvement, and polyarticular disease. Organ transplant recipients treated with cyclosporine or diuretics are also at increased risk of accelerated development of chronic tophaceous gout. Common sites for tophi include the olecranon, prepatellar bursae, ulnar surface of the forearm, Achilles tendons, over the fingers, and the helix of the ear. Large tophi over the hands may occur in association with crippling joint destruction. Tophi may ulcerate and exude a white chalky material composed of MSU crystals. Tophi typically progress insidiously, with the patient reporting increasing stiffness and pain in affected joints.

—*Renal disease:* Renal disease includes urolithiasis, urate nephropathy (deposition of MSU crystals in the interstitium), and uric acid nephropathy (deposition of MSU crystals in the collecting tubules). Uric acid stones account for 5% to 10% of all renal stones. The prevalence of urolithiasis is 22% in primary gout and 42% in secondary gout, and renal stones antedate arthritis in 40% of cases. Serum uric acid levels are directly related to the incidence of urolithiasis (found in nearly 50% of patients excreting >1,100 mg of uric acid daily). Urate nephropathy and uric acid nephropathy are difficult to differentiate clinically, and they are often referred to as gouty kidney. Uric acid nephropathy may present acutely in patients with malignancy treated with chemotherapy or radiation. Urate nephropathy is slowly progressive and associated with hypertension and proteinuria. A causal relationship between renal dysfunction in gout and hypertension is equivocal.

Uncommon Findings: Uncommon sites of initial involvement are the hands, shoulders, sternoclavicular joints, hips, spine, and sacroiliac joints. Initial presentation of gout may be polyarticular, especially in women. Aseptic necrosis of the hip has been reported as a manifestation of gout. Tophaceous involvement of the axial skeleton has been rarely noted. Tophaceous involvement of parenchymal organs, although rare, has been also been reported. Uncommonly, atypical gout arises in nodal OA with acute inflammatory swelling affecting the Heberden or Bouchard nodes. Such patients tend to be elderly females with renal insufficiency, often treated with diuretics.

Diagnostic Tests: At initial presentation, serum uric acid levels are elevated, although levels are normal in as many as 40% of patients experiencing an acute gouty attack. Nonetheless, the vast majority of patients with gout demonstrate an elevated uric acid level at some time. The serum creatinine level should be determined because it may influence subsequent therapy. During an acute attack, there is frequently leukocytosis, thrombocytosis, and elevated acute-phase reactant (ESR, CRP) levels.

—*Joint fluid:* Synovial fluid in acute gout is inflammatory, with high leukocyte counts (>2,000 cells/mm^3; WBC differential >75% neutrophils); occasionally, synovial leukocyte counts are very high (>50,000 cells/mm^3). MSU crystals are identified with the polarized light microscopy. Needle-shaped crystals, 5 to 25 μm, can be seen against a dark background. These are best identified with polarizing lenses and a red compensator, which reveals characteristic negatively birefringent crystals that appear yellow against a lilac background when parallel to the plane of the red compensator and blue when at right angles to it. In acute gout, urate crystals are usually intracellular (within neutrophils); between attacks, urate crystals may still be seen, but they tend to be extracellular. Only one or two drops of synovial fluid are necessary for crystal examination. Needle-shaped MSU crystals can also be seen under plain light microscopy. Demonstration of MSU crystals does not exclude pseudogout or septic arthritis because these conditions may coexist with gout. If septic arthritis is considered, Gram staining and culture should be performed. Exudate from gouty tophi can be examined for MSU crystals in a similar manner.

—*Urine tests:* A 24-hour collection for uric acid determination is useful for assessing the risk of renal stones and for planning therapy (if use of a uricosuric agent is contemplated).

Imaging: Radiographic examination in acute gout is most valuable in excluding other types of arthritis (e.g., septic arthritis, fracture). Radiographic abnormalities seen in long-standing gout are an asymmetric, erosive arthritis with characteristic "scooped-out" marginal erosions with sclerotic borders and often an overhanging edge of cortical bone. Periarticular osteopenia is absent, and the joint space is preserved until late in the disease.

Keys to Diagnosis: A history of podagra, dramatic onset of arthritis, history of episodic or prior arthritis with spontaneous resolution in 3 to 10 days, and the presence of tophi should all suggest a diagnosis of gout. For the diagnosis of acute gout, serum uric acid concentrations are neither sensitive (often not raised in acute attacks) nor specific. Definitive diagnosis rests on demonstration of MSU crystals within leukocytes in affected joints. A scooped-out marginal joint erosion with sclerotic borders and an overhanging edge also suggests gout.

Differential Diagnosis: The differential diagnosis depends on the stage of gout encountered.
—*Acute gout:* The differential diagnosis of acute gout is essentially that of acute inflammatory monarthritis and includes septic arthritis, reactive arthritis, ARF, pseudogout, and other crystalline arthropathies. Fever, leukocytosis, and localized erythema may lead to erroneous consideration of cellulitis or thrombophlebitis (when the distal lower extremity is involved).
—*Chronic tophaceous gout:* The differential diagnosis of chronic tophaceous gout includes other destructive arthropathies, RA, chronic CPPD crystal deposition disease, seronegative SpAs, and erosive OA. Tophi are often mistaken for rheumatoid nodules because of their appearance and location. Coexistence of gout and RA is exceedingly rare.

Therapy: The goal of therapy is to treat the acute attack of gout and prevent recurrent attacks and the complications of untreated gout. There is usually no justification for treating asymptomatic hyperuricemia. However, some physicians make exceptions when serum urate levels are very high (e.g., >12 mg/dL) and the risk of nephrolithiasis is substantial. In addition, allopurinol therapy may be indicated in the setting of malignancy, when the anticipation of tumor lysis results in acute overproduction of urate. Treatment options vary with the stage of gout encountered (Fig. 3).

—*Acute gout:* NSAIDs, corticosteroids (locally or systemically), or oral colchicine may be used (Fig. 3). NSAIDs are the preferred modality in acute gout because they have a rapid clinical effect and are usually well tolerated when used for 3 to 14 days or until the attack subsides. Nonetheless, NSAIDs may be associated with acute gastritis and renal toxicity and should be avoided in those with a history of GI intolerance, renal insufficiency, congestive heart failure, ascites, bleeding diathesis, or chronic anticoagulant therapy. Although indomethacin (1–2 mg/kg/day) is historically the most widely used NSAID for treatment of acute gout, other nonselective NSAIDs and COX-2 inhibitors have been effective at antiinflammatory doses. When

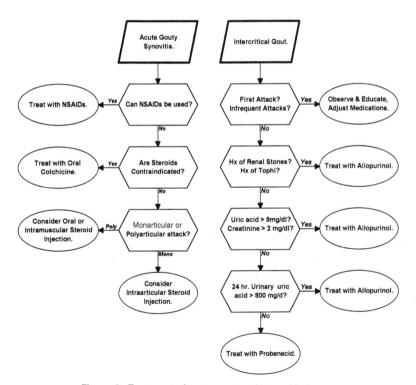

Figure 3. Treatment of acute gout and intercritical gout.

NSAIDs are contraindicated, corticosteroids are usually effective. They may be particularly useful in the elderly, in persons with renal insufficiency or congestive heart failure, and in organ transplant recipients—all situations in which NSAIDs and colchicine may be relatively contraindicated. Intraarticular preparations (e.g., methylprednisolone acetate) are particularly efficacious in monarticular gout. Oral or parenteral steroids are also effective in the treatment of monarticular and polyarticular gout. Historically, colchicine therapy has been used to control acute attacks. However, unacceptable GI toxicity (i.e., nausea, diarrhea) and delayed onset of action make this the least option in acute gout. In patients with normal renal function, colchicine can be administered orally with a dose of 1.2 mg initially, followed by 0.6 mg every 2 hours, until abdominal discomfort or diarrhea develops or a total dose of 8 mg has been administered. Most patients have some relief of arthritic symptoms by 18 hours, with joint inflammation subsiding in 48 hours. Colchicine's effect relates to the inhibition of microtubule formation and neutrophil chemotaxis. *Intravenous colchicine should not be used* (see Comments below). Antihyperuricemic measures (i.e., allopurinol) should not be initiated or continued until the acute attack is resolved because the duration of joint inflammation may be prolonged. Doses of allopurinol and colchicine must be adjusted with renal insufficiency.

—*Intercritical gout:* Once the acute attack has resolved, attention is directed at prevention and prophylaxis. The decision to initiate chronic pharmacotherapy is made in accord with the patient's wishes (Fig. 3). Those with one or few attacks may prefer to wait and treat the attack, when and if it arises. Those with multiple attacks should be offered the opportunity to prevent attacks with medical therapy. Prevention can be achieved by correcting hyperuricemia, either by eliminating identifiable causes of hyperuricemia (diuretic therapy) or by administering drugs that lower uric acid production or enhance its excretion. Complete avoidance of purine-rich foods (meats, yeast, alcohol, legumes, spinach, asparagus, cauliflower, and mushrooms) is impractical, ineffective, and rarely adhered to in clinical practice. Gout can be prevented or diminished by lowering serum uric acid levels with uricosuric agents (probenecid, sulfinpyrazone) or by inhibiting production of uric acid (allopurinol). Indications for pharmacologic lowering of serum uric acid include the inability to reverse secondary causes of gout, recurrent attacks of gout arthritis, chronic tophaceous gout, and an increased risk of nephrolithiasis. In general, use of uricosuric agents is limited to persons with normal renal function, decreased urinary urate excretion (<800 mg/day on a normal diet), and no evidence of tophi. They are contraindicated in the presence of renal stones and have no benefit in persons with low urinary volumes (<1 mL/min) and renal insufficiency (creatinine clearance <50 mL/min). Uricosuric agents carry the risk of developing urolithiasis, which can be decreased by ensuring high urinary volumes and by addition of sodium bicarbonate, 1 g three to four times per day. Two agents are available: probenecid (1–2 g/day) and sulfinpyrazone (50–400 mg twice daily). The dose should be gradually increased until serum uric acid levels are <6.0

mg/day. Therapy may be unsuccessful in some patients. Allopurinol effectively lowers uric acid levels in both overproducers and underexcreters of urate and is indicated in persons with overproduction of uric acid, renal stones, tophi, renal insufficiency, and extreme elevation of uric acid and those in whom uricosuric agents are contraindicated or are ineffective. Allopurinol is also indicated in the prophylaxis of tumor lysis syndrome. The usual dose of 300 mg/day must be reduced in the presence of renal insufficiency (200 mg/day for a creatinine clearance <60 mL/min, 100 mg/day for a creatinine clearance <30 mL/min). Beginning with small doses reduces the likelihood of precipitating an attack of acute gout. The chief side effect of allopurinol is a rash that develops in as many as 2% of patients and can occasionally be life threatening if exfoliative dermatitis develops (one in 1,000 cases). Chronic colchicine therapy (0.6–1.2 mg/day) may also be prophylactic against gouty attacks. The dose must be adjusted for renal insufficiency. Neuromyopathy or rhabdomyolysis is a rare side effect strongly associated with renal insufficiency.

Prognosis: Untreated, gout progresses over several years from the initial attack of acute gout through a period of intercritical gout to chronic tophaceous gout. More rapid progression may be seen in the presence of severe renal insufficiency. Early intervention can interrupt this progression. Tophi can regress completely with prolonged treatment. Occasionally, gout is difficult to manage, often because of multiple factors such as compliance, alcoholism, renal insufficiency, and the need for continued diuretic therapy.

Comment: The clinician should refrain from using intravenous colchicine to treat acute gout because of the risk of acute bone marrow suppression and hepatic, renal, and CNS toxicity, especially in those with renal impairment. Although the intravenous preparation is available in the United States, it is banned in many formularies and in many other countries, including the United Kingdom and Australia.

BIBLIOGRAPHY

Boomershine KH. Colchicine-induced rhabdomyolysis. *Ann Pharmacother* 2002;36:824–826.
Emmerson BT. The management of gout. *N Engl J Med* 1996;334:445–451.
Halla JT, Ball GV. Saturnine gout: a review of 42 patients. *Semin Arthritis Rheum* 1982;11:307–314.
Kim KY, Ralph Schumacher H, Hunsche E, et al. A literature review of the epidemiology and treatment of acute gout. *Clin Ther* 2003;25:1593–1617.
Rott KT, Agudelo CA. Gout. *JAMA* 2003;289:2857–2860.

HAND AND WRIST PAIN

Definition: Disorders of the wrist and hand are a common cause of medical consultation. Pain, swelling, dysfunction, or structural abnormalities may incite such an evaluation.

ICD-9 Codes: Hand pain, 719.44; Wrist pain, 719.43.

Anatomic Considerations: Sources of pain and swelling may include di-arthrodial joints, tendons, tenosynovium, bone, nerve, skin, or other soft tissue structures. A detailed physical examination is required to determine whether there is articular or nonarticular (periarticular) involvement.

Cardinal Findings: It is important to note the chronology of involvement so that acute, chronic, intermittent, additive, or migratory joint involvement may be identified. Musculoskeletal disorders often manifest a distinctive pattern of joint involvement (Fig. 4). For example, RA commonly involves the proximal

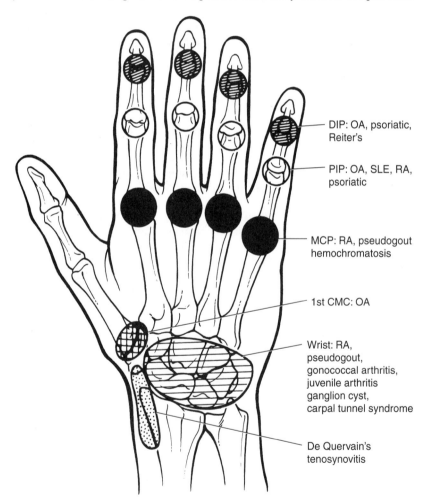

DIP: OA, psoriatic, Reiter's

PIP: OA, SLE, RA, psoriatic

MCP: RA, pseudogout hemochromatosis

1st CMC: OA

Wrist: RA, pseudogout, gonococcal arthritis, juvenile arthritis ganglion cyst, carpal tunnel syndrome

De Quervain's tenosynovitis

Figure 4. Sites of hand/wrist involvement and their disease associations.

interphalangeal, metacarpophalangeal, and wrist joints, whereas OA tends to involve the distal interphalangeal, proximal interphalangeal, or first carpometacarpal (base of the thumb) joints. A history of trauma should suggest the possibility of a fracture or a degenerative (OA) or overuse (CTS) condition. Patients should describe the functional limitations associated with their complaint. The medical history may disclose disorders with prominent musculoskeletal manifestations. For example, diabetics may develop flexion contractures of the fingers, the so-called syndrome of limited joint mobility.

Articular abnormalities often demonstrate obvious clinical findings. Bony, nodular enlargement of the distal interphalangeal (Heberden's nodes) or proximal interphalangeal (Bouchard's nodes) joints may suggest OA. By contrast, soft tissue swelling and effusion of the metacarpophalangeal or proximal interphalangeal joints, with or without swan-neck or boutonnière deformities, should suggest RA. Degenerative changes at the metacarpophalangeal joint may be related to OA (a rare manifestation of a common disease) or hemochromatosis (a common manifestation of a rare disease). Soft tissue abnormalities may include nodular swellings owing to ganglion cysts (see p. 185), rheumatoid nodules, nodules associated with MTX use, or gouty tophi. Nodular or fibrotic changes involving the flexor tendons may result in episodic "catch" or "trigger finger" when the finger is flexed and extended. Trigger fingers may be seen in both RA and OA. Thickening of the palmar fascia may result in a Dupuytren's contracture of the fourth or fifth flexor tendons with a fixed flexion deformity of the involved digits. Tendon rupture of the fingers results in an unopposed reducible malposition or deformity away from the involved side. Thus, rupture of the extensor tendons over the dorsum of the hand (as in RA) results in the fingers being held in a position of unopposed flexion. A common cause of periarticular wrist pain is de Quervain tenosynovitis (see p. 154) manifest as distal radial pain, with or without swelling, and a positive Finkelstein test (see p. 13). Examination of the hand and wrist should also reveal the presence of cutaneous abnormalities. Common skin lesions indicating a systemic disorder may include Gottron papules over the metacarpophalangeal joints (DM), erythema or hyperpigmentation over inflamed joints (RA), periungual erythema (SLE, myositis, scleroderma, Reiter's syndrome, psoriatic arthritis), vasculitic lesions (digital infarcts, painful Osler's nodes, Janeway lesions), psoriatic lesions (scaly plaques, nail pitting, onycholysis), nail abnormalities (psoriasis, Reiter's syndrome), sclerodactyly and distal digital pulp scars (scleroderma), and Raynaud's phenomenon. Neurologic examination should seek muscle atrophy (from disuse or neuromuscular disease), signs of CTS (Tinel's sign, thenar muscle wasting), and brachioradialis reflex (C5-6 innervation) and include careful sensory and motor examination of the hand and digits.

Diagnostic Testing: Testing should be guided by the results of the history and physical examination. Routine serologic testing and rheumatic screens or panels should be avoided. Nailfold capillaroscopy (see p. 88) should be done on all patients suspected of having Raynaud phenomenon or sclerodactyly. Nerve

Table 15
Differential Diagnosis of Wrist/Hand Pain

Periarticular
    de Quervain tenosynovitis
    Tenosynovitis (RA, gonococcal, gout)
    Trigger finger
    Dupuytren's contracture
    Syndrome of limited joint mobility (diabetes)
Articular
    RA (PIP, MCP, wrist)
    Osteoarthritis (DIP, PIP, 1st CMC joints)
    Psoriatic arthritis (DIP, PIP, MCP joints)
    Hemochromatosis (second and third MCP joints)
Bone
    Avascular necrosis (i.e., Kienbock's necrosis of the lunate)
    Fracture (e.g., Colles)
    Sarcoid (cystic lytic lesions)
    Periostitis (osteomyelitis, hypertrophic osteoarthropathy)
Neurologic/vascular
    Carpal tunnel syndrome
    Raynaud's phenomenon
    Subacute bacterial endocarditis with emboli
    Digital vasculitis (RA, SLE, cholesterol emboli)
    Reflex sympathetic dystrophy
Soft tissue
    Ganglion cysts
    Rheumatoid nodules
    Gouty tophi
    Clubbing (hypertrophic osteoarthropathy)

RA, rheumatoid arthritis; PIP, proximal interphalangeal; MCP, metacarpophalangeal; DIP, distal interphalangeal; CMC, carpometacarpal; SLE, systemic lupus erythematosus.

conduction velocity testing may be useful in evaluating a potential neuropathy or radiculopathy. Patients with acute or chronic monarthritis may benefit from synovial fluid aspiration and analysis, and those with undiagnosed chronic monarthritis may benefit from arthrocentesis or synovial biopsy to exclude indolent infection.

Imaging: Radiographs of the hands are seldom revealing with acute presentations and may only show soft tissue swelling. Nonetheless, they should be considered if there is a history of trauma, if the condition is chronic, if there are vasomotor changes suggesting reflex sympathetic dystrophy, or if a baseline assessment is needed for a chronic osseous/articular disorder. MRI is largely an investigative tool and should be reserved for situations in which osteonecrosis or osteomyelitis is being considered.

Therapy: Treatment is dictated by the underlying disorder.

HEMOCHROMATOSIS

ICD-9 Code: 275.0.

Definition: Hemochromatosis is a common hereditary disorder of excessive iron absorption and deposition causing tissue damage and organ dysfunction.

Etiology: Hemochromatosis is an autosomal recessive condition related to mutations in HFE, a gene located on the short arm of chromosome 6 that has homology to major histocompatibility complex class I molecules. HFE encodes a 348-amino-acid protein, known as the hereditary hemochromatosis protein, that functions in conjunction with β_2-microglobulin to regulate intestinal iron uptake. The disease has age-related incomplete penetrance and varied clinical expression. The defect causes increased intestinal absorption of iron, resulting in increased saturation of serum transferrin, elevated serum ferritin concentrations, and deposition in the liver, heart, some endocrine organs, and joints. Heterozygotes have increased iron stores but rarely develop clinical disease.

Demographics: Although present from birth, the peak age at symptom onset is 40 to 60 years. The female:male ratio is 1:5. Prevalence is 30 to 60/10,000. It is mostly seen in northern European populations; 10% of whites are heterozygous for the mutation.

Cardinal Findings: Multiple organ systems may be affected.
—*Liver:* Transaminases are elevated, with occasional hepatomegaly and tenderness and eventual cirrhosis.
—*Endocrine:* Diabetes is usually a late manifestation. Hypogonadism (loss of libido, impotence, testicular atrophy, gynecomastia) and skin pigmentation (related to increased melanin) are often seen.
—*Heart:* Cardiac involvement is uncommon but may present as a cardiomyopathy.
—*Arthropathy:* This may be a presenting feature. Joints typically involved include the second and third metacarpophalangeal and proximal interphalangeal joints, hips, knees, and spine. Joints may be mildly tender or swollen or clinically resemble OA; 50% have chondrocalcinosis. Iron deposition may cause pseudogout.

Diagnostic Tests: Screen with transferrin saturation (100 $\times$ serum iron/total iron binding capacity); if >50%, measure serum ferritin; in hemochromatosis, serum ferritin exceeds 200 ng/mL in males and 100 ng/mL in females. Ferritin behaves as an acute-phase reactant and levels may increase in the presence of inflammatory disease elsewhere. Diagnosis should be confirmed with liver biopsy. Noninvasive imaging with CT or MRI may be useful. Screen first-degree relatives because early detection and treatment can prevent clinical disease.

Keys to Diagnosis: Consider hemochromatosis in all cases of transaminitis and chondrocalcinosis and when an OA-like disease is seen in men in their fourth and fifth decade.

Therapy: Weekly phlebotomy is performed to deplete iron stores; maintenance phlebotomy should occur three to six times per year to keep the hematocrit <40%. The arthropathy is usually not reversible. Arthritis should be treated symptomatically.

BIBLIOGRAPHY

Braun J, Sieper J. Rheumatologic manifestations of gastrointestinal disorders. *Curr Opin Rheumatol* 1999;11:68–74.
Chi ZC, Ma SZ. Rheumatologic manifestations of hepatic diseases. *Hepatobiliary Pancreat Dis Int* 2003;2:32–37.

HEMOPHILIA

Synonyms: Hemophilia A (factor VIII deficiency), hemophilia B (factor IX deficiency).

ICD-9 Code: Hemophilia A, 286.0; hemophilia B, 286.1; hemarthrosis, 719.10.

Definition: Hemophilia A and B are congenital, X-linked recessive disorders of the coagulation cascade that may manifest with hemorrhage into weight-bearing joints, muscle, or soft tissues. Hemophilia A and B are clinically similar; hemophilia A accounts for >80% of cases. Disease severity is based on the amount of factor present (2% is severe, 2%–5% is moderate, and 5%–25% is mild). Factor levels >25% are rarely associated with hemorrhagic events.

Etiology: Hemophilia is caused by congenital deficiency of factors VIII or IX. Acquired deficiencies have been reported.

Pathology: Intraarticular blood does not coagulate because of the lack of prothrombin, fibrinogen, and tissue thromboplastin. Red blood cells may incite inflammation and may lead to synovial proliferation (without inflammatory cells), pannus, and cartilage damage. Hemosiderin is found in synovium and chondrocytes.

Demographics: Hemophilia A affects one in 10,000 males. Females are asymptomatic. Males are commonly affected and the first episode of bleeding occurs before the age of 5 years.

Cardinal Findings: Acute hemarthrosis may begin as stiffness or warmth that is followed by intense pain. Low-grade fever may occur. Intraarticular hemorrhage commonly affects the knees, ankles, and elbows and manifests as an acute, erythematous, warm mono- or oligoarthritis. Involvement of small joints (fingers, wrist, sternoclavicular) is unusual and should suggest other diagnoses. Repetitive hemarthrosis may cause secondary OA, deformity, or less commonly a chronic synovitis (with or without effusion). Other common sites of bleeding include muscle (resulting in myonecrosis or compartments syndrome), bone, CNS, or kidney (manifest as hematuria).

Complications: Transfusions and factor VIII therapy have resulted in HIV positivity, acquired immunodeficiency syndrome (AIDS), hepatitis B or C infection, and chronic liver disease. Septic arthritis rarely accompanies hemarthrosis. Nonetheless, staphylococcal, pneumococcal, and *Salmonella* septic arthritis have been well described in hemophilia.

Diagnostic Tests: Activated PTT is prolonged; prothrombin time and platelet counts are normal. Assays for factor VIII are commonly available, and titers are low during bleeding episodes. Synovial fluid shows a predominance of red blood cells.

Imaging: Radiographs may show soft tissue swelling, juxtaarticular osteopenia, joint space narrowing, and subchondral cyst formation. Marginal erosions may be seen with chronic disease. Widening of the femoral intercondylar notch is said to be characteristic of hemophilia.

Keys to Diagnosis: Look for a positive family history or antecedent diagnosis of hemophilia associated with hemorrhage into joints or soft tissues.

Differential Diagnosis: Hemorrhagic joint effusions may also be owing to von Willebrand's disease, vitamin K deficiency, platelet disorders, crystal-induced arthritis, trauma, fracture, ligament tear (cruciate), neuropathic arthritis, and pigmented villonodular synovitis. Acute hemophiliac hemarthrosis must be distinguished from septic arthritis, HIV-related arthropathies, and crystal-induced arthritis.

Therapy: Long-term use of aspirin and NSAIDs should be avoided. Acute bleeding can be treated with sufficient recombinant factor VIII to elevate levels to 40% to 50%. The dose is calculated from the patient's weight and factor VIII level. Ice, rest, analgesia, and joint extension (to avoid contractures) is advised. Do not attempt invasive procedures (e.g., arthrocentesis) until factor VIII levels are >50%. Arthrocentesis is indicated if infection is suspected. Septic arthritis may accompany an acute hemarthrosis. The therapeutic value of arthrocentesis to remove blood and red blood cells that may exacerbate inflammation is controversial. Intraarticular steroids should not be used. Major bleeding (e.g., CNS) requires chronic factor VIII levels >50% until resolved. Prophylactic administration of factor VIII (three times weekly) has been advocated for patients with recurrent or severe bleeding. Although seldom used, reports suggest that chronic inflammatory synovitis may benefit from penicillamine or gold therapy.

DISEASES

Surgery: Arthroscopic synovectomy is seldom required for chronic synovitis. Surgical procedures (e.g., total joint replacement) can be cautiously performed with adequate factor replacement.

BIBLIOGRAPHY

Avina-Zubieta JA, Galindo-Rodriguez G, Lavalle C. Rheumatic manifestations of hematologic disorders. *Curr Opin Rheumatol* 1998;10:86–90.

HENOCH-SCHÖNLEIN PURPURA

Synonyms: Anaphylactoid purpura, allergic purpura.

ICD-9 Code: 287.0.

Definition: Henoch-Schönlein purpura is a systemic, small-vessel vasculopathy affecting the skin (lower extremities), gut, and kidneys. Henoch-Schönlein purpura is classically characterized by the triad of nonthrombocytopenic purpura, arthralgia, and abdominal pain.

Etiology: The cause of Henoch-Schönlein purpura is unknown; it is labeled as allergic because peak onset is in the spring, often after upper respiratory infection by viruses or streptococci. It is sometimes a consequence of therapy (e.g., ampicillin, penicillin, erythromycin, quinidine, quinine).

Pathology: Biopsies demonstrate leukocytoclastic vasculitis (venulitis) in the skin or GI tract. IgA deposition, found in 70% of skin and 90% of renal lesions, is diagnostic. Renal biopsy specimen may show mesangial hypercellularity and segmental necrotizing glomerulonephritis.

Demographics: Age at onset is bimodal. Most cases affect children, usually between 2 and 11 years of age. The mean age at onset is 43 years for adults (range, 30–70). Males are affected more than females.

Cardinal Findings: Onset is usually heralded by persistent or intermittent palpable purpura or petechiae involving the lower extremities and buttocks, sometimes with dependent edema. Lesions often progress from red to purple to brown. They may coalesce to form large ecchymoses. Fever is seen in 50% of patients, and musculoskeletal manifestations (arthralgia/arthritis of ankles or knees) are present in 75% of patients. Intestinal disease is more common in children and manifests as diarrhea, cramping, GI bleeding, hematemesis, melena, or, rarely, intussusception. IgA nephropathy is more common in adults than children. Renal insufficiency is typically brief but may develop in 3% to 15% of patients.

Uncommon Manifestations: Skin involvement of the face, upper extremities, or torso; ulcerative lesions; bleeding gums; bowel perforation; renal insufficiency; headache; neuropathy; seizures; orchitis; hemoptysis; and cardiac arrhythmias have been reported.

Diagnostic Tests: Anemia, leukocytosis, elevated ESR, and abnormal urinalysis (hematuria, casts, proteinuria) are common.

Keys to Diagnosis: Consider the diagnosis of Henoch-Schönlein purpura with lower extremity palpable purpura and/or evidence of leukocytoclastic vasculitis and IgA deposition in the skin, gut, or kidney.

Differential Diagnosis: Cryoglobulinemia, PAN, Wegener's granulomatosis, bacterial endocarditis, SLE, or lymphoma should be considered.

Diagnostic Criteria: The ACR requires two of the following four criteria: age younger than 20 years at onset, palpable purpura, acute abdominal pain, or biopsy evidence of granulocytes in the walls of venules or small arterioles (leukocytoclastic vasculitis).

Therapy: Most patients (especially children) require only (a) supportive care (bed rest, hydration), (b) treatment of suspected infection, or (c) removal of the offending drug. Acetyl salicylic acid or NSAIDs are usually ineffective. Corticosteroids tend not to be effective with skin or renal disease and are reserved for CNS, testicular torsion, intestinal bleeding, or severe abdominal or joint pain. Treatment of renal disease is controversial.

Surgery: Surgery is reserved for those with uncontrolled abdominal hemorrhage and perforation.

Prognosis: Most patients show spontaneous improvement in 4 to 16 weeks. Relapse is seen in 5% to 10%. Prognosis depends on renal outcome. The mortality rate is 2%.

BIBLIOGRAPHY
Ballinger S. Henoch-Schonlein purpura. *Curr Opin Rheumatol* 2003;15:591–594.
Mukhopadhyay S, Mousa S, George BR, et al. Palpable purpura, polyarthritis and abdominal pain. *Med J Aust* 2004;180:121–122.

HEPATITIS: MUSCULOSKELETAL MANIFESTATIONS

ICD-9 Codes: Hepatitis A, 070.1; hepatitis B, 070.30; acute hepatitis C, 070.51; chronic hepatitis C, 070.54; lupoid hepatitis, 571.49; chronic active hepatitis, 571.49; drug-induced hepatitis, 573.3.

Definition: A variety of musculoskeletal disorders may be associated with hepatitis A virus (HAV), hepatitis B virus (HBV), or hepatitis C virus (HCV).

Etiology: The arthritis associated with acute HBV infection involves a serum sickness syndrome, with formation of circulating immune complexes. Immune complexes are deposited in joints and other parts of the body when the quantity of viral antigens approximates that of the antiviral antibodies. This is often transient, occurring as antigen levels fall and antibody levels rise, typically in the prodromal phase of clinical infection. In addition to arthritis, maculopapular rash, urticaria, and renal disease may result from formation of circulating immune complexes. In chronic HBV and HCV infections, formation of cryoglobulins (especially HCV) or induction of PAN can further lead to arthritic symptoms. Intermittent viremia may be responsible for chronic arthritis reported in both HBV and HCV infection. A direct viral cytopathogenic effect on the synovium has also been postulated in HBV infection.

Demographics

—*HAV:* Infection is transmitted enterally. The precise number of cases is not known; 30,000 cases/year are reported by the Centers for Disease Control and Prevention. Actual numbers are likely much higher because the illness is frequently subclinical (30%–50% of adults have serologic evidence of past exposure to HAV, but only 3%–5% recall a clinically compatible acute illness). Transient arthralgia has been reported in 10% of patients and is twice as frequent in icteric patients. Arthritis rarely occurs in HAV infection.

—*HBV:* Transmitted parenterally, sexually, and vertically, 200,000 cases of HBV occur annually in the United States, with 6% to 10% becoming chronic. Most cases occur in young adults, especially in high-risk groups such as parenteral drug users and some immigrant groups from endemic regions. Arthralgias develop in 25% of patients and frank arthritis in 10%; there is a slight male preponderance (1.5:1 male:female ratio).

—*HCV:* Antibodies to HCV are detected in 1.4% of the U.S. population. Prevalence is higher in developing countries (>3%). Transmission is primarily via contaminated blood. Risk factors include parenteral drug use, tattooing, blood transfusions, and hemodialysis. In 40% to 50%, no risk factors can be identified. Persistent infection occurs in 50% to 60% of patients. HCV-associated arthritis is uncommon. Arthritic syndromes associated with type II cryoglobulinemia are more commonly symptomatic.

Cardinal Findings

—*HAV:* Transient arthralgias may occur in acute infection. A transient serum sickness-like syndrome uncommonly occurs.

—*HBV:* The most common rheumatic syndrome in acute HBV infection is abrupt onset of a severe, symmetric polyarthritis in the prodromal phase. Simultaneous joint involvement is the usual pattern; occasionally a migratory or additive pattern is observed. The arthritis and rash are often short-lived and typically disappear with the onset of jaundice. Urticaria, petechiae, and maculopapular eruptions commonly accompany the arthritis. A similar syndrome, after HBV vaccination, has been reported. In 1% of cases of chronic

HBV infection, PAN may occur with necrotizing vasculitis, mononeuritis multiplex, and fever. HBV-associated glomerulonephritis is a variant of this condition.

—*HCV*: As many as one-third of patients with chronic HCV will have rheumatic complaints that may include an acute arthritis (rare), chronic RA-like arthritis affecting small joints and associated with low-titer positive RF and ESR elevations, and an intermittent mono/oligoarthritis (usually with cryoglobulins) of large and medium-sized joints. RA-like arthritis is typically nonerosive. Mixed cryoglobulinemia (type II cryoglobulins) has been strongly associated with chronic HCV infection (30%–90%) with associated membranoproliferative glomerulonephritis. Chronic HCV infection has been associated with Sjögren syndrome, psoriasis, or psoriatic arthritis, with sporadic reports occurring after interferon treatment.

Uncommon Findings
—*HAV*: Rarely, cryoglobulinemia may occur with purpura and arthritis. There are rare reports of inflammatory reactive arthritis after HAV vaccination.
—*HBV*: Cryoglobulinemia may occur. In persistent HBV infection, chronic polyarthritis may occur.
—*HCV*: Anti-HCV antibodies have been detected in 14% of patients with PAN.

Diagnostic Tests: See p. 73 for more information on serologic tests for hepatitis.
—*HAV* accounts for approximately 20% of cases of acute viral hepatitis in the United States. Anti-HAV IgM is found in acute HAV infection. Anti-HAV IgG indicates previous exposure to HAV. Serum transaminases rise in the prodromal phase and peak by the time jaundice develops. Other findings include leukopenia. In the icteric phase, many liver function abnormalities are noted, including hyperbilirubinemia and a prolonged prothrombin time, depending on the severity of the illness.
—*HBV* causes approximately 60% of cases of acute viral hepatitis in the United States. HBsAg is the first serologic marker to appear; anti-HBsAg follows. In chronic HBV infection, HB$_s$Ag (hepatitis B surface antigen) is detectable; anti-HB$_s$Ag is not. Serum transaminase levels vary and are often less than twice normal. Hyperbilirubinemia, if present, is usually mild. Serologic tests for ANA, RF, and native DNA are frequently positive in patients with acute or chronic HBV infection.
—*HCV* causes approximately 20% of cases of acute viral hepatitis in the United States (but HCV is responsible for 90% of posttransfusion hepatitis). IgG anti-HCV antibody is usually not seen until 2 to 6 months after acute infection. Biochemical abnormalities are typically mild; transaminase levels often wax and wane. More sensitive assays for HCV infection include ELISA, recombinant immunoblot assay, polymerase chain reaction (PCR), and branched DNA assay. Patients with HCV may be RF positive (75%) or ANA positive (>20%) or have anti–smooth muscle antibodies (>60%).

Differential Diagnosis

—*Acute arthritis:* Because arthritis occurs in the prodromal preicteric phase of hepatitis, clues to the correct diagnosis are few. Serum transaminases are frequently elevated, but the diagnosis is often made retrospectively, after jaundice develops. Nonetheless, acute polyarthritis, especially when accompanied by a serum sickness-like syndrome, should raise suspicion of acute viral hepatitis. Other viral infections presenting in a similar manner include rubella, mumps, Parvovirus B19, herpesviruses, HIV, enteroviruses, and a variety of arboviruses. At the outset, acute HBV infection may be mistaken for RA, SLE, rheumatic fever, Still's disease, or gonococcal or reactive arthritis.

—*Cryoglobulinemia:* Detection of cryoglobulins should prompt testing for viral hepatitis (HBV, HCV). Other causes of cryoglobulinemia include connective tissue diseases and myeloproliferative and lymphoproliferative disorders.

—*PAN:* Ten to 25% of cases of classic PAN are associated with chronic HBV or HCV infection.

Keys to Diagnosis: The availability of sensitive and specific assays for viral hepatitis has greatly simplified diagnosis. A high index of suspicion, especially when such risk factors for viral hepatitis as household exposure, blood transfusion, hemodialysis, and parenteral drug use are present, is the main key to establishing the correct diagnosis.

Therapy

—*Arthritis:* Acute arthritis is managed symptomatically with analgesics or NSAIDs. Chronic or intermittent arthritis may require additional measures. Many DMARDs cannot be used owing to hepatotoxic effects. Gold, hydroxychloroquine, and corticosteroids have been used with modest success. Recent studies suggest that TNF inhibitors may be used safely in patients with HCV and without flare of HCV infection, but further studies are needed. There are reports of HBV exacerbation and fulminant hepatitis occurring with TNF inhibitor use.

—*Cryoglobulinemia:* Interferon alpha has been used successfully in the management of HCV infection. In patients with HCV-associated cryoglobulinemia, interferon alpha can decrease the cryocrit and improve purpura, but symptoms often rebound after discontinuation of therapy. Purpura and arthritis can be managed with NSAIDs. If visceral organs such as the kidney and lung are involved, corticosteroids and cyclophosphamide may be required. Plasma exchange also has a role as a supplementary measure, especially with fulminant disease. Liver transplantation may be indicated in selected patients with chronic HCV infection.

—*PAN:* PAN associated with HBV infection is often problematic to treat because interferon alpha has immunostimulatory effects and glucocorticoid therapy can exacerbate HBV infection. Corticosteroids are often used initially for rapid control of the most life-threatening manifestations of PAN. This can be followed by antiviral regimens of vidarabine or interferon alpha combined with cyclophosphamide, with plasma exchange playing a supplementary role.

Prognosis

—*HAV:* Arthritis is usually transient and self-limited.

—*HBV:* Arthritis is usually self-limited but may occasionally become chronic with persistent HBV infection. HBV-associated PAN, when treated, had an 83% survival rate in one series, compared with an untreated 5-year survival rate of 13%.

—*HCV:* Arthritis is usually transient; rarely, it is chronic. HCV-associated cryoglobulinemia has a 70% 10-year survival rate overall; it is lower in patients who develop renal disease.

BIBLIOGRAPHY

Olivieri I, Palazzi C, Padula A. Hepatitis C virus and arthritis. *Rheum Dis Clin North Am* 2003;29:111–122.

Pyrsopoulos NT, Reddy KR. Extrahepatic manifestations of chronic viral hepatitis. *Curr Gastroenterol Rep* 2001;3:71–78.

Hereditary Periodic Fever Syndromes (see "Febrile Syndromes")

HIP PAIN

Definition: Hip pain is one of the most often misdiagnosed joint complaints, primarily because of the public misconception that the hip is located in either the gluteal or trochanteric region. True hip pain is sensed anteriorly and may radiate medially into the groin or to the anteromedial thigh. This is to be distinguished from the more common complaint of buttock pain that is often referred from the lumbosacral impingement of nerve roots. Trochanteric pain is sensed over the upper lateral thigh with point tenderness and usually indicates trochanteric bursitis (Fig. 5).

ICD-9 Code: 719.45.

Anatomic Considerations: Hip pain may originate in the femoral-acetabular joint or joint capsule, proximal femur or acetabulum, pelvic rami, surrounding bursae (e.g., trochanteric, ischiogluteal, iliopsoas), ligaments (e.g., inguinal, iliofemoral), and intraabdominal or vascular structures.

Etiology: Pain in the hip may result from traumatic, mechanical/degenerative, inflammatory, reactive, infectious, or neoplastic disorders affecting the joint or juxtaarticular structures.

Cardinal Findings: In elderly individuals, hip pain is commonly caused by OA of the hip, referred lumbosacral pain, trochanteric bursitis, or osteoporotic fractures. Young and middle-aged adults are often affected by trochanteric bursitis, adductor tendinitis, or inflammatory arthritis (e.g., RA, Reiter's). Hip pain in

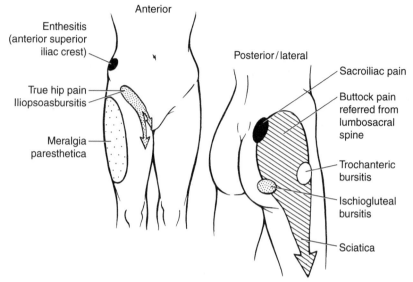

Figure 5. Origins of hip pain.

children is commonly caused by toxic synovitis of the hip, juvenile arthritis, or congenital anomalies of the joint. Toxic synovitis of the hip (see p. 381) is common in children 1 to 13 years of age and typically follows an upper respiratory infection. It manifests as an acute inflammatory arthropathy that is self-limiting and lasts 2 to 4 weeks. This condition responds well to rest and aspirin or NSAID therapy.

Referred pain accounts for many cases of hip pain. Whereas involvement of the T12–L1 nerve roots may result in buttock/trochanteric pain, L2-4 nerve roots may produce inguinal or anterior thigh pain (see Appendix E, p. 535). Thus, it is important to detect lumbosacral spine, vascular, or intraabdominal disorders that may masquerade as hip pain. Buttock pain may originate from the lumbosacral spine, sacroiliac joint, ischiogluteal bursa, or vascular insufficiency. Groin pain may be from true hip disease, iliopsoas bursitis, hernia, adductor tendinitis, pelvic fracture, osteitis pubis, ureteral stones, or pain referred from L2-4 nerve roots.

Trochanteric bursitis (see p. 259) manifests as lateral thigh pain, often with radiation downward to the knee. It is worsened by general activity, sleeping on the affected side, or sitting with the affected leg crossed.

Ischiogluteal bursitis will manifest as lower buttock pain, possibly with radiation down the leg. Pain is worsened by prolonged sitting with legs uncrossed and may be exacerbated by standing on tiptoes.

The iliopsoas bursa lies between the psoas muscle and hip joint capsule. Inflammation of the psoas bursa may manifest as pain in the groin or anterior thigh that is exacerbated by extension of the hip or flexion against resistance.

Patients may hold the joint in flexion to reduce pain. Iliopsoas bursitis is unaffected by rotation.

Acute monarticular presentations should lead the examiner to consider urgent noninflammatory (e.g., fracture) or inflammatory (e.g., septic arthritis) causes. Severe hip pain associated with weight bearing should suggest a fracture.

By virtue of its deep location, inspection and palpation is unlikely to yield diagnostic findings. Examination of periarticular bursae may disclose point tenderness over the greater trochanter laterally or ischial tuberosity posteriorly. Palpation and auscultation should identify abnormal bruits or pulsatile masses involving the abdominal aorta or iliac arteries. Palpable masses over the anterior groin may suggest a hernia or iliopsoas bursitis. Adductor tendinitis is common in young individuals who assume a straddling position (e.g., gymnasts, horseback riders) and manifests as pain in the groin or anterior thigh. Pain is elicited over the insertion of adductor musculature and is exacerbated by passive abduction or active adduction. Range of motion testing (flexion, internal and external rotation, abduction) may disclose true hip joint involvement because bursitis seldom causes true limitation of motion. True hip (and sacroiliac) disorders and range of motion are best assessed using the Patrick (or Fabere) test (see p. 12). Notably, nondisplaced fractures may demonstrate a normal range of motion until extremes in rotation are achieved. A pelvic tilt may indicate true hip disease, scoliosis, or a leg length discrepancy. Leg length discrepancies may be ascertained by comparative measurements from the anterior superior iliac crest to the lateral malleolus. Normally, there is <1 cm variation between limbs. A flexion contracture of the hip may indicate antecedent trauma or undiagnosed articular inflammation and is best diagnosed by the Thomas test (flexion of the contralateral hip results in involuntary flexion of the involved hip).

Diagnostic Testing: Laboratory testing should be guided by the clinical findings. The examiner should avoid using routine laboratory screening tests. Inflammatory or infectious conditions may be associated with nonspecific elevation of acute-phase reactants (e.g., ESR, CRP). If acute infectious arthritis is suspected, synovial fluid aspiration (under fluoroscopic guidance), culture, and analysis should be strongly considered.

Imaging: For nontraumatic acute presentations, radiographs are not indicated because they are seldom revealing. Those with trauma or who have undiagnosed chronic hip pain should undergo radiography of the hip and pelvis. Lumbosacral spine films should be obtained if there is a history of low back pain, if hip and pelvic radiographs are unrevealing, and if referred lumbosacral pain is suspected. MRI has largely replaced the bone scan in the evaluation of hip disorders and may be useful in the diagnosis of osteonecrosis, osteomyelitis, or early fractures not yet apparent by routine radiography.

Therapy: Depending on the condition, nonpharmacologic modalities of cold or warm compresses, immobilization, ambulatory-assist devices, physical therapy, and range of motion exercises may be indicated. Symptomatic control of

Table 16
Common Causes of Hip Pain

Arthritis
  Inflammatory: rheumatoid arthritis, spondyloarthropathy, septic arthritis, juvenile
    arthritis, toxic synovitis of the hip, sarcoidosis
  Noninflammatory: osteoarthritis, osteonecrosis, fracture (femur, acetabulum, pelvic
    rami), hemochromatosis, osteoid osteoma, hemarthrosis
Periarticular
  Inflammatory: septic bursitis, enthesitis, polymyalgia rheumatica, osteomyelitis
  Noninflammatory: trochanteric bursitis, iliopsoas bursitis, ischiogluteal bursitis, ad-
    ductor tendinitis
  Abdominal/genitourinary: aortic aneurysm, hernia, pelvic inflammatory disease, ureteral
    nephrolithiasis, retroperitoneal disorders, lymphadenopathy (inguinal, paraaortic)
  Bone: fracture (osteoporotic), Paget disease, osteitis pubis, osteomyelitis, osteoid os-
    teoma
  Referred pain: sciatica, degenerative disc disease, lumbar facet osteoarthritis, spinal
    stenosis, vascular insufficiency, meralgia paresthetica, sacroiliitis

pain may be achieved with NSAIDs or simple analgesics (e.g., acetaminophen). In selected instances, judicious use of local corticosteroid injections may be helpful in treating trochanteric or ischiogluteal bursitis. Surgery may be indicated for some pelvic, acetabular, or femoral fractures. Total hip replacement may be indicated in those with advanced joint damage and pain.

BIBLIOGRAPHY

DeAngelis NA, Busconi BD. Assessment and differential diagnosis of the painful hip. *Clin Orthop* 2003;406:11–18.
Newberg AH, Newman JS. Imaging the painful hip. *Clin Orthop* 2003;406:19–28.
Zacher J, Gursche A. Regional musculoskeletal conditions: 'hip' pain. *Best Pract Res Clin Rheumatol* 2003;17:71–85.

HUMAN IMMUNODEFICIENCY VIRUS: MUSCULOSKELETAL MANIFESTATIONS

ICD-9 Code: HIV, 042.0.

Definition: A variety of rheumatic syndromes may be associated with HIV-1 infection.

Etiology: Some rheumatic syndromes (e.g., septic arthritis and pyomyositis) may result from immunodeficiency secondary to CD4 T cell depletion. Others such as the lymphocytic infiltrative syndromes are a consequence of the host response to chronic antigenic stimulation by HIV-1. The diffuse infiltrative lymphocytosis syndrome has been associated with certain human leukocyte antigens (HLA): HLA-B45, HLA-B49, HLA-B50, HLA-DR5, and HLA-DR6. Infection with HIV-1 causes immune dysregulation manifest as abnormal cytokine production, which may be responsible for inflammatory arthritis. CD8-dependent diseases such as Reiter's syndrome and psoriasis seem to have a more aggressive course in HIV-1 infection.

Demographics: Forty million people are infected with HIV worldwide. Rheumatic problems usually occur later in the disease or in those with evidence of recent progression to AIDS. Epidemiologic studies on those with Reiter syndrome and psoriasis have yielded conflicting data. In general, rheumatic syndromes in the HIV-positive population seem to occur with the same frequency as in immunocompetent populations, although they may be more aggressive or demonstrate atypical features.

Clinical Subsets: Several distinct syndromes have been reported in HIV-positive patients.

—*Arthralgia/myalgia:* This syndrome occurs in one-third of patients with HIV, usually later in the disease. These symptoms are thought to be reactive in nature rather than owing to direct infection with the virus.

—*Inflammatory arthritis:* An RF-positive, symmetric, erosive polyarthritis rarely occurs in HIV-1 infection, despite CD4 T cell depletion. There are anecdotal reports of patients with RA developing HIV infection with improvement of synovitis. However, this occurrence is rare, and the relationship between RA activity and HIV infection remains unresolved. There are more than 25 reports of HIV and SLE in the medical literature.

—*Reiter's syndrome and psoriatic arthritis:* Onset is usually heralded by urethritis or enteritis and is later followed by skin and joint disease. Uveitis and sacroiliitis are rare. Cutaneous disease (psoriasis or keratoderma blenorrhagica) is very prominent. Keratoderma blenorrhagica, a papulosquamous eruption that occurs on the palms, soles, and penis, may be indistinguishable from pustular psoriasis. Oligoarticular arthritis (involving the knee or ankle), dactylitis, and enthesitis are common. Although features of SpA are often present, AS has not been associated with HIV or AIDS.

—*Diffuse infiltrative lymphocytosis syndrome:* This syndrome, a disorder resembling Sjögren syndrome, is caused by CD8 T cell infiltration with bilateral parotid gland enlargement (often massive), sicca symptoms (often minor), and prominent extraglandular sites of lymphocytic infiltration (lung, muscle, lymph nodes). CD8 T cell infiltration of the lung causes a lymphocytic interstitial pneumonitis presenting with dyspnea and can progress to fibrosis. Diffuse infiltrative lymphocytosis syndrome is associated with a very slow progression to AIDS.

—*Myopathy:* CD8 T cell infiltration may cause a myopathy indistinguishable from idiopathic PM, with elevated serum creatine kinase levels, proximal muscle weakness, and occasionally skin lesions characteristic of DM (heliotrope, Gottron papules, periungual erythema). HIV therapy with zidovudine (AZT) can cause a myopathy similar to PM but with less inflammatory infiltrate.

—*Vasculitis:* Sporadic reports in the literature describe HIV associated with hypersensitivity vasculitis (often a drug reaction), PAN, granulomatous angiitis, or primary angiitis of the CNS.

—*Musculoskeletal infections:* As in normal individuals, *S. aureus* infection accounts for >70% of cases of nongonococcal septic arthritis. Such patients often present with an acute monarthritis with systemic symptoms. Pyogenic sacroiliitis, primarily occurring in intravenous drug users, is also usually caused by *S. aureus.* With advanced CD4 T cell depletion, fungal (e.g., cryptococcal) and mycobacterial septic arthritis have been reported. The arthritis is generally monarticular and more indolent, with subtle inflammation. Juxtaarticular osteomyelitis is not an uncommon complication. Pyomyositis, or deep muscle abscess, typically presents with acute muscle pain (often in the thigh), with woody induration, swelling, and erythema; it is usually caused by *S. aureus.*

Diagnostic Tests: Abnormalities vary with the clinical picture. HIV-positive patients may have a low incidence of low-titer ANA and RF. Others have been described with cryoglobulins, APL antibodies, and false-positive VDRL results.
—*Arthritis:* Monarthritis or oligoarthritis with systemic features (e.g., fever) should prompt consideration of diagnostic arthrocentesis, synovial fluid analysis with cell count, and cultures for bacteria, fungi, and mycobacteria. Serologic tests (ANA, RF) and HLA-B27 testing are occasionally needed to diagnose inflammatory arthritis or Reiter syndrome.
—*Myopathy:* Serum creatine kinase, urine toxicology screen (i.e., cocaine), and withdrawal of zidovudine (if applicable) with repeat serum creatine kinase assay in 4 to 6 weeks should be considered. Persistent unexplained serum creatine kinase elevation should be investigated with EMG or muscle biopsy for evidence of inflammatory myositis. In pyomyositis, imaging studies (ultrasonography, CT, or MRI) are necessary for diagnosis and can be used for diagnostic aspiration, Gram stain, and culture.
—*Suspected vasculitis:* Biopsy of the most accessible or involved tissue (e.g., skin, nerve, liver, kidney) or angiography may be required to document vasculitis.
—*Diffuse infiltrative lymphocytosis syndrome:* Exocrine involvement can be documented by minor salivary gland biopsy or noninvasively with gallium-67 scans.

Therapy: Many patients with HIV infection can be safely treated with corticosteroids and a few selected agents detailed below. However, some immunosuppressive medications (e.g., MTX, azathioprine, cyclosporine, cyclophosphamide) should be avoided because they may further immunosuppress the patient and predispose to disease progression or infections.
—*Infectious musculoskeletal disease:* Antimicrobial therapy should be tailored to the causative organism. Septic joints should be serially aspirated. Inaccessible joints such as the sacroiliac require imaging-guided aspiration.
—*Reiter's syndrome or psoriatic arthritis:* Initially, optimize antiretroviral therapy. Consider using sulfasalazine (2–3 g/day in divided doses). Both in-

domethacin (75–150 mg/day) and hydroxychloroquine (400 mg/day) have proven beneficial and have anti-HIV effects as well. Effective treatment with thalidomide or TNF inhibitors (e.g., etanercept) has been described, although there is a concern about secondary infections.

—*Polymyositis (PM):* Can be safely treated with prednisone (0.5–1.0 mg/kg/day for 3 months and quickly tapered to minimum effective dose). Refractory patients may respond to intravenous gamma-globulin therapy.

—*Diffuse infiltrative lymphocytosis syndrome:* Frequently, this syndrome responds to antiretroviral therapy alone. Prednisone (20–40 mg/day) will rapidly decrease salivary gland size and improve lymphocytic interstitial pneumonitis. Taper to minimum effective dose. Patients seem to tolerate low-dose prednisone well.

—*Vasculitis:* High-dose corticosteroids may be necessary for those with systemic necrotizing vasculitis. Advanced HIV infection often precludes immunosuppressive therapy, but it has been used in some patients with life-threatening vasculitis.

Prognosis: The HIV stage often determines the prognosis. Patients with advanced HIV infection generally have a poorer response to therapy. Patients with diffuse infiltrative lymphocytosis syndrome generally respond well and are typically long-term nonprogressors. Vasculitis in HIV-1 has a poor prognosis. The protease inhibitors (relatively new, powerful antiretroviral drugs) can, in some instances, dramatically reverse clinical disease.

BIBLIOGRAPHY

Medina Rodríguez F. Rheumatic manifestations of human immunodeficiency virus infection. *Rheum Dis Clin North Am* 2003;29:145–161.

HYPERMOBILITY SYNDROME

Synonyms: Benign joint hypermobility syndrome.

ICD-9 code: 728.5.

Definition: The term *hypermobility syndrome,* coined by Ansell and Bywaters in 1967, denotes joint symptoms associated with excessive joint laxity, often in individuals with a strong family history of the same. This benign disorder excludes other causes of connective tissue laxity (Ehlers-Danlos syndrome, Marfan's syndrome, osteogenesis imperfecta) that may result in cutaneous, ocular, or cardiovascular complications.

Etiology: It appears to be a genetically linked disorder of connective tissue. This is suggested by a strong family history. Family members may be asymptomatic yet exhibit the same connective tissue findings on examination.

Pathology: Thin skin with reduction and disorganization of collagen fibers. Alterations in collagen content and type have been reported.

Demographics: Symptoms often begin in children and young adults but may persist throughout adulthood. It is most common in females (60%–85%). Young women often have a history of gymnastics, ballet, dancing, and contortionism and later develop hypermobility syndrome when they resume physical activity. Older individuals can be suspected as having hypermobility syndrome with the onset of premature OA.

Cardinal Features: Symmetric joint pain, stiffness, and fatigue may arise or be aggravated by use. Some experience brief subjective swelling. Overuse and traumatic syndromes occur and may include recurrent sprains, tendonitis, and dislocations. Affected joints include the hands, wrists, elbows, feet, knees, and low back. Localized and asymmetric forms are common. Patients should be examined for hyperextensible joints using Beighton maneuvers (Table 17). Scoliosis, genu valgum, pes planus, and excessive lateral motion of patella or proximal interphalangeal joints are evident on examination. A marfanoid habitus and hyperextensible skin are seen with hypermobility syndrome.

Uncommon Findings: Dysautonomia (autonomic nervous system dysfunction) with complaints of palpitations, chest pains, light-headedness, orthostatic

Table 17
Diagnostic Criteria for Hypermobility Syndrome

Beighton Criteria[a]: Screening maneuvers for hypermobility
1. Passive hyperextension of fifth metacarpophalangeal joint >90 degrees
2. Passive apposition of the thumb to flexor aspect of forearm
3. Hyperextension of the elbows >10 degrees
4. Hyperextension of the knee >10 degrees
5. Flexing the trunk and placing hands flat on the floor while keeping knees locked/extended

1998 Revised Brighton Criteria[b] for Benign Joint Hypermobility Syndrome
Major criteria
1. Beighton score ≥4 (of 9) current or historic
2. Arthralgia (≥4 joints) for at least 3 mo

Minor criteria
1. Beighton score of 1–3 (0–3 if >age 50 y)
2. Oligoarthralgia, back pain, spondylosis for ≥3 mo
3. Dislocation/subluxation in ≥1 joint more than once
4. Soft tissue rheumatism ≥3 lesions (bursitis, epicondylitis, tenosynovitis)
5. Marfanoid habitus
6. Abnormal skin striae, hyperextensibility of skin, papyraceous scarring
7. Drooping eyelids, myopia, or antimongoloid slant
8. Varicose veins or hernia or uterine/rectal prolapse

[a]Scores range from 0 to 9: 1 point for each side (metacarpophalangeal, thumb, elbow, knee joints) and 1 point for hands to floor. Diagnosis of hypermobility syndrome requires 4 or more points.
[b]Diagnosis requires two major criteria or one major and two minor or four minor criteria or two minor criteria with unequivocally affected first-degree relative. These criteria have only been established for adults older than the age of 16 years.

dizziness, and syncope is more common in hypermobility syndrome than matched control patients. Urinary stress incontinence may occur.

Complications: Although suggested by some studies, it is not clear whether patients with hypermobility have an increased rate of cardiac complications (mitral valve prolapse, other valvular lesions, aortic root disorders, abnormal electrocardiogram).

Imaging: Patients with benign joint hypermobility syndrome have a tendency for osteopenia and premature OA.

Diagnostic Criteria: Brighton criteria have long been used. Recent Brighton criteria expand the ability to make this diagnosis. Ethnic and age variations may allow for as many as 5% to 25% to achieve at least 4 points using the Brighton scale.

Keys to Diagnosis: Hypermobility syndrome is more common in young females. To diagnose the syndrome, Brighton criteria (at least 4 points, but higher is preferred) plus any of the following are required: a similar family history, joint complaints, ligamentous injuries, flatfeet, marfanoid habitus, or easy bruising. Children with fibromyalgia-like complaints should be evaluated for hypermobility syndrome.

Differential Diagnosis: Fibromyalgia, genetic disorders of joint laxity (Ehlers-Danlos syndrome, Marfan syndrome, osteogenesis imperfecta, homocystinuria, pseudoxanthoma elasticum), rheumatic fever, or acromegaly.

Therapy: Patients will benefit from reassurance. Maintenance of low body weight and moderate exercise to maintain extensor muscular and ligamentous support is advised. Modification of daily activities (especially those that provoke) and avoidance of repetitive joint stress are more effective than the use of simple analgesics or NSAIDs. Joint injections should be discouraged.

Prognosis: Some suggestion that patients with hypermobility syndrome are at risk of ligamentous and tendinous injury and may be at risk of premature OA.

BIBLIOGRAPHY

Gazit Y, Nahir AM, Grahame R, et al. Dysautonomia in the joint hypermobility syndrome. *Am J Med* 2003;115:33–40.

Graham R, Bird HA, Child A. The revised (Brighton 1998) criteria for the diagnosis of benign joint hypermobility syndrome (BJHS). *J Rheumatol* 2000;27:1777–1779.

Kirk JA, Ansell BM, Bywaters EGL. The hypermobility syndrome: musculoskeletal complaints associated with generalized joint hypermobility. *Ann Rheum Dis* 1967;26:419–425.

HYPERTROPHIC OSTEOARTHROPATHY

Synonyms: HOA, Acropachy, familial idiopathic hypertrophic osteoarthropathy, pachydermoperiostosis, Marie-Bamberger syndrome.

ICD-9 Code: 731.2.

Definition: Hypertrophic osteoarthropathy is a syndrome characterized by proliferation of skin and bone in the distal extremities. The complete hypertrophic osteoarthropathy syndrome includes clubbing of the fingers and toes, periostitis (with new bone formation on long bones), and arthritis. Not all patients have all manifestations.

Etiology: The primary form is of unknown etiology, but most likely has a genetic basis. Secondary forms are associated with pulmonary (cystic fibrosis, pulmonary fibrosis, cancer, chronic infection), cardiac (cyanotic congenital heart disease, patent ductus arteriosus, bacterial endocarditis), GI (inflammatory bowel disease, cancer, cirrhosis), or malignant disorders (lymphoma). Mechanisms underlying these associations are unknown.

Pathology: Long bones show various stages of new bone formation on cortical surfaces. Clubbed digits show increased numbers of fibroblasts, and collagenous tissue and synovial membranes may have proliferative features.

Demographics: The primary genetic form appears in children or young adults. Secondary forms are more likely to be seen in older patients.

Cardinal Findings: Clubbed digits (fingers and toes) have been described as having a drumstick-like appearance, with softening and mobility of the nail bed. Involvement of long bones may produce severe, incapacitating, or deep bone pain. Areas affected by periostitis are often painful and may be associated with overlying warmth or edema. Arthralgia or arthritis is often symmetric and involves the metacarpophalangeal, wrist, elbow, knee, and ankle joints. Joints may be warm and swollen with an effusion.

Uncommon Findings: Thickening of the skin (pachydermia) may alter facial features and produce coarse or leonine features. Pachydermia is uncommon in the secondary forms of hypertrophic osteoarthropathy. Thyroid acropachy, a rare manifestation of hyperthyroidism, may be associated with exophthalmos and pretibial myxedema.

Diagnostic Tests: Laboratory tests are not specific for hypertrophic osteoarthropathy but may reflect the underlying malignant or infectious disorder. The ESR is often elevated in secondary hypertrophic osteoarthropathy. Synovial fluid is often noninflammatory (WBCs <2,000 cells/mm^3).

Imaging: Radiographs of long bones show new bone formation (periostitis), especially in the extremities. Periostitis is common in the distal tibia or fibula, radius, or ulna. It is less common in the phalanges. Acroosteolysis may be seen; joint space narrowing or erosions are absent. Bone scanning may be useful.

Diagnostic Criteria: Digital clubbing and periostosis of tubular bones are required for the complete syndrome. Three incomplete forms are defined: (a) clubbing alone; (b) periostosis without clubbing but with any of the systemic illnesses associated with hypertrophic osteoarthropathy; and (c) pachydermia associated with any of the minor manifestations, including synovial effusions.

Differential Diagnosis: Skin resembles scleroderma. See causes for periostitis (p. 289).

Therapy: Clubbing alone requires no specific treatment. Secondary forms respond to removal or treatment of underlying thoracic disease. NSAIDs are used to treat symptoms.

Prognosis: In secondary forms, the outcome is dictated by the underlying disorder.

BIBLIOGRAPHY

Martinez-Lavin M, Matucci-Cerinic M, Jajic I, et al. Hypertrophic osteoarthropathy: consensus on its definition, classification, assessment and diagnostic criteria. *J Rheumatol* 1993; 20:1386–1387.

IMMUNODEFICIENCY

Synonyms: Common variable immunodeficiency; severe combined immunodeficiency; X-linked immunodeficiency.

ICD-9 Codes: Immunodeficiency, 279.3; common variable, 279.06; severe combined, 279.2.

Definition: Immunodeficiency diseases are a diverse group of disorders that result from quantitative or qualitative defects in specific parts of the immune system. They may be categorized as primary or secondary (Table 18).

Etiology: Primary immunodeficiencies often relate to focal defects in enzyme systems, cell surface molecules, or other factors critical to development or function of immunocompetent cells. Secondary immunodeficiencies represent impairments in the immune response related to use of immunosuppressive medications, systemic infections, and other conditions.

Demographics: The incidence of primary immunodeficiencies ranges from one in 10,000 to one in 100,000 population. They typically arise in children, and approximately 85% of cases are found in persons 15 years of age or younger. Because many of the primary immunodeficiencies are X-linked, boys substantially outnumber girls. Secondary immunodeficiencies are much more common than primary; in addition, they occur most commonly among older adults.

Cardinal Findings: The clinical hallmark of immunodeficiency is increased susceptibility to infection. However, some immunodeficiencies are associated with a variety of autoimmune and musculoskeletal manifestations. This is par-

Table 18
Immunodeficiency Diseases

Selected primary immunodeficiencies
  B cell (antibody/immunoglobulin) defects
    X-linked (Bruton) agammaglobulinemia
    Common variable immunodeficiency
    IgA deficiency
  Combined B cell and T cell defects
    Severe combined immunodeficiency
    Wiskott-Aldrich syndrome
  T cell defects
    DiGeorge syndrome
  Phagocyte defects
    Chronic granulomatous disease
  Complement deficiencies
Selected causes of secondary immunodeficiency
  Pharmacologic/therapeutic
    Corticosteroids
    Chemotherapeutic drugs
    Plasmapheresis
    Irradiation
  Lymphoproliferative disease
    Lymphoma/leukemia
  Infectious diseases
    HIV-1, HIV-2
    Influenza
  Systemic inflammatory diseases
    Systemic lupus erythematosus
    Rheumatoid arthritis
  Other diseases
    Protein-losing nephropathy/enteropathy
    Diabetes mellitus
    Solid tumors
    Malnutrition

HIV, human immunodeficiency virus.

ticularly true for antibody- or immunoglobulin-deficiency syndromes, which have been associated with an increased incidence of arthritis, SLE, immune thrombocytopenia, autoimmune hemolytic anemia, myositis, and vasculitis. The most common musculoskeletal manifestation is arthritis, which may occur in 35% of untreated patients with immunoglobulin deficiency. The arthritis is usually oligoarticular and affects the larger joints such as the knee. However, some patients have joint involvement resembling that of RA. In some patients, the arthritis may be related to infection with *Mycoplasma*. The presumed infectious etiology of the arthritis in these patients is supported by a decreased incidence among patients receiving therapy with γ-globulin.

Diagnostic Tests: The diagnosis of an immunodeficiency is established by demonstrating defects in particular components of the immune response. For immunoglobulin deficiencies, one should initially determine the serum immunoglobulin (IgG, IgA, IgM) levels (see p. 79). In rare cases, more elaborate testing may be required.

Keys to Diagnosis: Key to the diagnosis of an underlying immunodeficiency is a high degree of clinical suspicion. Patients typically have a history of recurrent infections that may also be excessively severe, respond poorly to therapy, or be caused by unusual organisms.

Therapy: Therapy of antibody deficiency syndromes consists of gammaglobulin, typically administered intravenously at 4-week intervals. This has almost entirely replaced such older forms of therapy as intramuscular gammaglobulin or prophylactic antibiotics.

Prognosis: With appropriate treatment, the prognosis of those with antibody deficiency diseases improves substantially and approaches normal.

BIBLIOGRAPHY

Cassidy JT, Burt A, Petty R, et al. Selective IgA deficiency in connective tissue diseases. *N Engl J Med* 1969;280:275–279.

Huston DP, Kavanaugh AF, Rohane PW, et al. Immunoglobulin deficiency syndromes and therapy. *J Allergy Clin Immunol* 1991;87:1–19.

Rosen FS, Cooper MD, Wedgwood JP. The primary immunodeficiencies. *N Engl J Med* 1995;333:431–440.

INCLUSION BODY MYOSITIS

ICD-9 Code: 728.89.

Definition: Inclusion body myositis is a form of idiopathic inflammatory myositis (IIM) (see p. 298) of unknown etiology. Inclusion body myositis has distinct differences from the more common forms of IIM, PM, and DM.

Pathology: Histopathologic analysis is the key differentiating feature between inclusion body myositis and other forms of IIM. On light microscopic analysis, there is an endomysial accumulation of mononuclear cells, particularly CD8$^+$ T cells (similar to the findings in PM). Other characteristic findings in muscle include vacuoles lined with basophilic granules, eosinophilic inclusions, abnormal microtubular filaments in nuclear and cytoplasmic inclusions, and ragged red fibers.

Demographics: Affected patients are usually older than 50 years old. The male:female ratio is 2:1 or higher. Inclusion body myositis represents 15% to 30% of IIM cases, which have a prevalence of five to 10 per million population.

Cardinal Findings: Symmetric proximal muscle weakness is typically present. Weakness is often slowly progressive and painless. In contrast to PM/DM, distal muscle weakness, and asymmetric involvement are more commonly seen in inclusion body myositis. In addition, 30% of patients may have an associated axonal neuropathy.

Diagnostic Tests: Muscle enzymes (e.g., creatine kinase) are elevated in inclusion body myositis as they are in IIM but usually less so in inclusion body myositis (as much as 10 times normal) than in PM/DM (as much as 50 times normal). Electromyography shows a myopathic pattern (similar to that of PM/DM). Nonetheless, muscle biopsy with electron microscopic analysis is required to make a diagnosis of inclusion body myositis.

Keys to Diagnosis: Often the diagnosis of inclusion body myositis is made when patients with presumed PM or DM either do not respond to steroid therapy or display atypical manifestations (e.g., asymmetry, distal muscle weakness, peripheral neuropathy). In such instances, inclusion body myositis should be suspected, and muscle biopsy repeated or reviewed with emphasis on electron microscopic findings.

Differential Diagnosis: The differential diagnosis of inclusion body myositis includes other types of IIM as well as other endocrinologic, metabolic, infectious, and toxic etiologies (see p. 249).

Diagnostic Criteria: Diagnostic criteria for inclusion body myositis have been proposed but not validated (Table 19).

Therapy: Patients are treated like patients with PM/DM. However, because of the poor response to corticosteroid or immunosuppressive therapies, many physicians do not pursue aggressive or alternative therapies in patients with inclusion body myositis with little or no response to corticosteroids.

Table 19
Proposed Diagnostic Criteria for Inclusion Body Myositis

Pathologic criteria
  Electron microscopy
    1. Microtubular filaments in the inclusions
  Light microscopy
    1. Lined vacuoles
    2. Intranuclear and intracytoplasmic inclusions
Clinical criteria
    1. Proximal muscle weakness (insidious onset)
    2. Distal muscle weakness
    3. Electromyographic evidence of generalized inflammatory myopathy
    4. Elevation of muscle enzyme levels (creatine kinase, aldolase)
    5. Failure of muscle weakness to improve with steroids
Definite IBM = pathologic electron microscopic criterion and clinical criterion 1 + 1 other clinical criterion
Probable IBM = pathologic light microscopic criterion 1 and clinical criterion 1 + 3 other clinical criteria
Possible IBM = pathologic light microscopic criterion 2 + any 3 clinical criteria

Prognosis: Inclusion body myositis is a slowly progressive disorder, and patients are less likely to respond to therapy than those with other types of IIM. Approximately 50% of patients have no response to corticosteroids; rare patients have a complete response.

BIBLIOGRAPHY

Rose MB. A prospective natural history study of inclusion body myositis: implications for clinical trials. *Neurology* 2001;57:548–550.
Sayers ME, Chou SM, Calabrese LH. Inclusion body myositis: analysis of 32 cases. *J Rheumatol* 1992;19:1385–1389.

INTESTINAL-BYPASS SYNDROME

Synonyms: Arthritis-dermatitis syndrome.

Definition: Arthritis and dermatitis develops in less than 30% of patients after intestinal (jejunoileal or jejunocolonic) bypass surgery for the treatment of morbid obesity. This syndrome has not been reported with newer bariatric techniques (vertical band gastroplasty).

Etiology: Symptoms result from blind loop bacterial overgrowth; treatment with antibiotics tends to alleviate symptoms. This may represent a form of reactive arthritis. The significance of circulating cryoglobulins and immune complexes is unknown.

Demographics: Women are more often affected than men.

Cardinal Findings: Acute onset occurs 1 to 30 months after bypass surgery. Patients may complain of intermittent diarrhea, bloating, cramping, low-grade fever, and malaise. Patients may have episodic or migratory arthralgia or nondeforming symmetric polyarthritis involving large and small joints. Joint effusions tend to be mildly inflammatory. Tendinitis and myalgias are common. Joint symptoms and GI symptoms do not run a parallel course. Cutaneous findings (66%–80%) often accompany arthritis and manifest as vesiculopustular lesions over the extremities or trunk. Less common are erythematous macules and urticarial or erythema nodosum–like lesions.

Uncommon Findings: Sacroiliitis, spondylitis, conjunctivitis, episcleritis, retinal vasculitis, serositis, Raynaud's phenomenon, dysarthria, hemolytic anemia, and thrombocytopenia can be seen.

Diagnostic Tests: CBC is normal or reveals mild leukocytosis. ESR is modestly elevated (20–60 mm/h). Cryoglobulins and circulating immune complexes are found in some patients.

Imaging: Radiographs may reveal only soft tissue swelling.

Differential Diagnosis: Gonococcal arthritis, Sweet's syndrome, erythema nodosum, ulcerative colitis, reactive arthritis, Behçet's syndrome, and Whipple's disease should be considered.

Therapy: Some patients respond to antibiotic therapy (tetracyclines, clindamycin, or metronidazole). Most require NSAIDs or low-dose corticosteroids (5–15 mg prednisone per day). Nonresponsive patients may respond to dapsone or may require corrective surgery (sphincteroplasty or reanastomosis).

BIBLIOGRAPHY

Fisch C. First presentation of intestinal bypass syndrome 18 yr after initial surgery. *Rheumatology* 2001;40:351–353.

JUVENILE ARTHRITIS

Synonyms: Juvenile Rhuematoid Arthritis (JRA); Juvenile Idiopathic Arthritis (JIA); Juvenile Chronic Arthritis (JCA).

ICD-9 Codes: Juvenile arthritis, 714.3; systemic juvenile arthritis, 714.3; polyarticular juvenile arthritis, 714.31; pauciarticular juvenile arthritis, 714.32.

Definition: Juvenile arthritis (JA) comprises a group of inflammatory arthropathies that affect children younger than the age of 16 years. Juvenile arthritis may be divided into four subsets that differ in their presentation (in the first 6 months) and outcomes: pauciarticular juvenile arthritis, juvenile spondylitis, polyarticular juvenile arthritis, and systemic-onset juvenile arthritis (Table 20).

Etiology: The cause of juvenile arthritis is unknown. Disordered immunoregulation has been reported, and some have suggested a role for latent viral infection, especially rubella. Increased numbers of patients with juvenile arthritis are seen among those with IgA deficiency and hypogammaglobulinemia. Future research in this area must study subsets separately because they are unlikely to share a common cause.

Pathology: Synovial inflammatory changes are similar to those seen in RA.

Demographics: Juvenile arthritis may affect children at any age from birth to 16 years. Onset is usually before the age of 9 years. Incidence rates are roughly 12 to 20 cases per 100,000 population. Females are more commonly affected than males, with the exception of juvenile spondylitis (males predominate) and systemic juvenile arthritis (equally affected) (Table 20).

Cardinal Findings: Presentations and manifestations vary with each disease subset.
—*Pauciarticular juvenile arthritis:* This is the most common variety of juvenile arthritis, accounting for >50% of cases. Onset is usually before 6 years of

Table 20
Comparison of Juvenile Arthritis Subsets

	Pauciarticular-Onset JA	Juvenile Spondylitis	Polyarticular-Onset JA	Systemic Onset JA
Frequency	50%	10%	30%	10%
Onset age (y)	1–10	9–16	3–16	3–16
Female:male	5:1	1:4	4:1	1:1
Joint pattern	Mono- or pauciarticular	Sacroiliitis or asymmetric oligoarthritis	Polyarticular, symmetric	Polyarticular
Extraarticular features	Rare	Psoriasis, enthesitis, inflammatory bowel disease	Rheumatoid nodules, weight loss	Fever, rash, lymphadenopathy, serositis, hepatosplenomegaly
Uveitis	10%–50%	10%	Rare	Rare
Laboratory findings	RF(−), 85% ANA(+)	50% are HLA-B27(+)	80% RF(−), 20% RF(+), 40% ANA(+)	Leukocytosis, ESR > 50 mm/h, anemia, increased LFTs, negative ANA & RF
Prognosis	Excellent for joints: guarded for eyes	? Risk of spondylitis and uveitis	Severe erosive arthritis in 50% of RF(−) patients	50% develop chronic arthritis; 20% severe erosive arthritis

age. Monarthritis or oligoarthritis (two to four joints) is seen in the first 6 months. The knee is most commonly and hip least commonly affected. Most achieve remission. However, there is a serious risk of uveitis in this subset. Blindness occurs in <10% of patients and can be prevented by early detection and treatment. Most patients are ANA positive.

—*Juvenile spondylitis:* This is also known as late-onset pauciarticular disease. Males are more commonly affected than females, and onset is usually between 9 and 16 years of age. Onset is typically characterized by pauciarthritis affecting the knee, ankle, or hip. Some patients have a family history of psoriasis or a SpA. Extraarticular features of an SpA rarely antedate and usually follow the onset of arthritis. HLA-B27 positivity is seen in nearly half, and sacroiliitis may be clinically or radiographically evident. Between 20% and 50% of these patients go on to develop a chronic SpA (see p. 358).

—*Polyarticular juvenile arthritis:* Nearly 30% of patients have involvement of five or more joints, often in a symmetric distribution similar to that seen in adult RA. RF positivity is seen in 20% to 30%, and ANA positivity is seen in 40% of patients with polyarticular disease. Constitutional features of low-grade fever, weight loss, and lymphadenopathy are occasionally seen. Rheumatoid nodules are only seen in RF-positive patients. This subset tends to have a chronic course and significant disability. More than 20% develop severe, erosive juvenile arthritis that is indistinguishable from seropositive adult RA.

—*Systemic-onset juvenile arthritis:* Also known as Still's disease, this subset accounts for 10% of cases. Manifestations include daily spiking (quotidian) fevers of $\geq102°F$; an evanescent, salmon-pink rash; arthritis; generalized lymphadenopathy; serositis; hepato- or splenomegaly; weight loss; myalgias; neutrophilic leukocytosis; anemia; increased ESR (often >50 mm/h); negative serologic tests for ANA and RF; and nonspecific elevations of hepatic enzymes. Systemic disease is seldom life threatening (i.e., pericardial tamponade or DIC), and prognosis is most often determined by the arthritis. Severe erosive, chronic, disabling arthritis develops in 20%. Juvenile arthritis is identical to AOSD (see p. 110), except for less prodromal sore throat in juveniles.

Uncommon Findings: Patients with polyarticular disease are at risk for micrognathia and growth retardation. Patients with systemic juvenile arthritis may develop pleuritis, pericarditis, myocarditis, DIC, amyloidosis, or salicylate hepatotoxicity.

Complications: Chronic nongranulomatous uveitis (see p. 386) occurs in 10% to 50% of patients with pauciarticular disease. There is a questionable association of uveitis with ANA positivity. Most patients are asymptomatic, but some manifest pain and altered vision. It tends to be bilateral, chronic, and progressive and may lead to band keratopathy, posterior synechiae, cataracts, glaucoma, visual loss, or blindness. All patients with pauciarticular and polyarticular juvenile arthritis should undergo slit-lamp examinations every 3 to 6 months to identify early inflammatory lesions.

Cervical arthritis, especially C2-3 apophyseal fusion, may be seen in patients with pauciarticular, polyarticular, or systemic disease.

Diagnostic Tests: There is no diagnostic laboratory test for JA. Extreme elevations of WBCs and ESR are typical in the systemic subset. RF positivity is seen in a minority of patients with polyarticular disease. ANA positivity is common in both pauciarticular and RF-positive patients with polyarticular disease. HLA-B27 assay (see p. 75) is seldom necessary to establish a diagnosis of juvenile spondylitis.

Imaging: Early radiographic changes may include soft tissue swelling, juxtaarticular osteopenia, or periostitis. Stunted or accelerated bone growth may be seen. With chronicity, loss of joint space and marginal erosions may develop. Fusion of cervical zygapophyseal joints (especially C2-3) may be seen. Atlantoaxial (C1-2) subluxation is less common than in RA.

Keys to Diagnosis: Juvenile arthritis should be suspected with development of a chronic (>6 weeks) inflammatory arthritis in a child. The diagnosis is further established by identifying the pattern of arthritis and associated extraarticular features.

Diagnostic Criteria: ACR criteria are shown in Table 21.

Differential Diagnosis: Other disorders may affect children in a similar fashion, including SLE, reactive arthritis, Lyme disease, DM, Kawasaki's disease, rheumatic fever, infantile-onset multisystemic inflammatory disease, and the vasculitides. Acute-onset inflammatory mon- or oligoarthritis should raise the possibility of septic arthritis, toxic synovitis of the hip, and especially staphylococcal, streptococcal, or gonococcal arthritis. Arthritis may herald the onset of neoplasia (e.g., leukemia, neuroblastoma) in children.

Therapy: A comprehensive approach to treatment must be initiated from the time of diagnosis and must involve the patient and family. Ongoing patient/family education should be interspersed with assessments by the physical therapist, ophthalmologist, dentist, and orthopaedist, if necessary. Patients should be enrolled in a program of active exercise, passive stretch, and periods of rest when the disease is most active. The goal of drug therapy is to reduce pain and inflammation, maintain optimal function, and avoid drug toxicity. This is particularly important with regard to corticosteroids, which should be avoided in children because growth retardation may be an unfortunate consequence.

—*NSAIDs:* Aspirin has historically been used to treat juvenile arthritis. Doses of 80 to 100 mg/kg per day are used to achieve serum levels between 18 and 25 mg/dL. Because of the risk of Reye's syndrome, aspirin should not be used in children suspected of having influenza, varicella, or other active viral infections. Aspirin and NSAIDs do not alter the course of disease but are effective in ameliorating joint pain and stiffness. Children with juvenile arthritis may be at increased risk of salicylate hepatotoxicity. In recent years, a variety of

Table 21
American College or Rheumatology Classification Criteria for the Diagnosis of Juvenile Rheumatoid Arthritis

1. Age at onset younger than 16 years
2. Arthritis in ≥1 joints: defined as swelling or effusion or at least 2 of the following:
   Limitation of range of motion
   Tenderness or pain on motion
   Increased heat
3. Duration of disease ≥6 wk
4. Type of onset of disease during the first 6 mo classified as
   a. Polyarthritis: ≥5 joints
   b. Oligoarthritis: ≤4 joints
   c. Systemic disease with arthritis and intermittent fever
5. Exclusion of other forms of juvenile arthritis

NSAIDs have gained popularity, and few are FDA approved for use in juvenile arthritis. Commonly used NSAIDs are dosed according to body mass and include ibuprofen (30–50 mg/kg/day) q.i.d., tolmetin (15–30 mg/kg/day) q.i.d., naproxen (10–20 mg/kg/day) b.i.d., and indomethacin (1–3 mg/kg/day) t.i.d. These agents are dosed based on body mass. Less than 50% of patients respond to NSAIDs alone. Multiple NSAIDs should not be used at the same time because this increases the risk of serious GI toxicity.

—DMARDs: MTX (10–15 mg/m^2/wk) or intramuscular gold (5 mg test dose, then 0.75–1.0 mg/kg/wk) is most commonly used in the treatment of chronic poly- or pauciarticular juvenile arthritis unresponsive to NSAID therapy and other conservative measures. Alternative DMARDs include hydroxychloroquine (5–7 mg/kg/day), D-penicillamine (5–10 mg/kg/day), auranofin (0.1 mg/kg/day), sulfasalazine (30–50 mg/kg/day), and cyclosporine. Patients with intractable systemic-onset arthritis (i.e., fever, rash) may benefit from long-term MTX therapy. Alternatively, patients may receive hydroxychloroquine, azathioprine, or cyclosporine to control their systemic manifestations. Etanercept has been approved for use in juvenile arthritis. Anakinra appears to be more effective than TNF inhibitors controlling the systemic manifestations of Still disease.

—Corticosteroids: Systemic steroids should be avoided unless absolutely indicated. Prednisone doses of 5 mg/day or more may result in growth retardation. Corticosteroid therapy should be reserved for intractable systemic disease, life-threatening pericarditis or pericardial tamponade, and visual compromise owing to iridocyclitis. Patients with refractory monarthritis or new joint contracture owing to synovitis may benefit from intraarticular corticosteroid injection(s).

—Eye disease: Inflammatory uveitis may respond to topical corticosteroid eyedrops and mydriatics. Systemic administration is seldom necessary. Secondary glaucoma may also require treatment.

BIBLIOGRAPHY

Burgos-Vargas R, Pacheco-Tena C, Vazquez-Mellado J. The juvenile-onset spondyloarthritides: rationale for clinical evaluation. Best Pract Res Clin Rheumatol 2002;16:551–572.
Olson JC. Juvenile idiopathic arthritis: an update. WMJ 2003;102:45–50.
Petty RE, Smith JR, Rosenbaum JT. Arthritis and uveitis in children. A pediatric rheumatology perspective. Am J Ophthalmol 2003;135:879–884.
Ravelli A, Martini A. Early predictors of outcome in juvenile idiopathic arthritis. Clin Exp Rheumatol 2003;21(5 suppl 31):S89–S93.
Schneider R, Passo MH. Juvenile rheumatoid arthritis. Rheum Dis Clin North Am 2002;28:503–530.

KAWASAKI'S DISEASE

Synonym: Mucocutaneous lymph node syndrome.

ICD-9 Code: 446.1.

Definition: Kawasaki's disease is an acute febrile illness of children.

Etiology: Although a variety of infectious organisms and other environmental agents have been proposed to be of etiologic relevance, none has been conclusively implicated. However, there is evidence of restricted clonality of T cells in patients with Kawasaki's disease, strongly suggesting an immune response to an as yet unidentified antigen.

Demographics: Most affected patients are under 5 years old, with many cases arising in infancy. There is a slight (~1.4:1) female preponderance. It is most common in Japan but is increasingly seen in China, the United States, and England. It is considered an uncommon disease, with an incidence of four to 15 cases per 100,000 younger than the age of 5 years.

Cardinal Findings: Typically, Kawasaki's disease presents acutely. After a few days of intermittent or consistent fever, patients develop conjunctival injection, swelling of the lips and oral mucous membranes, cervical lymphadenopathy, and rash. An erythematous macular rash may appear on the trunk, limbs, hands, or feet and may be accompanied by diffuse swelling. Skin lesions may resolve with desquamation. Coronary aneurysms may occur early in the first few weeks of disease. The prevalence of these lesions decreases from 20% to 10% to 5% at 1 month, 2 months, and 1 year, respectively. Aneurysms >8 mm in diameter are less likely to regress. Potential sequelae of coronary arterial involvement with Kawasaki disease include rupture and myocardial infarction. The mortality rate is ~0.1%.

Diagnostic Testing: Common abnormalities include leukocytosis, thrombocytosis, elevated transaminases, CRP, and ESR. Electrocardiogram abnormalities are common.

Diagnostic Criteria: Diagnostic features include: (a) fever for ≥5 days; (b) erythema of the palms or soles with edema or desquamation in the convalescent stage; (c) polymorphous truncal rash; (d) bilateral conjunctival injection; (e) erythema of the lips, strawberry tongue, or oral mucosa injection; and (f) acute nonpurulent cervical lymphadenopathy. A diagnosis of Kawasaki's disease requires that five of the six criteria be fulfilled or that four criteria be present with evidence of coronary aneurysm by echocardiography or angiography.

Therapy: Treatment is directed primarily at preventing development or progression of coronary aneurysms. The current standard therapy consists of high-dose intravenous gamma-globulin (2 g/kg IgG, administered as either a single dose or in split doses, e.g., 400 mg/kg for 5 days) in conjunction with aspirin (30–100 mg/kg/day). Aspirin may be continued in patients with persistent aneurysms until the lesions resolve.

BIBLIOGRAPHY

Burns JC. Kawasaki disease. *Adv Pediatr* 2001;48:157–177.

Kato H, Ichinose E, Kawasaki T. Myocardial infarction in Kawasaki disease: clinical analysis in 195 cases. *J Pediatr* 1986;108:923–927.

KIKUCHI'S DISEASE

Synonyms: Kikuchi-Fujimoto disease, histiocytic necrotizing lymphadenitis.

ICD-9 Code: 683.0.

Definition: A benign, rare disorder that affects young women (more so than men) with recurrent necrotizing lymphadenitis often associated with other systemic inflammatory or infectious disorders.

Pathology: Lymph node biopsies show histiocytic necrotizing lymphadenitis, fragmentation, necrosis, karyorrhexis zonation, and absence of neutrophils and predominance of histiocytes, T lymphocytes with many plasmacytoid monocytes. Immunohistochemistry may be necessary to distinguish Kikuchi's from malignant lymphoma.

Risk Factors: Kikuchi's disease may be seen in association with lupus, Still's disease, interstitial lung disease, hemophagocytic syndrome, mononeuritis, or infections (e.g., tuberculosis, HIV, Parvovirus, *Brucella*).

Cardinal Findings: Affects adolescents and young adults (<40 years) with painful cervical lymphadenopathy, often associated with fever, flu-like symptoms, weight loss, and night sweats, and uncommonly demonstrates arthritis or hepatosplenomegaly.

Diagnostic Tests: Tests are normal or show nonspecific elevations of ESR, CRP, and hepatic enzymes. Lactate dehydrogenase is usually elevated and 20% to 50% will show lymphopenia.

Differential Diagnosis: Lupus, infective lymphadenopathy, and lymphoma.

Therapy: Supportive care and corticosteroids are primarily used.

Prognosis: Kikuchi's disease is a self-limiting disease that will spontaneously remit in 4 to 6 months, although lymph nodes may persist longer.

BIBLIOGRAPHY

Chen YH, Lan JL. Kikuchi disease in systemic lupus erythematosus: clinical features and literature review. *J Microbiol Immunol Infect* 1998;31:187–192.

KNEE PAIN

Definition: The knee joint is the largest and most frequently affected peripheral joint. This primarily relates to its importance in ambulation and weight bearing and its numerous supportive periarticular structures.

ICD-9 Code: 719.46

Anatomic Considerations: The knee is often divided into the medial compartment, lateral (femorotibial) compartment, and patellofemoral compartment. Articular structures within these compartments include the synovium, synovial effusion, articular cartilage, meniscal cartilage, cruciate ligaments, and joint capsule. The term *internal derangement of the knee* implies mechanical damage to one of these structures. Outside the joint, periarticular structures that are common sources of pain may include a variety of bursae (e.g., anserine, prepatellar, superficial and deep infrapatellar), ligaments (e.g., collateral), tendons (e.g., semimembranosus, semitendinosus), bones (e.g., patella, femur, tibia), muscles (e.g., quadriceps), vessels (e.g., popliteal artery), and other soft tissue structures (e.g., popliteal cysts) (see Fig. 1, Section 1.2).

Etiology: Pain in the knee may result from traumatic, mechanical/degenerative, inflammatory, reactive, infectious, or neoplastic disorders affecting the joint or juxtaarticular structures.

Cardinal Findings: Knee pain in middle-aged and elderly individuals is likely caused by periarticular bursitis, traumatic or degenerative meniscal cartilage tears, or degenerative arthritis of the knee. In children, disorders commonly involving the knee may include Osgood-Schlatter disease (osteochondritis at the insertion of the patellar tendon on the tibial tubercle), benign growing pains, or juvenile arthritis. Young adults are most likely to complain of pain from chondromalacia patellae or trauma-induced internal derangement, with possible damage to menisci and cruciate or collateral ligaments.

It is important to ask about the presence of low back or hip pain with referred pain to, or below, the knee. A history of recent trauma may suggest fracture, internal derangement, bursitis, tendinitis, or even septic bursitis or arthritis. A history of remote, repetitive trauma and occupational or athletic contributions to knee pain should be sought. Although many individuals complain of fine or coarse joint crepitus, this is rarely associated with pain and thus has little diagnostic significance. However, pain associated with a sudden pop or snap may indicate severe ligamentous or tendinous injury or rupture. Most chronic articular disorders are accompanied by stiffness. However, prolonged morning stiffness (>1 hour) may indicate an inflammatory process.

Often patients complain of locking, buckling, or giving way. Such complaints suggests a meniscal tear but may also result from loose bodies, cruciate tear, severe quadriceps weakness, or patellar dislocation.

Acute monarticular presentations should lead the examiner to consider urgent noninflammatory (e.g., fracture) or inflammatory (e.g., crystal-induced or septic arthritis) causes.

Pain involving articular structures is likely to be diffuse and deep, whereas periarticular disorders may manifest focal or "point" tenderness. A careful search of periarticular bursae may disclose point tenderness, with or without local signs of inflammation, possibly indicating a bursal or tendinous condition. Palpation should also include examination of the popliteal fossa to detect any fluctuant mass indicating a Baker cyst. The examination should identify limb alignment or the presence of contracture. A contracture may indicate antecedent trauma or undiagnosed articular inflammation. Range of motion is best assessed with the patient supine. Hypermobility of the patella and hyperextension at the knee may indicate a hypermobility syndrome. Ligamentous laxity may lead to excessive medial, lateral, forward, or posterior "play" at the knee. A series of specific maneuvers (i.e., Drawer sign or McMurray test) may be used to detect damage to the meniscal cartilage or cruciate ligaments (see p. 12). Synovial effusion or proliferation is best palpated on either side of the patella and, if large enough, causes a "bulge sign" or distention of the suprapatellar pouch.

Diagnostic Testing: Laboratory testing should be guided by clinical findings. The examiner should avoid using routine laboratory screening tests. If an acute or chronic monarthritis exists, synovial fluid aspiration and analysis should be strongly considered (see p. 17).

Imaging: For nontraumatic acute presentations, radiographs are not indicated because they seldom reveal more than soft tissue swelling or effusion. Acute trauma and knee pain may benefit from imaging. The Ottawa knee rules propose who should undergo radiography. These include injury from trauma and age >55 years, tenderness at the head of the fibula or the patella, inability to bear weight for four steps, or inability to flex the knee to 90 degrees. Anteroposterior and lateral views of the knees should be obtained in those with trauma or who have undiagnosed chronic knee pain. If tolerable, weight-bearing films are preferred because they yield information on articular alignment and the degree of cartilage loss (resulting in uni- or bicompartmental joint space narrowing). Arthroscopy and MRI are powerful imaging tools best reserved for those with severe internal derangement of the knee. MRI may be indicated to diagnose osteonecrosis, osteomyelitis, pigmented villonodular synovitis, or early fractures not yet apparent by routine radiography.

Table 22
Common Causes of Knee Pain

Articular disorders
    Inflammatory: rheumatoid arthritis, gout, pseudogout, systemic lupus erythematosus, Reiter's syndrome, juvenile arthritis, sarcoidosis, and psoriatic, viral, or septic arthritis
    Noninflammatory: osteoarthritis, osteonecrosis, internal derangement, fracture, genu valgum
Periarticular disorders
    Inflammatory: septic bursitis, enthesitis, osteomyelitis
    Noninflammatory: fracture, prepatellar bursitis, infrapatellar bursitis, anserine bursitis, patellar tendinitis, patellar tendon rupture, quadriceps tendinitis, chondromalacia patella, fibromyalgia, Osgood-Schlatter disease, hypermobility syndrome, referred pain

---

Therapy: Depending on the condition, nonpharmacologic modalities of cold or warm compresses, immobilization, and quadriceps-strengthening exercises may be indicated. Symptomatic control of pain may be achieved with NSAIDs or simple analgesics (e.g., acetaminophen). In selected instances, infrequent use of local corticosteroid injections may enhance therapeutic results. Surgery (e.g., arthroscopy) may be indicated with acute internal derangement or fractures or chronically with advanced joint and cartilage damage.

BIBLIOGRAPHY

Calmbach WL, Hutchens M. Evaluation of patients presenting with knee pain. Part I. History, physical examination, radiographs, and laboratory tests. *Am Fam Physician* 2003; 68:907–912.
Jackson JL, O'Malley PG, Kroenke K. Evaluation of acute knee pain in primary care. *Ann Intern Med* 2003;139:575–588.

LEGG-CALVÉ-PERTHES DISEASE

Synonyms: Legg-Perthes disease; primary osteochondritis of the hip.

ICD-9 Code: 732.1.

Definition: A noninflammatory disorder caused by ischemic necrosis of the hip (capital femoral epiphysis), with subsequent collapse and/or remolding of the femoral head.

Etiology: Unknown but may be associated with vascular or thrombolytic disorders. Associations with deficiency of protein C or S and factor V Leiden deficiency or trauma have been reported.

Pathology: Core biopsies show fat necrosis and ischemic vascular changes.

Demographics: Boys are more frequently affected (male:female, 4:1). Usual age at onset is between 3 and 12 years. It is estimated that Legg-Calvé-Perthes disease affects one in 1,300 children.

Cardinal Features: Children usually present with painless limping, but with time, pain becomes evident, especially during exertion. On examination, unilaterally limited internal rotation and abduction of the hip is seen, although bilateral hip disease in ~10%. Lab tests (e.g., CBC, ESR) are normal.

Complications: Rarely there is delayed bone growth and short stature.

Imaging: Abnormalities depend on the stage and age of patient. Initially, an irregular and smaller epiphyseal plate, indistinct metaphysis and widening of the joint may be seen. With progression, the femoral head becomes fragmented, flattened, and sclerotic and is displaced laterally within the joint. Changes in the acetabulum has long-term implications on outcome and surgery. Preservation of the acetabulum offers the chance of maturational remodeling of the femoral head. Scintigraphy may be abnormal before radiography and early on shows decreased uptake, but with revascularization, uptake increases. In most centers, MRI remains the modality of choice in making the earliest diagnosis of femoral head disease and can identify ischemia, revascularization, and concurrent synovitis.

Keys to Diagnosis: Consider Legg-Calvé-Perthes disease in any child with hip pain or limp before puberty.

Treatment: Immediate orthopedic referral is recommended for patients with Legg-Calvé-Perthes disease. Mild cases may not require treatment. Loss of hip movement requires mechanical measures to keep the femoral head contained within the acetabulum (with weight-bearing abduction braces) such that with time and healing, the head is remolded by the intact acetabulum. This is best accomplished in those younger than age 6 years with >50% femoral head involvement.

Surgery: Recommended for advanced cases with pain and includes intertrochanteric rotational osteotomy.

Prognosis: Seventy to 90% of patients are active and pain free on long-term follow-up (20–40 years later). Function is often normal, although x-rays are not. Favorable outcomes were seen in younger children and earlier onset of healing. Those with disease onset after 6 to 8 years may have a poorer prognosis. The shape of the femoral head at the time of skeletal maturity best predicts the outcome.

BIBLIOGRAPHY

Lindsley CB, Asher MA, Olney BW. Legg-Perthes and other hip diseases in children. In: Hochberg MC, Silman AJ, Smolen JS, et al., eds. *Rheumatology*, 3rd ed. Edinburgh: Mosby, 2003:987–990.

Roposch A, Mayr J, Linhart WE. Age at onset, extent of necrosis, and containment in Perthes disease. Results at maturity. *Arch Orthop Trauma Surg* 2003;123:68–73.

LIVEDO RETICULARIS

ICD-9 Code: 782.61.

Definition: Livedo reticularis is a painless, cyanotic mottling of the skin in a fishnet pattern. It may affect extremities or trunk and is exaggerated by cold exposure. It may be associated with autoimmune diseases, vasculitis, Raynaud phenomenon, fibromyalgia, atheromatous disease, hyperviscosity syndrome, thrombotic conditions, and exposure to cold or heat.

Etiology: Livedo reticularis results from vasospasm or sluggish blood flow through the deep dermal arterioles. Thickening of the dermal capillary walls can ultimately result in ischemia or infarction of affected tissues.

Demographics: Livedo is common (and usually not associated with disease) in infants and fair-skinned children, especially at times of cold exposure.

Livedo reticularis is sensitive but not specific for connective tissue disorders. It occurs in SLE, Raynaud phenomenon, and APL syndrome. Sneddon syndrome is the historical association of livedo reticularis, a false-positive VDRL, and stroke in young women.

Diagnostic Testing: APL antibodies or vasculitis autoantibodies (i.e., ANCA) may be sought if warranted by the overall clinical presentation.

Keys to Diagnosis: Cutaneous findings are characteristic. A careful history, physical examination, and selected laboratory evaluation may disclose evidence of underlying cause. In cutaneous PAN, patchy livedo reticularis is associated with skin nodules.

Therapy: Therapy is directed toward any underlying illness. Few patients will require specific therapy for livedo reticularis.

BIBLIOGRAPHY
Picascia DD, Pellegrini JR. Livedo reticularis. *Cutis* 1987;39:429–432.

LOW BACK PAIN

ICD-9 Codes: Low back pain, 724.5; cervical OA, 721.0; neck pain, 723.1; lumbosacral OA, 721.3; degenerative disc disease, 722.6; lumbosacral strain, 846.0; herniated intervertebral disc, 722.2.

Definition: Low back pain is the most common acute musculoskeletal complaint in general practice. Although acute or episodic low back pain will affect as much as 75% of the adult population, most cases will resolve and ~10% of patients will develop chronic low back pain. The societal ramifications of low back pain in disability, psychosocial impact, and legal implications are enormous. It has been estimated that the total annual costs related to patients with low back pain exceed $24 billion.

Anatomic Considerations: Back pain can derive from many structures in the area of the lower back, including joints, bursae, ligaments, nerves, tendons, and muscles (Table 23).

Etiology: Inciting stimuli for pain in these structures can include acute trauma, repetitive trauma, degeneration, inflammation, bony hypertrophy, infection, and tumor. In ~90% of patients with low back pain, the etiology relates to a mechanical or degenerative cause; 10% have pain associated with a systemic illness. Inflammatory low back pain is a small subset of those with chronic low back pain but is distinguished by onset age of 15 to 30 years, pain worse in the morning, pain improved by activity, and elevated ESR or CRP levels.

Demographics: Overall, it is second only to upper respiratory ailments as the most common reason why patients seek medical attention. Low back pain is

Table 23
Differential Diagnosis of Back Pain

Soft tissue injury (affecting ligaments, muscles, and other nonosseous structures)
    Myofascial pain (injury sometimes referred to as sprain)
    Fibromyalgia
    Often secondary to trauma or overuse (mechanical pain)
Arthritis (e.g., affecting facet, uncovertebral, sacroiliac joints)
    Osteoarthritis (with or without osteophyte formation)
    Inflammatory arthritis
        Ankylosing spondylitis
        Other spondyloarthropathies
        Rheumatoid arthritis
        Septic arthritis
Intervertebral disc disease
    Herniation (of the nucleus pulposus)
    Infection (discitis)
Neurologic/spinal cord injury
    Cauda equina compression syndrome
    Radicular (nerve root) entrapment (sciatica)
    Spinal stenosis
    Tumors (intramedullary/extramedullary)
    Infection (meninges, epidural space)
    Syringomyelia
Bursitis
    Trochanteric
    Ischial
    Iliopsoas
Lumbosacral bone disease
    Spondylosis, spondylolysis, spondylolisthesis
    Fracture
    Diffuse idiopathic skeletal hyperostosis
    Osteoporosis (with compression fracture)
    Metastatic cancer
    Infections (vertebral body)
Pelvic bone disease
    Insufficiency fractures (e.g., sacral) caused by trauma or osteoporosis
    Metastatic cancer
    Infections (sacroiliac)
Other
    Abdominal/pelvic sources of pain
        Uterus
        Prostate
        Aorta
        Kidney
    Piriformis syndrome (pain from the piriformis muscle)

most prevalent in persons between 45 and 64 years of age. The annual incidence of low back pain is ~5%. Moreover, between 60% and 85% of the population experience this symptom at some time in their lives.

Evaluation: The primary objective in the assessment of a patient with low back pain is to make a timely diagnosis, relieve pain, and return the patient to regular activity as soon as possible. Secondarily, it is important to identify the uncommon, but serious, causes of low back pain, including the cauda equina syndrome, abdominal aortic aneurysm, fracture, infection, or tumor.

Because most patients with low back pain have a readily discernable cause, the workup need not be extensive. Generally, a history focusing on recent over-use, strain, or trauma will identify the inciting cause. In concert with a focused physical examination, this will also frequently identify the involved pathology. A thorough neurologic examination is indicated because it will not only define the severity of the problem but also provide some guidance for optimal ther-apy. In unusual cases or in patients without a clear inciting cause, a history and physical examination looking for systemic conditions associated with back pain (e.g., infection, tumor, autoimmune disease) are indicated.

Cardinal Findings: The vast majority of patients with low back pain have myofascial pain, i.e., pain originating in muscles, ligaments, or other soft tis-sues as opposed to bones or joints. The pain may occur acutely, with stress or related to excess lifting or turning. In addition, many patients experience sim-ilar symptoms recurrently or chronically, sometimes with minimal exertion. Patients with myofascial pain uncomplicated by spine or nerve involvement should have a normal neurologic examination. They may report tenderness on palpation of the paraspinous muscles, and a good deal of the pain probably de-rives from continuous contraction (spasm) of the paraspinous musculature. Several factors may predispose patients to development of myofascial injury, including occupational factors (work that requires repetitive lifting in the for-ward bent and twisted position), exposure to vibrations, deconditioning, obe-sity, and poor posture. Psychologic factors such as job dissatisfaction and de-pression are often associated with chronic low back pain. Variations in spinal posture such as scoliosis do not appear to increase the risk of low back pain.

Several joints in the lumbosacral spine and pelvis may be involved in low back pain. These joints can be affected by inflammatory (e.g., RA, AS) or, more commonly, by degenerative arthritis of the spine. However, radiographic changes consistent with OA are quite common, particularly with advancing age. Many patients with radiographic evidence of OA are asymptomatic, and even in patients with low back pain, finding degenerative arthritis on x-ray does not establish it as the source of pain in a given patient.

The intervertebral disc may be a source of low back pain. Classically, patients with discogenic pain have increased pain with maneuvers that increase intraab-dominal pressure (e.g., Valsalva maneuver, coughing, laughing). In addition, in contrast to spinal stenosis, patients may find relief by walking around. Degener-ation of the intervertebral disc is common with aging. Tears of the circumferential annulus fibrosus may allow herniation of the central nucleus pulposus. Mild bulging or protrusion of the disc into the spinal canal is common and can be demonstrated in approximately half of asymptomatic normal persons by sensi-tive techniques such as MRI. Therefore, demonstration of such findings does not prove that the disc is the source of the pain.

Patients with arthritis (particularly with bony spur formation), disc disease, and other pathophysiologic changes may have impingement on the spinal cord or nerve roots and consequent neurologic symptoms. If such lesions are central, they may cause spinal stenosis. More commonly, bony spurs near the neural foramina impinge on the exiting nerve root, resulting in radiculopathy. Depending on the severity, impairment of neurologic function may be demonstrable. Radicular pain originating in the lower lumbar nerve roots is commonly known as sciatica.

Sciatica, defined as pain that radiates from the gluteal region and down the posterolateral leg below the knee is often associated with mechanical impingement of nerve. Sciatica may be exacerbated by flexion or extension. Lumbar flexion- or sitting-induced pain may be caused by a herniated intervertebral disc (often involving L5 or S1 nerve roots). Extension- or standing-induced pain may be related to spinal stenosis. Both forms of sciatica should be treated with conservative measures, NSAIDs, and muscle relaxants. If these are ineffective, epidural injection with corticosteroids may be helpful.

Low back pain associated with anterior thigh (with or without groin) pain may be caused by hip disease, inguinal hernia, femoral neuropathy, tumor, aortic aneurysm, kidney disease, or retroperitoneal fibrosis. Anterior thigh pain may imply involvement of nerve roots L1-3 (see Dermatomes, p 535).

Low back pain associated with posterior thigh pain (above the knee) may be caused by lumbosacral strain or a herniated lumbar disc (usually L3-4).

Cauda equina syndrome is an uncommon and serious cause of low back pain and may be suggested by findings of incontinence and saddle anesthesia (e.g., cauda equina syndrome). Tumor may be suggested by fever, weight loss, or pain exacerbated by sleep or recumbency. Fracture may manifest as focal bone pain worsened by manual pressure or standing.

Diagnostic Testing: Laboratory testing is seldom needed to determine the cause of low back pain. ESR or CRP may provide nonspecific evidence of a systemic, inflammatory, or infectious process. HLA-B27 is only needed if a spondyloarthropathy is suspected

Imaging: Radiographs are not routinely recommended because of their low yield (i.e., most patients with low back pain do not have conditions visible on radiographs as the cause) and low specificity (as above, many older patients have findings of OA that may be of no consequence). Radiographs should be obtained if there is history of serious trauma, suspicion of malignant disease, suspicion of infection or fracture, or neurologic deficit. If abnormalities are seen on plain films, tomograms or CT scans may give further delineation. If neurologic impairments are suspected (e.g., spinal stenosis), MRI may be the imaging procedure of choice because it allows definition of bone, nerve, and soft tissue.

Therapy: Historically, patients with low back pain were put at strict bed rest for several weeks to rest the affected structures. However, more recent studies have shown that most patients with acute back pain do as well with continuing ordinary activities as well as bed rest or back-mobilizing exercises. No more than 2 days of bed rest is advised and should be followed by progressive mobilization and exercise. Treatment of back pain often involves several modalities. Local pain may respond well to cold or warm compresses and should be determined by patient preference. Many patients respond to NSAIDs or simple analgesics, such as acetaminophen. More potent analgesics such as narcotics may be necessary in the acute setting. However, many patients have chronic symptoms, and such agents must be used with caution. Because muscle spasm may be an important contributor to the pain, muscle relaxants are sometimes useful adjuncts. Spinal manipulation is effective for some patients. Although there has been anecdotal support for the analgesic efficacy of electrical stimulation (transcutaneous electrical nerve stimulation units), controlled trials have not shown it to be beneficial. Chronically, back-strengthening exercises may be of some value. Although they are widely used, lumbar belts have not been proven to be of benefit. Surgery is rarely indicated and should be reserved for those proven to have tumor, infections, fractures, or dislocations.

BIBLIOGRAPHY

Borenstein DG. A clinician's approach to acute low back pain. *Am J Med* 1997;102(suppl 1A):16S–22S.
Deyo RA, Weinstein JN. Low back pain. *N Engl J Med* 2001;344:363–370.

LYME DISEASE

ICD-9 Code: 088.81.

Definition: Lyme disease is a spirochetal tick-borne infection with acute and chronic sequelae capable of affecting the skin, heart, joints, and nervous system.

Etiology: The spirochete *Borrelia burgdorferi* causes Lyme disease and is transmitted by a variety of ticks. Transmission occurs after tick bites in ~10% of cases. The *Ixodes* species of deer ticks facilitate transmission in the endemic areas of the northeastern United States (*Ixodes dammini* and *Ixodes scapularis*) and on the Pacific Coast of the United States (*Ixodes pacificus*). In the mid-Atlantic United States and Texas, the lone star tick (*Amblyomma americanum*), and in endemic areas of Europe, the sheep tick (*Ixodes ricinus*), are vectors. The white-footed mouse is an intermediate reservoir host for immature stages of the tick.

Pathology: There is evidence that both persisting infection and parainfectious (reactive) etiologies contribute to the pathogenesis of Lyme disease. Perhaps secondary to molecular mimicry, persistence of the spirochete in tissues (CNS) leads to an intense inflammatory reaction. Patients with HLA-DR4 and HLA-DR2 are at higher risk to develop a chronic, erosive arthropathy mimicking seronegative RA. *B. burgdorferi* has been isolated by PCR from synovial fluid in untreated or partially treated disease. However, it is unclear whether chronic arthritis is from persistent infection or a reactive immunologic mechanism.

Demographics: In the United States, most Lyme disease cases have been reported in the northeast and around the Great Lakes (particularly in northern Wisconsin and Minnesota). Lyme disease is seasonal and determined by the feeding patterns of the tick nymphs, which are most active in the late spring and early summer. Lyme disease is distributed worldwide, with cases reported in Europe, China, Australia, Russia, and Sweden.

Cardinal Findings: Three stages of Lyme disease have been described (Fig. 6). However, many patients do not experience an orderly progression of disease

Clinical Features of Lyme Disease

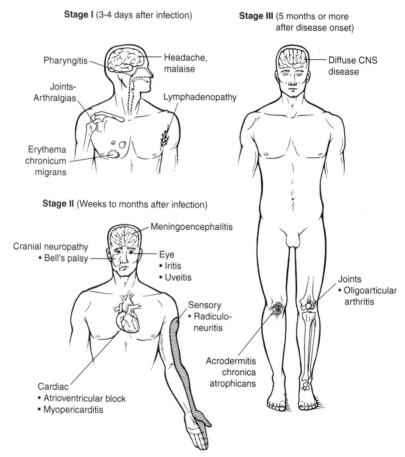

Figure 6. The protean manifestations of Lyme disease (symptoms and signs are sketched in appropriate locations based on early and late manifestations).

manifestations. Some patients may have overlapping features or skip stages entirely. The stages of Lyme disease serve only as a guideline to approximate a time course for the most common clinical symptoms.

—*Stage 1 (3 days to 4 weeks postinfection):* Constitutional symptoms of malaise, fatigue, and fever predominate. The hallmark manifestation of early Lyme disease is the rash of erythema chronicum migrans. Erythema chronicum migrans commonly occurs on an extremity or near an intertriginous zone (thigh, groin, axilla) at the site of the tick bite. Erythema chronicum migrans has a central zone of partial clearing surrounded by an annular area of erythema with an expanding margin that can enlarge to as much as 20 cm. Lesions may last as long as a month and can be asymptomatic, painful, or occasionally indurated. Secondary annular skin lesions may also develop in other locations. Diffuse arthralgias or myalgias are early musculoskeletal manifestations. Other nonspecific early symptoms may include headache, pharyngitis, conjunctivitis, regional lymphadenopathy, and testicular swelling.

—*Stage 2 (weeks to months post-infection):* Approximately 8% of people develop cardiac sequelae including atrioventricular heart block (first degree, Wenckebach, or complete), myopericarditis, and, rarely, cardiomyopathy. Neurologic features occur in 15% of patients and include meningoencephalitis, cranial neuropathies (in particular, Bell's palsy), and radiculoneuritis. Migratory myalgias, arthralgias, and bone or tendon pain may also be detected. Anterior and posterior uveitis and panophthalmitis have been rarely reported.

—*Stage 3 (>5 months after onset):* In the United States, episodic oligoarticular arthritis predominantly of the lower extremities is the most common late Lyme disease manifestation, occurring in 50% to 70% of patients. Knees frequently have large effusions and occasional popliteal cysts. Chronic neurologic sequelae may result in diffuse CNS symptoms that resemble organic brain syndromes. Demyelinating encephalopathy and chronic radiculoneuropathy are other late neurologic complications. Acrodermatitis chronica atrophicans (a sclerotic or atrophic skin change resembling morphea) is a late cutaneous manifestation seen in Europe but rarely in the United States.

Diagnostic Testing: Serologic studies for Lyme disease have been fraught with considerable difficulties and should only be done when Lyme disease is strongly suspected. Serologic diagnosis is suspected with an increase in IgG antibodies against *B. burgdorferi* and/or a specific IgM. Serologic increases do not begin until 2 to 4 weeks after infection. ELISA is the current standard for Lyme disease serology, with most confirmatory tests performed by Western blot. Significant intra- and interlaboratory variation in serologic assays coupled with substantial false-positive and false-negative results hinder interpretation of this test. Early antibiotics may abort or curtail antibody production. Additionally, significant cross-reactivity exists with *Treponema pallidum* and other spirochetes. In early Lyme disease, microscopic hematuria, proteinuria and elevated liver enzymes may be detected in addition to nonspecific indicators of acute inflammation such as an increased ESR and mild anemia. Inflammatory synovial fluid with an average of 25,000 WBCs/mm³ (mostly neutrophils) is commonly seen. In the setting of CNS Lyme disease, lymphocytic pleocytosis and mildly elevated CSF protein are commonly noted. *B. burgdorferi* antibodies may be greater in the CSF than serum in patients with neuroborreliosis. Skin biopsy of the leading edge of erythema chronicum migrans uncommonly reveals spirochetes.

Keys to Diagnosis: The characteristic erythema chronicum migrans rash (antedated by a tick bite) is most helpful diagnostically. Unfortunately, only 50% of afflicted individuals recall a tick bite, and erythema chronicum migrans may be missed or not occur at all. Lyme disease is a clinical diagnosis with laboratory confirmation.

Differential Diagnosis: Early Lyme disease should be distinguished from other causes of febrile arthritis syndromes with rash, including viral arthritis, rheumatic fever, SLE, and Still's disease. The Lyme disease rash may be mistaken for erythema multiforme. Later stages of Lyme disease may be confused with other causes of oligoarticular arthritis such as the spondyloarthropathies. The migratory nature of Lyme disease arthritis and involvement of tendons also may suggest gonococcal arthritis. Polyarthritis may be confused with RA. In the northeast, ehrlichiosis and babesiosis may be co-infections with overlapping clinical manifestations. Severe chronic fatigue and myalgias may indicate fibromyalgia rather than chronic Lyme disease (especially in nonendemic patients).

Therapy: Primary prevention of tick bites includes appropriate protective clothing, use of insecticides, and prompt tick removal. The value of preventive antibiotics after a tick bite in an endemic area versus removal of the tick followed by cautious surveillance is controversial. Preventive antibiotic therapy may be cost effective if the risk of Lyme disease is regionally >1% after a tick bite. Therapeutic recommendations based on the stage of Lyme disease and particular disease manifestations are shown in Table 24. Early manifestations without cardiac or neurologic symptoms may be appropriately managed with oral agents such as doxycycline. Mild cardiac disease, limited neurologic involvement (Bell palsy), and early arthritis may be effectively managed with oral antibiotic therapy. Significant joint, heart, or neurologic involvement requires intravenous therapy, most commonly with ceftriaxone. Significant arthropathy may also respond to intraarticular therapy with corticosteroids and rarely synovectomy. Transient use of cardiac pacing is indicated for symptomatic heart block. A clinical conundrum exists when patients, particularly those who have already received appropriate Lyme disease antibiotic therapy, experience chronic arthralgias and fatigue. Intravenous antibiotics are not cost effective in patients with positive serology whose only manifestations are myalgias and fatigue. There appears to be no value to prophylactic antibiotics for asymptomatic individuals, even in endemic areas. A Lyme vaccine was introduced in 1998, but was withdrawn in 2002 for poor sales, musculoskeletal side effects and litigation. Progress on a 2nd generation vaccine has been slow.

Table 24
Treatment of Lyme Disease

Disease Manifestations	Therapeutic Intervention
Early disease (stage I) Erythema chronicum migrans	Oral antibiotics for 3 wk (except as noted) Doxycycline 100 mg p.o. b.i.d.[a] or Amoxicillin 500 mg p.o. t.i.d. or Cefuroxime axetil 500 mg b.i.d. or Clarithromycin 500 mg b.i.d.[b] or Azithromycin 500 mg q.d. for 1 wk[b]
Carditis (stage 2) Mild (PR interval ≤0.30 s)	Doxycycline 100 mg p.o. b.i.d. for 3 wk or Amoxicillin 500 mg p.o. t.i.d. for 3 wk
Moderate or severe	Intravenous therapy for 2 wk Ceftriaxone 2.0 g i.v. q.d. or Cefotaxime 2.0 g i.v. q 4 h or Pen G 24 million units i.v. q.d.
Isolated Bell palsy (stage 2)	If lumbar puncture negative, consider oral regimens (as above)
Meningitis (stage 2)	Ceftriaxone 2.0 g i.v. q.d. for 3 wk or Penicillin G 24 million units i.v. q.d.
Arthritis (stage 3)	Doxycycline 100 mg p.o. b.i.d. for 4 wk or Amoxicillin with probenecid, both at 500 mg p.o. q.i.d. for 4 wk or Ceftriaxone 2.0 g i.v. q.d. × 2 wk

[a]Avoid in pregnant women and in children.
[b]Azithromycin or clarithromycin are not approved by the U.S. Food and Drug Administration for use in Lyme disease.

Prognosis: With appropriate antibiotic therapy within 4 weeks of disease onset, Lyme disease is a potentially curable infectious illness that may not result in chronic complications. Delayed recognition and therapeutic failure can result in persisting constitutional symptoms, arthralgias, and neurologic complications in as many as 34% of cases. An increasing number of late neurologic complications of Lyme disease have been reported. More sustained musculoskeletal impairment and a higher prevalence of verbal memory loss have been associated with late disease. Active persistent infection, particularly after appropriate antibiotic therapy, is an unlikely explanation for these findings. Careful clinical evaluation of these patients shows a high proportion with fibromyalgia or a poorly characterized chronic pain syndrome.

BIBLIOGRAPHY

Eppes SC. Diagnosis, treatment, and prevention of Lyme disease in children. *Paediatr Drugs* 2003;5:363–372.
Lightfoot RW, Luft BJ, Rahn DW, et al. Empiric parenteral antibiotic treatment of patients with fibromyalgia and fatigue and a positive serologic result for Lyme disease: a cost effectiveness analysis. *Ann Intern Med* 1993;119:503–509.

Shadick NA, Phillips CB, Logigian EL, et al. The long-term clinical outcomes of Lyme disease: a population-based retrospective cohort study. *Ann Intern Med* 1994;121:560–567.

Steere AC, Levin RE, Molloy PJ, et al. Treatment of Lyme disease. *Arthritis Rheum* 1994; 37:878–888.

Stanek G, Strle F. Lyme borreliosis. *Lancet* 2003;362:1639–1647.

MCARDLE'S DISEASE

Synonyms: Myophosphorylase deficiency.

ICD-9 Code: 271.0.

Definition: Inherited disorder of glycogen metabolism with a deficiency of myophosphorylase that impairs glycogen breakdown for energy utilization by muscle.

Pathogenesis: McArdle disease is caused by a deficiency of myophosphorylase and is a good example of a glycolytic disorder. Myophosphorylase deficiency impairs the ability of the muscle to metabolize glycogen as an energy source. This is particularly important during anaerobic muscle activity, when oxidative phosphorylation cannot be depended on because of reduced oxygen delivery to the muscle tissue.

Pathology: Absence of myophosphorylase activity on muscle biopsy.

Demographics: Typically is diagnosed early in life but occasionally is seen in neonates or goes unnoticed until adulthood.

Cardinal Findings: Primarily manifests as episodic, exercise-induced muscle pain, fatigue, cramps, and weakness, and symptoms are relieved by rest and often result in myoglobinuria. Some patients will experience fewer symptoms by ingesting glucose or fructose before exercise. Many patients describe a "second wind" phenomenon wherein after exercise and symptom onset, patients stop exercising briefly, only to restart exercise and then perform better. This represents a transition from glycolytic-dependent pathway to oxidative phosphorylation and release of glucose and free fatty acids as energy sources.

Uncommon Findings: Over time, some patients will develop chronic fixed proximal muscle weakness. McArdle's disease may cause rhabdomyolysis, thereby causing acute tubular necrosis and renal dysfunction. Gout and hyperuricemia may occur in patients with McArdle's disease.

Diagnostic Tests: The majority of patients have low-level muscle enzyme (CPK, aldolase) elevations in response to low-level physical activity. However, with exercise, these may increase 10-fold or more and result in myoglobinuria. Myoglobinuria and higher levels of muscle enzyme elevations should lead one to suspect rhabdomyolysis. Patients should undergo ischemic (or nonischemic) forearm exercise testing (see p. 81). Patients with McArdle disease demonstrate an inability to raise serum lactate levels in the exercised arm, whereas serum ammonia (and sometimes creatine phosphokinase) levels will rise. Myophosphorylase staining of the muscle tissue will confirm the diagnosis.

Keys to Diagnosis: Exercise-induced myalgia or cramping with a resultant myoglobinuria and increase in creatine phosphokinase. Diagnosis is confirmed by a lack of myophosphorylase activity on muscle biopsy or the inability to generate lactate with ischemic forearm exercise testing.

Differential Diagnosis: McArdle's disease needs to be differentiated from inflammatory myositis, and other causes of myopathy (see p. 249) including include myoadenylate deaminase deficiency, carnitine palmityl transferase deficiency (only after prolonged exercise), acid maltase deficiency (with early, severe respiratory involvement), and mitochondrial myopathies.

Therapy: Currently, no effective treatment is available for McArdle's disease, but accurate diagnosis is important to appropriately counsel patients regarding the need for prompt treatment of episodes of myoglobinuria. Creatinine-enriched dietary supplementation has been advocated by some.

BIBLIOGRAPHY

McArdle B. Myopathy due to defect in muscle glycogen breakdown. *Clin Sci* 1951;10:13–33.
Wolfe GI, Baker NS, Haller RG, et al. McArdle's disease presenting with asymmetric, late-onset arm weakness. *Muscle Nerve* 2000;23:641–645.

MIXED CONNECTIVE TISSUE DISEASE

Synonyms: Undifferentiated connective tissue disease or overlap syndrome.

ICD-9 Code: 710.9.

Definition: As initially described, MCTD is defined as having (a) a combination or overlap of clinical symptoms that are characteristic of systemic sclerosis, SLE, and inflammatory myositis (i.e., DM or PM) and (b) high titers of serum antibodies that react with nuclear ribonuclear proteins (or U1-RNP). Although MCTD was originally considered a unique disease state, that concept has come under question. Although such patients may have similar symptoms early in their disease, when followed over time, patients with MCTD evolve into a single identifiable rheumatic condition, most commonly scleroderma. Thus, the reason for designating these patients as having undifferentiated connective tissue disease. In addition, patients with MCTD do not seem to have a unique prognosis or disease course, and antibodies to ribonuclear proteins are not unique to MCTD; they are detectable in more than half of patients with SLE and in those with other autoimmune diseases. Few patients with MCTD will meet ACR criteria for more than one disorder.

Cardinal Findings: Probably more useful than the concept of a single MCTD is the appreciation that many patients have an overlap of signs and symptoms resembling several rheumatic diseases. Overlapping symptoms common to classically described MCTD and several rheumatic diseases include arthritis, dactylitis (sausage digits), Raynaud's phenomenon, sclerodactyly, dysphagia, inflammatory myositis, pleuritis/pericarditis, and interstitial lung disease.

Diagnostic Tests: Although such patients are uniformly positive for ANA and often have very high titers of U1-RNP antibodies, neither is specific for MCTD or other connective tissue diseases. Complement levels are normal, and no antibodies to native, double-stranded DNA are detected. Blood counts may reveal leukopenia or thrombocytopenia.

Keys to Diagnosis: Overlap in symptoms among the various rheumatologic conditions may lead to diagnostic uncertainty, particularly early in the disease course. It has been estimated that one-third of patients initially presenting with clear rheumatologic complaints cannot be diagnosed with a definitive rheumatologic disease. Such patients may initially be designated as having undifferentiated connective tissue disease (the term preferred to MCTD). Careful observation over time usually discloses whether the dominant disorder is scleroderma, SLE, or an inflammatory myopathy.

Therapy: Patients with an undifferentiated disease should be treated according to the symptoms or features present. Thus, many patients may be managed with NSAIDs or analgesic agents for their musculoskeletal complaints. In some, therapy is guided by more serious end-organ involvement. For example, patients with severe myositis may require high-dose corticosteroids, whereas those with chronic polyarticular synovitis may be treated according to a paradigm similar to that used for RA.

BIBLIOGRAPHY

Hoffman RW, Greidinger EL. Mixed connective tissue disease. *Curr Opin Rheumatol* 2000; 12:386–390.

Sharp GC, Irwin WS, Tan EM, et al. Mixed connective tissue disease—an apparently distinct rheumatic disease syndrome associated with a specific antibody to extractable nuclear antigen (ENA). *Am J Med* 1972;52:148–159.

MULTICENTRIC RETICULOHISTIOCYTOSIS

Synonyms: Lipoid dermatoarthritis, normocholesterolemic xanthomatosis.

ICD-9 Code: 272.8.

Definition: Multicentric reticulohistiocytosis is a rare disorder characterized by infiltration of lipid-laden histiocytes into various tissues. The typical clinical picture includes skin nodules and a chronic destructive polyarthritis.

Etiology: Although the cause is unknown, infectious agents such as mycobacteria have been suspected as an etiologic agent; none has been conclusively implicated. There are no known genetic associations.

Pathology: Multicentric reticulohistiocytosis is characterized by accumulation of histiocytes and multinucleated giant cells at affected sites.

Demographics: Multicentric reticulohistiocytosis is a rare disorder that is seen in middle-aged women more frequently than children.

Cardinal Findings: Multicentric reticulohistiocytosis often presents with a chronic, symmetric, polyarthritis affecting the proximal or distal interphalangeal joints of the hands and may be associated with joint destruction, particularly of the distal interphalangeal joints. Less commonly involved joints include the shoulders, knees, wrists, and hips. The skin nodules over the hands and elbows resemble rheumatoid nodules. Nodules may also occur on the ears, chest, face, and mucosal surfaces (e.g., lips, tongue, gingiva). Other skin lesions seen in multicentric reticulohistiocytosis (but not typical of RA) include small papules that occur in bead-like clusters about the nailfolds and xanthelasma.

Complications: A minority may be tuberculin positive or have an associated malignancy.

Diagnostic Tests: Less than one-third of patients have an elevated ESR or hypercholesterolemia. Patients are seronegative for RF and ANA. Synovial fluid findings are variable and may reveal inflammatory or noninflammatory fluid.

Keys to Diagnosis: The diagnosis of multicentric reticulohistiocytosis is made by biopsy of the affected synovium or skin lesions. Multinucleated giant cells in these lesions characteristically contain large amounts of periodic acid–Schiff staining material, indicating lipid accumulation. There are no diagnostic laboratory tests. Multicentric reticulohistiocytosis needs to be distinguished from RA and other chronic inflammatory arthritides such as psoriatic arthritis.

Therapy: Therapeutic agents that have been used for this disorder include corticosteroids and cytotoxic drugs such as cyclophosphamide. The small number of affected patients precludes large therapeutic trials. Although spontaneous remission has been reported, particularly among children, the disease in most patients has a progressive course.

BIBLIOGRAPHY

Santilli D. Multicentric reticulohistiocytosis: a rare cause of erosive arthropathy of the distal interphalangeal finger joints. *Ann Rheum Dis* 2002;61:485–487.

MULTIPLE SCLEROSIS

ICD-9 Code: 340.0.

Definition: Multiple sclerosis is a immunologically mediated disease characterized by demyelination within the CNS. The typical clinical presentation is neurologic events separated in time (recurrent or relapsing) and space (arising from distinct parts of the brain, brainstem, and spinal cord).

Demographics: Multiple sclerosis occurs predominantly among whites of northern European descent. The prevalence of multiple sclerosis varies dramatically with longitude. Multiple sclerosis occurs in approximately 20 per 100,000 persons living in the southern United States and increases as one moves north; the prevalence exceeds 125 per 100,000 in Canadians. Although there is a small genetic predisposition to multiple sclerosis (monozygotic twins have a concordance of approximately 25%), environmental exposure to an unidentified antigen at a young age appears to be important. Peak onset age is 20 to 40 years. Women are affected twice as often as men.

Cardinal Findings: The characteristic clinical presentation of multiple sclerosis is neurologic defects separated in space and time. Most defects arise acutely, with 75% occurring within a few days. Typically, the defects persist for 6 to 8 weeks, and many resolve spontaneously. In most patients, this is followed by a recurrence of neurologic defects. The most common presenting symptoms include weakness in one or more limbs (50%), numbness in the limbs (45%), optic neuritis (20%), unsteady gait or ataxia (15%), and diplopia (10%). A useful clinical clue to the diagnosis of multiple sclerosis is that the symptoms reflect involvement of the white matter of the CNS. Thus, symptoms seen primarily with gray matter damage in the CNS (e.g., loss of consciousness, seizures, syncope, dementia, muscle atrophy, pain) are uncommon. Physical examination may reveal evidence of optic (e.g., internuclear ophthalmoplegia) or spinal cord involvement (e.g., a positive Babinski reflex, dysfunctional sphincter).

Diagnostic Tests: Standard laboratory and serologic tests are of little value. CSF studies (see p. 55) may reveal normal cell counts or show a mild mononuclear pleocytosis, mildly increased CSF protein, increased CSF IgG index or synthetic rate (90%), or evidence of CSF oligoclonal bands or myelin basic protein (>85%). In addition, visual evoked potentials or brainstem evoked potentials may help confirm the diagnosis of multiple sclerosis.

Imaging: The diagnosis of multiple sclerosis may be supported by imaging studies. Perhaps the most important advance has been the availability of MRI. Areas of demyelination, or plaques, are readily revealed by MRI. However, some patients (e.g., those with predominant spinal cord involvement) may have entirely normal scans. Although consistent with multiple sclerosis, white matter lesions on MRI may also be seen in other conditions, including hypertensive vasculopathy, SLE with CNS involvement, and various infections (e.g., Lyme disease, HIV, human T-cell lymphotropic virus type 1).

Therapy: Conservative measures should include evaluation by physical and occupational therapy. Interferon beta 1-a and beta 1-b and glatiramer acetate have been approved for use in multiple sclerosis and are considered first-line agents. Corticosteroids are also effective first-line drugs, especially with optic-neuritis. Second-line agents include intravenous gamma-globulin, azathio-prine, methotrexate, and cyclophosphamide.

BIBLIOGRAPHY

Rolak LA. The diagnosis of multiple sclerosis. *Neurol Clin* 1996;14:27–43.

MYASTHENIA GRAVIS

ICD-9 Code: 358.0.

Definition: Myasthenia gravis is an autoimmune disorder of the neuromuscular junction. It is characterized clinically by muscle weakness and immunologically by autoantibodies directed against the postsynaptic acetylcholine receptor. These autoantibodies are pathogenic, causing increased turnover and decreased surface expression of the acetylcholine receptor, which results in decreased muscle depolarization and weakness.

Etiology: Although most cases of myasthenia gravis are idiopathic, some patients have associated thymomas or thymic hyperplasia. Myasthenia gravis may also occur as a rare reaction to D-penicillamine therapy.

Demographics: Myasthenia gravis is rare, with a prevalence of approximately 14 per 100,000, and has a bimodal distribution. There is a slight female predominance among patients with disease onset in the second and third decades, and a male predominance among patients older than 50 years of age. There is a genetic predisposition, partly related to expression of the HLA-B8 and DR3 alleles.

Associated Conditions: Many patients with myasthenia gravis, particularly those with younger onset of disease, have associated thymomas (10% of patients) or thymic hyperplasia (70%). Myasthenia gravis is also associated with other autoimmune diseases, including thyroid disease (15% of patients), RA (4%), and SLE (2%).

Cardinal Findings: The characteristic clinical picture of myasthenia gravis is muscle weakness that worsens with repetitive use and improves with rest. Ocular muscle involvement is most common, and two-thirds of patients present with symptoms such as ptosis and diplopia. Symptoms typically worsen after strain and at the end of the day. Approximately 15% of patients have myasthenia gravis that remains limited to the ocular muscles. For the remainder, the disease progresses to involve the oropharyngeal (i.e., dysphagia, dysphonia, dysarthria) and limb muscles. When it affects the respiratory muscles, myasthenia gravis can be fatal. For approximately two-thirds of patients, maximum muscle weakness occurs in the first year of disease. Exacerbations may be associated with various factors such as emotional stress, infection, and thyroid disease. In addition, medications that affect neuromuscular transmission (e.g., aminoglycoside antibiotics, neuromuscular blockers, class I antiarrhythmics) may also exacerbate myasthenia gravis.

Diagnostic Tests: The diagnosis of myasthenia gravis may be accomplished by several means. Pharmacologic testing or the Tensilon test uses a short-acting acetylcholinesterase inhibitor (e.g., edrophonium) and may reveal dramatic improvement in muscle strength. Pharmacologic testing may be falsely negative in some patients with myasthenia gravis, particularly children.

Increased serum concentrations of antibodies directed against the acetylcholine receptor are seen in approximately 65% of patients with myasthenia gravis limited to ocular musculature and 85% of patients with more generalized myasthenia gravis. Anti–acetylcholine receptor antibody tests are available from reference laboratories. The presence of anti–acetylcholine receptor antibodies is relatively specific, although false-positive results may be seen in patients with SLE and among healthy relatives of patients with myasthenia gravis.

Finally, electrophysiologic studies may aid in the diagnosis of myasthenia gravis by demonstrating characteristic abnormalities (e.g., decremental responses on repeated muscle stimulation).

Differential Diagnosis: Myasthenia gravis may be mistaken for Eaton-Lambert syndrome (commonly a paraneoplastic syndrome that affects the presynaptic segment of the neuromuscular junction), inflammatory myositis (i.e., PM, DM, inclusion body myositis), other myopathies, multiple sclerosis, and chronic fatigue syndrome.

Therapy: Myasthenia gravis therapy must be individualized. Long-acting anticholinesterase drugs (e.g., pyridostigmine) are the mainstay of therapy for most patients. Thymectomy is indicated in many patients with myasthenia gravis, particularly those with thymoma. Thymectomy may not be advisable for those for whom the risks of surgery may outweigh the potential benefit, including the elderly and those with purely ocular muscle involvement. Various immunomodulatory agents also have a role as therapeutic agents for patients with myasthenia gravis. Corticosteroids, often used initially at high doses (e.g., 1 mg/kg), achieve a response in ~75% of patients. Other immunomodulatory therapies that have been used include intravenous γ-globulin, plasma exchange, azathioprine, cyclosporine, and cyclophosphamide.

BIBLIOGRAPHY

Drachman DB. Myasthenia gravis. N Engl J Med 1994;330:1797–1803.
Finley JC, Pascuzzi RM. Rational therapy of myasthenia gravis. Semin Neurol 1990;10:70–85.

MYOPATHY

Synonyms: Metabolic diseases of muscle, metabolic myopathies, statin-induced myopathy, drug-induced myopathy.

ICD-9 Codes: Myopathy, 359.9; alcoholic, 359.4; amyloid, 359.6; toxic, 359.4; Tarui disease, 271.2; deficiency of carnitine, 277.81; carnitine palmityl transferase, 791.3.

Definition: Myopathy is a generalized term applied to a heterogeneous group of disorders that affect muscle. Inflammatory muscle disease is considered elsewhere (see p. 298). The differential diagnosis of weakness and myopathy is expansive. The metabolic myopathies include disorders of skeletal muscle caused by alterations in biochemical pathways and divided into disorders of glycogenolysis, lipid metabolism, and mitochondrial myopathies.

Etiology: Most of these disorders have a genetic basis and show an autosomal recessive pattern of inheritance. Hypokalemic periodic paralysis is an autosomal dominant disorder. Mitochondrial myopathies show a maternal pattern of transmission because all mitochondrial DNA is derived from the mother. A small number of cases are acquired and are attributable to other underlying disorders such as cirrhosis, renal failure, metabolic disorders, or drugs.

Pathology: Light microscopic examination of the muscle biopsy specimen may demonstrate lipid deposition (shown on oil red O stain) in lipid storage myopathies. Mitochondrial abnormalities may also be seen on routine microscopic examination, and the presence of irregular, ragged red fibers suggests a mitochondrial disorder. On electron microscopic examination, increased collagen deposition may be observed in patients with glycogen storage diseases. However, biopsy specimens from some patients may appear normal.

Demographics: Most primary inherited cases become apparent in children and adolescents but may occur later in life.

Cardinal Findings: These disorders impair muscle function on demand and often manifest as fatigue, aches, cramps, and myalgia and may result in myoglobinuria, rhabdomyolysis, or fixed weakness in some. In most, symptoms only develop when muscular activity or nutritional defect unmasks the underlying defect. Most patients show muscle weakness. Some are able to perform normal daily activities without problems but become symptomatic at higher levels of exercise.

Myopathy Subsets

DISORDERS OF GLYCOGENOLYSIS

—*McArdle's disease:* Caused by a myophosphorylase deficiency (see p. 242)
—*Tarui's disease:* Caused by a phosphofructokinase deficiency, Tarui's disease has features similar to those of McArdle's disease, but there may also be nau-

sea, vomiting, and a hemolytic anemia. Most patients are diagnosed as adults and may or may not recall exercise intolerance when younger. Patients with phosphofructokinase deficiency cannot utilize glucose, and thus high carbohydrate meals may exacerbate exercise intolerance.

—*Acid maltase deficiency:* An autosomal recessive disease with three phenotypes. It may manifest before 2 years of age as Pompe's disease with infantile weakness, hypotonia, heart failure, and early death. A second variety begins in early childhood with truncal, proximal, and respiratory muscle weakness. Last, a milder adult subset may begin in the third or fourth decade, with muscle weakness and a pattern indistinguishable from polymyositis or limb-girdle muscular dystrophy. Acid maltase deficiency causes a vacuolar myopathy, and biochemical studies are necessary to prove the diagnosis.

—*Others:* Episodic myopathy may occur as a result of deficiency of lactate dehydrogenase, aldolase, B-enolase, phosphorylase b kinase, or phosphoglycerate mutase. Brancher enzyme deficiency causes chronic proximal myopathy in children or older adults. Debrancher enzyme deficiency causes distal, rather than proximal, myopathy in the third to fourth decade of life.

—*Myoadenylate deaminase deficiency:* Myoadenylate deaminase is a muscle-specific isoenzyme and is involved in the purine nucleotide cycle production of fumarate. It is characterized by exercise-related cramps in children and rarely leads to myoglobinuria. May be associated with delayed motor and speech development, hypotonia, or cardiomyopathy. Muscle enzymes are normal or high, but there is a lack of myoadenylate deaminase activity on histochemical staining of muscle. On ischemic forearm exercise testing, these patients are unable to generated an increase in serum ammonia levels.

DISORDERS OF LIPID METABOLISM

—*Carnitine deficiency:* Deficient transfer of long-chain free fatty acids to the mitochondria results from carnitine deficiency. Muscle weakness begins in childhood and may be associated with myalgias, proximal weakness, respiratory muscle weakness, cardiomyopathy, myoglobinuria, increased creatine phosphokinase, hypoketotic hypoglycemia, and increased lipid in muscle.

—*Carnitine palmityltransferase deficiency:* An autosomal recessive disorder, carnitine palmityltransferase deficiency typically affects males, with exercise intolerance, myalgias, cramps, stiffness, and myoglobinuria. Attacks are triggered by exercise or fasting. Creatine phosphokinase and ischemic exercise tests are usually normal. Diagnosis is based on biochemical analysis of enzyme activity in muscle. Some of these patients develop rhabdomyolysis and renal failure, which is reversible if appropriately treated.

MITOCHONDRIAL MYOPATHIES

Mitochondrial myopathies include a variety of disorders that result in alterations of mitochondria structure, number, or size. These may arise in children as limb myopathy, with or without ophthalmoplegia. Patients exhibit exercise intolerance, proximal or extraocular muscle weakness, myoclonus, salt craving, ataxia, sensorineural hearing loss, or peripheral neuropathy. Mitochondrial myopathies may arise in the adult as exercise intolerance, generalized or proximal weakness, and with normal or elevated creatine phosphokinase levels. Some may be acquired after exposure to mitochondrial toxins such as zidovudine or clofibrate.

STATIN MYOPATHY

Myopathy has been reported to occur with cerivastatin, lovastatin, and simvastatin much more commonly than with pravastatin or atorvastatin. Dose-dependent myotoxic effects (including myalgia, myositis, or rhabdomyolysis) of statins occurs in 1% to 7% of patients. A 2002 FDA review of statin safety suggested that the fatal rhabdomyolysis rate was 0.15 cases per every 106 prescriptions. Cerivastatin was removed from the market after 31 cases of fatal rhabdomyolysis and 52 deaths worldwide. Those at risk were on higher doses and took concomitant gemfibrozil. Other factors that may contribute to statin myopathy include age, renal insufficiency, biliary obstruction, preexisting myopathic disorders (e.g., hypothyroidism), and use of other myotoxic drugs or drugs that induce the cytochrome P-450 enzyme CYP3A4. Mechanisms are not fully delineated, but statins inhibit the formation of mevalonate and ultimately ubiquinone (coenzyme Q_{10}). Ubiquinone deficiency may further inhibit mitochondrial adenosine 5′-triphosphate production and myocyte function. There is no evidence that ubiquinone supplementation will have any clinical benefit in these patients. Treatment hinges on early recognition and drug cessation when appropriate.

Diagnostic Tests: Serum potassium, magnesium, and creatine kinase should be measured. Some, but not all, metabolic myopathies are associated with elevated creatine phosphokinase levels; normal values do not exclude these disorders. Defects in the glycogenolytic pathway such as myophosphorylase deficiency may be detected with the forearm ischemic exercise test (absence of the normal increase in postexercise serum lactate levels is diagnostic). Myoglobin should be measured in urine if rhabdomyolysis is suspected.

Biopsy: A muscle biopsy may be required to establish the diagnosis. Some metabolic syndromes are associated with elevated levels of muscle enzymes, but many do not show any abnormality or have findings only during episodes of rhabdomyolysis; in these cases, measurement of enzymatic activities in the biopsy specimen is usually required. Special handling of tissues is necessary to achieve accurate enzymatic determinations, and consultation with the pathology laboratory that will perform the analysis is essential to ensure that the specimen is collected correctly. The amount of tissue required for enzymatic analysis necessitates an open, rather than a needle, biopsy.

Keys to Diagnosis: Muscle biopsy and measurement of muscle enzyme levels are usually required to establish the diagnosis in a patient with episodic or

DISEASES

exercise-induced weakness or rhabdomyolysis. Secondary cases might be detected by routine blood and urine testing for metabolic imbalances.

Therapy: Specific treatments are not always required. However, because the patient may be advised to modify diet and exercise to minimize problems, establishing the diagnosis is very important. For example, patients with carnitine palmityltransferase deficiency should be advised to avoid fasting and strenuous exercise; carbohydrate loading before moderate exercise may be useful.

Carnitine deficiency may be treated by dietary supplements (as much as 4 g/day of carnitine), and anecdotal reports suggest the utility of L-carnitine, coenzyme Q_{10}, or menadione in patients with mitochondrial myopathies.

Acute rhabdomyolysis, which may occur in some of these syndromes, constitutes a medical emergency, requiring aggressive hydration, mannitol (for urine dilution) and alkalinization of urine to avoid permanent renal damage.

Prognosis: Most patients can pursue normal daily activities and do not develop progressive problems. Precautions regarding diet and exercise are an important component of a successful outcome.

BIBLIOGRAPHY

Martin A, Haller RG, Barohn R. Metabolic myopathies. *Curr Opin Rheumatol* 1994;6:552–558.
Rosenson RS. Current overview of statin-induced myopathy. *Am J Med* 2004;116:408–416.
Wortmann RL, DiMauro S. Differentiating idiopathic inflammatory myopathies from metabolic myopathies. *Rheum Dis Clin North Am* 2002;28:759–778.

NECK PAIN

Definition: Neck pain is a relatively common complaint, affecting approximately one-third of the population at some time in their lives.

ICD-9 Code: 723.1.

Anatomic Considerations: Neck pain can derive from several structures within the neck, including cervical vertebral, zygapophyseal joints, ligaments, tendons, muscles, or spinal cord and nerve roots. Pain originating in the neck may be referred to other locations, including the suboccipital and interscapular regions or shoulder and arm. Whereas cervical rotation is primarily caused by craniocervical and C1-2 articulations, flexion and extension are largely accomplished at the C5-6 and C6-7 articulations.

Etiology: Precipitating causes for pain in these structures include degenerative arthritis, inflammatory arthritis, bony hypertrophy, trauma, muscle spasm, fibromyalgia, myelopathy, infection (e.g., osteomyelitis, septic discitis), and tumor (primary or metastatic) (Table 25). Systemic causes of neck pain are suggested by the findings of fever, chills, sweats, weight loss, and pain not relieved by rest or recumbency.

Table 25
Differential Diagnosis of Neck Pain

Soft tissue injury (sprain)
   Traumatic (e.g., whiplash)
   Secondary to strain or overuse
   Associated with other diseases (e.g., osteoarthritis)
Arthritis
   Osteoarthritis (with or without osteophyte formation)
   Inflammatory arthritides
Ankylosing spondylitis and other spondyloarthropathies
   Juvenile arthritis (juvenile rheumatoid arthritis)
   Rheumatoid arthritis
Neurologic
   Radicular (nerve root) entrapment (i.e., radiculopathy)
   Spinal stenosis
   Syringomyelia
Bone disease
   Fracture/dislocation
   Diffuse idiopathic skeletal hyperostosis
   Osteoporosis (with compression fracture)
   Metastatic cancer
   Infections of bone (osteomyelitis)
Other
   Discitis
   Meningitis
   Thyroiditis
   Fibromyalgia myofascial pain syndrome

Cardinal Findings: Acute onset of neck pain is often related to injury to muscle or other soft tissues. Such pain may be caused by direct trauma, indirect trauma (e.g., rapid deceleration, whiplash), or overuse. This is sometimes referred to as cervical strain. In this condition, neurologic examination should be normal. Patients often try to resist motion and will keep their head/neck in a fixed, single position. On palpation, paraspinal spasm may be evident. Acute neck pain may also result from infection, fracture, vertebral collapse, or meningitis. Chronic cervical pain (e.g., cervical OA) may also be exacerbated by any cause of soft tissue strain or spasm, thereby magnifying the patient's overall perception of pain. Common causes of chronic neck pain also includes fibromyalgia, inflammatory arthritis (e.g., RA, AS), or bony metastases.

Patients with neck pain should be evaluated by assessing for range of motion (flexion, extension, lateral bending, lateral rotation), muscle spasm, tender trigger points (indicating myofascial pain syndrome or fibromyalgia), focal vertebral tenderness, and neurologic deficit. A detailed neurologic examination is indicated for all patients with neck pain, primarily to identify radicular causes or myelopathy. Patients with myelopathy have symptoms in all extremities, weakness, hyperreflexia, and a Babinski sign.

On examination, the anatomic source of pain should be sought. Nonradiating axial pain usually originates in facet joints or cervical disc disorders. Radicular pain denotes radiation to an extremity in a dermatomal distribution (see Appendix E, p. 535). Radicular pain may be inflammatory, traumatic, or degenerative in origin and manifests with weakness, loss of reflexes, and abnormal nerve conduction velocities. Focal axial pain should raise suspicion of neoplasia, mass, or infection.

Complications: Neurologic findings may result from cervical myelopathy, radiculopathy, or spinal cord trauma or transection after trauma (especially in patients with AS). Cervical myelopathy may be seen in patients with RA with C1-2 subluxation owing to destruction of the transverse ligament or erosion of the odontoid. Subaxial subluxation (usually at C4-5, C5-6) may result from apophyseal joint damage at these levels. Myelopathy should be suggested by either upper extremity weakness, paresthesias, hyperactive reflexes, or the Lhermitte sign (the induction of paresthesias or electric sensations down the thoracic spine on cervical flexion). Patients with OA of the neck may form bony spurs or ligamentous hypertrophy that may cause impingement of the spinal cord or nerve root. If such lesions are central, they may result in spinal stenosis. More commonly, bony spurs near the neural foramina impinge on the exiting nerve root, resulting in radiculopathy. Depending on the severity, there may be demonstrable impairment of neurologic function.

Diagnostic Testing: There are no specific diagnostic tests. HLA-B27 may be helpful in young adults who manifest features of spondyloarthropathy.

Imaging: Routine radiographs are not routinely recommended but may be indicated for patients with trauma, chronic complaints, suspected malignancy, or infection or if neurologic deficit is found. C1 and C2 abnormalities are common in RA and lower cervical segments (C4-7) are often involved in OA. Scintigraphy, CT, and MRI may provide the extent of disease and structures involved. MRI is indicated in the evaluation if neurologic impairments are suspected (e.g., cervical spinal stenosis). Nerve conduction studies are indicated if a radiculopathy or upper extremity neuropathy is suspected.

Therapy: Several modalities may be used. Education and physical therapy are important and often overlooked. Many patients respond to NSAIDs or simple analgesics. Because muscle spasm may be an important contributor to the pain, muscle relaxants are sometimes useful adjuncts. Some patients with cervical soft tissue injury report good pain relief with short-term use of a soft cervical collar and intermittent isometric exercise. Surgical interventions are seldom indicated and usually not effective. Surgical stabilization may be indicated for patients with severe C1-2 subluxation or with marked cephalad migration of the odontoid and a neurologic deficit.

Prognosis: Most neck pain is benign. However, patients with neurologic deficits tend to have greater morbidity. Because most neck pain is mechanical in nature, at least half will improve within 4 to 6 weeks with conservative measures. More than 70% will be asymptomatic within 3 months.

BIBLIOGRAPHY

Devereaux MW. Neck and low back pain. *Med Clin North Am* 2003;87:643–662.
Sweezey RL. Chronic neck pain. *Rheum Dis Clin North Am* 1996;22:411–437.

NEUROPATHIC ARTHRITIS

Synonyms: Charcot arthritis.

ICD-9 Code: 713.5 (diabetic, 250.6; syphilitic, 094.0; syringomyelic, 336.0).

Definition: Neuropathic joint disease (Charcot arthritis) is a chronic, exaggerated form of degenerative arthritis caused by loss of proprioception to involved joints.

Etiology: Loss of proprioception leads to repetitive trauma to unprotected joints and subsequent osteoarthritic change. Alternatively, sympathetic neurovascular reflexes may lead to hyperemia and active bone resorption. Common causes include diabetic neuropathy, tabes dorsalis (syphilis), and syringomyelia. Other causes include CPPD crystal deposition disease, recurrent intraarticular steroids, alcoholic neuropathy, amyloidosis, congenital indifference to pain, meningomyelocele, yaws, and spinal dysraphism. As many as one-third of patients have no demonstrable neurologic disorder.

Pathology: Pathologic changes are similar to those of OA. Pannus may be seen. There may be coincident and dramatic bony disintegration and new bone formation.

Demographics: Demography depends on the underlying condition. Neuroarthropathy occurs in 0.1% to 0.5% of diabetics, 4% to 10% of patients with tabes dorsalis, and >30% of those with syringomyelia.

Cardinal Findings: There may be large joint effusion, synovitis, joint instability, dislocation, and bony fragments with marked crepitus. Progression is variable. Two modes of presentation have been described:
1. Acute neuropathic arthropathy (atrophic/resorptive form) is rare and manifests as acute-onset inflammatory monarthritis of non–weight-bearing joints, with associated swelling, warmth, and pain. It may be misdiagnosed as infectious or crystal-induced arthritis.
2. Chronic neuropathic arthropathy is the more commonly recognized form. There is often an insidious chronic history of joint problems, usually involving weight-bearing joints. Joints are typically swollen from effusion or exaggerated osteoarthritic changes. Joints are usually not painful, and there is a loss of deep tendon reflexes.

Patterns of joint involvement differ according to etiology.

—*Diabetic neuroarthropathy:* The tarsometatarsal joint is commonly affected (less commonly, the ankle and metatarsophalangeal joint). Overlying soft tissue swelling and ulceration may be seen. The pain is often less than expected for the degree of deformity and osseous change.

—*Tabes dorsalis:* The knee and hip are most commonly affected, often with a genu varum deformity. A large, unstable knee may be accompanied by an Argyll Robertson pupil or an absent knee jerk reflex. Axial disease has been described.

—*Syringomyelia:* This degenerative condition affects the spinal cord, resulting in weakness and atrophy of the upper extremities with loss of reflexes and thermal anesthesia. Neuroarthropathy may affect the shoulders, elbows, and cervical spine.

Complications: Spontaneous fractures, dislocation, and osteomyelitis may occur.

Diagnostic Tests: Laboratory tests reflect the underlying disorder. Synovial fluid is either noninflammatory or hemorrhagic. Inflammatory effusions are uncommon and should prompt a search for other causes (e.g., crystal arthritis).

Imaging: During the acute phase, changes are nonspecific and include soft tissue swelling. Early changes resemble OA. Later, large osteophytes, new bone formation, bony fragmentation, dislocation, and subluxation may occur. Damage to periarticular structures may lead to malalignment and may contribute to subluxation and deformity. Bone scans show markedly abnormal uptake but are seldom required for diagnosis. Bone scan and MRI may be useful in diagnosing coexistent osteomyelitis or occult fracture.

Keys to Diagnosis: Diagnosis should be suspected in (a) diabetics with foot pain; (b) patients with exaggerated severe OA of the knee; (c) spontaneous fracture after little or no trauma; and (d) severe scoliosis with destructive radiographic changes (search for syringomyelia or syphilis).

Therapy: The underlying disorder should be treated, which may prevent further damage. Weight reduction, immobilization, and use of orthotics may be helpful. Pain medication and NSAIDs are not required in most. Intraarticular steroids are contraindicated.

Surgery: Arthrodesis and joint replacement have a high failure rate and are generally contraindicated. Amputation may rarely be necessary for advanced disease complicated by infection.

BIBLIOGRAPHY

Ellman MH. Neuropathic joint disease (Charcot joints). In: Koopman WJ, ed. *Arthritis and allied conditions: a textbook of rheumatology,* 13th ed. Baltimore: Williams & Wilkins, 1997:1641–1659.
Gupta R. A short history of neuropathic arthropathy. *Clin Orthop* 1993;296:43–49.

NEUROPATHY

ICD-9 Code: 356.9.

Classification: Several patterns of peripheral neuropathy are relevant to rheumatologic disorders: (a) mononeuropathy involvement of one nerve, (b) mononeuritis multiplex-sequential peripheral nerves are affected usually in an asymmetric fashion, and (c) polyneuropathy-symmetric involvement of multiple sensory and/or motor nerves.

Etiology: Rheumatologic diseases most commonly associated with peripheral neuropathy include the vasculitides (particularly PAN), cryoglobulinemia, RA, SLE, Sjögren's syndrome, and amyloidosis. Vasculitis leading to mononeuritis multiplex, for example, commonly results in a mixed sensorimotor axonal neuropathy. Lyme disease may lead to a facial nerve (Bell's) palsy and, less commonly, a sensory radiculoneuritis. Peripheral neuropathy may also result from compression, trauma, or injury of a nerve root as it emerges from the spinal cord (radiculopathy), in the brachial plexus (plexopathy), or more distally (focal nerve entrapment) (Table 26). Entrapment neuropathies are often caused by noninflammatory mechanical trauma but may also be owing to abnormal nerve compression, such as median nerve mononeuropathy (CTS) in a patient with wrist synovitis (e.g., RA) or progressive degenerative conditions (e.g., diabetes mellitus).

Pathology: Mononeuritis multiplex results from vasculitis and vascular ischemia of the vessels supplying the nerve (vasa nervorum). In amyloidosis, polyneuropathy is believed to be caused by amyloid deposition in or around nerves that alter nerve conduction. Sensory polyneuropathy sometimes seen in Sjögren's syndrome may be caused by small vessel vasculitis and dorsal root

Table 26
Entrapment Neuropathies

Syndrome Name/Site	Nerve Involved	Common Noninflammatory Causes
Carpal tunnel (CTS)	Median	Repetitive trauma, pregnancy, hypothyroidism, acromegaly
Cubital tunnel	Ulnar	Excessive leaning on elbows (i.e., patients with severe COPD)
Saturday night palsy	Radial	Postanesthesia, sleeping upon an improperly positioned arm while intoxicated
Meralgia paresthetica	Lateral cutaneous nerve of thigh	Obesity, pregnancy, rapid weight gain/loss, tight pants
Head of fibula	Common peroneal	Diabetes, habitual leg crossing
Tarsal tunnel	Posterior tibial	Severe foot deformity, trauma

DISEASES

ganglionitis. Entrapment neuropathy results from nerve compression, leading first to sensory and then motor deficits.

Cardinal Findings: Painful burning dysesthesia and motor weakness are the hallmark symptoms of peripheral neuropathy. Muscle atrophy, paresthesia, and frank sensory deficits may follow. Foot drop (lower extremity symptoms occur more commonly than upper extremity ones) or wrist drop in a patient who is systemically ill with multiple organ disorder may indicate mononeuritis multiplex owing to PAN or another form of systemic vasculitis.

Diagnostic Testing: Electrodiagnostic evaluation by EMG (see p. 69) and sensory/motor nerve conduction studies (see p. 90) helps to pinpoint the areas affected and may elucidate the specific type of abnormality. In peripheral neuropathy, EMG usually show fibrillation potentials and positive sharp wave owing to muscle denervation. Nerve conduction studies show reduced amplitudes with relatively normal sensory and motor conduction velocity. In mononeuritis multiplex, biopsy of the sural nerve is often performed to look for evidence of vasculitis in the vasa nervorum. The nerve itself may show axonal degeneration and, occasionally, patchy demyelination. Other laboratory studies potentially helpful in confirming the cause of an underlying inflammatory disorder should be dictated by the history and physical examination. Useful studies may include CBC, serum creatinine, urinalysis, chest x-ray, ANA, RF, cryoglobulins, hepatitis serology, immunoelectrophoresis, and ANCA.

Keys to Diagnosis: A comprehensive neurologic examination with particular attention to the sensory components of the examination is essential. Diminished vibratory and position sense are sensitive indicators of early peripheral neuropathy.

Therapy: If the neuropathy is caused by an active inflammatory process (e.g., a vasculitis), then systemic corticosteroids alone or in combination with immunosuppressive agents are frequently indicated, with the dosage dictated by the specific disorder and its severity. Compressive lesions such as CTS may respond well to local measures (e.g., splinting) or surgical release. Physical modalities and rehabilitative services, including appropriate use of splints, braces, and occupational and physical therapy, are frequently very appropriate. Infrequently, agents such as tricyclic antidepressants or carbamazepine are used to alleviate neuropathic pain.

Prognosis: The course and prognosis are highly influenced by the underlying pathologic mechanisms and systemic response to antiinflammatory therapy, if indicated.

BIBLIOGRAPHY

Alexander EL. Neurologic disease in Sjogren's syndrome: mononuclear inflammatory vasculopathy affecting central/peripheral nervous system and muscle. *Rheum Dis Clin North Am* 1993;19:869–908.

Hadler NH. Nerve entrapment syndromes. In: Koopman WJ, ed. *Arthritis and allied conditions: a textbook of rheumatology*, 13th ed. Baltimore: Williams & Wilkins, 1997:1859–1866.

Sigal LH. The neurologic presentation of vasculitic and rheumatologic syndromes. *Medicine (Baltimore)* 1987;66:157–180.

Tervaert JWC, Kallenberg C. Neurologic manifestations of systemic vasculitides. *Rheum Dis Clin North Am* 1993:19:913–940.

NONARTICULAR DISORDERS (BURSITIS, TENDINITIS, ENTHESITIS)

Synonyms: Soft tissue rheumatism, overuse syndrome, bursitis; tendinitis, enthesitis.

ICD-9 Codes: Bursitis, 727.3; tendinitis, 726.9; Achilles tendinitis, 726.71; enthesitis, 726.9.

Definition: The term *nonarticular disorders* refers to pain and dysfunction attributed to structures that surround and support joints and by their proximity are often mistaken for arthritis. Pain originating in nonarticular structures is perhaps the most frequent musculoskeletal complaint seen in general practice. Nonarticular structures include the numerous bursae, tendons, and ligaments present throughout the body. In many cases, injury secondary to repetitive overuse or trauma may cause inflammation and pain. However, some of these structures can become inflamed secondary to a systemic condition such as RA or gout.

—*Bursae:* Numerous bursae (>150) are present throughout the body. They are typically located between muscles or between muscle and bone and contain scant amounts of synovium-like fluid. Their function is to allow smooth gliding between adjacent surfaces and to provide some buffer against injury. Inflammation of a bursa, or bursitis, usually results from trauma (particularly, repetitive trauma), overuse, or other types of direct injury. Bursitis may also be associated with systemic diseases (e.g., gout, pseudogout, RA). An inflamed or injured bursa often enlarges with fluid and can become a source of pain. Bursae can also become infected, usually with organisms (e.g., *S. aureus*) introduced from overlying skin.

—*Tendons:* Tendons can be a source of pain typically related to such biomechanical causes as overuse or repetitive injury. As is true for bursae, when tendinitis is the origin of pain, tenderness can usually be elicited by palpation and specific range-of-motion testing on physical examination. A number of tendons travel through a fibrous tube or sheath. Inflammation of the lining of this sheath is known as tenosynovitis. Tenosynovitis may result from direct trauma, repetitive-use injury, systemic inflammatory diseases, or infection. Stenosis and/or inflammation of a tendon sheath may interfere with smooth movement of the tendon. A "trigger finger" occurs when the flexor tendons of the hand cannot pass smoothly through the fibrous tunnels of the fingers and become caught. Other conditions of pain and entrapment related to tenosynovial involvement include de Quervain's tenosynovitis, carpal and tarsal tunnel syndrome. When tendon injury or inflammation becomes chronic, rupture of the tendon may result.

—*Ligaments:* Ligaments attach one bone to another and thereby provide structural integrity to the skeleton. Injury to ligaments usually results from excessive force being applied. Such sprains range in severity from mild partial tears to complete disruption of the ligament with resultant laxity.

—*Entheses:* The place where ligaments and tendons insert into bone (the enthesis) may also be the site of inflammation. Enthesitis may result from trauma but may also be associated with systemic inflammatory diseases such as the seronegative spondyloarthropathies (see p. 166)

Etiology: Most forms of nonarticular pain are caused by direct trauma, repetitive-use injury, systemic inflammatory or crystal-induced diseases, or infection.

Demographics: Tendinitis, bursitis, and overuse syndromes are very common, affecting young, middle-aged, and older adults. Traumatic conditions are more common in young adults. Males are slightly more often affected than females. The prevalence of bursitis is estimated to be 2%.

Cardinal Findings: Often, a focused history and physical examination can readily pinpoint the specific cause of the patient's complaint. However, it may sometimes be difficult to differentiate these soft tissue syndromes from arthritis or other processes. Often tendinitis, bursitis, or enthesitis can be identified as producing "point tenderness" and may exhibit pain on active, but not passive, motion. Examples of nonarticular pain are presented below.

—*Subacromial (subdeltoid) bursitis.* The subacromial bursa, the largest bursa in the body, lies between the deltoid muscle and the rotator cuff musculature of the shoulder (see p. 25 and p. 349). It may become inflamed in association with rotator cuff dysfunction or independently. Diagnosis of subacromial bursitis is usually made by demonstration of tenderness on direct palpation (the bursa lies immediately below the acromion).

—*Bicipital tendinitis:* Bicipital tendinitis often presents with pain localized to the anterior aspect of the shoulder. Pain often derives from the proximal end of the long head of the biceps, which runs through a tendon sheath in the bicipital groove of the humerus at the shoulder (see p. 25). Direct palpation of an inflamed tendon often generates pain. Pain may also be elicited by forced supination and flexion of the forearm against resistance. Rupture of the tendon of the long head of the biceps results in appearance of a bulge in the upper arm.

—*Olecranon bursitis:* The olecranon bursa lies directly over the olecranon process at the elbow. Olecranon bursitis is a common condition, particularly among older persons. Although it may be associated with conditions such as RA, gout, pseudogout, and infection with *S. aureus* (septic bursitis), most cases are idiopathic or result from minor repetitive trauma to the area. Tenderness on palpation and swelling owing to effusion are the key findings on physical examination. A useful clue to help differentiate olecranon bursitis from elbow synovitis is that pain related to olecranon bursitis increases as the forearm is fully flexed against the upper arm (which stretches the bursa) and diminishes with the elbow in full extension. By contrast, with true elbow synovitis, patients often hold the elbow in the neutral position (i.e., ~30 degrees of flexion); full flexion or full extension both increase pressure within the synovium and cause pain.

—*Tennis elbow:* Inflammation of the common tendon of the extensor muscles of the forearm as it inserts on the lateral epicondyle of the humerus is known as "tennis elbow." This form of lateral epicondylitis often results from overuse (e.g., repetitive pronating or supinating of the wrist, in extension, against force). Physical examination often revels tenderness over the lateral epicondyle.

—*Medial epicondylitis:* Sometimes referred to as golfer's elbow, medial epicondylitis is less common than lateral epicondylitis. Pain over the insertion of the common flexor tendon at the medial epicondyle is the key to diagnosis. In addition to these conditions, other causes of elbow pain include synovitis of the elbow joint and ulnar nerve entrapment (with tenderness on palpation of the ulnar nerve groove and signs of ulnar neuropathy).

—*Wrist tenosynovitis:* Common in patients with RA, wrist tenosynovitis may be difficult to distinguish from synovitis of the underlying radiocarpal joint. Unilateral tenosynovitis may be seen in patients with disseminated gonococcal infection or gout.

—*de Quervain tenosynovitis:* Inflammation of the abductor pollicis longus or extensor pollicis brevis on the radial aspect of the wrist is referred to as de Quervain tenosynovitis (see p. 27 and p. 195).

—*Trochanteric bursitis:* There are several bursae in the area of the greater trochanter of the femur. These bursae are positioned between the trochanter (the bony prominence felt on the lateral aspect of the upper thigh), the gluteus medius and minimus muscles, and the fascia lata. Trochanteric bursitis is a common cause of pain in the region of the hip (see hip pain, p. 207). It occurs mostly among older persons and is more common in women. It may be associated with other conditions that can affect gait, such as OA of the hip, knee, or lumbar spine; leg length discrepancy; and obesity. The typical presentation is chronic, intermittent pain over the lateral aspect of the hip. The pain may radiate inferiorly or superiorly and may be confused with hip pain of other causes. The diagnosis is usually established by demonstration of excessive tenderness on palpation over the trochanter. In addition to NSAIDs and local corticosteroid injections, therapy directed at correcting associated conditions may provide relief.

—*Ischial bursitis:* Inflammation of the ischial bursa presents as pain over the ischial tuberosity (the bony prominences beneath the gluteal muscles) that is exacerbated by prolonged sitting on hard surfaces (see p. 208). Ischial bursi-

DISEASES

tis was previously referred to as "weaver's bottom." Iliopsoas bursitis presents with groin pain just anterior to the hip joint and lateral to the femoral vessels.

—*Meralgia paresthetica:* Compression neuropathy of the lateral femoral cutaneous nerve commonly presents with burning pain in the anterolateral aspect of the hip and thigh (see p. 208). It is commonly seen in patients who are pregnant, diabetic, or obese.

—*Anserine bursitis:* The anserine bursa is located just inferior and medial to the knee (see p. 24). Anserine bursitis is common, particularly among overweight women. Pain can be elicited by palpation directly over the bursa and is often exacerbated by stair climbing. Other bursae are located below the medial and lateral collateral ligaments and may be a source of pain.

—*Prepatellar bursitis:* Often manifesting as swelling and tenderness superficial to the patella, prepatellar bursitis (known previously as "housemaid's knee") is associated with trauma to the front of the knee, as with kneeling. Tendinitis of the patellar tendon may also produce anterior knee pain. It is typically aggravated by athletic activities and has been referred to as "jumper's knee." In children, particularly 10- to 16-year-old boys, pain over the insertion of the patellar tendon into the tibia may indicate Osgood-Schlatter disease (avulsion of the tibial tubercle).

—*Chondromalacia patellae:* Characterized by knee pain, crepitus, and degenerative cartilage changes on the underside of the patella, chondromalacia patellae occurs primarily in young adults, particularly women. The pain of chondromalacia patella is exacerbated by knee flexion against force, for example with stair climbing. Such movements pull the patella close against the femoral condyles. In addition, patients may complain of pain and stiffness with prolonged inactivity that is relieved with motion. Pain attributable to chondromalacia patella can often be elicited by pushing the patella against the femur, particularly at the lateral aspect. This condition is also known as patellofemoral pain syndrome and patellofemoral tracking abnormality. Relative weakness of the medial thigh muscles that allows lateral drift of the patella and abnormal tracking movements may contribute to the pathophysiology. Furthermore, in addition to NSAIDs and avoidance of overuse, exercises aimed at strengthening the medial thigh muscles (e.g., bicycling) may be a useful therapeutic intervention. In more severe or refractory cases, surgical intervention (e.g., release of the lateral retinaculum, realignment of the vastus medialis oblique muscle) may be indicated in some patients.

—*Adams-Baker's cyst:* Patients with synovitis of the knee may develop Adams-Baker cysts (also known as Baker's cysts or popliteal cysts). In this condition, fluid accumulates within the posterior compartment of the knee. Although effusion and swelling may be asymptomatic initially, continued accumulation often causes pain. In addition, the fluid may dissect inferiorly, between the muscles of the calf. This may result in a clinical presentation resembling deep venous thrombosis, and ultrasonography may be necessary to differentiate the two. Various conditions (RA, OA, mechanical derangement of knee) are associated with popliteal cysts. Synovial fluid accumulation in the cyst is caused by a ball-valve mechanism, whereby synovial fluid is forced from the anterior to the posterior aspect of the knee and cannot freely flow back. This may be the result of proliferative synovium (e.g., in RA or other forms of inflammatory arthritis), a torn meniscus, or a fold of synovium (known as a plica). Therapy is directed at the appropriate underlying condition. Inflammatory conditions can sometimes be treated, and the cyst resolved, by local injection of corticosteroids into the joint rather than the cyst.

—*Achilles tendinitis:* The Achilles tendon may become painful from a variety of causes, including direct trauma (e.g., with improper footwear), repetitive overuse (e.g., with athletic activity), and systemic inflammatory diseases (e.g., AS, Reiter syndrome). Pain on palpation is often appreciated at the bony insertion of the tendon. With chronicity, the tendon can become "bumpy" with irregular swellings and have crepitus with motion. There are also bursae superficial to and deep to the Achilles tendon that can become inflamed and be a source of pain. Although not typically associated with pain, xanthomas or rheumatoid nodules along the Achilles tendon can be seen in patients with hypercholesterolemia or RA, respectively.

—*Plantar fasciitis:* Plantar fascia can be a source of substantial pain. Plantar fasciitis (see p. 290) may be associated with trauma, and some patients have an associated spur on x-ray. This condition is also associated with SpA.

—*Costochondritis:* Pain may arise from the costochondral junctions. The term Tietze's syndrome is commonly used to describe cases of costochondritis in which there is not only substantial tenderness on examination but also swelling. The first and second costochondral junctions are most commonly affected.

Diagnostic Tests: Laboratory tests are seldom useful because these are clinical diagnoses.

Imaging: In general, radiographs are of limited value in patients with tendinitis and bursitis. As these soft tissue injuries become chronic, they may be associated with local deposition of calcium, resulting in conditions such as calcific tendinitis and periarthritis.

Keys to Diagnosis: Nonarticular pain should be suspected when there is a history of trauma or repetitive movement associated with the onset of symptoms. "Joint" pain without abnormalities localized to the joint on examination should lead the clinician to search for nonarticular (periarticular) sources of joint pain.

Differential Diagnosis: The site of involvement determines the differential diagnosis. In general, a careful history and physical examination are necessary to distinguish true arthritis from tendinitis, bursitis, and enthesitis. Whenever inflammatory findings exist, infectious, crystal-induced, and inflammatory conditions should be considered.

Therapy: Therapy for local soft tissue injuries typically involves several modalities. NSAIDs are commonly used, either at their lower analgesic doses or at higher antiinflammatory doses. Topical therapies (e.g., local heat and/or cold) may offer some benefit. Physiotherapy is an important part of the treatment of these conditions. Because many relate to overuse, rest and protection of the affected area are often beneficial acutely. Subsequently, physiotherapy is aimed at preventing recurrence of the condition by optimizing range of motion, improving flexibility, and maximizing the strength of the surrounding musculature. In some cases, local injection of corticosteroids can effectively ameliorate the inflammation and thus decrease pain.

BIBLIOGRAPHY

Biundo JJ, Mipro RC, Fahey P. Sports-related and other soft-tissue injuries, tendinitis, bursitis and occupation-related syndromes. *Curr Opin Rheumatol* 1997;9:151–154.

NSAID GASTROPATHY

ICD-9 Codes: Gastritis, 535.5; gastroesophageal reflux disease, 530.81.

Definition: The use of NSAIDs is associated with several important adverse effects in the GI tract, particularly gastric ulceration. NSAID-associated GI side effects are the most frequently reported adverse drug effect in the United States.

Etiology: NSAIDs inhibit cyclooxygenase (COX), the enzyme that converts arachidonic acid into prostaglandin. Inhibition of prostaglandin, which normally protects the gastric mucosa, is the major mechanism underlying NSAID gastropathy. Most NSAIDs are also acidic compounds and accumulate at high local concentrations in the gastric mucosa; this potentiates their effects. Other mechanisms may also be involved.

Risk Factors: Important patient risk factors for NSAID gastropathy include (a) history of peptic ulcer disease, (b) history of any GI bleeding, (c) serious comorbid disease (e.g., functionally compromised cardiopulmonary disease), and (d) advanced age (>60 years old). Other risk factors include anticoagulation (e.g., warfarin) and the use of corticosteroids (although apart from NSAIDs, corticosteroids are not a clinically significant cause of GI toxicity). In some series, patients with dyspeptic symptoms (e.g., heartburn) and those self-medicated with over-the-counter antacids were also at increased risk of NSAID gastropathy.

Several risk factors for gastropathy relate to the NSAID itself, including dose (higher doses and multiple NSAID use confers a greater risk), duration of therapy (longer treatment is associated with higher risk), and choice of NSAID. NSAIDs can be roughly ranked in order of the risk of gastropathy, from somewhat higher risk (aspirin, piroxicam, indomethacin, naproxen, sulindac) to somewhat lower risk (diclofenac, etodolac, ibuprofen, nabumetone, meloxicam) to the lowest risk (celecoxib, rofecoxib, valdecoxib). Differences in the propensity to cause NSAID gastropathy may relate to differential inhibition of COX-1 and COX-2 isoenzymes. Low-dose aspirin (81 mg/day) is associated with significant risks for ulceration and bleeding. Nonacetylated NSAIDs (e.g., salsalate) are inefficient COX inhibitors (100-fold less than aspirin); they are rarely associated with gastropathy. Last, patients on NSAIDs may become infected with *Helicobacter pylori*, and the use of NSAIDs in patients infected with *H. pylori* will enhance the infection related inflammation and ulcers.

Demographics: The prevalence of NSAID gastropathy increases with age and in association with the risk factors outlined above. The prevalence and significance of NSAID gastropathy can be analyzed in several ways. Studies have shown that within the first 3 months of treatment with NSAIDs, 10% to 20% of patients develop a new gastric ulcer, and 4% to 10% develop a new duodenal ulcer. Because these were endoscopic studies and the ulcers seen were sometimes quite small, this may be an overestimate of clinically significant problems. In the United States, NSAID gastropathy results in ~70,000 hospitalizations and 7,000 deaths each year. Between 20% and 40% of all patients who present with upper GI bleeding have been found to be taking NSAIDs chronically. Symptomatic GI ulceration occurs in 2% to 4% of patients taking a NSAID for more than 1 year. However, this may be an underestimate because most NSAID gastropathy is asymptomatic, which makes estimation of its true prevalence difficult. In addition, the widespread use of NSAIDs (>13 $\times$ 10^6 people in the United States use NSAIDs chronically) underscores this serious health problem.

Cardinal Findings: NSAID-related gastric ulcer occurs twice as commonly as duodenal ulcer. In addition to frank ulceration, erosions may also be seen. Asymptomatic bleeding is a substantial problem because >50% of patients with NSAID gastropathy are asymptomatic (compared with approximately 25% of patients with non–NSAID-related gastropathy). Esophagitis may be related to, or exacerbated by, NSAID use. Anorexia, unexplained weight loss, orthostatic dizziness, or anemia may be early signs of occult NSAID-induced GI bleeding.

Complications: Bleeding is the most common complication. Because many ulcers are asymptomatic, it may be unexpected. Ulcers can be severe, leading to complications such as perforation or cardiovascular collapse owing to blood loss.

Differential Diagnosis: Idiopathic peptic ulcer disease is now considered to be secondary to infection with *H. pylori*. In a patient taking NSAIDs, it may be difficult to distinguish idiopathic from NSAID-related gastropathy. This is particularly true among older persons; advanced age is a risk factor for both NSAID gastropathy and *H. pylori* (the prevalence of this infection exceeds 50% in patients >60 years old). Several characteristics of *H. pylori*—related peptic ulcer disease may allow it to be differentiated from NSAID gastropathy: (a) most patients with *H. pylori* have a duodenal rather than gastric ulcer, (b) gastritis is seen, and (c) recurrence is very common unless the infection is treated. Nonetheless, patients found to have peptic ulcer disease are often tested for *H. pylori*, even if the peptic ulcer disease is suspected of being related to NSAID use. Such patients are usually treated to eradicate the infection in addition to receiving antiulcer treatment.

Keys to Diagnosis: Patients receiving NSAIDs who have GI symptoms should be suspected of having gastropathy. Because many patients with gastropathy are asymptomatic, a high degree of clinical suspicion is needed, particularly in patients with one or more risk factors for NSAID gastropathy.

Diagnostic Tests: Upper GI radiographic studies are used in patients with symptoms and in asymptomatic patients with evidence of bleeding. Regular testing of the stool for occult blood is a reasonable health maintenance procedure for patients receiving NSAIDs, although it is seldom positive in those with significant GI bleeding. Endoscopy allows definitive assessment of esophagogastroduodenal pathology. CBC may reveal significant blood loss.

Therapy: NSAID gastropathy therapy usually involves NSAID discontinuation. In patients with dyspepsia who do not have peptic ulcer disease or other serious GI pathology, it may be possible to relieve the symptoms by lowering the NSAID dose, switching to a different NSAID, or adding antacids such as H2-histamine blockers (e.g., ranitidine, cimetidine, famotidine). In patients with peptic ulcer disease, the NSAID should be stopped, and treatment with H2 blockers instituted. The healing rate for NSAID-related peptic ulcer disease after stopping NSAIDs approximates that of idiopathic peptic ulcer disease; 95% to 100% of gastric and duodenal ulcers are healed within 8 weeks of therapy with H2 blockers. If it is considered necessary to continue NSAIDs, healing of ulcers becomes slower and less complete (80%–90% healed with 12 weeks of H2 blocker therapy). In such patients, proton pump inhibitors (e.g., omeprazole, lansoprazole) are more effective. The size of the ulcer is a major factor in healing; larger ulcers (>0.5 cm) heal more slowly and less completely than smaller ones.

Prevention of NSAID gastropathy is an important consideration. First, NSAIDs should be avoided unless absolutely required for disease control. Although it is not cost-effective to treat all patients receiving NSAIDs, patients with one or more important risk factors for NSAID gastropathy may be offered treatment with a COX-2 inhibitor with or without gastroprotective agents such as misoprostol (200 mg q.i.d.) or proton pump inhibitors (e.g., omeprazole). COX-2 selective NSAIDs have reduced NSAID gastropathy but are not clinically superior to nonselective NSAIDs.

BIBLIOGRAPHY

Fendrick AM. *Helicobacter pylori* and NSAID gastropathy: an ambiguous association. *Curr Rheumatol Rep* 2001;3:107–111.
Fries JF. NSAID gastropathy: the second most deadly rheumatic disease? Epidemiology and risk appraisal. *J Rheumatol* 1991;18(suppl 28):6–10.
Hawkey CJ, Kanasch JA, Szczeparski L, et al. Omeprazole compared with misoprostol for ulcers associated with nonsteroidal antiinflammatory drugs. *N Engl J Med* 1998;338:727–734.
Straus WL. Gastrointestinal toxicity associated with nonsteroidal anti-inflammatory drugs. Epidemiologic and economic issues. *Gastroenterol Clin North Am* 2001;30:895–920.

OSGOOD-SCHLATTER DISEASE

Synonyms: Tibial apophysitis.

ICD-9 Code: 732.4.

Definition: Osgood-Schlatter disease is a traction apophysitis of the distal patellar tendons insertion at the tibial tuberosity. Larsen-Johansson disease is a similar to Osgood-Schlatter disease but involves the insertion of the patellar tendon on to patella.

Pathogenesis: Repetitive traction on the secondary ossification center of the tibial tuberosity.

Demographics: Osgood-Schlatter disease is a common sporting injury that occurs in 4% of adolescents. It typically affects athletic adolescents; boys more frequently than girls. Onset age is younger in girls (10–11 years) than boys (13–14 years).

Cardinal Findings: Pain over the tibial tubercle worsened with exercise or extension against resistance. Symptoms may be worse with squatting, jumping, or using stairs. Localized pain, with or without swelling, may be found over the tubercle. Bony hypertrophy may persist after pain subsides. Rarely tibial tubercle avulsion fractures occur. The prognosis is favorable for most.

Imaging: If symptoms are chronic, imaging is indicated and often shows soft tissue swelling or hypertrophy and fragmentation of the tubercle (which is normally irregular in contour in young people). Chronic symptoms may be further imaged by CT or MRI.

Differential Diagnosis: Patellar subluxation, patellar tendonitis, Larsen-Johansson disease.

Therapy: Rest, activity avoidance or ice after activity, and quadriceps strengthening exercises are all helpful. Splinting or casting is discouraged. Pain management with simple analgesics or NSAIDs may be useful. Surgery may be indicated if symptoms persist into adulthood.

DISEASES

BIBLIOGRAPHY

Bloom OJ. What is the best treatment for Osgood-Schlatter disease? *J Fam Pract* 2004; 53:153–156.

Hogan KA. Overuse injuries in pediatric athletes. *Orthop Clin North Am* 2003;34:405–415.

OSTEITIS CONDENSANS ILII

ICD-9 Code: 733.5.

Definition: Osteitis condensans ilii refers to an increase in bone density (sclerosis) located on the inferomedial aspect of the ilium adjacent to the sacroiliac joint. It is often bilateral, symmetric, and triangular. Sacroiliac and spinal abnormalities (i.e., erosions) are not found.

Etiology: The cause is unknown. It may be owing to increased mechanical stress across the sacroiliac joint during pregnancy. It is usually associated with pregnancy but has also been reported in those with hydroxyapatite crystal deposition disease.

Demographics: It is primarily seen in young multiparous women.

Cardinal Findings: Only rarely are the radiographic findings symptomatic with pain.

Imaging: Radiographs show ill-defined ilial sclerosis that may resolve or persist.

Differential Diagnosis: Sacroiliitis and AS characteristically affect the sacroiliac joint with erosions, pseudowidening, or ankylosis. Degenerative changes in the sacroiliac joint may be confused with osteitis condensans ilii.

Therapy: None is indicated.

OSTEOARTHRITIS

Synonyms: OA, degenerative joint disease, osteoarthrosis.

ICD-9 Codes: 715.9 (multiple sites); hand, 715.4; hip, 715.5; knee, 715.6; spine, 721.90.

Definition: OA is the most common arthropathy seen in adults. This noninflammatory condition arises from degenerative changes and progressive loss of cartilage with resultant hypertrophic changes in surrounding bone.

Etiology: Cause is unknown. Mechanical (e.g., trauma, repetitive stress), biochemical, and inflammatory factors contribute to its pathogenesis. A genetic predisposition exists for women with OA of the distal interphalangeal joints (Heberden nodes).

Pathology: Biochemical changes in cartilage result in a loss of water content, loss of proteoglycan and collagen, and a decreased number of chondrocytes, changes that soften cartilage and make it more prone to damage. Grossly, there is evidence of cartilage damage, with fissuring, pitting, ulceration, and (eventually) denuded bone. Adjacent to cartilage loss is the development of reactive or hypertrophic bone, most often manifest as osteophyte (or spur) formation. Underlying subchondral bone may remodel and show sclerosis or bony cysts. The synovium in OA may be normal or show mild to moderate inflammatory changes, similar to those seen in RA, although not as intense. It is possible that intermittent inflammatory synovial disease may further contribute to degeneration of articular cartilage.

Demographics: OA has a prevalence of 12% in the U.S. population and is most common in those older than age 65. Radiographic changes of degenerative joint disease are seen in >80% of those older than age 75. OA is most common in women. Isolated hip OA is most common in men. All races are affected.

Risk Factors: OA is either primary/idiopathic or secondary. Secondary causes of OA include trauma, obesity, congenital or metabolic disorders (Wilson's disease, alcaptonuria, hemochromatosis), inflammatory arthritis (i.e., RA, septic arthritis), neuropathic arthritis, and hemophilia. Obesity increases the risk of knee OA (especially in women) but does not increase risk of hand or hip OA. With structurally normal knees, there is no added risk of OA in long-distance runners. There is an inverse relationship between OA and bone mass.

Cardinal Findings: Most patients note the insidious onset of pain in affected joints. This mechanical or degenerative pain is worsened by activity and improved with rest. It is maximal at the end of the day or during the night and may interfere with sleep. Stiffness tends to be minor in the morning, yet it recurs during periods of sedentary rest throughout the day and is described as "gel phenomenon." Inflammatory swelling or effusions are unusual. Instead, bony swelling (or hypertrophy) may develop and interfere with normal range of motion. Bony hypertrophy is most obvious in the distal interphalangeal joints (Heberden's nodes), proximal interphalangeal joints (Bouchard's nodes), and first carpometacarpal joints (base of the thumb), often in a symmetric fashion. Heberden's nodes are primarily found in women. Once the hypertrophic changes have fully evolved in affected hand joints, the pain often subsides. Beyond the hand, asymmetric joint disease is most common and typically affects the hip, knees, metatarsophalangeal joints, and cervical and lumbar spine. Shoulders, elbows, ankles, and tarsal joints tend to be spared unless traumatic or occupational events predispose the patient to degenerative changes in these joints. For example, tarsal OA is a common finding in ballerinas. Coarse crepitus may be felt in joints of those with moderate to severe OA.

—*Primary generalized OA (nodal OA):* Occurring predominantly in middle-aged women, primary generalized OA affects the distal and proximal interphalangeal joints, first carpometacarpal joint, knee, metatarsophalangeal joint, hips, and spine.

—*Chondromalacia patellae:* Chondromalacia patellae is a form of degenerative arthritis that affects the patellofemoral joint and is often caused by malalignment of the patella within the intercondylar groove. The underside of the patellar cartilage develops degenerative features and manifests with pain that is worsened by walking, running, squatting, or climbing stairs. Such patients are often treated conservatively with NSAIDs, analgesics, and quadriceps-strengthening exercises.

—*Inflammatory OA:* Erosive or inflammatory OA typically affects postmenopausal women with inflammatory changes and erosions at nodal sites, the proximal or distal interphalangeal joints. Medial or lateral subluxation at the proximal or distal interphalangeal joint is common in this variant of OA. Radiographic changes include loss of joint spaces, sclerosis, and osteophytes, with erosions and occasional ankylosis. In the fingers, these central erosions and peripheral osteophytes may give rise to a "seagull" sign on radiography. Inflammatory OA must be distinguished from psoriatic arthritis. Uncommonly, inflammation arising in Heberden or Bouchard nodes may be caused by gout. This usually occurs in older women on diuretics with renal insufficiency.

Uncommon Findings: OA uncommonly affects the MCP (usually the second and third) joints but, if present, may be idiopathic or secondary to trauma or hemochromatosis (see p. 199).

Diagnostic Testing: Laboratory tests (e.g., CBC, ESR, SMA12) tend to be normal for age. Serologic testing for ANA and RF is not necessary. Synovial fluid is usually amber, clear, and noninflammatory (WBCs <2,000 cells/mm^3), with normal viscosity.

Imaging: Conventional radiography may help establish OA as a diagnosis. Typical radiographic changes include loss of joint space, subchondral sclerosis, bony cysts, and reactive osteophytes. Articular erosions and osteoporosis are rare. It is important to note that radiographic findings do not correlate with clinical symptoms.

Keys to Diagnosis: Two primary patterns are seen: (a) patients with Heberden and Bouchard nodes (with or without first carpometacarpal hypertrophy) or (b) patients with a noninflammatory asymmetric oligo- or monarthritis affecting the hip, knee, metatarsophalangeal joints, or spine.

Differential Diagnosis: Disorders commonly confused with OA include psoriatic arthritis, Reiter syndrome, hemochromatosis, osteonecrosis, gout, pseudogout, or hydroxyapatite deposition disease.

Therapy: The primary goals of therapy are to relieve pain and maintain function. The initial approach to treatment should always include patient and family education regarding the nature of the disorder and the prognosis. Physical and occupational therapy should be periodically encouraged to optimize joint protection, mobility, and function. Use of weight loss, splinting, ambulatory assist-devices, and vocational rehabilitation should also be considered.

Several studies have shown that regular low-impact aerobic exercise (i.e., stationary bicycling, swimming) and isometric exercise can substantially reduce pain, increase mobility, and (in some patients) even retard progression to joint replacement surgery.

Initial pharmacologic attempts at pain control should rely on the use of safe therapies, such as nonnarcotic analgesics (e.g., acetaminophen), topical therapies (e.g., ice, heat, capsaicin cream), and nonacetylated salicylate (e.g., salsalate). Low-dose NSAIDs may be used if not contraindicated. Patients who do not respond well to these conservative measures may try other or higher dose NSAIDs, add other analgesic agents (e.g., propoxyphene, tramadol, nightly tricyclic antidepressants), or be considered for intraarticular injection. Use of strong narcotics and oral corticosteroids should be discouraged.

Intraarticular corticosteroid injection may provide temporary or sustained relief of pain. Intraarticular injection of hyaluronate (usually given as a series of three to five weekly injections) has a modest to moderate effect in patients with OA of the knees. Because of equivocal results, joint lavage is not routinely recommended for the treatment of knee OA. Intraarticular hyaluronic acid injections.

Glucosamine and chondroitin sulfate have been advocated by lay individuals as beneficial. Recent reports suggest this combination has a modest effect on pain and long-term use may be associated with a delay in cartilage loss over time in the knees.

Surgery: For those with advanced disease, joint replacement surgery may dramatically improve the quality of life. Surgery should be considered for patients who experience intractable/refractory pain, loss of function or mobility, and radiographic evidence of advanced degenerative changes in the joint. Arthroplasty (joint replacement surgery) is routinely recommended for advanced OA involving the hip or knee. More than 265,000 knee and >165,000 hip replacements are performed yearly in the United States. Relative contraindications to arthroplasty include obesity, multiple medical disorders (that impart a high perioperative risk of death), and a lack of motivation or inability to participate in a postoperative rehabilitation program.

BIBLIOGRAPHY

Bradley JD, Brandt KD, Katz BP, et al. Comparison of an antiinflammatory dose of ibuprofen, an analgesic dose of ibuprofen and acetaminophen in the treatment of patients with osteoarthritis of the knee. *N Engl J Med* 1991;325:87–91.

Felson DT. The epidemiology of knee osteoarthritis: results from the Framingham Osteoarthritis Study. *Semin Arthritis Rheum* 1990;20:42–50.

Hochberg MC, Altman RD, Brandt KD, et al. Guidelines for the medical management of osteoarthritis. Part I: Osteoarthritis of the hip. Part II: osteoarthritis of the knee. *Arthritis Rheum* 1995;38:1535–1546.

Roddy E, Doherty M. Guidelines for management of osteoarthritis published by the American College of Rheumatology and the European League Against Rheumatism: why are they so different? *Rheum Dis Clin North Am* 2003;29:717–731.

Wang CT. Therapeutic effects of hyaluronic acid on osteoarthritis of the knee. A meta-analysis of randomized controlled trials. *J Bone Joint Surg Am* 2004;86A:538–545.

OSTEOCHONDROMATOSIS, SYNOVIAL

ICD-9 Code: 727.82.

Definition: Synovial osteochondromatosis is a benign monarticular process characterized by intraarticular calcific bodies that mainly affects large arthrodial joints.

Etiology: Although the majority of cases are idiopathic, synovial osteochondromatosis has also been suggested to be associated with other preexisting articular conditions, such as OA, RA, neuropathic arthropathy, osteonecrosis, and trauma.

Pathology: Metaplastic changes in the synovium result in the formation of cartilaginous bodies that protrude into the joint space. Bone formation in the cartilage and calcification subsequently develop. Detachment from the synovium leads to multiple intraarticular loose bodies. Although considered benign from a clinical standpoint, clonal proliferation has been demonstrated within lesions, suggesting a neoplastic process. However, malignant transformation to chondrosarcoma appears to be a very rare event.

Demographics: Men are affected about twice as often as women. Diagnosis is usually made between 20 and 40 years of age.

Cardinal Findings: The knee is affected in ≥50% of cases. Other joints commonly involved include the hip, elbow, and shoulder. Small joints are uncommonly involved. Patients typically complain of pain in the affected joint, sometimes associated with loss of motion or catching. Physical examination findings are nonspecific.

Diagnosis/Imaging: The diagnosis is almost always made by radiography, with characteristic multiple, rounded, intraarticular calcified nodules of similar size. The diagnosis can be confirmed by MRI, particularly in cases in which calcification is less prominent.

Differential Diagnosis: Synovial sarcoma, gout, CPPD crystal deposition disease, hydroxyapatite disease, scleroderma (with calcinosis).

Therapy: Surgical removal of symptomatic intraarticular bodies, via arthroscopy if possible, is the standard treatment.

BIBLIOGRAPHY

Ozark L, Demos T, Lomasney L, et al. Synovial osteochondromatosis. *Orthopedics* 2000; 23:513–516.

OSTEOMYELITIS

ICD-9 Codes: Acute osteomyelitis, 730.0; chronic osteomyelitis, 730.1.

Definition: Osteomyelitis is infection of bone and bone marrow.

Etiology: Most cases occur by either hematogenous or contiguous spread from local soft tissue infections or by direct inoculation (e.g., trauma). The highly vascular metaphysis (in children) or diaphysis (in adults) is a frequent site of hematogenous spread. Contiguous spread is more likely to occur in areas of vascular compromise. Acute hematogenous osteomyelitis is commonly caused by *S. aureus, Streptococcus* spp, and *H. influenzae*. Cases caused by contiguous spread may involve mixed aerobic and anaerobic organisms. Infections caused by prosthetic devices may be caused by coagulase-negative staphylococci, *S. aureus*, or gram-negative bacteria.

Pathology: In acute osteomyelitis, involved bony tissues show suppurative infiltrates, vascular congestion, edema, and thrombosis. Chronic osteomyelitis involvement shows devitalized bony tissues or fibrotic replacement.

Demographics: In infants and children, almost all cases are from hematogenous spread. Adults may develop infection from hematogenous dissemination or local spread. Local extension is more likely to involve bone in individuals with significant comorbidity such as diabetes or RA.

Risk Factors: Diabetes, RA, sickle cell disease, intravenous drug use, hemodialysis, trauma, recent fractures, prosthetic implants, and vascular insufficiency are risk factors.

Cardinal Findings: Acute signs of inflammation, such as erythema, swelling, and pain, may be localized over affected areas. However, many patients lack localizing signs and present instead with deep bony pain that may be referred some distance from the lesion. Contiguous spread to bone should be suspected around chronic soft tissue infections that may have draining sinuses. Fever is common but not universal. Single or multiple sites may be involved; children usually have multiple lesions. Tubular bones are commonly affected in children, and the vertebral column is frequently involved in adults.

Diagnostic Tests: Bone biopsy and culture are required for definitive diagnosis; cultures of sinus tracts do not reliably indicate the causative organism. Blood cultures can be useful but are positive in only a minority of cases. Leukocytosis and elevated ESR and CRP levels may be seen.

Imaging: Radiographs may show soft tissue swelling, periosteal elevation, cortical lucencies (with or without surrounding sclerosis), and destruction or erosion of the metaphysis, epiphysis, or diaphysis. Chronic osteomyelitis may be suggested by areas of osteolysis, periostitis, or sequestration. Scintigraphy and MRI may be used to define the extent of the osteomyelitis and are most useful in assessing chronic osteomyelitis.

Key to Diagnosis: Bone pain or radiographic abnormalities in patient with localized infection or possible bacteremia should suggest consideration of osteomyelitis. Osteomyelitis is more likely to occur in immunosuppressed hosts or those with comorbid risk factors.

Differential Diagnosis: Chronic soft tissue infections (cellulitis, abscesses) can be present without bone involvement. In such cases, radionuclide imaging studies (early) or plain radiographs (late) can be useful to suggest whether underlying bone is abnormal. Osteonecrosis and other causes of bony infarcts may be mistaken for osteomyelitis.

Therapy: If the organism is identified by bone biopsy/culture or blood culture, treatment with the appropriate antibiotic, administered parenterally, is required for 4 to 6 weeks.

Surgery: Surgical treatment may be required in chronic osteomyelitis for debridement of nonvital tissues or to drain abscesses. Hyperbaric oxygen therapy is a useful adjunct in cases of vascular insufficiency.

Prognosis: Outcome depends greatly on the time to diagnosis and the comorbidity. Children may recover completely; at the other end of the spectrum, adults with limb infections may require amputation.

BIBLIOGRAPHY

McGuire JH. Osteomyelitis and infections of prosthetic joints. In: Isselbacher KJ, Braunwald E, Wilson JD, et al., eds. *Harrison's principles of internal medicine,* 13th ed. New York: McGraw-Hill, 1994:558–560.

OSTEONECROSIS

Synonyms: Avascular necrosis, aseptic necrosis, ischemic necrosis of bone.

ICD-9 Code: 733.40.

Definition: Osteonecrosis is the ischemic death of bone and bone marrow, clinically manifest as bone pain with distinctive radiographic sequelae.

Etiology: Although a variety of states predispose to osteonecrosis, it may be idiopathic. Underlying mechanisms may include disruption in normal osseous blood flow, thrombosis, fat emboli, endothelial injury, hypercoagulability, increase in intraosseous pressure, and local alterations in tissue architecture (i.e., trauma) or bone stock (osteomalacia).

Risk Factors: Numerous associations have been described, including (in decreasing order of frequency) trauma (with or without adjacent fracture), high-dose corticosteroids, chronic alcoholism, renal failure, organ transplantation, SLE and other connective tissue diseases (e.g., PM), thrombotic states (e.g., sickle cell anemia, hemoglobinopathies), radiation injury, pancreatitis, gout, pregnancy, hyperlipidemia, and caisson disease (decompression sickness in divers).

Pathology: Sequence of events includes cell death, eosinophilic reticulated necrosis, mesenchymal and capillary ingrowth, resorption of bone, collapse, and deposition of new woven bone on ischemic/necrotic trabecular bone.

Demographics: The underlying condition or cause determines the demographics. Osteonecrosis may account for nearly 10% of total hip replacements (>165,000) done in the United States each year. Most commonly seen in third to sixth decades of life, osteonecrosis is more common in men than women (perhaps owing to trauma or alcohol).

Cardinal Findings: Osteonecrosis most commonly affects the proximal femoral head (men), more so than the distal femoral condyles (women). Less common sites include the proximal humeral head, talus, lunate bone of the wrist (Kienböck disease), and tarsal bones. Once clinically recognized, the symptoms and radiographic changes are progressive.

Diagnostic Tests: Laboratory tests have value only in documenting an underlying cause of osteonecrosis.

Imaging: Plain radiographs usually suffice to make a diagnosis. Table 27 demonstrates the correlation between symptoms and typical imaging changes in the course of osteonecrosis. Common early findings on radiographs include alteration in the normal trabecular pattern, with lytic or sclerotic change. Later findings include a crescent sign (subchondral crescent-shaped lucency), collapse, loss of joint space, and secondary osteoarthritic changes (osteophytes). Scintigraphy (bone scan) using technetium-99m may show asymmetric changes, whose nature depends on the stage of disease. The early infarctive stage shows no uptake or a "cold" spot that may be present before the radiographs change. Later, during the reparative stages, the bone scan may show increased areas of uptake. MRI may be more sensitive than bone scanning in picking up earlier lesions but may yield a false-negative result in the first 2 to 3 weeks. The earliest finding is nonspecific marrow edema, later followed by marrow necrosis with changes in cortical bone.

Table 27
Staging of Osteonecrosis of the Femoral Head

Stage	Symptoms	X-ray	Other Imaging
0	No pain	Normal	Normal bone scan, MRI
1	Minimal or no pain	Normal	Abnormal MRI or bone scan
2	Minimal pain, night pain	Sclerosis or cyst formation; no collapse, normal joint space	Abnormal MRI and bone scan
3	Intermittent groin/thigh pain, limitation of motion	Early subchondral collapse (crescent sign), no flattening, normal joint space	Unnecessary
4	Increasing pain, antalgic limp	Flattening of femoral head, normal joint space	Unnecessary
5	Increasing pain, severe loss of motion	Flattening of femoral head, joint space narrowing and acetabular changes	Unnecessary

Keys to Diagnosis: Complaints of vague bone pain (at the ends of long bones), possibly worse at night, in patients with an identifiable risk factor (e.g., steroid use) should suggest osteonecrosis. Remember that clinical symptoms precede radiographic evidence of osteonecrosis by months. The earliest and most reliable diagnosis is made by MRI.

Differential Diagnosis: Monarticular OA, fracture, transient osteoporosis of the hip, osteoidosteoma, sickle cell crisis, osteomyelitis, and primary or metastatic tumor should be considered.

Therapy: Treatment varies according to the stage of disease and whether an underlying cause is identified. For instance, abstinence from alcohol, lowering or discontinuing corticosteroid therapy, lipid-lowering therapy, or avoidance of sickle cell crises may benefit some.

Conservative measures should be aimed at maintaining strength, avoiding contractures or debility (with the assistance of physical and occupational therapy), and pain management.

Pain can be managed with analgesic agents (e.g., acetaminophen) or NSAIDs. Intraarticular steroids are not advisable. Pain may be alleviated with ambulatory assist devices (crutches, cane, or walker).

Surgery: Early stages may benefit from debridement of necrotic bone with subsequent bone grafting. Core decompression, with or without biopsy, is controversial and may be indicated in osteonecrosis of the femoral head when applied early. Joint replacement may be indicated for intractable pain with moderate to severe radiographic changes.

Total joint replacement, unilateral endoprosthesis, and rotational osteotomy have been used to treat advanced painful disease.

Prognosis: Although some patients with osteonecrosis do not progress to bony collapse, most exhibit progressive pain, debility, and radiographic change and may require surgical intervention. Joint replacement surgery for osteonecrosis is less successful than that for other disorders because of a younger population and other comorbid conditions that may result in weaker bone stock.

BIBLIOGRAPHY

Chang CC, Greenspan A, Gershwin ME. Osteonecrosis: current perspectives on pathogenesis and treatment. *Semin Arthritis Rheum* 1993;23:47–69.
Mankin HJ. Nontraumatic necrosis of bone (osteonecrosis). *N Engl J Med* 1992;326:1473–1479.

OSTEOID OSTEOMA

Definition: A benign tumor usually affecting long bones.

ICD-9 Code: M9191/0

Pathology: Lesions are typically small (<1.5 cm), round, and characterized as a central core (or nidus) of highly vascularized immature bone and osteoid tissue.

Demographics: One of the more common benign tumors of bone. More frequently affects young boys (3:1 male:female ratio). Typically affects older children and young adults (7–25 years). It is rare after age 30.

Cardinal Findings: Most patients present with localized dull pain or aching, often maximal at night, worse with alcohol ingestion and are not relieved by rest but may be improved by NSAIDs or aspirin. Most common sites include long bones (femur, tibia) and less commonly in the hands or feet. These arise in the shaft or near metaphysis and are particularly common in the neck of the femur or intertrochanteric region.

Uncommon Findings: Intraarticular osteoid osteomas may present as chronic monarthritis with synovitis. Uncommonly they are found in vertebral bodies as a cause of low back pain.

Imaging: Early on, plain radiographs are often normal but with time, a central nidus of osteolysis appears as a radiolucent core and is surrounded by a halo of reactive/sclerotic bone. The diagnosis may be made earlier with the use of scintigraphy (increased uptake) or CT. A normal bone scan excludes osteoid osteoma. MRI may be helpful in intracortical lesions but is not superior to the methods cited.

Keys to Diagnosis: Chronic focal pain, worse at night, should prompt imaging evaluation. There are no diagnostic laboratory tests. It can be detected by radiography, scintigraphy, or CT. Diagnosis can be confirmed by CT-guided needle biopsy or, preferably, MRI-guided biopsy and ablation

Differential Diagnosis: It must be differentiated from osteomyelitis, Brodie's abscess of bone, stress fracture, and other tumors of bone (i.e., osteosarcoma, osteoblastoma).

Therapy: Aspirin, nonselective NSAIDs, and COX-2 inhibitors are often effective at improving symptoms. MRI-guided, percutaneous interstitial laser ablation (photocoagulation) is becoming the less invasive treatment of choice. Where interventional methods are not available, surgery may be effective. Some lesions will regress without ablation or excision.

BIBLIOGRAPHY

Dixon J. Tumors of bone. In: Hochberg MC, Silman AJ, Smolen JS, et al., eds. *Rheumatology*, 3rd ed. Edinburgh: Mosby, 2003:2186–2187.
Westhovens R, Dequeker J. Musculoskeletal manifestations of benign and malignant tumors of bone. *Curr Opin Rheumatol* 2003;15:70–75.

OSTEOPOROSIS

ICD-9 Codes: Generalized, 733.0; postmenopausal, 733.1.

Definition: Osteoporosis is a reduction in bone density, or osteopenia, that affects all skeletal components. Altered bone density results in increased fragility and may lead to fractures with minimal trauma.

Etiology: Many causes have been identified (Table 28) including excess glucocorticoids (Cushing's or iatrogenic), deficiencies of sex steroids in men and women, lack of gravitational force (immobilization or space flight), or nutritional deficiencies (calcium, vitamin D), which may result from dietary lack or malabsorption. Estrogen deficiency mediates enhanced bone loss through production of cytokines including IL-1.

Pathology: Bone mineral and organic phases are structurally normal and present in normal proportions. The primary defect is in the total quantity of bone, such that trabeculae and cortical areas show decreased thickness.

Demographics: Over 10 million Americans are affected by osteoporosis and 34 million are at risk. Postmenopausal women represent the largest patient group. Men older than age 60 may show decreasing bone density, although increased fracture risk does not appear until after age 70. Patients of all ages who are treated with glucocorticoids have accelerated bone loss. The risk of vertebral compression fracture and hip fracture in postmenopausal white women is

Table 28
Risk Factors for Development of Osteoporosis

Age
Female gender
Hypogonadal (both genders)
Postmenopausal (females)
Small skeletal mass
White race
Lifestyle habits: tobacco, alcohol, lack of exercise, malnutrition
Medications: glucocorticoids, phenytoin, thyroid preparations, heparin
Comorbid conditions: hyperparathyroidism, hyperthyroidism, diabetes mellitus, malabsorption syndromes, Cushing syndrome, rheumatoid arthritis

nearly 20%. Black individuals tend to have greater bone density and are thus at a much lower risk of osteoporotic fractures.

Cardinal Findings: At the outset, osteoporosis is clinically silent. In later stages, fracture may occur in the vertebral bones, with resulting wedge-shaped deformities that can cause radiating pain and contribute to formation of an exaggerated kyphosis, known as the dowager's hump. Other sites at risk of fracture include the forearm (Colles fracture) and the hip. Fractures in osteoporotic ribs may be induced by coughing and can cause considerable pain. Cortical bone stress fractures may occur in the lower extremities or feet.

Uncommon Manifestations: Vertebral fractures can rarely cause spinal cord compromise.

Diagnostic Tests: Osteoporosis may be suspected based on routine conventional radiography, although this is an insensitive measure of bone density. Nonetheless, fractures can be seen on standard radiographs. Bone densitometry (e.g., DEXA scan) measurements are diagnostic (see p. 66). Tests should include two sites: the hip and lumbar spine. Measurement of serum calcium and phosphate levels and liver/renal chemistries are important to determine underlying conditions. Elevated serum calcium or unexpectedly low densitometry measurements should be followed by measurement of parathyroid hormone and, possibly, an endocrinologic evaluation (e.g., thyroid function tests). Men with osteoporosis should have testosterone levels checked. Biochemical markers of bone turnover are available but not routinely done.

Keys to Diagnosis: An early diagnosis can be made (before fractures occur) if an individual in the at-risk population (Table 28) is identified and routinely assessed by bone densitometry or radiographic studies.

Differential Diagnosis: Fractures should be distinguished from pathologic fractures and their underlying abnormalities (i.e., bony metastases). Primary hyperparathyroidism causes accelerated bone loss in primarily cortical bone, especially the hip. Osteomalacia may be associated with low levels of 25-hydroxyvitamin D and phosphate. Bone biopsy may be required for definitive diagnosis of osteomalacia. Heritable disorders of connective tissue, including Marfan's and Ehlers-Danlos syndromes, are often associated with osteoporosis.

Therapy: The primary goal of therapy should be prevention of fractures.

—*General measures:* Lifestyle adjustments should include cessation of tobacco use and of excessive intake of alcohol. Weight-bearing exercise is recommended. Frail and elderly patients with high fracture risk should have a living situation that does not require use of stairs, and ambulation aids should be used if necessary.

—*Drugs:* Calcium (1,000–1,500 mg/day) and vitamin D supplementation are recommended for all. In postmenopausal women, long-term hormone replacement with conjugated estrogens (with or without progesterone) is effective but has been associated with other unacceptable (cardiovascular, breast cancer) risks. Other options include the use of raloxifene (selective estrogen receptor modulator), weekly oral bisphosphonates (i.e., alendronate, risedronate), or calcitonin (available as a nasal spray or subcutaneous injection). Calcitonin has the added benefit of analgesic properties, which may be useful for treatment of painful fractures. The recent release of daily subcutaneous injections of teriparatide (synthetic parathyroid hormone) has added to the arsenal against osteoporosis. The use of sodium fluoride is controversial. Combinations of these therapies may not produce additive effects.

The 1997 ACR guidelines on steroid-induced osteoporosis suggest

1. Use the lowest effective steroid dose.
2. Use topical or inhaled steroids when possible.
3. An adequate intake of calcium ≥1,500 mg/day.
4. Vitamin D (800 IU/day or 50,000 IU three times weekly) or calcitriol (0.5 μg/day).
5. Quit smoking.
6. Limit alcohol consumption.
7. Begin a daily weight-bearing exercise program.
8. Use calcium, vitamin D, and hormone replacement therapy unless contraindicated.
9. When hormone replacement therapy is contraindicated or refused, use bisphosphonates or calcitonin.
10. Patients on steroids with osteoporotic fracture and normal bone mineral density should be evaluated for other causes of fracture.
11. Bone mineral density should include assessment of lumbar spine and femoral neck; if only one site, use the lumbar spine in men and women younger than 60 years of age and the femoral neck in those older than age 60.
12. Repeat bone mineral density scan in 6 to 12 months.
13. Educate the patient.

Surgery: Surgery is rarely required except to stabilize fractures. Early detection of vertebral collapse may be managed with vertebroplasty (high pressure infusion of cement into collapsed vertebra) or kyphoplasty (vertebral height restored using an intravertebral balloon followed by cement) to relieve pain and restore vertebral morphology. Bone biopsy is occasionally required to confirm that other conditions (osteomalacia, hyperparathyroidism, Paget disease, metastatic disease) are not present.

Prognosis: Fractures (especially hip fractures) in elderly patients are associated with significant morbidity and mortality. Improved awareness and a wide range of available treatments for osteoporosis may significantly change the course of this disease.

BIBLIOGRAPHY

Brown SA, Rosen CJ. Osteoporosis. *Med Clin North Am* 2003;87:1039–1063.
Garfin SR. New technologies in spine: kyphoplasty and vertebroplasty for the treatment of painful osteoporotic compression fractures. *Spine* 2001;26:1511–1515.
McClung MR. Bisphosphonates. *Endocrinol Metab Clin North Am* 2003;32:253–271.
Saag KG. Glucocorticoid-induced osteoporosis. *Endocrinol Metab Clin North Am* 2003; 32:135–157.

OSTEOSARCOMA

Synonyms: Osteogenic sarcoma.

ICD-9 Code: M9180/3.

Definition: Osteosarcoma is a primary bone malignancy characterized by proliferating sarcomatous spindle cells producing osteoid.

Demographics: The incidence approaches two cases per million population. Osteosarcoma predominantly affects children and adolescents. Males are more commonly afflicted than females. Adults with Paget's disease (<1%) or those who have had previous bone irradiation are also at increased risk.

Cardinal Findings: Intermittent pain progresses to chronic, deep pain in an affected extremity. Firm, fusiform swelling of an extremity is accompanied by loss of movement in the adjacent joint. Primary tumor develops in the metaphyseal region of long bone. Approximately half of cases involve the distal femur or proximal tibia. The lung is the most common site of metastasis.

Keys to Diagnosis: Nonarticular extremity pain and swelling in an older child should suggest osteosarcoma.

Imaging: Plain radiography shows mixed sclerotic and lytic lesions with periosteal reaction and soft tissue mass. Occasionally a "sunburst" pattern of new bone formation is seen.

Therapy: Amputation or limb-sparing surgery with pre- and postoperative chemotherapy is used most commonly. Osteosarcoma is radioresistant.

Prognosis: Despite an aggressive disease course with a high risk of metastasis, a 5-year relapse-free survival rate as high as 40% to 80% has been reported in some series. Poor prognosis occurs with axial involvement, lesions larger than 15 cm, marked elevations of lactate dehydrogenase and alkaline phosphatase, in males, and those younger than 10 years of age. The best prognosis occurs with proximal tibial involvement, age older than 20 years, and in females.

BIBLIOGRAPHY

Clark CR, Bonfiglio M. *Orthopaedics: essentials of diagnosis and treatment.* New York: Churchill Livingstone, 1994.

PAGET'S DISEASE

Synonyms: Osteitis deformans.

ICD-9 Code: 731.0.

Definition: Paget's disease is a focal bone disorder in which the bone turnover rate is increased. It can affect single bones or multiple bones simultaneously.

Etiology: No cause is known, although a viral etiology has been postulated.

Pathology: In the earliest stage, increased bone resorption produces a purely lytic picture. This is followed by an intermediate stage in which active bone resorption and new bone formation (reactive sclerosis) occur in close proximity. Bony trabeculae may show thickening. Late in the disease, static sclerotic bony changes occur without further remodeling.

Demographics: The prevalence of Paget's disease is ~3% in those older than age 40. Studies have suggested a higher prevalence in more temperate climates.

Cardinal Findings: With the widespread use of automated laboratory test profiles, Paget's disease in most patients is detected in the asymptomatic stage by the finding of an elevated alkaline phosphatase. Bone pain and deformities can occur, distribution of which depends on the specific skeletal elements that are involved. Pain is described as deep, constant, and worse at night and may be aggravated by heat. Deformities include elongation of the long bones, causing bowing of the legs. The skull may also increase in size with resultant frontal bossing. Unstable pagetic bone may result in pathologic fractures after minimal trauma.

Uncommon Findings: Because of the high blood flow through newly formed bone, skin overlying the affected area may be warm. In severe cases, heart failure or decreased mentation may occur because of the high-output state. Hearing loss or vertigo may accompany impingement on the eighth cranial nerve. There is a small increased risk of giant cell tumors and osteogenic sarcoma.

Diagnostic Tests: Elevated alkaline phosphatase level suggests the diagnosis. Urinary excretion of hydroxyproline is increased and may be useful in following disease activity (Table 29). Bone biopsy is rarely indicated to exclude the presence of bone tumor.

Imaging: If bone pain is present, radiographs of these areas may be diagnostic. Long bones show the various stages of the disease from osteolysis to excessive bone formation. Thickening of the cranial bones may be seen on a skull film. Because the lumbar spine and sacrum are commonly affected, radiographs of these sites may be useful even in the absence of symptoms. Radionuclide bone scanning helps to determine the extent of skeletal involvement.

Differential Diagnosis: Some of the lytic lesions may suggest metastatic disease. Bony changes associated with hyperparathyroidism might be considered, but in Paget's disease the serum calcium levels are usually normal.

Therapy: Asymptomatic patients require no treatment. Bony pain, spinal involvement, deformities, or uncomfortable warmth are indications for medical therapy. Bisphosphonates (e.g., etidronate, alendronate, and pamidronate) are useful in reducing bone turnover and exert relatively long-lasting effects. Hyperphosphatemia is a possible side effect that can be corrected by lowering the dose. Bisphosphonates must be taken on an empty stomach to facilitate absorption. Calcitonin, another useful agent, is available as a nasal spray. Pain control may be better with calcitonin than with diphosphonates, but the effects of this agent are short-lived. Thus, flares are more frequent when the drug is stopped.

Surgery: Correction of deformities, including total joint replacements, appears to have the same success rate as in patients without Paget's disease.

Prognosis: Medications that alter the disease course make cures possible in some patients.

Table 29
Paget Disease: Key Points

- Alkaline phosphatase is high
- Calcium level is normal
- Urine hydroxyproline is high
- Decreased/increased bone on x-ray
- Treatment with bisphosphonates, calcitonin

BIBLIOGRAPHY

Hamdy RC. Clinical features and pharmacologic treatment of Paget's disease. *Endocrinol Metab Clin North Am* 1995;24:421–433.
Kanis JA. Treatment of Paget's disease-an overview. *Semin Arthritis Rheum* 1994;23:254–255.
Klein RM, Norman A. Diagnostic procedures for Paget's disease: radiologic, pathologic, and laboratory testing. *Endocrinol Metab Clin North Am* 1995;24:437–449.

PALINDROMIC RHEUMATISM

ICD-9 Code: 719.30.

Definition: A term originally coined in the 1942, palindromic rheumatism refers to episodes of arthritis and/or periarticular inflammation that wax and wane.

Cardinal Findings: As initially described, articular and periarticular symptoms typically last a few days or more before spontaneously resolving. Monarticular involvement is more common than polyarticular. Joint effusions are inflammatory.

Complications: Approximately one-third of patients with palindromic rheumatism will go on to develop RA. Approximately half of the patients retain the waxing and waning involvement, and a minority will experience remission.

Treatment: Therapy of palindromic rheumatism is often guided by both the severity and the persistence of symptoms. Many patients receive therapy with NSAIDs. Corticosteroids, often in the form of intraarticular injections or short oral courses, have been used in severe or refractory cases. Second-line agents, with the use of DMARDs such as hydroxychloroquine, have also been used.

BIBLIOGRAPHY

Guerne P, Weisman M. Palindromic rheumatism: a part of or apart from the spectrum of rheumatoid arthritis. *Am J Med* 1992;93:451–460.

PANNICULITIS

Synonyms: Erythema nodosum, Weber-Christian disease.

ICD-9 Code: 729.30.

Definition: Panniculitis is inflammation within subcutaneous fat.

Etiology: Panniculitis can be caused by a variety of systemic diseases and is classified according to histopathologic criteria in four major groups: septal, lobular, mixed, and with vasculitis (Table 30). Panniculitis seldom occurs in asso-

Table 30
Major Types of Panniculitis

Disease	Histologic Subtype	Peak Age	M:F Ratio	Key Features
Erythema nodosum	Septal	25–40	1:3	Acute process, anterior tibia; resolves without scarring
Weber-Christian disease	Lobular	37	3:7	Fever, multiple sites, visceral involvement
Lupus panniculitis (lupus profoundus)	Mixed	27	1:9	Lesions on face, upper arms, buttocks, breasts; may ulcerate with scarring

ciation with hypersensitivity vasculitis or PAN. The pathogenesis involves a dynamic process of inflammation evolving from a neutrophilic infiltrate to eventual fibrosis.

Pathology: Skin/fat biopsy findings reflect the age of the lesion. Neutrophils are seen early, followed by macrophage infiltration and the formation of granulomata. Fibrosis is seen late.

Demographics: Panniculitis is rare; prevalence is less than one per 100,000. It occurs in the third to fifth decades (Table 30).

Cardinal Findings: Features common to all panniculitides include tender subcutaneous nodules. Associated phenomena are common and depend on the underlying clinical syndrome. In erythema nodosum (see p. 170), tender nodules appear on the anterior tibial surface and evolve into ecchymotic lesions that typically regress in 4 to 6 weeks without scarring. Weber-Christian disease is characterized by multiple recurrent subcutaneous nodules, fever, arthralgia, myalgia, and occasional abdominal pain; eventually fibrosis occurs. Lupus erythematosus panniculitis (lupus profundus) is seen in less than 3% of patients with SLE, with tender nodules that may ulcerate occurring on the face, arms, buttocks, or breasts. In PAN, small vessel vasculitis may cause panniculitis. Some patients with pancreatic disease develop subcutaneous fat necrosis (lobular panniculitis) with polyarthritis. Lobular panniculitis has also been associated with α_1-antitrypsin deficiency.

Keys to Diagnosis: Panniculitis should be suspected with tender subcutaneous nodules that are often red and may turn violaceous. Fibrosis is seen in late cases. Ulceration is rare.

Diagnostic Tests: Choice of tests depends on the clinical picture but may include pharyngeal culture for streptococcal infection, chest radiograph, skin test for tuberculosis, and serum tests for amylase, lipase, and α_1-antitrypsin. Skin/fat biopsy is usually not necessary to diagnose erythema nodosum but may be helpful in other forms of panniculitis.

Therapy: Therapy is directed at underlying disease, if detected. In idiopathic cases, management is symptomatic: bed rest and elevation of extremity (if involved). NSAIDs may be useful, and oral corticosteroids are effective in most. Immunosuppressive agents are reserved for recurrent/ recalcitrant disease.

Prognosis: Prognosis depends on underlying disease. Most cases of erythema nodosum resolve in 4 to 6 weeks. Weber-Christian disease is typically chronic, with death in 10% to 15% of cases. In lupus profundus, the course often does not follow systemic disease activity.

BIBLIOGRAPHY

Callen JP. Miscellaneous disorders that commonly affect both skin and joints: panniculitis. In: Sontheimer RD, Provost TT, eds. *Cutaneous manifestations of rheumatic diseases.* Baltimore: Williams & Wilkins, 1996:266–273.

PARASITE-RELATED ARTHROPATHY

ICD-9 Code: 711.80.

Definition: The onset of an acute reactive inflammatory arthropathy, spondyloarthropathy (SpA), and, less commonly, myositis or vasculitis in the setting of an acute or chronic parasitic infection.

Etiology: Parasites are a rare cause of reactive arthritis, but it is more common in environments where these organisms commonly cause human disease. Parasites associated with this syndrome include *Strongyloides stercoralis, Giardia lamblia,* filariasis; *Schistosoma,* and *Taenia saginata.* Rare reports have occurred with infections owing to *Toxocara, Toxoplasma gondii, Echinococcus, Dirofilaria, Loa loa, Onchocerca, Cyclospora cayetan,* and *Cryptosporidia.*

Demographics: These events are more common among those who reside in (or visit) the tropics or areas of epidemic parasitic infections.

Cardinal Findings: After a known/identifiable infectious event, several modes of presentation have been seen and include acute reactive oligoarthritis, monarthritis, SpA, sacroiliitis, or, less commonly, asymmetric polyarthritis or rheumatoid-like polyarthritis.

Uncommon Findings: It may cause myositis (e.g., *Toxoplasma, Trichinella, Taenia, Leishmania, Microsporidia,* and *Echinococcus* infection) or infectious/parainfectious vasculitis (especially *Schistosoma, L. loa, Ascaris lumbricoides, Pneumocystis, Trypanosomiasis, Toxocara, Trichomonas, Trichinella,* and *Gnathostoma*).

Complications: A Mazzotti reaction occurs with treatment of onchocerciasis (filarial infection). Patients manifest arthralgia, fever, rash, lymphadenopathy, hypotension and tachycardia , possibly from eosinophil degranulation in response to killed organisms.

Diagnostic Tests: Eosinophilia is found in some but not all. Microbiologic identification is necessary for diagnosis and treatment.

Diagnostic Criteria (proposed): Must have more than six of the following: inflammatory arthropathy; residence in or travel to epidemic area; no radiographic changes; identification of parasite; lack of response to standard antiinflammatory therapy; good response to antiparasite therapy; inflammatory synovial fluid; elevated ESR; and eosinophilia.

Keys to Diagnosis: Parasite-induced arthritis should be suspected whenever there is an acute onset arthritis, enthesitis, myositis, or vasculitis in endemic areas or developing countries or in those who have recently traveled to such regions. Diagnosis is based on microbiologic or immunologic identification of infection with a known pathogen.

Therapy: A poor response to therapy with NSAIDs or prednisone should raise suspicion of a parasitic reactive process in a susceptible host. Most will require eradication of the parasite with an appropriate agent.

BIBLIOGRAPHY

Bocanegra TS, Vasey FB. Musculoskeletal syndromes in parasitic diseases. *Rheum Dis Clin North Am* 1993;19:505–513.
Peng SL. Rheumatic manifestations of parasitic diseases. *Semin Arthritis Rheum* 2002; 31:228–247.

PARVOVIRUS B19

Synonym: "Fifth's disease" or erythema infectiosum.

ICD-9 Code: Fifth's disease, 057.0; arthropathy associated with viral diseases, 711.5.

Definition: Human Parvovirus B19 is the most common viral cause of arthralgias and polyarthritis in adults. Fifth's disease is also seen in children.

Pathology: Parvovirus has tissue tropism for red blood cell progenitors. Parvovirus B19 has been isolated from bone marrow and synovium of affected individuals by molecular biologic techniques. Viral persistence may possibly explain those with chronic arthropathy.

Demographics: Parvovirus B19 is nearly endemic among school children. As many as 60% of adults in the United States demonstrate serologic evidence of past infection. Periodic outbreaks occur most commonly in late winter and spring. Young to middle-aged adult women are at highest risk of Parvovirus B19 arthropathy.

Cardinal Findings: Children typically manifest a bright red "slapped cheek" rash and may be diagnosed with erythema infectiosum. Less commonly, a lacy erythematous eruption may be seen on the torso or extremities. The rash may be accompanied by mild constitutional symptoms and low-grade fever. Some children may be asymptomatic.

Adults infected with Parvovirus B19 develop a flu-like illness. A mild maculopapular rash of the extremities may be seen. Arthralgia or arthritis is seen in 20% of patients. An acute polyarthritis is less common and may persist for weeks to months in some. Symmetric arthritis affecting the knee, proximal interphalangeal joint, wrist, or ankles may resemble early RA.

Uncommon Findings: Chronic arthropathy is a rare result of Parvovirus B19 infection. Although RA and SLE may occur after Parvovirus B19 infection, but no causal relationship is established. Other complications of Parvovirus B19 include aplastic crises, hemolytic anemia, bone marrow suppression in patients with immunodeficiency, and hydrops fetalis.

Keys to Diagnosis: Abrupt-onset symmetric polyarthritis in young women exposed to children infected with erythema infectiosum should suggest Parvovirus B19 infection.

Diagnostic Testing: Anemia may result from diminished red blood cell production. High-titer anti-IgM antibodies on ELISA help to confirm the diagnosis. However, IgM is only elevated for approximately 2 to 3 months after an attack. Positive Parvovirus B19 IgG antibody is consistent with previous exposure but does not help establish a diagnosis because of the high prevalence of seroconversion in the general population. RF and ANA are usually absent or transiently detected in low titer. Radiographic erosions are uncommon.

Therapy: Analgesics are given for joint pain in adults. NSAIDs may occasionally be helpful. Temporary supportive care is required for many because infection is self-limiting. For rare patients with persistent polyarthritis, therapy is similar to that used for RA.

Prognosis: In most patients, symptoms resolve within a couple of weeks. A subset of individuals develop protracted or intermittent musculoskeletal symptoms that may last months. Many patients meet classification criteria for RA at some point in the disease course.

BIBLIOGRAPHY

Gran JT, Johnsen V, Myklebust G, et al. The variable clinical picture of arthritis induced by human Parvovirus B19: report of seven adult cases and review of the literature. *Scand J Rheumatol* 1995;24:174–179.

Naides SJ, Scharosch LL, Foto F, et al. Rheumatologic manifestations of human Parvovirus B19 infection in adults: initial two-year clinical experience. *Arthritis Rheum* 1990;33:1297–1307.

Periodic Fever Syndromes (see Febrile syndromes)

PERIOSTITIS

ICD-9 Code: 730.30.

Definition: Periostitis refers to radiographic elevation of the periosteum in response to injury, inflammation, or infection.

Pathology: Periostitis is often associated with increased vascularity and local blood flow. Early round cell infiltration into the outer or fibrous layer is followed by deposition of new bone on the original cortical bone. Periosteal new bone is less dense pathologically and radiographically.

Associated Disorders: Hypertrophic pulmonary osteoarthropathy (primary or secondary), osteomyelitis, thyroid acropachy, psoriatic arthritis, RA, Reiter syndrome, juvenile arthritis, DISH, syphilis, tuberculosis, leukemia, lymphoma, plasma cell dyscrasias, neurofibromatosis, drugs (hypervitaminosis A, fluorosis, prostaglandin E, IL-11), or venous stasis may be associated.

Cardinal Findings: Periostitis may be asymptomatic or painful. It tends to be painful during the early or acute stage. Pain may be described as deep, aching, or burning. There may be palpable tenderness, local warmth or swelling, with or without associated pitting edema.

Diagnostic Tests: Characteristic changes include less dense, new bone formation that is elevated, running parallel to cortical bone and may appear linear, layered, or spiculated.

Imaging: Periostitis is best imaged by conventional radiography but may be identified by scintigraphy or CT. Periosteal elevation is frequently found near (in decreasing frequency) the diaphysis, metaphysis, or epiphysis of long bones, especially the tibia, fibula, radius, metacarpals, or metatarsals.

Therapy: Treat the underlying disorder. Limb elevation, local ice, or NSAIDs may be effective in managing pain.

BIBLIOGRAPHY

Resnick D, Niwayama G. Enostosis, hyperostosis and periostitis. In: Resnick D, Niwayama G, eds. *Diagnosis of bone and joint disorders,* 2nd ed. Philadelphia: WB Saunders, 1988:4073–4139.

PIGMENTED VILLONODULAR SYNOVITIS

ICD-9 Code: 719.2.

Definition: Pigmented villonodular synovitis is a benign tenosynovial or articular proliferative synovial neoplasm, frequently containing hemosiderin-laden cells.

DISEASES

Etiology: A nonmalignant tumor of unknown etiology. It may be preceded by trauma in a minority of cases. Malignant transformation is rare.

Demographics: The diffuse articular form is rare, with equal gender distribution. A localized tenosynovial form is more common, with a slight female predominance. Peak onset is during the third to fourth decade.

Cardinal Findings: Diffuse pigmented villonodular synovitis often presents insidiously as monarthritis of a lower extremity, especially the knee. Long-standing discomfort and swelling may be confused with chronic inflammatory arthropathies. Localized tenosynovial pigmented villonodular synovitis occurs as a painless nodular lesion, often next to a finger joint, and may be confused with a giant cell tumor of the tendon sheath. Recurrence is common.

Diagnostic Testing: Routine studies are normal. Synovial fluid is frankly bloody or xanthochromic. Plain radiographs of diffuse disease show a soft tissue mass often associated with effusion, bone erosions, or cartilage loss. T2-weighted MRI shows a diminished signal in areas of pigmented villonodular synovitis owing to increased hemosiderin (iron) content. Definitive diagnosis may be established by synovial biopsy or at the time of surgical resection. Diffuse pigmented villonodular synovitis has coarse villi and is locally invasive to the bone. Grossly, the diffuse lesion is yellow to dark brown.

Keys to Diagnosis: Bloody synovial fluid and characteristic MRI appearance suggests pigmented villonodular synovitis. It needs to be distinguished from soft tissue tumors, giant cell tumor, and osteochondromatosis.

Therapy: Surgical resection is used in most cases; 30% to 50% recur. External and intraarticular irradiation has met with varying success.

BIBLIOGRAPHY

Davidson A, Bentley G. Pigmented villonodular synovitis following arthroscopic laser surgery of the knee. *Arthroscopy* 2001;17:412–414.

PLANTAR FASCIITIS

Synonyms: Subcalcaneal heel pain, calcaneal bursitis.

ICD-9 Code: 728.71.

Definition: Plantar fasciitis is acute or chronic pain from the plantar surface of the heel and plantar fascia, worsened by weight bearing or local manual pressure. Often there are associated calcaneal spurs or bursitis.

Etiology: Plantar fasciitis may be idiopathic or posttraumatic with resultant inflammatory change owing to overuse or reinjury. It may result from obesity, reduced dorsiflexion, work-related weight-bearing, athletic activity, prolonged walking, improper shoes, structural instability, or direct trauma to the heel. Plantar fasciitis may also be associated with the spondyloarthropathies (SpA).

Pathology: There is local degenerative change in the origin of the plantar fascia with traction periostitis of the medical calcaneal tubercle. With repetitive stress, microtears develop, resulting in inflammation involving the bursa, plantar fascia, and enthesis (attachment sites on the calcaneus).

Demographics: Plantar fasciitis is most common between 40 and 60 years of age. Most patients have calcaneal spurs or history of trauma. In young patients, suspect trauma or an SpA.

Associations: It may be associated with inflammatory conditions (SpA, RA, SLE), structural abnormalities (pes valgus, flexible flat foot), overuse (long distance running, prolonged standing, aerobic dance), obesity, poor footwear, diabetes, calcaneal spurs, Dupuytren's contracture, Achilles tendinitis, or metabolic bone disease.

Cardinal Findings: Intense, sharp, aching, or burning heel pain tends to be unilateral and worse in the morning; it may improve with time and ambulation. However, pain may be exacerbated by prolonged standing or walking. Tenderness can be elicited by palpation over the inferior calcaneus near the insertion of the plantar fascia. Pronation (eversion) may worsen pain.

Diagnostic Tests: HLA-B27 may be positive in suspected SpA.

Imaging: Radiographic calcaneal spurs may not be present. Sharp, demarcated spurs tend to be degenerative. Soft, fluffy, cloudy, ill-defined spurs are typically inflammatory and may indicate a SpA (see p. 358). Periostitis is sometimes seen.

Keys to Diagnosis: Ask about activities that may provoke pain (e.g., running) and examine shoes. Diagnosis is based on history, tenderness on palpation, or radiographic spurs.

Differential Diagnosis: SpA, fat atrophy of the heel pad, calcaneal stress fracture, tarsal tunnel syndrome, plantar fascia rupture (from local steroid injections), or nerve entrapment of the abductor digiti quinti should be considered.

Therapy: Rest, weight loss, reduction of activity/ambulation, heel pads or heel cup orthoses, arch supports, analgesics, and NSAIDs are advised and useful. Examine shoes for appropriate heel and arch support, wear, or instability. A therapist can teach proper stretching exercises for Achilles tendon (dorsiflexion of ankle) and plantar fascia (dorsiflexion of great toe) to be done twice daily. Local injection (may be painful) of corticosteroids (10–20 mg prednisolone) should be tried when conservative measures fail. Surgery (partial plantar fascia release) is rarely necessary.

BIBLIOGRAPHY

Williams SK, Brage M. Heel pain-plantar fasciitis and Achilles enthesopathy. *Clin Sports Med* 2004;23:123.

Young CC, Rutherford DS, Niedfeldt MW. Treatment of plantar fasciitis. *Am Fam Physician* 2001;63:467–474, 477–478.

POEMS SYNDROME

Definition: A rare multisystem disorder associated with plasma cell dyscrasias.

Pathogenesis: Pathogenesis is unknown. Elevated serum concentrations of the proinflammatory cytokines IL-1, IL-6, and TNF-α and of the metalloproteinases TIMP and VEGF have been reported.

Cardinal Findings: The acronym POEMS represents the key features, including

—*Plasma cell dyscrasia with polyneuropathy:* Plasmocytomas often present as sclerotic bony lesions. A severe, sensorimotor inflammatory polyneuropathy is uncommon.

—*Organomegaly:* Hepatomegaly and lymphadenopathy are present in 67%; splenomegaly is seen in 33% of patients.

—*Endocrinopathy:* Hypothyroidism, hypogonadism with gynecomastia, amenorrhea, impotence, or hyperprolactinemia may be seen.

—*Monoclonal gammopathy:* IgG or IgA monoclonal paraproteinemia may be seen.

—*Skin changes:* Scleroderma-like skin changes are common, but changes may also include hyperpigmentation, hypertrichosis, hyperhidrosis, and angiomas.

—*Other features:* Fever, anorexia, and thrombocytosis occur. Rare associations include Castleman disease or vasculitis.

Therapy: Initially, most patients are treated with corticosteroids. Cyclophosphamide and other immunomodulatory agents have been used in refractory cases.

POLYARTERITIS NODOSA (FIG. 7)

Synonyms: Polyangiitis, periarteritis nodosa, systemic necrotizing vasculitis (PAN is part of this larger disease spectrum).

ICD-9 Code: 446.0.

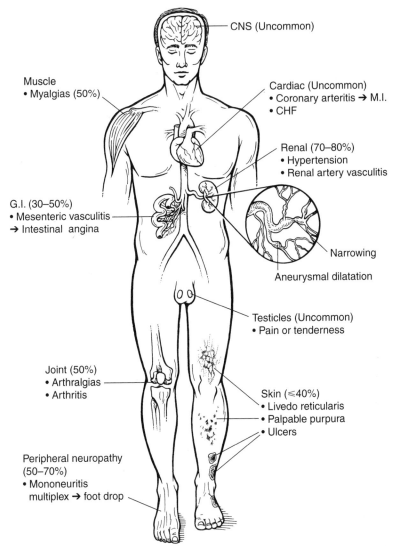

CNS (Uncommon)

Muscle
• Myalgias (50%)

Cardiac (Uncommon)
• Coronary arteritis → M.I.
• CHF

Renal (70–80%)
• Hypertension
• Renal artery vasculitis

G.I. (30–50%)
• Mesenteric vasculitis
→ Intestinal angina

Narrowing
Aneurysmal dilatation

Testicles (Uncommon)
• Pain or tenderness

Joint (50%)
• Arthralgias
• Arthritis

Skin (≤40%)
• Livedo reticularis
• Palpable purpura
• Ulcers

Peripheral neuropathy
(50–70%)
• Mononeuritis
  multiplex → foot drop

Figure 7. Manifestations of polyarteritis nodosa. Drawing of a visceral angiogram with classic vasculitis findings.

Definition: PAN is a systemic necrotizing vasculitis that affects medium and small muscular arteries of the skin, kidneys, muscle, GI tract, and peripheral nerves. Microscopic polyangiitis is also described because it is a PAN variant and affects smaller sized arteries. Microscopic polyangiitis is distinguished from PAN by manifesting pulmonary capillaritis, alveolar hemorrhage, and P-ANCA positivity.

Etiology: PAN is systemic vasculitis of uncertain etiology. Although there is no consistent infectious cause; PAN has been associated with hepatitis B antigenemia, especially in intravenous substance abusers. Hepatitis C has been described in both PAN and microscopic polyangiitis.

Pathology: Immune complexes deposited in the vascular endothelium activate complement, attracting inflammatory cells. The cellular infiltrate contains both neutrophils and mononuclear cells. Release of proteolytic enzymes and oxygen free radicals results in destruction of the entire vessel wall with fibrinoid necrosis. Eosinophils and granuloma are very rare.

Demographics: PAN and microscopic polyangiitis are uncommon disorders. Median onset age is 40 to 60 years, with a 2:1 male predominance.

Cardinal Findings: Significant constitutional symptoms may predominate early and include fever, weight loss, and severe malaise. Arthralgias/myalgias (50%) and severe abdominal pain often herald disease onset. In PAN, visceral organ manifestations (in order of decreasing frequency) include (Fig. 7):
—*Renal (70%–80%):* Impaired renal function, proteinuria, and hypertension are secondary to renal artery involvement.
—*Nerve (50%–70%):* Peripheral neuropathy is common and often manifests early in the disease as mononeuritis multiplex (vasculitis of the vasa nervorum) and may present as foot drop. Distal sensorimotor polyneuropathy and late CNS involvement leading to encephalopathy also occur.
—*GI (25%–70%):* Severe abdominal pain with intestinal angina is common. GI hemorrhage, perforation, cholecystitis, pancreatitis, intrahepatic aneurysm rupture, and appendicitis have all been reported.
—*Cardiac (<10%):* Although coronary vasculitis is common at postmortem, symptomatic coronary vasculitis and cardiac disease are uncommon in PAN.
—*Skin (40%):* Livedo reticularis, nodules, nonspecific maculopapular eruptions, and ulcerations are seen. Subcutaneous skin lesions are typical in the more limited form, cutaneous PAN.

Uncommon Findings: PAN seldom involves the cerebral or pulmonary vasculature. Palpable purpura is also uncommon. In contrast, microscopic polyangiitis often involves the lung and heart.

Complications: Infarction of the bowel leading to hemorrhage and/or perforation is one of the most feared complications. Congestive heart failure and myocardial infarction are occasionally seen. Microscopic polyangiitis can be accompanied by rapidly progressive glomerulonephritis.
Microscopic polyangiitis: Microscopic polyangiitis and PAN share a similar onset and range of signs and symptoms. Microscopic polyangiitis commonly manifests with palpable purpura, alveolar hemorrhage, symptomatic cardiac

involvement but is less likely to have hypertension, neuropathy, or hepatitis B. Distinctive pathology includes pulmonary capillaritis, necrotizing segmental glomerulonephritis, and P-ANCA serologies (Table 31). Although the prognosis is good, those with alveolar hemorrhage are at risk of early death.

Diagnostic Testing: Nonspecific inflammatory markers include elevated ESR or CRP, leukocytosis, anemia of chronic disease, and thrombocytosis. In the setting of renal disease, an abnormal urinalysis with proteinuria, granular or red blood cell casts, and declining creatinine clearance is frequently seen. Hypocomplementemia (low C4, C3) and circulating immune complexes are inconsistently detected; the latter are not recommended because of their poor sensitivity and specificity. Evidence of HBV or HCV infection should be sought. An angiogram of the mesenteric or renal arteries may strongly suggest PAN if vascular tapering, microaneurysms, and beading are noted. A histologic diagnosis is made by biopsy of a medium-sized muscular artery. Biopsies are best performed in clinically involved tissues and may include a sural nerve (with foot drop or neuropathy), a muscle (with myopathy or myalgia), or, less preferably, a symptomatic testicle. Renal biopsy is not helpful because specimens seldom exhibit characteristic abnormalities. Microscopic polyangiitis is associated with P-ANCA.

Keys to Diagnosis: PAN may be a diagnostic challenge. Histopathologic evidence of medium-vessel vasculitis or a pathognomonic angiogram in the appropriate clinical setting confirms a clinical diagnosis.

Diagnostic Criteria: The 1990 ACR criteria include (a) weight loss of at least 4 kg; (b) livedo reticularis; (c) testicular pain or tenderness; (d) myalgias, weakness, or leg tenderness; (e) mononeuropathy or polyneuropathy; (f) diastolic blood pressure >90 mm Hg; (g) BUN >40 mg/dL or creatinine >1.5 mg/dL; (h) HBV antigen or antibodies in serum; (i) arteriographic abnormalities (e.g., occlusions or aneurysms); and (j) small- or medium-sized artery biopsy speci-

Table 31
Comparison of Polyarteritis Nodosa and Microscopic Polyangiitis

	PAN	MPA
Neuropathy	50%-70%	<35%
Hypertension	Common	Uncommon
Alveolar hemorrhage	Absent	20%–30%
Glomerular disease	Absent (vascular nephropathy)	Segmental necrotizing glomerulonephritis
Hepatitis B	Uncommon	Absent
P-ANCA	10%	80%

PAN, polyarteritis nodosa; MPA, microscopic polyangiitis; P-ANCA, perinuclear antineutrophil cytoplasmic antibody.

DISEASES

men demonstrating PMN leukocytes. The presence of at least three of these features yields an 82% sensitivity and 87% specificity for the diagnosis of PAN.

Differential Diagnosis: Alternative forms of systemic vasculitis with overlapping features include Wegener granulomatosis, microscopic polyangiitis, Churg-Strauss angiitis, hypersensitivity vasculitis, and angiitis secondary to amphetamine or cocaine abuse. The vasculitides are compared in Appendix F (see p. 537). Medium-vessel arteritis may be a feature of many connective tissue and idiopathic inflammatory disorders (RA, SLE, cryoglobulinemia, Behçet's syndrome). Occult malignancy, infective endocarditis, cholesterol emboli syndrome, and left atrial myxoma are also in the differential diagnosis. Hairy cell leukemia has been associated with PAN-like picture.

Therapy: In PAN, high-dose corticosteroids are the first line of treatment and are generally begun with at least 1 mg/kg in divided doses. Addition of such cytotoxic agents as cyclophosphamide and less commonly azathioprine is often justified, both for steroid sparing and for disease refractory to steroids alone. Some studies suggest improved survival with the use of cyclophosphamide. MTX has not been studied. Although trials are in progress, TNF inhibitors (infliximab, etanercept) have nonetheless been used with success in some patients with refractory PAN and Wegener granulomatosis. The aggressiveness of therapy is based on the tempo of the disease and the extent of visceral involvement. Addition of plasma exchange to the therapeutic regimen is not of proven benefit. Antiviral therapy with interferon alpha should be considered in patients with PAN with evidence of active HBV infections. The benign course of limited cutaneous PAN supports conservative therapy for this variant.

Prognosis: PAN is associated with very high morbidity and substantial mortality. Untreated, mortality is >90%, but with corticosteroids, it decreases to 50%. The survival advantages of cytotoxic therapy are controversial. Most mortality is owing to renal failure, GI perforation/hemorrhage, and cardiac involvement. Patients who survive the initial manifestations of PAN are at high risk of infectious complications because of the potent immunosuppressive therapy necessary to control the disease. Chronic cardiac and/or renal disease are other long-term sequelae.

BIBLIOGRAPHY

Langford CA. Treatment of polyarteritis nodosa, microscopic polyangiitis, and Churg-Strauss syndrome: where do we stand? *Arthritis Rheum* 2001;44:508–512.
Langford CA. Vasculitis. *J Allergy Clin Immunol* 2003;111(suppl):S602–S612.
Lhote F, Guillevin L. Polyarteritis nodosa, microscopic polyangiitis and Churg Strauss syndrome: clinical aspects and treatment. *Rheum Dis Clin North Am* 1995;21:911–948.
Lightfoot RW, Michel BA, Bloch DA, et al. The American College of Rheumatology 1990 criteria for the classification of polyarteritis nodosa. *Arthritis Rheum* 1990;33:1088–1093.
Soto O, Conn DL. Polyarteritis nodosa and microscopic polyangiitis. In: Hochberg MC, Silman AJ, Smolen JS, et al., eds. *Rheumatology*, 3rd ed. Edinburgh: Mosby, 2003:1611–1621.

POLYMYALGIA RHEUMATICA

ICD-9 Code: 725.0.

Definition: Polymyalgia rheumatica is an inflammatory disorder of older white adults that causes pain and stiffness in the proximal musculature.

Etiology: The cause is unknown. It has a strong association with some HLA markers, especially HLA-DR4. As in RA, the genotype HLA-DRB1*04 more commonly occurs in polymyalgia rheumatica than in the general population. Seasonal clustering of polymyalgia rheumatica and a preponderance in people of northern latitudes may provide etiopathogenetic clues.

Pathology: No well-defined pathologic lesion has been identified in either muscle or surrounding joints. Arthroscopic synovial biopsy of the shoulders in affected patients has shown low-grade synovitis, suggesting a link with large-joint arthritis.

Demographics: The prevalence of polymyalgia rheumatica approaches that of RA in older populations. It is almost twice as common in women as in men, and it occurs preferentially in adults of northern European ancestry. It is rare in nonwhites. Approximately 85% of patients with polymyalgia rheumatica are older than 60 years of age. It is estimated that there are 400,000 to 700,000 patients with polymyalgia rheumatica in the United States. The annual incidence for those older than 50 years is 59 cases per 100,000.

Cardinal Findings: Onset before the age of 50 is highly unusual. Symptoms may begin abruptly or insidiously as pain, stiffness, and tenderness in the neck, hip, and shoulder girdle. Prolonged morning stiffness is also characteristic. Associated constitutional symptoms often include anorexia, fatigue, weight loss, low-grade fevers, and occasional night sweats. Synovial swelling is seen in 20% to 35% and may occur in the wrists, knees, and small joints of the hands. Polymyalgia rheumatica commonly overlaps with late-onset RA.

Complications: Progression from polymyalgia rheumatica to giant cell arteritis is seen in 10% to 13% of patients with polymyalgia rheumatica. Nonetheless, blind temporal artery biopsies should not be done in these patients. Progression to RA is seen in >15%, thus distinguishing between polymyalgia rheumatica and RA is difficult.

Diagnostic Testing: A moderately to markedly elevated ESR (usually >60 mm/h) or CRP is highly characteristic. Anemia of chronic disease, leukocytosis, reactive thrombocytosis, and decreased albumin are also common. Alkaline phosphatase and hepatic enzymes may be elevated. Factor VIII/von Willebrand factor and other endothelium-derived proteins also may be elevated in patients with polymyalgia rheumatica, but testing is not clinically indicated.

Radioisotope scans have identified synovitis in large joints but are not of any diagnostic value.

Keys to Diagnosis: Look for abrupt onset of soreness in the shoulder and hip girdle muscles with stiffness, fatigue, and elevated ESR in an older white person. Polymyalgia rheumatica may present as fever of unknown origin or an occult cause for anemia or weight loss.

Differential Diagnosis: A myriad of other systemic inflammatory, infectious, and neoplastic disorders can present with similar protean symptoms. Hypothyroidism is a frequent consideration. Polymyalgia rheumatica is differentiated from inflammatory myopathy (DM and PM) by the absence of frank muscle weakness or characteristic skin and other nonmusculoskeletal findings. Unlike fibromyalgia, polymyalgia rheumatica has significant evidence of systemic inflammation, with laboratory testing abnormalities.

Therapy: Initial treatment with low- to moderate-dose corticosteroid (prednisone, 10–20 mg/day) is highly effective in relieving symptoms. A significant response to prednisone within 2 to 3 days may be diagnostically helpful. Once symptoms are well controlled, corticosteroids may be tapered by approximately 1 to 2 mg/mo. Studies show that only 24% to 40% of patients are able to wean off prednisone after 24 months of therapy, and no suitable alternative for steroids has been proven. Although steroid-sparing agents are sometimes considered, none (e.g. MTX) are of proven value. Hydroxychloroquine has occasionally been used to treat polymyalgia rheumatica coupled with late-onset RA. NSAIDs may be added to help control mild inflammatory symptoms once the prednisone dose is 10 mg/day or less.

Prognosis: Although it may impose substantial disability, polymyalgia rheumatica itself is not a life-threatening illness. Nonetheless, considerable morbidity may result from long-term corticosteroid therapy.

BIBLIOGRAPHY

Bird HA, Esselinckx A, Dixon ASJ, et al. An evaluation of criteria for polymyalgia rheumatica. *Ann Rheum Dis* 1979;38:434–439.
Calvo-Romero JM. Giant cell arteritis. *Postgrad Med J* 2003;79:511–515.
Chuang T-Y, Hunder GG, Ilstrup DM, et al. Polymyalgia rheumatica: a ten year epidemiologic study. *Ann Intern Med* 1982;97:672–680.
Hazleman BL. Polymyalgia rheumatica and giant cell arteritis. In: Hochberg MC, Silman SJ, Smolen JS, eds., et al., *Rheumatology*, 3rd ed. Edinburgh: Mosby, 2003:1623–1633.

POLYMYOSITIS/DERMATOMYOSITIS

Synonyms: Idiopathic inflammatory myopathy (IIM), PM/DM, inflammatory myositis.

ICD-9 Code: DM, 710.3; PM, 710.4.

Definition: PM and DM are types of IIM. Other less common causes of IIM, such as inclusion body myositis (see p. 219), are listed in Table 32. IIM is characterized clinically by proximal muscle weakness, histopathologically by inflammation and damage to skeletal muscle, and serologically by elevated concentrations of muscle-derived proteins (e.g., creatine kinase).

Etiology: There is no known cause for these conditions. Somewhat distinct histopathologic findings suggest that DM, PM, and inclusion body myositis may have different causes. A number of cases of IIM, particularly DM, occur in patients with malignancies (see below).

Pathology: Histopathologic analysis of muscle tissue shows a mononuclear cell infiltrate, consisting predominantly of lymphocytes that surround or invade muscle fibers. Muscle fiber necrosis, degeneration, phagocytosis, and regeneration are also seen; atrophy, fibrosis, and fat replacement are late findings. In typical PM, the predominant cells are cytotoxic $CD8^+$ T cells that are endomysial in location. In typical DM, the infiltrates are predominantly perimysial and consist of $CD4^+$ T cells and B cells. Deposition of complement fragments (e.g., the membrane attack complex) in the muscle microvasculature causes vascular injury, leading to vasculitis and perifascicular atrophy. Proinflammatory cytokines IL-1α, IL-1β, TNF-α, transforming growth factor-β, and chemokines monocyte migration inhibitor factor, monocyte chemoattractant protein-1, CCR2A/B are increased in PM/DM.

Genetics: Some cases of DM are associated with the major histocompatibility complex alleles HLA-DR3 and DRw52. (*Note:* This genotype is associated with formation of antibodies to aminoacyl-tRNA synthetase; see below.)

Table 32
Idiopathic Inflammatory Myopathies

I.   Polymyositis/dermatomyositis
  A. Adult polymyositis
  B. Adult dermatomyositis
  C. Dermatomyositis associated with malignancy
  D. Juvenile dermatomyositis (or, less commonly, juvenile polymyositis)
  E. Overlap (i.e., dermatomyositis or polymyositisassociated with another autoimmune disease, particularly systemic lupus erythematosus or scleroderma)
II. Inclusion body myositis
III. Miscellaneous
  A. Dermatomyositis sine myositis (amyopathic dermatomyositis, i.e., patients with the characteristic dermatomyositis skin lesions without associated muscle inflammation)
  B. Myositis associated with infection
  C. Focal myositis (e.g. orbital myositis)
  D. Myositis associated with drugs or toxins
  E. Granulomatous myositis (e.g., in sarcoidosis, mycobacterial infection)

Demographics: The overall prevalence of PM and DM is five to 10 cases per million population. Whereas PM is more common (1.5:1) than DM in adults, the reverse is true in children. Peak incidence occurs between 40 and 60 years of age. The female:male ratio is 2:1. Familial aggregation is rare (thus, a family history of muscle problems should suggest an alternative diagnosis).

Cardinal Findings: IIM may affect skeletal muscle, skin, and other sites.

—*Muscle:* Most patients present with symmetric, proximal muscle weakness. Involvement of the large muscles of the legs and arms may compromise activities such as climbing stairs, getting in and out of a car, rising from the tub or toilet, and raising arms over the head. Neck weakness may cause difficulty raising the head while recumbent. Less than half of patients complain of myalgia at the onset. Pharyngeal skeletal muscle may be involved, causing upper pharyngeal dysphagia, dysphonia, nasal regurgitation, and the risk of aspiration. Some patients have involvement of the respiratory muscles (e.g., diaphragm or intercostals), which may result in dyspnea, respiratory failure, or even death.

—*Skin:* Patients with several characteristic cutaneous manifestations and inflammatory myositis are said to have DM. Gottron papules are raised, scaly, erythematous or violaceous, nontender lesions commonly seen over the metacarpophalangeal joints, proximal interphalangeal joints, or knees; they are seen in more than 70% of patients with DM. The heliotrope rash is a purplish ("violaceous") rash over the eyelids, often accompanied by periorbital edema. An erythematous or violaceous "V-neck" or "shawl" pattern rash is often noted in sun-exposed areas, affecting the upper chest, upper back, and base of the neck. Periungual erythema and dilated nailfold capillaries may be seen. Nailfold capillaroscopy (see p. 88) may show capillary dilatation or hemorrhage similar to that seen in scleroderma. "Mechanic's hands" (hyperkeratosis and scaling over the fingers) and calcinosis (soft tissue calcification) are uncommon. Calcinosis is more common in children.

—*Other findings:* Cardiac involvement (e.g., dysrhythmia, electrocardiographic changes) may be detected in 50% of patients but is infrequently symptomatic. Pulmonary involvement is less common and includes respiratory muscle weakness and interstitial lung disease. Some patients display constitutional symptoms including fever, weight loss, anorexia, and malaise.

Complications: Pulmonary involvement (aspiration pneumonia, interstitial lung disease, bronchiolitis obliterans, respiratory failure) is the most common cause of death. Cardiomyopathy is a rare but serious complication of PM/DM. Persistently active disease may cause substantial muscle loss and irreversible weakness. Patients with myositis may also develop "overlap disease" or MCTD with features of scleroderma, RA, or lupus.

Rhabdomyolysis is a potentially life-threatening complication of PM/DM but may occur as a result of trauma, hyperthermia, excessive muscle activity, hereditary muscle enzyme defects, myotoxic drugs (e.g., cocaine, statins), muscle hypoxia, metabolic and endocrine disorders, or infectious myositis. Patients often complain of muscle pain, profound weakness, and red-brown or "tea-colored" urine (from myoglobinuria) and are found to have marked muscle enzyme elevations. Early diagnosis is necessary to avoid electrolyte and renal disorders (myoglobin is toxic to renal tubules). Treatment includes aggressive hydration and mannitol diuresis, alkalinization, or dialysis.

Juvenile DM: DM is much more common (20:1) than PM in children. The peak age of onset is 5 to 14 years, and it is associated genetically with the major histocompatibility complex HLA-B8 and DR-3 alleles. Classically, the DM rash, which closely resembles rashes in the adult, precedes muscle involvement. There are several important differences between adult and childhood DM. Coexistent vasculitis, ectopic calcification of subcutaneous tissue or muscle, and lipodystrophy are more common in children with DM than adults. It has been suggested that measurements of aldolase may be more useful than creatine kinase in childhood myositis. In contrast with adult DM, childhood DM is rarely associated with malignancy. With successful therapy, children with DM return to normal strength and function more frequently than adults.

PM/DM and Malignancy: The possible association of IIM with malignancy has been debated in the medical literature for nearly a century. Studies have been hampered by small numbers of patients. Approximately 9% of PM and ≥15% of DM cases are associated with malignancy. The cancer may precede, follow, or be diagnosed concurrently with the myositis. In ~20% of DM cases, the tumor behaves as a paraneoplastic syndrome, with the activities of the two conditions apparently linked. The cancers observed are the same as those seen in the general population (i.e., in the United States, lung and breast cancer; in Japan, gastric cancer), although it has been suggested that ovarian cancer is seen with greater frequency. Most investigators recommend that only a thorough, directed history, physical examination, and laboratory evaluation (appropriate for the patient's age and gender) be performed. No evidence supports more extensive testing (e.g., imaging studies, tumor markers); such investigations are expensive and unlikely to yield useful data.

Diagnostic Criteria: See Table 33.

Diagnostic Tests

—*Markers of muscle damage:* Elevation in serum creatine kinase (see p. 61) reflects skeletal muscle injury; creatine kinase is the most commonly used diagnostic test in PM/DM. Its advantages include (a) sensitivity (elevations in creatine kinase are observed in at least 70%–90% of cases); (b) relative specificity for skeletal muscle (although creatine kinase is also found in brain and myocardium); (c) correlation of creatine kinase levels with disease activity (increases may be seen weeks before a clinical flare; normalization correlates with successful treatment); and (d) dynamic range (increases in creatine kinase with PM/DM are often 20–50 times normal). *Note:* Normal creatine kinase levels vary with gender (higher in men) and race (higher in blacks).

Table 33
Diagnostic Criteria for PM/DM (Bohan and Peter)

Criterion	Definition
Muscle weakness	Symmetric proximal muscle weakness (limb girdle muscles and anterior neck flexors) progressing over weeks to months, with or without dysphagia or respiratory muscle involvement
Muscle histology	Inflammatory cellular infiltrate, often perivascular, with myofiber necrosis
Serum enzymes	Elevation in serum of skeletal-muscle enzymes, particularly creatine kinase aldolase; lactate dehydrogenase, aspartate aminotransferase, and alanine aminotransferase may also be elevated
Electromyography	Electromyographic evidence of low-amplitude polyphasic motor unit potentials, fibrillation, positive sharp waves, insertional activity
Rash (DM)	Gottron papules, heliotrope rash, erythematous patchy rash on sun-exposed areas

PM or DM is definite when the patient has 4 of 5 criteria, probable when 3 criteria are present, and possible when 2 are present. Patients with DM must have a characteristic rash.
PM, polymyositis; DM, dermatomyositis.

Other tests that reflect muscle injury include aldolase (also relatively specific), lactate dehydrogenase, aspartate aminotransferase, and, less commonly, alanine aminotransferase.

—*EMG:* EMG (see p. 69) is very useful for confirming the diagnosis of PM/DM. It is abnormal in >90% of patients and can help exclude other potential causes of muscle weakness (e.g., neuropathy). EMG findings characteristic of PM/DM include myopathic motor unit potentials (small units, early recruitment), a myopathic interference pattern (full, low amplitude), and spontaneous insertional activity (fibrillations, positive sharp waves, complex repetitive discharges, but not fasciculations). Nerve conduction velocity studies should be normal. EMG is also used in longitudinal follow-up of disease activity in patients with PM/DM. It can be useful in determining whether new symptoms of weakness relate to a recurrence of inflammatory activity or some other cause (e.g., steroid myopathy). Practical considerations for EMG include (a) doing muscle enzyme determinations before EMG because the procedure may elevate them and (b) doing EMG unilaterally to allow biopsy to be done on the contralateral side.

—*Muscle biopsy:* Specimens may be required to confirm the diagnosis. Needle biopsies may provide sufficient tissue for examination, but definitive open surgical biopsies are commonly used. The biopsy yield may be improved by previous localization of involved muscle by EMG or MRI (see below). Proper procedures for handling the tissue should be discussed with the pathologist who will receive the specimen.

—*MRI:* MRI is a relatively new approach to the evaluation of IIM. T1-weighted images provide detail of muscle anatomy, but T2-weighted images are better for detecting inflammation. Fat-suppressed T2 (STIR) images may also be useful. MRI is not routinely recommended in evaluating PM/DM because it is expensive, and the results have not yet been correlated with histopathologic findings.

—*Autoantibodies:* ANA is positive in 50% to 80% of patients with PM/DM (thus, it usually does not help in evaluating any single patient). Autoantibodies to some aminoacyl-tRNA synthetases are characteristic of some subsets of IIM; for example, anti-Jo-1 (anti-histidyl-tRNA synthetase) and anti-PL-7 (anti-threonyl-tRNA synthetase) (see myositis-specific autoantibodies, p. 86). These antibodies are found in 25% to 30% of patients (more with PM than DM). Patients with the antisynthetase syndrome are characterized by interstitial lung disease, polyarticular arthritis (particularly of the small joints of the hands), Raynaud phenomenon, fever, acute onset, and mechanic's hands.

—*Other tests:* Acute-phase reactants (e.g., CRP and ESR) are elevated in ~50%.

Differential Diagnosis: The differential diagnosis of IIM includes various neuromuscular, metabolic, endocrinologic, infectious, and other causes of muscle weakness (Table 34). The evaluation of weakness and myopathy (see p. 249) is discussed elsewhere.

Therapy: Early recognition and treatment of PM/DM are critical. Delays in treatment increase the chance of irreversible muscle damage and decrease the likelihood of a full recovery. Glucocorticosteroids are the mainstay of therapy. Initial doses are usually 1 to 2 mg/kg or more of prednisone (e.g., 40 mg twice daily). These high doses are used for weeks to months to achieve disease control and lower serum muscle enzyme levels. Steroids may then be tapered over the next 2 to 3 months while the patient's symptoms (weakness) and muscle enzymes are carefully monitored. The response to steroids is often slow and may take 8 to 12 weeks. Approximately 25% of patients have a complete response, 60% a partial response, and 15% no response to an initial prednisone trial. In patients with no response or partial response to prednisone, second-line agents are commonly used to improve outcome and limit exposure to steroids. MTX (15–25 mg/wk) or azathioprine (1 to 2 mg/kg/day) are most commonly used, often in combination with prednisone initially. High-dose immunoglobulin (intravenous IgG, 2 g/kg) has been successful, but response is transient. The role of biologic therapies (i.e., anakinra, TNF inhibitors, rituximab) has not been defined in PM/DM.

—*Steroid myopathy:* Steroids can cause a myopathy, which becomes a consideration in patients receiving long-term therapy with these drugs. EMG or muscle biopsy (shows type II fiber atrophy) are often required to distinguish steroid myopathy from active IIM.

—*Physical therapy:* In addition to pharmacologic therapy, treatment of patients with PM/DM may include physiotherapy to improve functional status and facilitate rehabilitation.

Table 34
Differential Diagnosis of Polymyositis/Dermatomyositis

Neuromuscular disease
  Myasthenia gravis
  Guillain-Barré syndrome
  Eaton-Lambert syndrome
  Muscular dystrophy
  Mitochondrial myopathy
  Muscle necrosis (e.g., from to trauma, rhabdomyolysis)
Metabolic muscle disease
  Myophosphorylase deficiency (McArdle's disease)
  Lipid storage disease
  Myoadenylate deaminase deficiency
Endocrinopathies
  Hypo- or hyperthyroidism
  Hypercortisolism (Cushing's disease)
  Hypo- or hyperparathyroidism
  Hypokalemia (including periodic paralysis)
  Diabetes mellitus
Toxic myopathy caused by drugs
  Ethanol
  Corticosteroids
  Colchicine
  Chloroquine
  Cocaine
  HMG-CoA reductase inhibitors ("statins")
  Cyclosporine
Drugs associated with IIM
  Zidovudine (AZT)
  D-Penicillamine
  Statins
Infections
  Viruses
    Human immunodeficiency virus
    Human T-lymphotropic virus-1
    Coxsackie
    Picorna
    Influenza
  Bacteria
    Suppurative anaerobic staphylococci and streptococci (tropical pyomyositis)
    Lyme disease
    Clostridial myonecrosis
    Mycobacteria (tuberculosis, leprosy)
  Parasite
    Trichinosis
    Toxoplasmosis
    Cysticercosis
    Trypanosoma cruzi (Chagas disease)
  Fungi
    Candida

HMG-CoA, 3-hydroxy-3-methylglutaryl coenzyme A.

BIBLIOGRAPHY

Allison RC, Bedsole DL. The other medical causes of rhabdomyolysis. *Am J Med Sci* 2003;326:79–88.

Joffe MM, Love LA, Leff RL, et al. Drug therapy of the idiopathic inflammatory myopathies: predictors of response to prednisone, azathioprine and MTX and a comparison of their efficacy. *Am J Med* 1993;94:379–387.

Lundberg IE, Dastmalachi M. Possible pathogenic mechanisms in inflammatory myopathies. *Rheum Dis Clin North Am* 2002;28:799–822.

Sigurgeirsson B, Lindelöf B, Edhag O, et al. Risk of cancer in patients with dermatomyositis or polymyositis; a population based study. *N Engl J Med* 1992;326:363–367.

Sontheimer RD. Dermatomyositis: an overview of recent progress with emphasis on dermatologic aspects. *Dermatol Clin* 2002;20:387–408.

Targoff IN. Laboratory testing in the diagnosis and management of idiopathic inflammatory myopathies. *Rheum Dis Clin North Am* 2002;28:859–890.

PREGNANCY AND ARTHRITIS

Definition: The hormonal alterations accompanying pregnancy may affect disease activity in patients with several rheumatic conditions. In addition, anatomic changes associated with pregnancy may produce musculoskeletal symptoms.

Disease Improvement: Amelioration in the activity of RA has been noted anecdotally for more than half a decade. It has been reported that most patients with RA experience improvement in their arthritis during pregnancy. In approximately half of the cases, the improvement occurs in the first trimester, although some patients improve only in the third trimester. The improvement in symptoms is almost always transient; recurrence of arthritis after delivery is the rule. Other disorders reported to improve during pregnancy include psoriasis, psoriatic arthritis, and sarcoidosis.

Disease Exacerbation: Patients with other rheumatic diseases may have increased activity during pregnancy. Although there is some controversy, a large body of literature suggests that many patients with SLE experience a flare during pregnancy. Controversy comes from the fact that any group of patients with SLE, not only pregnant ones, observed over a 9-month period, is likely to include many with flares of disease during that period. Nevertheless, it does appear that some patients with SLE flare during their third trimester and in the immediate postpartum period. Moreover, patients with an increased level of disease activity before pregnancy appear to be susceptible to flare during pregnancy. Thus, many rheumatologists recommend that patients wait until their disease has been quiescent for at least 6 months before becoming pregnant. This is also relevant because many medications used to treat severe SLE are contraindicated during pregnancy. Patients with lupus also have a higher incidence of spontaneous abortion, prematurity, and intrauterine death. Distinguishing between a lupus renal flare and preeclampsia may be difficult. Although the data are less clear, other diseases reported to worsen during pregnancy include PM and DM.

Back Pain: Changes in posture related to pregnancy are thought to play some role in the high prevalence of low back pain among pregnant women. Approximately 50% of pregnant women complain of low back pain during pregnancy, typically during the late second and third trimesters. Pain is usually sacral or lumbar. Excess lumbar lordosis, direct pressure on the spine, the weight of the fetus, and pelvic ligament laxity have all been suggested as potential contributing factors. Lastly, poor sleep may lead to secondary fibromyalgia.

Therapy: Most pharmacologic agents are best avoided during pregnancy. However, if necessary, corticosteroids may be used throughout pregnancy. Acetaminophen and NSAIDs may also be used, but NSAIDs should be discontinued beyond the 30th week to avoid premature closure of the ductus arteriosus. Drugs contraindicated during pregnancy include MTX, leflunomide, penicillamine, gold, cyclophosphamide, and cyclosporine. Use of azathioprine during pregnancy is controversial. It appears that corticosteroids, sulfasalazine, and hydroxychloroquine may be used safely, if necessary, during pregnancy. Although newer agents, anakinra and the TNF inhibitors, have not been systematically studied in pregnant women, these are a class B pregnancy risk and pregnant women have sporadically been exposed to these medicines without overt toxicity or teratogenicity.

BIBLIOGRAPHY

Cecere FA, Persellin RH. The interaction of pregnancy and the rheumatic diseases. *Clin Rheum Dis* 1981;2:747–768.

PSORIATIC ARTHRITIS

ICD-9 Code: Psoriatic arthritis, 696.0; cutaneous psoriasis 696.1.

Definition: Psoriatic arthritis is an inflammatory arthropathy that usually occurs with established cutaneous psoriasis, with or without nail changes. Most have mild-moderate, manageable arthritis, but some exhibit progressive, erosive, or disabling arthritis.

Etiology: No etiologic agent or reactive process has ever been proven. Some contribution to disease by stress, trauma, heat-shock proteins, and infection with *Streptococcus* or *Staphylococcus* has been implicated because patients often attribute worsening of their signs and symptoms to such factors. Genetic associations with psoriatic arthritis are heterogeneous. Cutaneous psoriasis is associated with HLA-B13, HLA-B17, HLA-37, and HLA-Cw6. By contrast, HLA-B39 and HLA-B27 have been associated with psoriatic sacroiliitis and spondylitis. HLA-Cw6, HLA-Bw38, HLA-DR4, and HLA-DR7 have been linked with peripheral arthropathy.

Pathology: Histopathology of psoriatic synovitis is similar to that seen in other inflammatory arthritides such as RA. There is usually a lack of intrasynovial immunoglobulin and RF production, and a greater propensity for fibrous ankylosis, osseous resorption, and heterotopic bone formation.

Demographics: Psoriatic arthritis may develop in 5% to 20% of patients with psoriasis. Risk increases with a family history of SpA or extensive nail pitting. Skin involvement precedes joint involvement in the majority of patients, sometimes by a decade or longer. Age at onset is usually between 30 and 55 years. Most forms of psoriatic arthritis affect men and women equally; however, psoriatic spondylitis has a male:female ratio of 2.3:1.

Disease Subsets: Six variants of psoriatic arthritis have been described. These variants are not mutually exclusive, and patients may possess overlapping features. From the standpoint of therapeutic outcomes, there are essentially three distinct phenotypes: oligoarticular peripheral arthritis, polyarticular peripheral arthritis, and spondylitis.

1. Asymmetric oligoarthritis is seen in 30% to 40% of patients and involves large and small joints. Sausage digits (dactylitis) of the fingers or toes may be present. Skin disease may be minimal or overlooked.
2. Distal interphalangeal arthritis is seen in 10% to 15% of patients. A strong association with nail changes (nail pitting) exists.
3. RA-like polyarthritis (25%–50% of patients) with symmetric arthritis but lacks serum RF or nodules. Patients with polyarticular disease tend to have greater morbidity, less response to therapy, and a worse outcome than patients with oligoarticular disease.
4. Psoriatic spondylitis is seen in approximately 20% of patients with psoriatic arthritis, 50% of whom are HLA-B27 positive.
5. Arthritis mutilans, seen in ≤5% of patients, presents as destructive, erosive polyarthritis affecting the hands and feet. It often leads to deformity and disability.
6. HIV-associated psoriatic arthritis: The severity of psoriatic arthritis appears to be enhanced by coexistent HIV infection. Such patients often have aggressive cutaneous psoriasis, severe pauciarticular or polyarticular arthritis, impressive enthesitis, and poor correlation with CD4 lymphocyte counts. Spondylitis and uveitis are rare.

Cardinal Findings: Psoriatic arthritis typically has an insidious onset and a progressive course. The arthritis may manifest as axial or peripheral joint stiffness, pain, or swelling. Peripheral arthritis may present as a chronic, asymmetric oligoarthropathy, a symmetric distal interphalangeal polyarthritis, or a rheumatoid-like (metacarpophalangeal and proximal interphalangeal joints) polyarthritis. Inflammatory sausage-like swelling of the digits (dactylitis) involving the fingers or toes is common. Psoriatic spondylitis is seen in 20% of patients and manifests as spinal stiffness, pain, or limited range of motion affecting the lumbosacral more than cervical spine. Enthesitis (inflammation where tendon inserts on bone) often manifests as pain in the heel, greater trochanter, or anterior iliac crest. The degree of psoriatic skin disease correlates poorly with the extent of arthritis. A careful examination of the scalp, buttocks, umbilicus, genitalia, and nails (fingers and toes) may reveal psoriatic lesions. Typical nail lesions may include pitting, onycholysis, subungual hyperkeratosis, and transverse ridging. Eye disease (conjunctivitis, iritis, episcleritis, or keratoconjunctivitis sicca) occurs in as many as 30% of patients.

Complications: This is a risk of limited spinal mobility and spinal fracture in patients with spondylitis and ankylosis. Aortic insufficiency is rarely symptomatic.

Diagnostic Tests: Inflammatory indices such as increases in the ESR or CRP are less commonly observed in patients with psoriatic arthritis than in patients with RA. Hyperuricemia may be found in patients with extensive skin involvement and often correlates with the severity of cutaneous psoriasis. Synovial fluid has an inflammatory picture, with typical WBC counts ranging from 2,000 to 40,000 cells/mm^3, and a neutrophil predominance.

Imaging: Radiographic changes include soft tissue swelling, erosions, and periostitis. Distal interphalangeal disease or arthritis mutilans may develop a typical "pencil and cup" deformity resulting from erosive change and formation of reactive, heterotopic bone in the phalanges. Psoriatic spondylitis is characterized by asymmetric sacroiliitis and spondylitis with asymmetric, nonmarginal, "bulky" syndesmophytes (bridging osteophytes between vertebrae). Acroosteolysis, paravertebral ossification, and pericapsular calcification are uncommon.

Keys to Diagnosis: Look for psoriatic cutaneous or nail changes in association with one of the recognized articular subsets. Carefully examine scalp, ears, buttocks, nails, and umbilicus for psoriatic lesions.

Diagnostic Criteria: None are validated.

Differential Diagnosis: Cutaneous psoriasis should be distinguished from seborrheic dermatitis, fungal infection, exfoliative dermatitis, eczema, Gottron papules, keratoderma blennorrhagica, and palmoplantar pustulosis. Psoriatic arthritis should be distinguished from erosive OA, gout, RA, pauciarticular juvenile arthritis, AS, and Reiter syndrome.

Therapy: Treatment should be aimed at reducing pain, swelling, and stiffness while preserving optimal function and halting disease progression. The foundation of therapy should include patient education, joint protection, a rational program of exercise and rest, physical therapy, occupational therapy, and dietary and vocational counseling. Treatment of skin disease may include sunlight, topical agents (e.g., corticosteroids), or methoxypsoralen and PUVA. Specific articular therapies may include

—*NSAIDs:* NSAIDs may modify symptoms in some, but they do not suppress
    disease progression. All NSAIDs are equally efficacious and possess similar

toxicity profiles. However, some advocate indomethacin and diclofenac as having greater efficacy in the SpAs. Antiinflammatory (higher) doses may be necessary to control inflammation, although an increased risk of GI and renal toxicity may result.

—*Corticosteroids:* Corticosteroid therapy is infrequently used as an intraarticular steroid injection (for uncontrolled mon- or oligoarthritis), intralesional steroid to control enthesitis (i.e., Achilles tendinitis, plantar fasciitis), or topical steroid for treatment of conjunctivitis or uveitis. Use of oral low-dose prednisone (5–10 mg/day) should be reserved for severe, uncontrolled peripheral arthritis. Oral steroids are seldom effective in patients with psoriatic spondylitis. Withdrawal of oral steroids may incite a flare of skin disease and should be avoided in pustular psoriasis.

—*Slow-acting antirheumatic drugs:* These drugs are indicated when initial NSAID treatment attempts are unsuccessful or contraindicated. Sulfasalazine and MTX have been tested and advocated for use in psoriatic arthritis. Placebo-controlled trials of sulfasalazine (2 g/day) indicate greatest efficacy in patients with peripheral arthritis and enthesitis. It is uncertain whether patients with long-standing erosive disease, spondylitis, sacroiliitis, or ankylosis will respond to sulfasalazine. MTX at doses of 7.5 to 20 mg/wk, orally, subcutaneously, or intramuscularly is often effective in the treatment of both cutaneous and articular psoriasis. Higher doses and prolonged use have been associated with unacceptable hepatotoxicity and cirrhosis. Unlike RA, liver biopsy should be considered in those receiving a cumulative dose >1,500 mg and those with persistently abnormal hepatic enzymes. Cyclosporine (3–5 mg/kg/day) has a narrow therapeutic window and an increased risk of toxicity (GI, renal, hypertension) but may be very effective in controlling cutaneous and articular disease in patients unresponsive to conventional measures.

—Patients have also benefited from treatment with gold salts (i.e., Myochrysine), hydroxychloroquine, azathioprine, or etretinate (no longer available). Sulfasalazine should be considered for HIV-associated psoriatic arthritis.

—*Biologic agents:* Recently, there have been notable successes in psoriasis and psoriatic arthritis with the TNF inhibitors. Etanercept and infliximab have been studied in greater detail, and adalimumab has also been studied. Both cutaneous and articular (axial and peripheral) manifestations improved dramatically and treatment has been well tolerated. These agents can be considered with spondylitis or refractory peripheral arthritis.

Monitoring: Monitoring is tailored to the disease severity and the medications used. For example, patients with stable psoriatic spondylitis receiving indomethacin may need evaluation every 3 to 6 months, while a patient with uncontrolled, severe polyarthritis on MTX or cyclosporine may require monthly assessment.

Surgery: Surgery should be considered when pain and immobility markedly interfere with the patient's lifestyle. Total joint replacement is commonly performed in the hip or knee. The success of arthroplasty may be limited by post-surgical heterotopic bone formation. Surgical correction of spinal deformities or fusion is generally not advised.

BIBLIOGRAPHY

Antoni C, Kavanaugh A, Kirkham B, et al. The infliximab multinational psoriatic arthritis controlled trial. *Arthritis Rheum* 2002;46:S381.
Bulbul R, Williams WV, Schumacher HR Jr. Psoriatic arthritis. Diverse and sometimes highly destructive. *Postgrad Med* 1995;97:97–108.
Clegg DO, Reda DJ, Mejias E, et al. Comparison of sulfasalazine and placebo in the treatment of psoriatic arthritis: a Department of Veterans Affairs Cooperative study. *Arthritis Rheum* 1996;39:2013–2020.
Mease P, Goffe B, Metz A, et al. Etanercept in the treatment of psoriatic arthritis and psoriasis: a randomised trial. *Lancet* 2000;356:385–390.
Vasey FB. Seronegative spondyloarthropathies: psoriatic arthritis. In: Schumacher HR Jr, ed. *Primer on the rheumatic diseases*. Atlanta: Arthritis Foundation, 1996:161–163.

PULMONARY/RENAL SYNDROMES

Definition: A number of distinct conditions are characterized by significant pulmonary and renal involvement (Table 35). Typically, they present with hemoptysis related to alveolar hemorrhage and extensive alveolar infiltrates on chest radiograph. Renal involvement in these syndromes is usually a form of proliferative glomerulonephritis and may be asymptomatic at initial presentation. Nephritis often manifests with hematuria, proteinuria, and, in some cases, azotemia. Although the pathogenesis of the various conditions may be quite distinct, their presenting signs and symptoms tend to be similar and do not usually allow differentiation. Nevertheless, optimal treatment of these various diseases may differ; thus, an early specific diagnosis may favorably influence the outcome.

Table 35
Differential Diagnosis of Pulmonary/Renal Syndromes

Goodpasture's syndrome (anti–glomerular basement membrane antibody disease)
Systemic lupus erythematosus
Vasculitis
  Wegener's granulomatosis
  Churg-Strauss syndrome
  Microscopic polyarteritis
  Hypersensitivity vasculitis
Rapidly progressive glomerulonephritis
Cryoglobulinemia
Infection (e.g., subacute bacterial endocarditis)
Diffuse thromboembolic disease
Congestive heart failure

Etiology: See Table 35.

Disease Associations: The presence of symptoms in other organ systems may provide clues to the correct diagnosis. For example, patients with Wegener's granulomatosis may have nasal airway involvement or sinusitis in addition to the pulmonary and renal signs. Patients with SLE who have severe renal and pulmonary disease often have additional manifestations of lupus in other organ systems. Patient demographics sometimes also provide diagnostic clues. Goodpasture's syndrome tends to occur in white men in their twenties. SLE affects women 10 times as commonly as men, primarily during their child-bearing years. Wegener's granulomatosis and cryoglobulinemia tend to affect older persons more commonly than SLE and Goodpasture syndrome. However, males and females of all races and ages can be affected by each of these conditions.

Biopsy: Wegener's granulomatosis is characterized by granulomatous vas-culitis in affected tissues. Goodpasture's syndrome is characterized by anti-bodies to the GBM. Immunofluorescent staining of biopsy specimens from the lungs and kidneys of patients with Goodpasture's syndrome reveals a charac-teristic linear pattern of antibody deposition at the basement membrane. In contrast, diseases such as SLE and cryoglobulinemia are characterized by im-mune complex formation. Biopsy of affected tissues may reveal a "lumpy-bumpy" pattern of immunofluorescence in these conditions, consistent with immune complex formation.

　　Histopathology, particularly of renal lesions, may provide important di-agnostic clues. For example, cryoglobulinemia may be associated with pathognomonic findings on electron microscopic analysis of renal biopsy specimens. The renal pathologic findings of SLE are not seen commonly in other diseases and, in the correct clinical setting, can provide strong support for diagnosis of SLE.

　　There is an important caveat to the use of biopsy specimens to provide a di-agnosis in patients with pulmonary/renal presentations. Obtaining biopsies, particularly pulmonary biopsies, may be difficult and also dangerous in some cases. For example, in both Wegener's granulomatosis and Goodpasture's syn-drome, transbronchial biopsy has a low diagnostic yield and has been associ-ated with uncontrolled bleeding and death. If necessary, open lung biopsy is preferred.

Diagnostic Testing: Laboratory studies are often useful in evaluating patients with pulmonary/renal syndromes. Routine types of laboratory studies may not help to pinpoint the cause, but they can be quite important in defining the severity of end-organ involvement. For example, patients with most of these conditions have a hypoproliferative anemia, consistent with the anemia of chronic disease. In addition, those with significant blood loss from the lungs or kidneys may have a superimposed iron deficiency anemia. Urinalysis will re-veal hematuria, pyuria, and proteinuria, and serum creatinine will reflect the extent of renal impairment. These indices are useful not only in establishing renal involvement, but also in following the course of the disease and the response to therapy. Arterial blood gases are important for establishing the severity of pulmonary compromise and the need for specific therapies such as supplemental oxygen. Serum complement protein (C3, C4) levels reflect activation of the complement cascade. They tend to be depressed in conditions characterized by immune complex formation, such as SLE and cryoglobulinemia, and normal or elevated in other conditions.

Specific immunologic laboratory testing can be of great help in defining the etiology underlying a pulmonary/renal syndrome. Anti-GBM antibodies are seen in >95% of patients with Goodpasture's syndrome and are rarely seen in other conditions. In the correct clinical setting, the presence of cryoglobulins in the serum offers strong support for this diagnosis. Routine use of an ANA without regard for clinical symptoms or signs may be of little help in establishing the diagnosis of SLE. However, when used in selected patients (e.g., a young woman with a pulmonary/renal syndrome and a malar rash), ANA results have greater predictive value. Other tests, such as anti-DNA and anti-Sm antibodies, are more specific for SLE. Finding ANCA may help establish the diagnosis of a pulmonary/renal syndrome. Finding a C-ANCA or antiproteinase-3 antibody offers strong support for the diagnosis of Wegener granulomatosis. P-ANCA antibodies may suggest the presence of other vasculitic conditions associated with pulmonary and renal involvement, including Churg-Strauss syndrome, microscopic polyarteritis, and idiopathic crescentic glomerulonephritis.

Therapy: Treatment generally consists of nonspecific therapies in conjunction with specific immunomodulatory therapies. Interventions such as red cell transfusion, supplemental oxygen, tight control of blood pressure, appropriate therapy with antibiotics, and others may be critical to the patient's outcome. Immunomodulatory interventions generally include corticosteroids, plasmapheresis, and cytotoxic drugs such as cyclophosphamide and azathioprine. The choice of agents, dosage, and other variables may differ among the various pulmonary/renal syndromes.

BIBLIOGRAPHY

Jara LJ, Vera-Lastra O, Calleja MC. Pulmonary-renal vasculitic disorders: differential diagnosis and management. *Curr Rheumatol Rep* 2003;5:107–115.
Schwarz M, Fontenot AP. Drug-induced diffuse alveolar hemorrhage syndromes and vasculitis. *Clin Chest Med* 2004;25:133.

RAYNAUD'S PHENOMENON

Synonyms: Raynaud's disease.

ICD-9 Code: 443.0.

Definition: Raynaud's phenomenon is paroxysmal, reversible vasospasm of small arteries that may be triggered by cold exposure or stress. When it occurs in the absence of another underlying connective tissue disease, the term primary Raynaud's syndrome or Raynaud's disease is used.

Etiology: Structural and functional alterations of blood vessels are probably contributory. Arteries are usually narrowed (see Pathology section), so even normal vasospastic responses may occlude the lumen. Other data suggest changes in mediators of vascular tone, such as endothelin. Underlying causes for these abnormalities are unknown.

Pathology: Digital arteries show proliferation of subintimal tissues and fibrotic change. Small thrombi may form on the altered intimal surfaces. Luminal narrowing or occlusion can occur in these small vessels as well as in larger arteries. Vasculitis is not present.

Demographics: It occurs predominantly in females, accounting for at least 80% of those with Raynaud's phenomenon. Raynaud's disease may appear in younger women than the corresponding syndrome occurring in association with other connective tissue disorders. Almost all patients with systemic sclerosis have Raynaud's phenomenon.

Associated Conditions: Raynaud's phenomenon may be associated with diffuse and limited (CREST) systemic sclerosis, SLE, MCTD, antiphospholipid (APL) syndrome, RA, polymyositis (PM), cryoglobulinemia, and Sjögren syndrome.

Cardinal Findings: The classic "white, blue, and red" changes do not occur in all cases. Initially, severe blanching, or white, results from vasospasm and lack of arterial perfusion. This phase is uncommon and is followed by the commonly observed blueness caused by venous pooling and tissue cyanosis. On rewarming, reactive painful hyperemia causes redness in the fingers or hand. The hands are most commonly affected, but the feet and the tips of the nose and ears also can be involved.

Patients with primary Raynaud's phenomenon have a normal physical examination and only manifest physical findings in the distal extremities. Such patients usually have normal nailfold capillaries (see p. 88) and a low risk of developing other connective tissue diseases. Patients with secondary Raynaud's phenomenon clearly demonstrate evidence of the underlying connective tissue disorder (e.g., sclerodactyly, malar rash, arthritis). Nailfold capillaroscopy should be abnormal and the prognosis is guarded.

Uncommon Findings: Distal finger pad ulcerations and scarring are uncommon. In extreme cases, gangrene and autoamputation may develop.

Diagnostic Tests: The diagnosis is made largely on clinical data (history, physical examination). In patients without evidence of an associated connective tissue disorder (e.g., scleroderma, SLE), measurement of ANA may be useful in predicting the risk of developing such disorders.

Imaging: Changes in small capillaries can be viewed by nailfold capillaroscopy, which may provide prognostically important information. Radiographs show osteolysis of distal phalanges. Angiography is rarely required to distinguish Raynaud phenomenon from occluding blood clots or cholesterol emboli.

Keys to Diagnosis: Cold-induced pain, pallor, or cyanosis of digits is an important clue.

Differential Diagnosis: Atherosclerotic occlusion of small vessels occurs in older individuals, has a male predominance, and is less likely to be symmetric. Thromboangiitis obliterans (Buerger's disease) involves lower extremities more often than the hands and is usually accompanied by claudication. Heavy cigarette smoking can cause symptomatic vasospasm; obtaining a careful tobacco use history is important for all patients. Other causes of blue digits include cryoglobulinemia, hyperviscosity states, and APL syndrome.

Therapy: The hands and feet should be kept warm with gloves and other coverings that may be required both at night and during the day. Ulcerated finger tips may require protective bandages or guards. Tobacco should be discontinued, and particular medications (e.g., beta-blockers, ergotamine, amphetamines) should be avoided. Biofeedback training may be effective. A few pharmacologic agents, such as long-acting forms of nifedipine, are useful and well tolerated; blood pressure should be closely monitored. Antiplatelet therapy (e.g., ASA, dipyridamole) is advisable in some. Topical nitrates may help with digits, but their use may be limited by headaches. Difficult cases may require chronic vasodilator therapy. Although there has been anecdotal use of bosentan (endothelin receptor antagonist) and epoprostenol (prostacyclin) for severe, refractory digital ulcers, this requires further study because these agents are cost prohibitive and potentially toxic.

Surgery: Truncal or digital sympathectomy may be attempted if local measures and drugs are ineffective. Digital ischemic ulcers are best treated with local wound care measures rather than with surgical intervention. Gangrenous fingertips should be allowed to self-demarcate whenever possible.

Prognosis: For patients with secondary Raynaud's, outcome is related to the underlying disease. Raynaud's phenomenon has such a high prevalence in scleroderma (see p. 344) that it does not identify a prognostic subset. Patients may have an increased chance of developing other connective tissue disorders if Raynaud's phenomenon is accompanied by abnormal periungual capillaries, puffy fingers, pitting of the nails, or serum autoantibodies.

BIBLIOGRAPHY

Cutolo M, Grassi W, Matucci et al. Raynaud's phenomenon and the role of capillaroscopy. *Arthritis Rheum* 2003;48:3023–3030.

Hummers LK, Wigley FM. Management of Raynaud's phenomenon and digital ischemic lesions in scleroderma. *Rheum Dis Clin North Am* 2003;29:293–313.

REACTIVE ARTHRITIS

Synonyms: Reiter's syndrome, sexually acquired reactive arthritis.

ICD-9 Code: 099.3.

Definition: Reactive arthritis is an acute inflammatory arthritis occurring 1 to 4 weeks after an infection. It is characterized by a postinfectious onset, asymmetric oligoarthritis, and extraarticular sites of inflammation, often in association with HLA-B27. The arthritis is usually self-limited but may be chronic and disabling.

Etiology: HLA-B27 positivity is seen in 75% to 80% of whites with reactive arthritis, but only 50% of African Americans. HLA-B27 (see p. 75) is associated with increased disease susceptibility and severity and risk of spinal ankylosis and uveitis. Arthritogenic bacteria have been associated with reactive arthritis, possibly with molecular mimicry between bacterial antigens and HLA-B27. Whereas postdysenteric reactive arthritis may arise in HLA-B27–negative patients, postvenereal onset is often HLA-B27 related.

Pathology: Characteristic findings include inflammatory synovitis, inflammation and erosions at the insertion of ligaments and tendons (entheses), excessive production of heterotopic bone at sites of inflammation, and cutaneous pathology similar to that observed in psoriasis. Subclinical intestinal inflammation of the terminal ileum or colon occurs in 60% of patients and may parallel the clinical status and response to therapy.

Demographics: Reactive arthritis is the most common cause of inflammatory arthritis in young men. In Minnesota, the age-adjusted incidence for males (<50 years) was 3.5 cases per 100,000 men. Recent studies suggest that its frequency is decreasing in the HIV era, possibly because of increased use of condoms. Peak onset is during the third decade, but reactive arthritis may also be seen in children. Male:female ratio is 5:1 or 6:1 or higher. Women may go undiagnosed because of occult genitourinary disease and less severe arthritis. Postvenereal disease is more common in males, yet the postdysenteric syndrome affects men and women equally. With epidemic dysentery owing to arthritogenic strains, 5% of infected individuals and 20% of infected HLA-B27–positive individuals develop reactive arthritis.

Infectious Triggers: The most common pathogens known to induce reactive arthritis are enteric (*Shigella, Salmonella, Yersinia,* and *Campylobacter*) or urogenital/postvenereal (*Chlamydia, Ureaplasma,* HIV) pathogens. With enteric infections, the diarrheal illness resolves before the onset of arthritis (usually 1–4 weeks later). Patients with Reiter's syndrome who are HLA-B27 negative may have epidemic dysentery. Between 2% and 6% of patients develop Reiter's syndrome after epidemic dysentery owing to *Shigella* (*Shigella flexneri*) and *Salmonella* (*Salmonella typhimurium*). In most instances, no infectious cause can be identified.

—*Chlamydia trachomatis:* More than 50% of patients with Reiter's syndrome have antibodies to *C. trachomatis*. Rheumatic features of *Chlamydia* infections are similar to those described in classic Reiter's syndrome, except less than 50% are B27 positive, 15% have no urogenital features, and >50% develop chronic arthritis. Diagnosis is suggested by persistent mono- or oligoarthritis; genitourinary symptoms; positive serologic tests, cultures, or PCR evidence of chlamydial infection; and a response to antibiotic therapy.

—*HIV and reactive arthritis:* Although Reiter's syndrome has been described in patients with AIDS, studies have not shown an increased risk of Reiter's syndrome in HIV-positive populations matched for other risk factors. Most patients with AIDS with reactive arthritis are HLA-B27 positive and present with incomplete Reiter's syndrome with either (a) an additive, asymmetric polyarthritis or (b) an intermittent oligoarthritis. Dactylitis, conjunctivitis, urethritis, enthesitis, and fasciitis are common. These patients tend to have severe chronic disease and poor response to NSAIDs. Immunosuppressive drugs (i.e., MTX, azathioprine) should be avoided in such patients.

Cardinal Findings: The triad of arthritis, urethritis, and conjunctivitis defines Reiter's syndrome. However, <33% manifest the full triad. Most patients present with an acute, additive, lower extremity oligoarthritis. A careful history may reveal antecedent infection or extraarticular features to suggest the diagnosis.

—*Onset (within 1–4 weeks of exposure):* Onset is heralded by extraarticular features. Genitourinary involvement may manifest as dysuria, urethral discharge, prostatitis, cervicitis, or vaginitis. Fever, anorexia, malaise, fatigue, weight loss, and ocular symptoms (conjunctivitis or uveitis) are also common during onset.

—*Arthritis:* Typically an acute, asymmetric, additive, and ascending inflammatory oligoarthritis, involvement of the lower extremity (knees, ankles, and toes) is most common. The toes or fingers may be affected by dactylitis, resulting in a sausage digit. RA-like polyarthritis is uncommon.

—*Axial disease:* Symptomatic inflammatory back pain is present in ~50% of individuals. However, radiographic changes are seen in <20% of affected individuals. Sacroiliitis and spondylitis are seen in those with chronicity.

—*Enthesitis:* Inflammation at the insertion sites of tendon or ligament onto bone is called enthesitis. These sites are often painful but seldom swollen.

Common sites include the heel (insertion of Achilles tendon and plantar fascia), sausage digits, symphysis pubis, ischium, iliac crest, greater trochanter, and chest wall (see p. 166).

—*Mucocutaneous:* A sterile urethritis (in <33% of patients) may be transient in men and asymptomatic in women. Genitourinary symptoms are seen in postdysenteric or postvenereal reactive arthritis. Common findings also include circinate balanitis, cervicitis, and painless lingual or palatal oral ulcerations. Circinate balanitis is painless and may present as vesicles, shallow ulcerations, or plaques on the glans or shaft of the penis. Keratoderma blennorrhagica appears as painless, papulosquamous lesions on the soles or palms. Nail changes typically manifest as onycholysis, yellowish discoloration, or subungual hyperkeratosis.

—*Ocular:* Conjunctivitis, uveitis, or keratitis is seen in most patients. Conjunctivitis tends to be bilateral or unilateral, recurrent, and painful; it lasts days rather than weeks. Acute anterior uveitis often occurs with established disease and may follow a chronic or relapsing course.

Uncommon Findings: Cardiac conduction disturbances, myocarditis, aortitis, aortic regurgitation, amyloidosis, CNS involvement, serositis, and pulmonary infiltrates are rarely seen.

Diagnostic Tests: Most patients exhibit elevated ESR and CRP levels. Thrombocytosis, leukocytosis, hypoproliferative anemia, and elevated hepatic enzymes may also be seen. The synovial fluid is inflammatory (mostly neutrophils).

Culture of arthritogenic organisms is uncommon. Culture or serologic proof of infection is not necessary but may indicate the need for antibiotic therapy in *Yersinia-* or *Chlamydia*-induced arthritis. HIV testing is not routinely recommended; it should be reserved for those engaged in high-risk behavior.

HLA-B27 testing is seldom necessary. Very few HLA-B27–positive individuals develop reactive arthritis. Thus, HLA-B27 has a low predictive value. HLA-B27 may prove useful in patients with early incomplete features of reactive arthritis.

Imaging: Radiographs may show soft tissue swelling, joint space narrowing, or erosions in the peripheral and sacroiliac joints. Formation of reactive new bone is characteristic and may result in periostitis, enthesitis, or poorly defined intraarticular erosions. Radiographic changes are often most striking in the foot, ankle, and knee. Poorly defined, inflammatory heel spurs are found at the insertion of the plantar aponeurosis.

Axial involvement most often manifests as sacroiliitis. In chronic reactive arthritis, 40% to 60% have radiographic evidence of bilateral, asymmetric, or unilateral sacroiliitis. Ileal sclerosis and ankylosis are late findings. Asymmetric paravertebral ossification with nonmarginal syndesmophytes (bulky osteophytes) is common. Bone scan, CT, and MRI are sensitive in detecting early occult sacroiliitis but are rarely indicated.

Keys to Diagnosis: An asymmetric, inflammatory oligoarthritis with enthesitis (heel pain), nail, genitourinary, or ocular findings raise suspicion of reactive arthritis.

Diagnostic Criteria: ACR criteria require peripheral arthritis of more than 1-month duration and association with urethritis or cervicitis. These criteria show a sensitivity of 84.3% and a specificity of 98.2%.

Differential Diagnosis: Reactive arthritis should be distinguished from septic (especially gonococcal) arthritis, gout, sarcoidosis, erythema nodosum, seronegative RA, and ARF. Distinction from the other SpA (see p. 358) and other reactive arthritides (e.g., *Yersinia, Chlamydia*) may be difficult. Overlap of reactive arthritis and psoriasis or enteropathic arthritis may occur.

Therapy: Treatment should be aimed at patient education, joint protection, maintenance of function, relief of pain, suppression of inflammation, and, when appropriate, eradication of infection. Inactivity and immobilization should be discouraged, and stretching and range-of-motion exercises should be encouraged.

Treatment with NSAIDs improves symptoms but does not alter the course of chronic inflammatory disease. Indomethacin, sulindac, naproxen, diclofenac, enteric-coated salicylate, and phenylbutazone are approved by the FDA for use in AS and Reiter syndrome. Phenylbutazone is no longer available, primarily because of the risk of aplastic anemia. Indomethacin, in antiinflammatory doses (2–3 mg/kg), is commonly used in the treatment of reactive arthritis. The sustained-release form is effective in the treatment of morning stiffness. Other NSAIDs and COX-2 inhibitors also have been used. Long-term NSAID therapy is indicated as long as clinical evidence of inflammation (arthritis, enthesitis) persists.

Corticosteroids are relatively ineffective in the routine management of reactive arthritis. However, intraarticular or perilesional (tendons or entheses) injections or topical corticosteroids may benefit some patients.

DMARD therapy is indicated in patients with chronic reactive arthritis unresponsive to NSAIDs. Azathioprine, MTX, and sulfasalazine have shown efficacy in uncontrolled trials. In a multicenter, placebo-controlled trial, sulfasalazine (2 g/day) was effective in treating the peripheral arthritis of Reiter's syndrome. There are anecdotal reports of efficacy with TNF inhibitors in reactive arthritis.

Antibiotic therapy may be indicated in patients with culture-, serology-, or PCR-proven *Yersinia*- or *Chlamydia*-induced arthritis. Several reports suggest >3 months of antibiotic therapy (doxycycline or lymecycline) for patients with *Chlamydia*-induced arthritis. Recent reports suggest conflicting evidence favoring long-term benefit to antibiotic therapy. Reactive arthritides caused by *Salmonella* and *Shigella* do not respond to antibiotic therapy. Patients with idiopathic reactive arthritis will not benefit from antibiotic treatment.

Prognosis: In most patients, the initial episode of arthritis is self-limiting and lasts weeks to months. Many patients experience recurrent attacks, often after prolonged disease-free intervals. Less than 30% of patients exhibit a chronic arthritis. Severe disability occurs in <15% of patients and may be secondary to persistent lower extremity arthritis, aggressive axial involvement, or blindness. Death is rare and is usually from cardiac complications or amyloidosis.

BIBLIOGRAPHY

Cush JJ, Lipsky PE. Reiter's syndrome and reactive arthritis. In: Koopman WJ, ed. *Arthritis and allied conditions: a textbook of rheumatology,* 13th ed. Baltimore: Williams & Wilkins, 1997:1209–1227.

Flores D, Marquez J, Garza M, et al. Reactive arthritis: newer developments. *Rheum Dis Clin North Am* 2003;29:37–59.

Laasila K, Laasonen L, Leirisalo-Repo M. Antibiotic treatment and long term prognosis of reactive arthritis. *Ann Rheum Dis* 2003;62:655–658.

Mease PJ. Disease-modifying antirheumatic drug therapy for spondyloarthropathies: advances in treatment. *Curr Opin Rheumatol* 2003;15:205–212.

REFLEX SYMPATHETIC DYSTROPHY

ICD-9 Code: 733.7.

Synonyms: Shoulder-hand syndrome, Sudeck's atrophy, algodystrophy, causalgia.

Definition: Reflex sympathetic dystrophy is diffuse persistent pain, usually in an extremity, often associated with vasomotor disturbances, trophic changes, and limitation or immobility of joints. Causalgia, a different syndrome, refers to a traumatized peripheral nerve with resultant pain along the distribution of that nerve.

Etiology: Many diseases have been associated with reflex sympathetic dystrophy: trauma, fractures (especially Colles fracture), hemiplegia (prevalence of reflex sympathetic dystrophy 12%–21%), arterial thrombosis, peripheral nerve injury (3%), acute coronary artery disease (5%–20%), painful rotator cuff lesions, herpes zoster with postherpetic neuralgia, and spinal cord disorders. It is idiopathic in 25% of cases. Pathogenesis is obscure. Reflex sympathetic dystrophy may be a disorder of pain signaling and regulation as well as a persisting neural injury generating pain signals with reflex neurologic mechanisms involved. It has been proposed that primary afferent nociceptor neurons develop α_1-adrenoreceptors, making them responsive to norepinephrine released by sympathetic nerve terminals. This may in part explain the reduction in pain by α_1-antagonists. Central mechanisms of neuronal hyperresponsivity may also be a factor, especially at later stages of this syndrome.

Pathology: Skin and subcutaneous tissue are usually normal. Affected bone is hyperemic with patchy osteoporosis. There may be synovial proliferation and inflammation.

Demographics: In adults, there is a slight female predominance. It is reported to occur at all ages, most commonly between 40 and 60 years. In children, 80% of patients are female, often with lower extremity involvement.

Cardinal Findings: Three overlapping stages have been recognized in reflex sympathetic dystrophy, although the validity and usefulness of this approach has been questioned. The acute stage lasts 3 to 6 months and is characterized by intense limb pain, tenderness, swelling, and vasomotor disturbances (cyanosis or erythema, hyperhidrosis). The dystrophic (or subacute) stage lasts 6 to 12 months, during which acute symptoms resolve (often incompletely) while atrophic changes in the skin evolve and chronic aching or burning pain persists. Skin becomes dry and may be edematous or develop a brawny thickening. In the atrophic stage, skin and subcutaneous atrophy and contractures predominate.

—*Site:* Reflex sympathetic dystrophy is usually unilateral and affects the upper extremity more so than the lower extremity. It may involve the entire hand or foot. It may be bilateral in 25% of cases.

—*Pain:* Pain is often constant, burning, and severe early on. Chronic aching pain or myofascial limb pain may be present.

—*Appearance:* There are swelling, trophic skin changes, signs of vasomotor (Raynaud's phenomenon, temperature variation), and sudomotor (sweating) instability. Pitting or nonpitting edema is usually present.

—*Tenderness:* Exquisite tenderness occurs, especially in periarticular tissues. Allodynia (pain induced by light touch) and hyperpathia (persistent pain after light pressure) are characteristic.

—*Neurologic changes:* Tremor, incoordination, weakness, or sensory changes may occur.

Uncommon Findings: Nail changes and segmental involvement (one to two digital rays of the hand or foot) or involvement of knee, hip, portions of bone, or the femoral head can be seen.

Diagnostic Tests: Common lab tests (CBC, chemistry, ESR) are not useful.

Imaging: Plain radiography shows patchy or mottled osteopenia; however, this is neither sensitive nor specific. Late cases have a ground-glass appearance. Cortical breaks and crumbling erosion may also be noted. Scintigraphy is the most useful objective test. Three-phase bone scan shows asymmetry in all three phases, increased or decreased blood flow, pool, and uptake phases.

Keys to Diagnosis: Look for pain and swelling in a distal extremity with trophic skin changes and vasomotor instability, often with a history of trauma (especially fracture), myocardial infarction, hemiplegic stroke, or peripheral nerve injury.

Therapy: Early diagnosis or prevention is important, especially in high-risk individuals (trauma, myocardial infarction, hemiplegia). Treat the underlying problem, if one is identified. Once a diagnosis of reflex sympathetic dystrophy is established, initiate therapy early: analgesia, local heat, ice, physical therapy, and stress-loading and desensitization programs. Pharmacologic maneuvers include sympathetic blockade, followed by sympathectomy in those who respond (70%–80% improve). Oral α_1-antagonists (phenoxybenzamine, prazosin, terazosin, doxazosin) may be useful. Systemic corticosteroids (e.g., prednisone 20–60 mg/day for 4–6 weeks) may be useful in patients with "hot" bone scans, especially early in the disease. Treatment with calcitonin and topical ketamine has been studied. Recalcitrant disease may require chronic pain management. Rarely, amputation has been resorted to; even this measure may leave the patient with phantom limb pain.

Prognosis: Overall, 50% of patients still have significant pain or disability after 2 years.

BIBLIOGRAPHY

Schwartzman RJ, Popescu A. Reflex sympathetic dystrophy. *Curr Rheumatol Rep* 2002; 4:165–169.

RELAPSING POLYCHONDRITIS

ICD-9 Code: 733.99.

Definition: Relapsing polychondritis is a rare disease characterized by inflammation and destruction of the cartilage. It affects auricular cartilage in 85% of patients and may also affect nasal cartilage (50% of patients), laryngotracheal cartilage (50% of patients), and other organ systems.

Etiology: Although the etiology is unknown, there is both cellular and humoral immune reactivity to cartilage, particularly types IX and XI. In addition, CD4$^+$ T cells play an important role in the disease process, and the prevalence of HLA-DR4 is higher in patients than in controls.

Demographics: Relapsing polychondritis is a rare disorder. Although it has been described in many age groups, its incidence peaks in the fifth decade. There is no sexual predominance, and whites are most commonly affected.

Cardinal Findings: Ear pain, erythema and swelling, which may occur after minor trauma, is the initial complaint in nearly half of affected patients. Although the pinna of the ear may be grossly inflamed, the lower ear lobule is unaffected because it lacks underlying cartilage. Persistent or recurrent inflammation can lead to complete destruction of the cartilage, leaving a floppy or scarred pinna. Inflammation may also cause occlusion of the external auditory canal and hearing loss (~30% of patients). As many as one-third of patients may experience auditory or vestibular abnormalities secondary to vasculitis of the internal auditory artery. Nasal and laryngotracheal cartilage may be affected (in ~50% of patients). Nasal cartilage destruction may result in a "saddle nose" deformity. A saddle nose deformity may also be seen in Wegener granulomatosis, syphilis, or leprosy. Laryngotracheal involvement, which may present as hoarseness, stridor, or local tenderness, may be life threatening if the airway is involved.

Other organ involvement includes ocular (50%; iridocyclitis, retinal vasculitis, extraocular muscle paresis, periorbital edema, scleritis, episcleritis, conjunctivitis), articular (50%; chronic, seronegative, nonerosive, inflammatory oligoarthritis), vascular (10%; vasculitis of arteries of all sizes), and renal (10%; segmental proliferative glomerulonephritis).

Uncommon Findings: Aortic insufficiency, aortitis, and coexistent connective tissue disorders (e.g., vasculitis, JRA, SLE, Sjögren syndrome, Reiter syndrome) may occur. The overlap of Behçet's syndrome and relapsing polychondritis has been termed MAGIC syndrome (see p. 131).

Diagnostic Testing: There is no diagnostic test for relapsing polychondritis. Supportive, nonspecific findings include increased ESR, anemia of chronic disease, and hypergammaglobulinemia. Antibodies to type II collagen are found in 50% of patients. Pulmonary function tests, including flow volume curves, should be performed for baseline assessment and with respiratory symptoms.

Imaging: Tomograms and CT may help determine the presence and severity of laryngotracheal involvement.

Keys to Diagnosis: Diagnosis is based on the constellation of appropriate clinical findings. Biopsy is often not needed but may be done in atypical cases. Histopathologic confirmation of cartilage inflammation and destruction supports the diagnosis and may help exclude other diagnoses.

Differential Diagnosis: Wegener's granulomatosis, infection (e.g., fungal, mycobacterial, spirochetal), vasculitis, and malignancy should be considered.

Treatment: Therapy depends on the severity and extent of disease. In a minority of patients, NSAIDs and mild analgesics may suffice. Patients with more severe or refractory disease often require corticosteroids. Some patients (e.g., those with severe vasculitis, renal, or respiratory disease) may require high-dose oral corticosteroids or immunosuppressives (MTX, cyclophosphamide, cyclosporine). Laryngotracheal involvement associated with airway compromise may require surgical intervention such as excision or stenting.

Prognosis: The severity of involvement in particular organ systems determines the prognosis. Overall, a 5-year survival rate of 74% has been reported. Death is usually owing to infection, vasculitis, malignancy, or airway collapse.

BIBLIOGRAPHY

Barretto SN, Oliveira GH, Michet CJ Jr, et al. Multiple cardiovascular complications in a patient with relapsing polychondritis. *Mayo Clin Proc* 2002;77:971–974.

Letko E, Zafirakis P, Baltatzis S, et al. Relapsing polychondritis: a clinical review. *Semin Arthritis Rheum* 2002;31:384–395.

REMITTING SERONEGATIVE SYMMETRIC SYNOVITIS WITH PITTING EDEMA (RS3PE)

Definition: Remitting inflammatory arthritis of hands and feet affecting primarily the elderly. The etiology is unknown. One-half of patients are HLA-B7 positive.

Demographics: Older males, >50 years of age, are predominantly affected.

Cardinal Findings: Abrupt onset of marked dorsal swelling of the hands (or feet) with pitting edema, wrist synovitis, and flexor finger tendinitis. Most cases remit in a year; fewer cases develop into RA, SpA, or malignancy.

Therapy: Good response to low-dose prednisone, NSAID, or hydroxychloroquine therapy.

BIBLIOGRAPHY

Finnell JA, Cuesta IA. Remitting seronegative symmetrical synovitis with pitting edema (RS3PE) syndrome: a review of the literature and a report of three cases. *J Foot Ankle Surg* 2000;39:189–193.

RHEUMATOID ARTHRITIS

ICD-9 Code: RA, 714.0; Felty syndrome, 714.1; rheumatoid vasculitis, 447.6; rheumatoid nodules, 729.89.

Definition: RA is a chronic, progressive, systemic inflammatory disorder in which the joints are the primary target. The classic presentation of RA is a symmetric polyarthritis, particularly of the small joints of the hands and feet. Early arthritis is often accompanied by constitutional symptoms such as fatigue.

Etiology: The etiology of RA is unknown. The pathophysiology of RA is presumed to relate to a persistent immunologic response of a genetically susceptible host to some unknown antigen, possibly an infectious agent. Many infections have been suggested as the cause of RA (including mycobacteria, streptococci, *Mycoplasma, Yersinia,* rubella, Epstein-Barr virus). Despite the resemblance of RA to known infectious arthritides (e.g., Lyme disease) and extensive investigations, no agent has been conclusively implicated.

Genetics: Family studies demonstrate a genetic predisposition to the development of RA. The concordance rate for monozygotic twins is approximately 25% (i.e., if one twin has RA, there is a 25% chance that the other will develop RA). First-degree relatives of patients with RA develop RA at a rate approximately four times that of the general population. The most clearly defined genetic association with RA is with particular alleles of the class II major histocompatibility complex genes. Some HLA-DR molecules (e.g., HLA-DR4, HLA-DR1, which are currently designated HLA-DRB1*0401, 0101, 0404, etc.) are associated with the development and severity of RA (see p. 76).

Pathology: The most characteristic pathologic changes in RA occur in the joints. RA can affect any diarthrodial joint (i.e., joints having cartilage overlying bone, and a joint cavity lined by a synovial membrane that contains synovial fluid). With the onset of arthritis, the normally thin synovial lining layer hypertrophies and becomes edematous and infiltrated with mononuclear cells. Below the synovial layer are organized accumulations of predominantly CD4+ helper T cells and antigen-presenting cells (dendritic cells and macrophages). Lymphoid follicles and germinal centers are also seen; in these areas, large amounts of immunoglobulin, including RF, are produced. Substantial vascular changes (e.g., angiogenesis) reflect activation of the endothelium of the synovial blood vessels. Fibroblast activity is reflected by increased synthesis of extracellular matrix components. This inflamed synovium distends the joint space, erodes into subchondral bone, and destroys cartilage. Such alterations are not pathognomonic of RA and may be seen in the other inflammatory arthritides. However, the intensity of such changes is characteristic of RA. The synovial fluid in RA is inflammatory in nature and contains large numbers of neutrophils. Rheumatoid nodules show palisading histiocytes arrayed about an area of central necrosis. Although uncommon, vasculitis of small- or medium-sized vessels has been reported.

Immunologically, several components of the immune system contribute to the pathogenesis of RA. Several lines of evidence indicate that activated CD4+ helper T cells orchestrate the immune response in RA. In addition to T cells, cells of the monocyte/macrophage lineage play an important role, both by interacting with T cells and by elaborating a plethora of proinflammatory cytokines. Many manifestations of RA derive from the effects of proinflammatory cytokines, particularly IL-1, TNF-α, and IL-6. B cells are hyperactive as antigen-presenting cells and by secreting RF (usually IgM-RF, which binds to the Fc portion of IgG) that contributes to RA damage by forming immune complexes. Last, defects in apoptosis may perpetuate these findings.

Demographics: The prevalence of RA is remarkably consistent; throughout the world, it affects approximately 1% of the population. Exceptions include the scarcity of RA in rural sub-Saharan Africa and a higher prevalence of RA (>5%) among some Native American populations. In all populations, women are affected approximately three times as often as men. The prevalence of RA increases with age, and sex differences diminish among older patients. RA develops most commonly during the fourth and fifth decades of life. Peak onset age (80% of cases) is between 35 and 50 years.

Risk Factors: The greater prevalence of RA among women argues for an effect of sex hormones on the disease. This is supported by the tendency of RA to improve during pregnancy and with oral contraceptive use. Smoking may contribute to disease risk and risk of extraarticular manifestations. Historical evidence supports some environmental exposure as a risk factor for RA. Thus, unlike other types of arthritis such as OA and gout, it does not appear that RA existed before the industrial age.

Cardinal Findings: RA is a clinical diagnosis, easily made by history and examination.

—*Onset:* For approximately two-thirds of patients, the onset of RA is insidious; symmetric arthritis develops over the course of weeks to months. Approximately 10% to 15% of patients have a fulminant onset of polyarticular arthritis, and the diagnosis of RA is established more easily. Arthritis is often accompanied by prolonged morning stiffness affecting the joints that typically lasts an hour or more. Many patients also have constitutional symptoms such as fatigue, anorexia, and low-grade fever.

—*Joints:* Although the cardinal signs of inflammation (pain, swelling, erythema, warmth) may be seen early in the disease course or during flares, erythema and warmth may be absent in chronic RA. Warmth is often a subtle finding and erythema may be short-lived. Pain referred to the joint originates predominantly from the joint capsule, which is abundantly supplied with pain fibers and is exquisitely sensitive to distention. Factors that contribute to swelling of the joint include accumulation of synovial fluid and hypertrophy of the synovium. Initially, the patient may voluntarily restrict motion in response to pain. With progression of disease, tendon shortening and destruction of periarticular supporting structures may cause irreversible joint deformities (e.g., swan-neck deformity). Bony ankylosis (destruction of joints with collapse and bony overgrowth) tends to occur in some joints, particularly the wrist and ankle. Loss of function is critical to the patient because it is associated with interference with the ability to perform activities of daily living and substantial morbidity.

Although RA can affect any diarthrodial joint, there is a distinct predilection for particular joints, such as the small joints of the hands (Table 36). Some joints may be of particular concern to patients; for example, arthritis of the hands and wrists interferes substantially with daily life and often prompts patients to seek medical advice.

—*Deformities:* Damage to articular and periarticular (i.e., tendons, ligaments) structures may result in deformities (Fig. 8), including swan-neck deformity (manifest as hyperextension at the proximal interphalangeal joints and flexion at the distal interphalangeal joints of the fingers); boutonnière deformity (flexion at the proximal interphalangeal joint and hyperextension at the distal interphalangeal joint), ulnar drift (deviation of the metacarpophalangeal

Table 36
Joint Involvement in Rheumatoid Arthritis

Involved Joint	Frequency of Involvement (%)
Metacarpophalangeal	85
Wrist	80
Proximal interphalangeal	75
Knee	75
Metatarsophalangeal	75
Ankle (tibiotalar + subtalar)	75
Shoulder	60
Midfoot (tarsus)	60
Hip	50
Elbow	50
Acromioclavicular	50
Cervical spine	40
Temporomandibular	30
Sternoclavicular	30

joint and fingers ulnarly), piano-key deformity (with manual compression, prominent up and down movement of the ulnar styloid, caused by damage at the radioulnar joint), bent-fork deformity of the wrist (owing to collapse of the carpal bones with subluxation at the carpometacarpal joints, which results in a step-down appearance over the dorsum of the wrist), and hallux valgus (valgus deformity affecting the first metatarsophalangeal joints, with medial displacement at the metatarsophalangeal joint and outward deviation of the first toe bilaterally).

—*Extraarticular manifestations:* Although arthritis may be its most prominent clinical feature, RA is indeed a systemic disease. Many patients have a variety of extraarticular manifestations (Table 37). Extraarticular manifestations tend to occur in patients with high titers of RF in the serum. Some manifestations, for example, subcutaneous rheumatoid nodules, are common (30% of patients with RA) but usually do not require specific intervention. Rheumatoid nodules are commonly seen over the ulna, olecranon, fingers, and Achilles tendon or in the olecranon bursa. Rheumatoid nodules are only seen in patients with RF (often in high titers) and may be confused with gouty tophi, ganglion cysts, tendon xanthomas, or nodules associated with rheumatic fever, leprosy, MCTD, or multicentric reticulohistiocytosis. Pulmonary manifestations of RA are also common (some pathologic changes may be seen almost universally at autopsy) but infrequently become clinically apparent. Some extraarticular manifestations (e.g., vasculitis, Felty syndrome) are rare but often require specific therapy (see Rheumatoid Vasculitis, p. 333 and Felty's Syndrome, p. 175).

Complications: Joint destruction and deformities are the most common complications of RA. These changes can substantially impair the patient's mobility

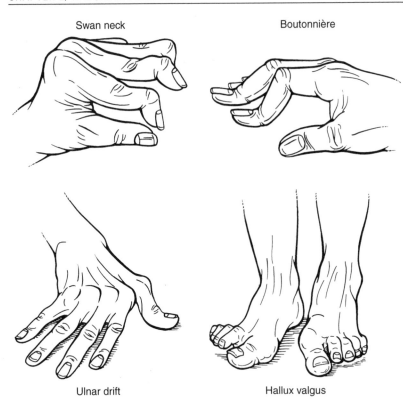

Figure 8. Deformities in rheumatoid arthritis.

as well as the ability to perform activities of daily living (e.g., preparing food, bathing, dressing). Extraarticular manifestations of RA may also cause complications (e.g., symptomatic pleural or pericardial effusion, vasculitic damage). Subluxation of upper cervical vertebrae is commonly seen on radiographs but is usually asymptomatic. Rarely, C1-2 subluxation results in spinal cord compression with permanent neurologic deficit.

Death: Patients with RA have an increased mortality rate and reduced survival by 10 to 18 years. This results from a lifetime of systemic inflammation and its contributory effects on the development of cardiovascular disease, infection, renal disease, neoplasia, and the development of additive comorbidities. Patients with RA have a nearly twofold increased rate of myocardial infarction, heart failure, and cardiovascular accident. Interestingly, patients treated with MTX show better survival and a lower rate of deaths caused by cardiovascular disease. Patients with RA have a lower rate of colon cancer but are at increased risk of lymphoma, with more than a twofold rate that increases with severely active disease. Last, patients with RA are at risk of serious infec-

Table 37
Extraarticular Manifestations of RA

Organ System	Manifestations
Constitutional	Fever, anorexia, fatigue, weakness, lymphadenopathy
Cutaneous	Rheumatoid nodules, vasculitis
Ocular	Sjögren syndrome (keratoconjunctivitis sicca), scleritis, episcleritis
Cardiovascular	Pericarditis, pericardial effusion
Pulmonary	Pleuritis, pleural effusion, interstitial fibrosis, rheumatoid nodules in the lung, Caplan syndrome (nodular pulmonary infiltrates in patients with RA with pneumoconiosis)
Hematologic	Anemia of chronic disease, thrombocytosis, eosinophilia, Felty syndrome (RA associated with neutropenia and splenomegaly)
Gastrointestinal	Sjögren syndrome (xerostomia), amyloidosis, vasculitis
Neurologic	Entrapment neuropathy, myelopathy/myositis
Renal	Amyloidosis, renal tubular acidosis, interstitial nephritis
Metabolic	Osteoporosis

RA, rheumatoid arthritis.

tions. Pneumonia is the leading cause of death due to infection. Risk for serious infections is primarily related to RA severity/debility, comorbidities, corticosteroid use, and surgery. With each morbid/mortal risk, RA severity appears to contribute to this risk more so than the DMARD or immunosuppressive therapies employed.

Diagnostic Tests: No laboratory test is diagnostic for RA; rather, the presence of various laboratory findings provide support for a clinically suspected diagnosis.

Rheumatoid factor (RF) is the laboratory test most closely associated with RA. RF (see p. 95) is an autoantibody (usually IgM) that binds to the Fc portion of IgG and is present in 75% to 85% of patients with RA. Thus, nearly 20% of patients with RA are seronegative for RF. Moreover, by definition, 5% of the general population test positive for RF, and nearly 20% of healthy elderly persons may be RF positive. In addition, RF is seen in a number of conditions other than RA, including Sjögren syndrome, cryoglobulinemia, SLE, bacterial endocarditis, mycobacterial disease, hepatitis, and lymphoproliferative malignancies. Because RA is present in approximately 1% of the population, random screening using RF would be expected to generate a large number of false-positive results. In patients with RA, high-titer RF is associated with aggressive disease, as evidenced by development of bony erosions, extraarticular involvement, and functional disability. Recently developed ELISA assays for anti-cyclic citrullinated peptide (CCP) antibodies (anti-CCP) add further to the profile provided by RF. Although anti-CCP antibodies appear to have nearly the same sensitivity (45%–70%) as RF, they appear to be more specific for RA (>95%) and are found earlier in the disease course and among those at risk of more severe outcomes.

Other laboratory tests that can be useful in supporting the diagnosis of RA include synovial fluid analysis, measurement of acute-phase reactants (ESR and CRP), and the CBC. In RA, synovial fluid is expected to be inflammatory with negative results on microbiologic culture and crystal analysis. Elevation in the ESR or CRP level provides a surrogate measure of active inflammation and may be useful in establishing a diagnosis, estimating the prognosis, and gauging the response to therapy. The most common abnormality in the CBC in patients with RA is a normochromic, normocytic anemia (anemia of chronic disease). Thrombocytosis may also be seen with uncontrolled inflammation. Nonspecific mild (two-fold) elevation of alkaline phosphatase is seen sporadically.

Imaging: Several imaging studies are used in assessing patients with RA. Early in the disease course, plain radiographs may show only soft tissue swelling or joint effusion. As the disease progresses, more abnormalities appear. Juxtaarticular osteopenia is characteristic of RA and other chronic inflammatory arthritides. Loss of articular cartilage and bony erosions may develop after months of active disease. Nearly 70% of patients will develop bony erosions within the first 2 years of disease. The presence of erosions in the first 2 years portends a progressive course. Erosions may be seen in virtually any joint but are most common in the metatarsophalangeal, metacarpophalangeal, and wrist joints. Plain radiographs are useful in helping to establish prognosis and in assessing joint damage longitudinally and when surgery is considered. MRI may demonstrate erosions much earlier than conventional radiography and offers superior detail in depicting the articular structures. However, its cost precludes widespread use in routine assessment of patients.

Keys to Diagnosis: Because it is the most common type of chronic inflammatory arthritis, RA should be a major consideration in patients with such a presentation. Early diagnosis and prompt treatment are critical. The presence of three or more swollen joints for >12 weeks associated with a symmetric pattern, prominent involvement of the small joints of the hands and feet, and the presence of subcutaneous nodules, serum RF, or cyclic citrullinated peptide antibodies adds further support to the diagnosis.

Diagnostic Criteria: Classification criteria for RA are shown in Table 38. Note that patients do not have to have a positive test for RF to be diagnosed with RA. However, seronegative patients must have other characteristic clinical features to be diagnosed as RA.

Differential Diagnosis: Acutely, RA is often confused with reactive arthritis, Reiter's syndrome, viral arthritis (e.g., Parvovirus B19, Epstein-Barr virus, HBV), Lyme disease, and the articular onset of other connective tissue disorders (e.g., PM, scleroderma, SLE). Chronically, RA needs to be distinguished from other forms of chronic, polyarticular, inflammatory arthritis: SLE, Lyme disease, psoriatic arthritis, polyarticular gout or pseudogout, Reiter's syndrome, reactive arthritis, enteropathic arthritis, erosive/inflammatory OA,

Table 38
1987 Revised Criteria for the Classification of Rheumatoid Arthritis

1. Stiffness in and around the joints lasting ≥1 h before maximal improvement
2. Arthritis of ≥3 joint areas, simultaneously, observed by a physician
3. Arthritis of the proximal interphalangeal, metacarpophalangeal, or wrist joints
4. Symmetric arthritis
5. Rheumatoid nodules
6. A positive test for serum rheumatoid factor
7. Radiographic changes characteristic of rheumatoid arthritis (erosions and/or periarticular osteopenia in hand and/or wrist joints)
A person can be classified as having rheumatoid arthritis if ≥4 criteria are present at any time
Criteria 1–4 must be present for at least 6 wk
Criteria 2–5 must be observed by a physician

scleroderma, rheumatic fever, and inflammatory myositis. There is a negative association between RA and gout.

Prognosis: Until the 1980s, RA was considered predominantly a benign disease; it was thought that many patients would go into spontaneous remission. Now it is realized that RA is a chronic progressive disease associated with substantial morbidity and accelerated mortality. Patients with severe RA have been shown to have a limited survival rate, comparable with that of patients with three-vessel coronary disease or advanced Hodgkin disease. This has had important implications for the approach to therapy of RA. Several studies have shown that early diagnosis and early use of DMARDs can favorably alter outcomes. Risk factors for worse outcome in RA are shown in Table 39.

Therapy: The goals of therapy for patients with RA are (a) relief of pain, (b) preservation of functional status, (c) reduction of inflammation, (d) control of systemic involvement, (e) protection of articular and extraarticular structures, (f) control of disease progression, and (g) avoidance of complications related to

Table 39
Features of Rheumatoid Arthritis Associated with Aggressive Disease

Functional disability (inability to perform activities of daily living)
Lower socioeconomic status/less education
Arthritis of numerous joints (e.g., >20)
Rheumatoid nodules (and other extraarticular manifestations)
Elevated acute-phase reactants (e.g., erythrocyte sedimentation rate, C-reactive protein)
High positive titers of rheumatoid factor
Anti-cyclic citrullinated peptide antibodies
Specific HLA-DR alleles (e.g. HLA-DR4)
Radiographic evidence of bony erosions

therapy. The types of therapeutic interventions include pharmacologic agents (including oral, parenteral, and topical agents) and nonpharmacologic agents (Table 40).

In previous years, therapy of RA was guided by the therapeutic pyramid. In this scheme, which was based on the assumption that RA was predominantly a benign disease with spontaneous remissions, therapy began with NSAIDs. Other agents, such as injectable gold salts, were added in a stepwise fashion as patients clearly failed treatment with NSAIDs. Today RA is recognized as a chronic progressive disease wherein damage can occur early in the disease, and, thus, therapy of RA has become more aggressive.

A critical decision point in the approach to therapy of patients with RA is an estimation of the severity of disease and its expected prognosis. Patients with several prognostic factors consistent with a worse outcome (Table 39) may be considered to have "aggressive" disease. Patients with RA who lack these features may be considered as having "slowly progressive" disease. These categories are not static; many patients initially labeled slowly progressive may later develop more aggressive disease features and thus fall into the category of aggressive RA. Close follow-up and repeated evaluations are crucial for patients with RA. At these follow-up evaluations, the patient should be assessed for (a) activity of the disease, (b) changes in functional status, (c) response to

Table 40
Common Therapies for Patients with Rheumatoid Arthritis

Pharmacologic	Nonpharmacologic
Analgesics	Ambulatory assist devices
Nonnarcotic	Physiotherapy
Antidepressants	Splints/orthotics
Narcotic	Occupational therapy
NSAIDs	Patient education
Topical agents (e.g., capsaicin)	Exercise/rest
Corticosteroids	Orthopaedic surgery
DMARDs	Synovectomy
Methotrexate	Tendon repair
Hydroxychloroquine	Joint reconstruction
Sulfasalazine	Joint fusion (arthrodesis)
Leflunomide	Joint replacement
Injectable gold salts	
Cyclosporine	
D-Penicillamine	Biologics
Azathioprine	Anakinra
Cyclophosphamide	Infliximab
Auranofin	Etanercept
Minocycline	
Adalimumab	

NSAIDs, nonsteroidal antiinflammatory drugs; DMARDs, disease-modifying antirheumatic drugs the therapeutic interventions (e.g., control of pain and inflammation), and (d) development of adverse effects related to therapy.

Patients with slowly progressive disease are often treated with NSAIDs (see Appendix A, p. 527). Some patients may require oral corticosteroids (e.g., prednisone ≤10 mg/day) or intraarticular steroids in one to two joints. DMARDs may be used in patients with slowly progressive RA, particularly those with incomplete relief from NSAIDs, analgesics, and nonpharmacologic therapies. Hydroxychloroquine, sulfasalazine, and MTX are commonly used in patients with slowly progressive disease.

Patients with aggressive RA may also receive NSAIDs; however, higher antiinflammatory doses may be used. Low-dose oral steroids and intraarticular steroid injections are commonly used. DMARDs are used very early in the disease course for patients with aggressive RA. MTX (with concomitant folate) is the most commonly used DMARD in such patients. Other DMARDs have also been used with success in RA (Table 40, Appendix B, p. 529).

DMARDs form the mainstay of therapy for many patients with RA (see Appendix B, p. 529). The choice of individual agent depends on several factors including (a) the severity and activity of disease, (b) comorbidity in the patient (e.g., MTX is not the drug of choice in an alcoholic patient), (c) cost and convenience issues. Many patients with RA fail to remain on any given DMARD long term because of either therapeutic inefficacy or development of adverse effects.

Many advocate combination DMARDs therapy in an effort to enhance efficacy while minimizing toxicity. Acceptance and use of combination therapy have grown in the past decade whereas MTX has been shown to be an effective "anchor" drug when used at effective doses (15–20 mg/wk) in addition to select DMARDs or biologics. Such combinations have demonstrated superior efficacy without augmenting toxicity. Hence, there are many studies showing that any of the following effective combination regimens can be safely used in patients with active uncontrolled RA: (a) MTX + hydroxychloroquine, (b) MTX + hydroxychloroquine + sulfasalazine, (c) MTX + sulfasalazine + prednisolone, (d) MTX + leflunomide, (e) MTX + infliximab, (f) MTX + etanercept, (g) MTX + adalimumab, (h) MTX + anakinra, and (i) MTX + rituximab. In nearly all these studies, patients with a suboptimal response to MTX alone were then given the combination regimen to achieve greater results. Some of these are quite inexpensive (MTX + hydroxychloroquine or sulfasalazine), whereas others are quite costly (MTX + TNF inhibitor). These combination regimens have also been shown to be particularly effective in retarding radiographic damage or progression. This is especially true for the MTX + TNF inhibitor combinations. Promising regimens under investigation will employ monoclonal antibodies directed at B cells (rituximab) and modulators of costimulation (CTLA4-Ig or abatacept) to treat aggressive RA.

Surgery: A number of orthopaedic surgical interventions have revolutionized the care of the patient with RA (Table 40). Surgical outcomes have improved consistently in recent years and offer many patients the chance for substantial improvement in functional status and quality of life. Indications for surgery include (a) impending tendon rupture, (b) marked functional limitation, and (c) severe pain related to extensive joint damage (see Appendix G p. 541).

BIBLIOGRAPHY

Alarcon GS. Epidemiology of rheumatoid arthritis. *Rheum Dis Clin North Am* 1995;21:589–604.
Arnett FC, Edworthy SM, Bloch DA, et al. The ARA 1987 revised criteria for the classification of rheumatoid arthritis. *Arthritis Rheum* 1988;31:315–324.
Choi HK, Hernan MA, Seeger JD, et al. Methotrexate and mortality in patients with rheumatoid arthritis: a prospective study. *Lancet* 2002;359:1173–1177.
Doran MF, Crowson CS, Pond GR, et al. Frequency of infection in patients with rheumatoid arthritis compared with controls: a population-based study. *Arthritis Rheum* 2002; 46:2287–2293.
Kavanaugh A, Keystone EC. The safety of biologic agents in early rheumatoid arthritis. *Clin Exp Rheumatol* 2003;21(suppl 31):S203–S208.
Pincus T, Brooks RH, Callahan LF. Prediction of long-term mortality in patients with rheumatoid arthritis according to simple questionnaire and joint count measures. *Ann Intern Med* 1994;120:26–34.
Pincus T, Yazici Y, Sokka T, et al. Methotrexate as the "anchor drug" for the treatment of early rheumatoid arthritis. *Clin Exp Rheumatol* 2003;21(suppl 31):S179–S185.
Solomon DH, Karlson EW, Rimm EB, et al. Cardiovascular morbidity and mortality in women diagnosed with rheumatoid arthritis. *Circulation* 2003;107:1303–1307.
Turesson C, O'Fallon WM, Crowson CS, et al. Extra-articular disease manifestations in rheumatoid arthritis: incidence trends and risk factors over 46 years. *Ann Rheum Dis* 2003; 62:722–727.

RHEUMATOID VASCULITIS

ICD-9 Code: 447.6.

Definition: Rheumatoid vasculitis is inflammation of blood vessels in patients with RA. Vasculitis is considered a serious extraarticular manifestation of RA.

Etiology: Immune complexes, probably containing RFs, are passively deposited on blood vessel walls. All patients manifesting rheumatoid vasculitis have strongly positive titers of IgM-RF. Most of these RF-containing complexes also fix complement, which contributes to tissue damage.

Pathology: In small- to medium-sized vessels, the lesion may include an infiltrate consisting of both mononuclear and polymorphonuclear cells, and fibrinoid necrosis. In small vessels of the skin, leukocytoclastic vasculitis may be seen.

Demographics: Rheumatoid vasculitis is usually associated with aggressive and long-standing RA. The incidence in males is somewhat higher than in females. The vast majority of patients are positive for IgM-RF; cases of putatively seronegative patients may be associated with IgG-RF, which is not detected by routine clinical assays. This complication of RA appears to be decreasing in incidence. Limited cutaneous lesions are more common than severe necrotizing complications, which are rare. Autopsy studies suggest that the true incidence of vasculitis is higher, although most cases are subclinical and not detected during life.

Cardinal Findings: Nailfold lesions are most common and include prominent periungual vessels, localized infarction, splinter hemorrhages, and tender macules of the fingertips (which may be dark red or brown). Palpable purpura has been described. Larger vessel involvement often manifests as leg ulcers. Nerve involvement presents most commonly as a mononeuritis multiplex syndrome (e.g., with wrist or foot drop). Involvement of larger arteries, resulting in infarction of the myocardium, bowel, lung, and so on, is seen rarely.

Diagnostic Tests: Patients are universally seropositive with high titers of IgM-RF. ESR and CRP are usually very elevated. Complement levels (C3, C4) are usually decreased. Leukocytosis, anemia of chronic disease, cryoglobulinemia, and P-ANCA may be present. Nerve conduction velocity testing may indicate a mononeuritis multiplex.

Key to Diagnosis: A diagnosis of rheumatoid vasculitis should be questioned if the patient does not have severe seropositive RA of long-standing duration. However, active synovial inflammation does not correlate with the onset or activity of the vasculitis. In cases of specific organ or tissue involvement such as a mononeuritis syndrome, biopsy of the affected tissue (in this case the nerve) may be very useful in establishing a diagnosis. A skin biopsy should be performed if palpable purpura is seen.

Differential Diagnosis: Clinical and pathologic lesions may resemble those seen in association with subacute bacterial endocarditis, PAN, Wegener's granulomatosis, or cholesterol emboli syndrome.

Therapy: Leukocytoclastic vasculitis does not require aggressive therapy. Aggressive therapy with cyclophosphamide is reserved for rheumatoid vasculitis involving medium- to large-sized vessels. Cyclophosphamide may be administered as a daily oral dose or as an intermittent intravenous bolus infusion. Concomitant treatment with moderate doses of prednisone is required. Anecdotal reports of TNF inhibitor treatment of rheumatoid vasculitis have been favorable. The duration of therapy is unclear, although some require maintenance therapy for years. Foot and wrist drops are managed with splints.

Prognosis: Outcome depends on the organ system involved. Patients whose vasculitis is limited to fingertip lesions generally do well, whereas involvement of major nerves or arteries in organs such as the heart is associated with a poorer prognosis. The use of cyclophosphamide has had a major impact on reducing associated morbidity and mortality.

BIBLIOGRAPHY

Bacon PA, Kitas GD. The significance of vascular inflammation in rheumatoid arthritis (review). *Ann Rheum Dis* 1994;53:621–623.
Bacon PA, Moots RJ. Extra-articular rheumatoid arthritis. In: Koopman WJ, ed. *Arthritis and allied conditions: a textbook of rheumatology,* 13th ed. Baltimore: Williams & Wilkins, 1997:1071–1088.

ROTATOR CUFF DYSFUNCTION

Synonyms: Rotator cuff tendinitis, impingement syndrome.

ICD-9 Codes: Rotator cuff tear, 727.61; rotator cuff dysfunction NOS, 726.10.

Definition: Rotator cuff dysfunction refers to a spectrum of pathologic changes in the rotator cuff tendons, ranging from mild inflammation or tendinitis to a complete tear. Associated pathologic changes have given rise to names such as impingement syndrome and frozen shoulder. Many patients also have subacromial bursitis in conjunction with rotator cuff dysfunction. Rotator cuff dysfunction is the most common cause of shoulder complaints among the elderly, accounting for >75% of cases. This is notable because shoulder problems are the second most common musculoskeletal complaint in general practice.

Anatomic Considerations: Four muscles and their tendons constitute the rotator cuff apparatus. These muscles (the supraspinatus, infraspinatus, subscapularis, and teres minor) originate on the scapula, pass through a tunnel of ligaments on the underside of the acromion process, and insert on the trochanters of the humerus. They function to abduct, internally rotate, and externally rotate the humeral head. This allows free upper extremity movement in many different planes. The rotator cuff tendons also form the roof of the glenohumeral joint, being contiguous with its fibrous capsule. The rotator cuff tendons are separated from the overlying deltoid muscle by the subacromial bursa.

Pathology: Pathologically, it can be demonstrated that the rotator cuff tendons tend to degenerate with advancing age, which provides some explanation for the increasing prevalence of rotator cuff problems with advancing age. Intrinsic degeneration may be exacerbated by chronic overuse (e.g., manual labor involving repetitive shoulder movements against force) or by arthritis in adjacent joints (e.g., RA affecting the acromioclavicular or glenohumeral joints). Rotator cuff dysfunction in many persons represents a continuum of disease. Initial involvement with mild tendinitis may progress, resulting in a complete tear of the rotator cuff tendons. In addition, mild tendinitis may cause the patient to favor the affected arm, diminishing movements of the affected muscles. This allows the deltoid to pull the humeral head higher in the glenohumeral fossa, which in turn reduces the area of the space through which the rotator cuff tendons must pass. This may result in impingement of the rotator cuff against the acromion, which can cause further pain and worsen the entire process. If this is allowed to become chronic, tendon shortening may ensue, greatly diminishing movement of the shoulder. This frozen shoulder syndrome has also been referred to as adhesive capsulitis. However, because adhesions are not typically a part of the pathologic process, restrictive capsulitis has become the preferred term.

Demographics: Those at risk include the elderly, those with inflammatory arthritis of the shoulder (e.g., RA), diabetics, alcoholics, athletes with repetitive over-head or throwing movement, carpenters, welders, and painters.

Cardinal Findings: In some cases, particularly in younger persons (e.g., baseball pitchers), injury to the rotator cuff is acute. More commonly, pain related to rotator cuff dysfunction arises insidiously and often becomes chronic.

Patients with rotator cuff dysfunction characteristically complain of shoulder pain. The pain is usually somewhat difficult for the patient to localize more specifically, other than perhaps saying it is deep. Many patients complain of waking at night because of the pain. It is often worsened by movements that require specific use of the affected muscles. However, patients may compensate and perform movements that normally use the rotator cuff muscles by using other motions. For example, patients may avoid upper extremity abduction while hair brushing. Patients often report pain performing activities that require rotator cuff muscles (e.g., tying an apron behind the back or tucking a shirt into the back of the pants).

Physical examination for rotator cuff function should assess active and passive range of motion of the shoulder and test the muscles individually for pain or weakness. Patients with rotator cuff dysfunction typically have no difficulty with forward flexion or extension of the shoulder. Many have problems with abduction. Normally, the first 15 degrees of abduction is initiated by the deltoid. Abduction from there through 90 degrees depends mostly on the supraspinatus. (Above 90 degrees there is little further abduction; rather, the trapezius and rhomboid muscles tilt the scapula and bring it toward the midline.) Patients with rotator cuff dysfunction frequently have pain on, or limited range of, active abduction. If it is severe, e.g., in someone with long-standing disease and restrictive capsulitis, passive movements (i.e., done by the examiner) may be limited or result in pain. Some consider patients with impaired range of active motion but normal range of passive motion to have evidence of impingement. The other rotator cuff muscles can also be a source of pain and should be assessed. The subscapularis internally rotates the humeral head. This can be tested by having the patient hold the elbow against the side, with 90 degrees of elbow flexion, and try to move the hand medially against the examiner's resistance. External rotation is mediated by the infraspinatus and teres minor. It can be tested as for internal rotation, except the examiner provides resistance against the patient's attempt to move the hand laterally. In some cases, it may be possible to differentiate tendon inflammation from a complete tendon tear; the former being associated with pain, the latter with both pain and weakness. However, in practicality, it is difficult to differentiate between the two.

Complete tear of the rotator cuff is usually an acute posttraumatic event. Patients also complain of shoulder pain and weakness and may have a positive drop arm test (see p. 12).

Diagnostic Tests: No laboratory tests are helpful in diagnosing rotator cuff disease.

Imaging: Imaging modalities, although usually unnecessary to establish rotator cuff dysfunction as the cause of shoulder pain, may be helpful in determining the need for surgery or in unusual cases. Plain radiographs are not usually helpful because bony abnormalities are not commonly a critical part of the pathology. Commonly, the humeral head appears to be displaced slightly superiorly in the glenohumeral fossa. Some patients have acromioclavicular joint hypertrophy, which may contribute to impingement. Ultrasonography may define abnormalities in the rotator cuff, but the interpretation and utility of the study depend to a large extent on the experience of the ultrasonographer. MRI allows exquisite detail of the relevant tissues. It has replaced arthrography in the diagnosis of complete rotator cuff tendon tears.

Treatment: The treatment of rotator cuff disease may incorporate rest in acute settings. The use of hot packs, ice packs, ultrasonography, analgesic agents, or NSAIDs may be helpful in some individuals. However, aggressive physiotherapy with range-of-motion exercises and strengthening of the rotator cuff muscles is a critical component of therapy for all. Injection of the subacromial bursa with corticosteroids can provide substantial relief, particularly in patients with evidence of subacromial bursitis.

Surgery: Surgery is indicated in particular circumstances. For example, in patients with evidence of impingement, acromioplasty can increase the available space and decrease symptoms. In past years, some patients with frozen shoulder underwent surgical release. However, because this intervention did not appear to affect the ultimate outcome for these patients, most patients are now treated conservatively.

BIBLIOGRAPHY

Bland JH, Merrit JA, Boushey DR. The painful shoulder. *Semin Arthritis Rheum* 1977;7:21–47.
Dalton SE. The conservative management of rotator cuff disorders. *Br J Rheumatol* 1994;33:663–667.
Dinnes J, Loveman E, McIntyre L, et al. The effectiveness of diagnostic tests for the assessment of shoulder pain owing to soft tissue disorders: a systematic review. *Health Technol Assess* 2003;7:1–166.
Kavanaugh A, Eshagi N, Cush J, et al. Rotator cuff dysfunction in patients with rheumatoid arthritis. *J Clin Rheumatol* 1995;1:274–279.
Tennent TD, Beach WR, Meyers JF. A review of the special tests associated with shoulder examination. Part I: the rotator cuff tests. *Am J Sports Med* 2003;31:154–160.

RUBELLA ARTHRITIS

Synonyms: Rubella is also known as German measles.

ICD-9 Code: 056.71.

Definition: Rubella arthritis is a previously common childhood exanthem that may lead to arthritis in affected adults or children.

Etiology: Chronic rubella arthritis is caused by infection with an RNA virus. The rubella virus has been isolated from synovial fluid and peripheral blood. Although persistence of viral antigen may be detected, the pathogenic importance of this remains unclear.

Demographics: Rubella arthritis most commonly affects young women who are exposed to school-age children. It develops in approximately one-third of natural infections. Arthritis also has been described after rubella vaccination, which uses a live attenuated virus. Previous vaccine strains were more commonly associated with arthropathy than those used currently. Despite widespread vaccination, sporadic outbreaks are reported in hospitals, prenatal clinics, and colleges.

Cardinal Findings: The classic morbilliform rash can precede or accompany joint symptoms. Nonspecific constitutional symptoms may briefly antedate the rash and include malaise, fever, anorexia, upper respiratory tract infection, lymphadenopathy, and eye pain. Symmetric inflammatory arthritis, which occurs more often in adults than children, affects both small and large joints, including the proximal interphalangeal joints, wrist, and knees. Carpal tunnel syndrome or tendinitis may develop. Joint symptoms may be the sole manifestation in adults. Arthropathy generally remits by 1 month but may last as long as a year in some. Atypical neurologic sequelae, such as radiculoneuritis affecting an arm or leg, have been described after vaccine administration.

Diagnostic Tests: Diagnosis is confirmed serologically by hemagglutination inhibition, complement fixation, or ELISA. RF is elevated in <25% of patients. Synovial fluid is moderately inflammatory. The virus is occasionally isolated from respiratory secretions.

Keys to Diagnosis: Look for abrupt-onset arthritis with classic rash after exposure to infected children or vaccination and diagnostic confirmation by serologic tests.

Therapy: There is no specific therapy other than analgesics and occasionally NSAIDs. Symptoms are self-limiting except in rare cases.

BIBLIOGRAPHY

Smith CA, Petty RE, Tingle AJ. Rubella virus and arthritis. *Rheum Dis Clin North Am* 1987;13:265.

SAPHO (SYNOVITIS, ACNE, PUSTULOSIS, HYPEROSTOSIS, OSTEITIS) SYNDROME

Synonyms: Palmoplantar pustulosis, sternocostoclavicular hyperostosis, pustulotic arthrosteitis, chronic recurrent multifocal osteomyelitis, acne arthritis or acne-associated SpA, and hidradenitis suppurativa–associated arthritis.

Definition: SAPHO syndrome comprises a variety of disorders manifesting reactive osteitis, arthritis, and chronic cutaneous pustular lesions.

Etiology: The cause is unknown. SAPHO syndrome is often considered to be reactive owing to pustulosis, osteitis, and clinical similarities with the SpA.

Pathology: Hyperostotic bony lesions, osteitis, and inflammatory synovitis are seen.

Demographics: This very rare disorder affects males and females equally. Most cases are reported in Japan. Far fewer cases are seen in whites, predominantly from Scandinavia and France. Most frequently it affects adults between 20 and 60 years of age.

Cardinal Findings: Painful, nodular swelling of skeletal lesions characterized by development of early erosive and late hyperostotic changes in the joints of the anterior chest wall or axial skeleton. Skeletal disease develops after established pustulosis (i.e., palmoplantar pustulosis, acne conglobata, acne fulminans, hidradenitis suppurativa, pustular psoriasis). The anterior chest wall and axial skeleton are preferentially targeted. Affected amphiarthroses (saddle joints) of the anterior chest wall include the sternoclavicular, manubriosternal, and sternocostal joints. Peripheral involvement of the hands and feet is uncommon. Spondylodiscitis and enthesitis are sometimes seen. Chronic relapsing pustular lesions may affect palms or soles (palmoplantar pustulosis), intertriginous areas (hidradenitis), or face, trunk, and extremities (acne).

Diagnostic Tests: Mild to moderate elevation of the acute-phase reactants and increased leukocyte counts are common. Serum RF is usually absent, and HLA-B27 is positive in <30% of patients.

Differential Diagnosis: Other SpA, DISH, fluorosis, retinoid therapy, ochronosis, alcaptonuria, and hypoparathyroidism should be considered.

Imaging: Early in the disease, radiographs show erosive changes in the anterior chest wall joints, sometimes accompanied by subchondral sclerosis and periostitis. With chronicity, subchondral sclerosis and hyperostosis ensue. Bony ankylosis is uncommon. Spondylodiscitis is the most common axial finding and is suggested by erosions of the vertebral plates with reactive vertebral sclerosis. Sacroiliitis is seen in as many as one-third of patients. Bone scans reveal increased uptake in affected skeletal areas.

Therapy: Topical and systemic therapies are directed at the underlying pustular disorder. The musculoskeletal manifestations are often difficult to treat, although most individuals exhibit some response to systemic antibiotics, NSAIDs, and oral or intraarticular corticosteroids. Sulfasalazine and colchicine have been suggested but not tested extensively. Recent use of parenteral pamidronate or TNF inhibitors appears promising.

Surgery: Resection of the proximal clavicular head or synovectomy may be necessary to control pain.

BIBLIOGRAPHY

Cush JJ, Lipsky PE. Reiter's syndrome and reactive arthritis: hyperostotic syndromes associated with cutaneous pustular lesions. In: Koopman WJ, ed. *Arthritis and allied conditions: a textbook of rheumatology*, 13th ed. Baltimore: Williams & Wilkins, 1997:1222–1223.
Kahn MF, Chamot AM. SAPHO syndrome. *Rheum Dis Clin North Am* 1992;18:225–246.

SARCOIDOSIS

Synonyms: Boeck's sarcoid, uveoparotid fever, Loefgren's syndrome.

ICD-9 Code: Systemic, 135.0; sarcoid arthritis, 713.7.

Definition: Sarcoidosis is a chronic systemic inflammatory disorder of unknown etiology characterized by noncaseating granulomata at involved sites.

Etiology: Although exposure to an infectious organism or some other environmental agent has long been hypothesized to be etiologically relevant to the disease, none has been conclusively implicated. A variety of infectious agents (particularly intracellular pathogens such as fungi) can induce similar histopathologic changes, but none has been reliably recovered from sarcoid lesions. Similar changes may also be seen in association with malignancy.

Pathology: Based on histopathologic studies, activated CD4$^+$ helper T cells are considered to play a central role in the orchestration of sarcoid inflammation. Although commonly considered a pulmonary disorder, the disease process affects many other organ systems. Indeed, approximately one-half of patients with sarcoidosis present initially with constitutional symptoms such as fever or symptoms related to inflammation at extrathoracic sites, including musculoskeletal complaints. Extrathoracic involvement is also common throughout the course of the disease. For example, approximately 10% to 15% of patients with sarcoidosis have arthritis.

Demographics: Sarcoid typically affects young and middle-aged adults. There is a slight female preponderance. Prevalence is highest among African Americans (~40 per 100,000) and whites of northern European extraction (~60 per 100,000). It has been suggested that patients with sarcoidosis carrying the HLA-B8 allele may be more prone to develop erythema nodosum and acute arthritis, whereas patients with sarcoidosis positive for HLA-DR3 may be more likely to develop the chronic form of arthritis.

Cardinal Findings: Sarcoid often affects multiple organ systems.
—*Pulmonary:* Although some patients may never report pulmonary symptoms, >90% show abnormalities on chest radiographs. Characteristic abnormalities have been classified into three types: type I, bilateral hilar lymphadenopathy, sometimes associated with right paratracheal lymphadenopathy; type II, lymphadenopathy as in type I plus pulmonary infiltrates; and

type III, pulmonary infiltrates without lymphadenopathy. Patients with type I chest radiographic findings achieve spontaneous remission much more frequently than those with types II and III and typically require far less therapeutic intervention.

—*Musculoskeletal:* The most common musculoskeletal complaint of sarcoidosis is arthritis, which affects 10% to 15% of patients. Sarcoid arthritis may occur in two distinct patterns, and arthritis arising early in the disease course (e.g., within the initial 6 months) differs from that occurring later. Early arthritis, which is the more common type and may be the initial symptom of sarcoidosis, typically manifests as oligoarthritis of the ankles and, less commonly, the knees. In addition to true arthritis, patients may also have tenosynovitis and periarticular swelling. If joint effusions are present, they are often noninflammatory. Early sarcoid arthritis is often self-limited, lasting for days to months, and the prognosis is excellent. For example, most patients with Loefgren's syndrome (defined as acute arthritis, erythema nodosum, and bilateral hilar lymphadenopathy), which occurs in a subset of patients with early disease, achieve spontaneous remission. Late sarcoid arthritis typically occurs >6 months after disease onset. Although it may manifest as monarthritis, it typically presents as an oligoarthritis, with two or three joints involved. In decreasing order of frequency, affected joints include the knees, ankles, and proximal interphalangeal joints. In addition to synovitis, patients may have periarticular swelling. When this occurs in the fingers (dactylitis or sausage digit), it may resemble the findings seen in the seronegative SpA, such as Reiter's syndrome. Although it may also be transient, late sarcoid arthritis persists more frequently than does early arthritis, which has implications for the therapeutic approach. Last, although joint x-rays in early sarcoid arthritis are typically normal, changes may be noted in late arthritis, including cystic changes in the middle of the phalanges.

—*Dermatologic:* Approximately one-third of patients with sarcoidosis have one of the varied dermatologic manifestations of this disease. Erythema nodosum often occurs early in the disease course and typically remits spontaneously. It is associated with early arthritis, occurring in two-thirds of such patients. Late arthritis is not associated with erythema nodosum but rather with some of the more chronic dermatologic manifestations of sarcoidosis, including plaques, papules, and nodular and scaly lesions. Lupus pernio lesions are characteristic of sarcoidosis and appear as chronic, indurated papules or plaques, red-brown to purple in color, swollen, shiny skin lesions over the lips, cheeks, ears, and mid-face and are more common in African-American women.

—*Other:* Other extrathoracic manifestations of sarcoidosis are relevant from a rheumatologic standpoint because they may mimic various inflammatory diseases. Ocular involvement, especially uveitis, may develop in >20% of sarcoid patients. Uveitis is associated with a variety of systemic inflammatory disorders (see p. 386). Sarcoid involvement of the exocrine glands of the head (e.g., parotid, lacrimal) may resemble the findings of

Sjögren's syndrome. Sarcoidosis of the skeletal muscles, although it may be asymptomatic, may present with a clinical picture resembling inflammatory myositis. Finally, sarcoid may also affect the liver, the central (Bell's palsy) and peripheral nervous systems, the lymphoid organs, and the kidney.

Diagnostic Testing: No single clinical test is diagnostic of sarcoidosis. Nonspecific findings include leukopenia, lymphopenia, anemia, and increased hepatic enzymes or alkaline phosphatase. Hypercalciuria and hypercalcemia are seen in <10% of patients.

—*Kveim test:* Historically, this was used to make a diagnosis. Material obtained from a sarcoid granuloma was injected intradermally, and the patient was assessed for development of a delayed-type hypersensitivity reaction. However, the sensitivity and specificity of this test were disappointing, and it is no longer acceptable to inject tissue from one patient into another for diagnostic purposes. Thus, this test is no longer performed.

—*Angiotensin-converting enzyme:* Serum levels reflect macrophage activity in granulomata and are elevated in ~60% of patients with sarcoidosis. However, elevation in angiotensin-converting enzyme level is not specific for sarcoidosis as it is in other conditions (see p. 31). Moreover, because they reflect macrophage activity, they are most commonly elevated in patients with substantial active pulmonary involvement. Thus, angiotensin-converting enzyme levels are a poor screening diagnostic tool for unselected populations and for patients with less typical presentations.

Imaging: Chest radiographic abnormalities are commonly seen. Many investigators believe that the presence of bilateral and right paratracheal lymphadenopathy is both consistent with the diagnosis of sarcoidosis and associated with a benign prognosis to the extent that further diagnostic intervention may not be warranted. Gallium scans may show uptake in the chest, lymph nodes, and parotid glands during periods of active disease.

Keys to Diagnosis: The diagnosis of sarcoidosis is usually achieved by the constellation of clinical findings, exclusion of diseases with similar conditions, and (if indicated) demonstration of noncaseating granulomata in histopathologic specimens.

Differential Diagnosis: Diseases with clinical presentations similar to that of sarcoidosis include infectious diseases (e.g., mycobacteria, fungi), lymphoproliferative neoplasms, foreign body reactions, Sjögren's syndrome, SpA, and SLE.

Therapy: The therapy for sarcoidosis varies and is usually driven by the most severe organ involvement. In many cases, therapy focuses on pulmonary involvement, although involvement of other organs (e.g., uveitis) sometimes mandates aggressive treatment. Corticosteroids, often at relatively high doses (≥40 mg/day), have been the therapeutic mainstay for severe sarcoidosis.

Early sarcoid arthritis, because it is often self-limited, is usually treated with NSAIDs and simple analgesics. Intraarticular injection of steroids may be helpful in those with oligoarthritis. In refractory cases, a variety of agents have been tried, including colchicine, MTX, other DMARDs, and TNF inhibitors. Oral corticosteroids are seldom indicated solely for sarcoid arthritis, but patients treated with steroids for other manifestations may show dramatic improvement in their arthritis. Uncontrolled studies show TNF inhibitors to be inconsistently effective in pulmonary sarcoid but effective in those with extrapulmonary disease.

BIBLIOGRAPHY

FitzGerald AA, Davis P. Arthritis, hilar adenopathy, erythema nodosum complex. *J Rheumatol* 1982;9:935–938.
Giuffrida TJ, Kerdel FA. Sarcoidosis. *Dermatol Clin* 2002;20:435–447.

SCHMORL'S NODES

Synonyms: Cartilaginous nodes.

ICD-9 Code: Unspecified, 722.30; lumbar or lumbosacral, 722.32; thoracic, 722.31.

Definition: Schmorl's nodes are cartilaginous extrusions of disc material (nucleus pulposus) through the vertebral endplate into the body of the vertebrae. They are often incidental asymptomatic findings on radiographs.

Etiology: Schmorl's nodes may be idiopathic or associated with disorders that weaken or disrupt vertebral endplates or body (e.g., intervertebral osteochondrosis, Scheuermann's disease, trauma, hyperparathyroidism, osteoporosis, infection, neoplasm).

Demographics: Schmorl's nodes are more common in men than women.

Cardinal Findings: Schmorl's nodes are often asymptomatic but may produce local mechanical pain. They are most frequently found at the lower endplate in the lower thoracic and upper lumbar vertebrae.

Uncommon Findings: Thoracic kyphosis may be seen in young individuals with Scheuermann's disease.

Diagnostic Tests: Conventional radiography is used.

Imaging: On radiographs, vertebral lesions appear as radiolucent (round or irregularly shaped) areas surrounded by sclerosis. They may also be visualized by CT or MRI.

Differential Diagnosis: Intervertebral osteochondrosis, Scheuermann's disease, trauma, hyperparathyroidism, osteoporosis, infection, and neoplasm should be considered.

Therapy: Usually no therapy is required. Analgesic agents may be used for pain.

SCLERODERMA

Synonyms: Progressive systemic sclerosis (PSS); diffuse scleroderma (CREST syndrome is discussed on p. 150).

ICD-9 Code: Scleroderma, 710.1; with lung involvement, 517.2.

Definition: Scleroderma is a multisystem disorder characterized by skin thickening and vascular abnormalities. In addition to skin, the most commonly affected organs are lung and kidney. Three major disease subsets are recognized, based on the extent of skin disease. Limited disease is defined as skin fibrosis in distal extremities and some areas of the face and neck. Limited disease is also known as CREST syndrome. Diffuse disease includes patients with skin abnormalities extending to the proximal extremities (i.e., above the elbow or knee) and trunk. Localized disease manifests as patches (morphea) or bandlike (linear scleroderma) areas of skin thickening.

Etiology: Causes of scleroderma remain mysterious. Immunologic abnormalities are suggested by the presence of characteristic autoantibodies such as ANA, anticentromere, and anti-Scl-70 antibodies. Early dermal changes include lymphocytic infiltrates consisting primarily of T cells, but the major abnormality is collagen accumulation with fibrosis. In addition, other striking abnormalities are seen in small- to medium-sized blood vessels, which show immunologically bland fibrotic change. The theory that the vasculature is the primary target is supported by significant experimental data. In addition to these intrinsic abnormalities, the association of scleroderma-like syndromes with epidemic exposures to toxins (e.g., toxic oil syndrome, eosinophilia-myalgia syndrome) suggests that an environmental trigger may start the process in a susceptible individual.

Pathology: Small arteries in the skin, lung, and kidney show proliferation of subintimal tissues and fibrotic change. Small thrombi may form on the altered intimal surfaces. Luminal narrowing or occlusion characterize these small vessels, with a lesser role by vasospasm. Increased accumulation of fibrotic tissue, primarily collagen, is seen in the dermis and is accompanied by loss of normal skin appendages such as hair follicles. Skeletal muscle and myocardium may show atrophy of the muscle fibers and replacement by fibrotic tissue. Infrequently, histologic myositis is seen.

Demographics: Scleroderma is a rare disease. Approximately 80% of patients are females, and one-half present before the age of 40. Some studies suggest a higher incidence and severity of disease in black females than in whites. A much higher prevalence is seen in the United States than in northern Europe or in Asia, a difference that at present remains unexplained.

Cardinal Findings: A variety of organ systems may be involved in scleroderma.
—*Skin:* Skin changes are the hallmark of this disease in most patients. Skin thickening is most noticeable in the hands, which in early stages may appear swollen or puffy. The skin is not easily pinched into small folds and may be indurated or bound down to underlying tissues. Normal skinfolds (e.g., over the knuckles) may be obliterated, and hair no longer grows over sclerodermatous skin. In the diffuse form, proximal extremity, truncal, and facial skin thickening is seen. The area around the mouth is often affected, with thinning of the lips and an inability to open the mouth fully. The lack of facial wrinkling may make patients appear younger than their actual age. Skin changes are often accompanied by Raynaud phenomenon (see p. 312), and fingertips may be cool and dusky, with loss of the usual digital pulp. With time, hyperkeratosis develops under the nails, which may be another clue to Raynaud phenomenon. Digital pits or scarring of the distal digital pulp is characteristic; some patients may have open ulcerations. Subcutaneous calcinosis can manifest as hard white lesions that uncommonly ulcerate with exudation of chalky material from open ulcers (see p. 135). Rarely, patients are seen without skin changes but with organ (usually GI) involvement only (scleroderma sine scleroderma).
—*Musculoskeletal:* Arthralgias and joint stiffness are common. Uncommonly, patients may initially display rheumatoid-like synovitis, with subsequent development of sclerodermal skin findings. Palpable tendon friction rubs are best felt over the flexor and extensor surface of the wrists, knees, or above the ankles and produce a palpable grating sensation with movement. Tendon friction rubs may be seen early in diffuse disease and are associated with increased incidence of organ involvement. Muscle weakness may be from muscle atrophy, fibrosis, or less commonly frank myositis.
—*GI:* Esophageal dysmotility with substernal dysphagia is common. Incompetence of the gastroesophageal sphincter leads to symptomatic reflux esophagitis. Common symptoms are heartburn and a sensation that food or pills are lodged in the chest behind the sternum. Involvement of the small bowel is less common and can produce a malabsorptive or blind loop syndrome. Colon abnormalities may contribute to constipation. Wide-mouthed diverticula commonly occur in the large intestine.
—*Cardiopulmonary:* Insidious development of interstitial lung involvement is common early in the course of diffuse disease and may lead to a restrictive defect seen on pulmonary function testing. If fibrosis is present, auscultatory dry rales may be appreciated on examination. By contrast, patients with limited scleroderma may develop acute-onset pulmonary hypertension late in the disease. Increased pulmonary pressures can contribute to right-sided heart failure.
—*Renal:* Kidney involvement, most common in the diffuse form, is an ominous finding and important cause of death in diffuse scleroderma. Renal (or hypertensive) crisis may herald the onset of rapidly progressive renal failure. This syndrome includes very high blood pressure, headaches, visual disturbances, and heart failure. Renal crisis risk factors include cold exposure,

steroid use, dehydration, rapid progression of skin disease, and pregnancy. Microscopic hematuria may be observed, and microangiopathic hemolytic anemia is usually present. Before the use of the angiotensin-converting enzyme inhibitors, this syndrome was uniformly fatal. The more widespread use of angiotensin-converting enzyme inhibitors has dramatically reduced the numbers of renal deaths in diffuse scleroderma. More than half of patients with renal crisis do well and avoid long-term dialysis; <20% die of this infrequent complication.

—*Eyes/mouth:* Secondary Sjögren's syndrome occurs in a significant number of patients with scleroderma who are usually anti-SSA antibody positive and exhibit dry eyes and dry mouth.

—*Thyroid:* Hypothyroidism, present in approximately one-fourth of patients, is often clinically unrecognized. The thyroid gland shows fibrotic change. Hyperthyroidism is rare.

Uncommon Manifestations: Exudative pleural or pericardial effusions are rare. Intestinal pseudo-obstruction has been reported. Primary biliary cirrhosis appears to be increased in patients with the limited variant of scleroderma.

Diagnostic Tests: The diagnosis is made largely by history and physical examination. Laboratory information may provide supportive or prognostic information. More than 90% of patients are positive for ANAs. The nucleolar ANA pattern is common in patients with diffuse scleroderma, and the centromere pattern is characteristic of the limited (CREST syndrome) variant. Antibodies to Scl-70 are directed against topoisomerase-1 and are associated with the diffuse form. Patients tend to have either anticentromere (limited disease) or anti-Scl-70 (diffuse disease) antibodies but not both. Nailfold capillaroscopy (see p. 88) should be performed early in patients with Raynaud's phenomenon or suspected scleroderma to help define the prognosis. Periodic pulmonary function testing, including the force vital capacity and diffusion capacity (DL_{CO}), is indicated in patients with diffuse disease and is an effective measure of interstitial lung disease. Routine hemogram, chemistries, and urinalysis are most often indicated as part of drug monitoring.

Imaging: Chest radiographs should be performed to evaluate pulmonary symptoms and may aid in diagnosis of pulmonary fibrosis. High-resolution CT scans may be used to further evaluate pulmonary fibrosis and may show a honeycomb (with pulmonary fibrosis) or ground-glass (with alveolitis) appearance. Esophageal studies such as barium swallow with a cine-esophagram can identify lower esophageal dysmotility.

Keys to Diagnosis: Tightening of the skin, especially of the hands (sclerodactyly), associated with Raynaud's phenomenon strongly suggests scleroderma, either limited or diffuse.

Differential Diagnosis: Eosinophilic fasciitis (see p. 169) is a scleroderma variant in which skin tightening is most common in the extremities but spares the hands, feet, and face and is not associated with Raynaud's phenomenon. Tight skin may also be caused by exposure to vinyl chloride, solvents, rapeseed oil, bleomycin, pentazocine, and tryptophan (eosinophil-myalgia syndrome). Pseudosclerodactyly refers to waxy or tight skin changes seen with diabetes or hypothyroidism. Scleromyxedema causes waxy tightening of the extremities and trunk. It is often associated with myopathy, monoclonal gammopathy, lymphoma, arthritis, neuropathy, and Sjögren's syndrome. The cause is unknown.

Diagnostic Criteria: A classification schema for scleroderma has been proposed that includes patients with diffuse or limited forms of the disease while excluding other syndromes such as eosinophilic fasciitis (Table 41). However, it is estimated that 10% of patients in clinical practice who appear to have scleroderma do not fulfill these criteria.

Therapy: Treatment of Raynaud's phenomenon should include care to keep hands and feet warm with gloves or other coverings; these may be required at night as well as during the day. Tobacco should be discontinued and beta-blockers should be avoided. Biofeedback training or stress reduction techniques may be effective in limiting frequency or severity of the vasospastic episodes. Major dental procedures or appliances present a problem because of limitation of mouth excursion. Gastric reflux measures should be instituted, including elevating the head of the bed and avoiding late evening meals.
—*Raynaud phenomenon:* Vasodilating agents may be used, especially long-acting calcium channel blockers such as nifedipine. High blood pressure is best treated with angiotensin-converting enzyme inhibitors.
—*Corticosteroids:* In the early stages of diffuse disease, when hands appear puffy or edematous, low doses of prednisone may be useful. However, data suggest that high doses of corticosteroids can lead to renal crisis or failure. Thus, steroids should be avoided in most patients.
—*Penicillamine:* Data from several uncontrolled studies show a reduction in skin thickening with penicillamine treatment. Beneficial effects on pulmonary and GI abnormalities have also been reported in retrospective stud-

Table 41
Proposed Criteria for the Classification of Patients with Scleroderma

A. Major criteria
    Proximal scleroderma: skin thickening/induration proximal to the metacarpophalangeal (or metatarsophalangeal) joints, in areas including face, neck, proximal extremities, and trunk
B. Minor criteria
    1. Sclerodactyly
    2. Digital pitting scars or loss of terminal digital pulp
    3. Bibasilar pulmonary fibrosis seen on standard chest radiograph

A diagnosis of scleroderma requires 1 major or 2 minor criteria.

DISEASES

ies. Thus, penicillamine is generally recommended in patients with early disease who manifest progressive skin changes, pulmonary compromise, or renal disease. A recent study did not show any clinical difference between low-dose (250–750 mg/day) and high-dose (1,000–1,500 mg/day) penicillamine. Unfortunately, a placebo-treated group was not included.

—*Others:* Use of other immunosuppressive drugs is not promising; no controlled trials suggest their benefit. Some investigators anecdotally advocate the use of cyclophosphamide with progressive pulmonary fibrosis and cyclosporine for rapidly advancing early disease. Agents such as chlorambucil, MTX, recombinant human relaxin, extracorporeal photopheresis, antithymocyte globulin, interferon alpha, minocycline, and Potaba (potassium aminobenzoate) have been tried but remain unproven. The efficacy and safety of autologous stem cell transplantation in scleroderma is under study.

Surgery: Surgery is not generally indicated. Renal transplants have been relatively successful, and few patients have received heart or lung transplants.

Prognosis: The outcome is most closely related to the extent of significant organ involvement, especially lung and kidney. In one study, 5-year survival in patients without organ involvement was >90%; patients with pulmonary or renal involvement had survival rates of 70% and 50%, respectively. Patients with diffuse skin involvement show shorter survival times than those with limited involvement. Patients with diffuse disease are at risk of early progressive end-organ damage, and those with limited disease are at a small but significant risk of developing pulmonary hypertension or small bowel malabsorption.

BIBLIOGRAPHY

Denton CP, Black CM. Management of systemic sclerosis. In: Hochberg MC, Silman AJ, Smolen JS, et al., eds. *Rheumatology,* 3rd ed. Edinburgh: Mosby, 2003:1493–1506.
Masi AT, Rodnan GP, Medsger TA Jr, et al. Preliminary criteria for the classification of systemic sclerosis (scleroderma). *Arthritis Rheum* 1980;23:581–590.
Mayes MD. Scleroderma epidemiology. *Rheum Dis Clin North Am* 1996;22:751–764.

SEPTIC BURSITIS

ICD-9 Code: Bursitis not otherwise specified, 727.3 (code first underlying infection if present).

Definition: Septic bursitis is a bacterial infection of the bursal space, most commonly involving the olecranon and prepatellar areas.

Etiology: Most cases are caused by inoculation of skin flora into the bursal space by local trauma. Some occupations (e.g., carpet laying, roofing) may be predisposed to inflammatory or septic bursitis.

Pathology: Changes of acute and chronic inflammation in the bursa and adjacent tissues.

Demographics: Most series have a predominance of males, possibly because of occupational hazards. Normal individuals without underlying comorbid conditions can be affected.

Cardinal Findings: The classic presentation is an acute, painful, warm swelling in the periarticular region. Because the joint is not involved, range of motion is usually unaffected. Fever is usually not present.

Diagnostic Tests: Because of the focal acute inflammatory presentation, bursal aspiration should be performed with a large-bore needle (18 or 19 gauge). Cultures of bursal fluid are diagnostic. The bursal fluid WBC can be variable and does not correlate well with the severity of infection. Even relatively low WBC values can be seen with active bacterial infection; thus, cultures are important in all suspected cases. Bursal fluid is more superficial than synovial fluid; care should be taken to avoid the joint space.

Keys to Diagnosis: Acute onset of periarticular swelling should raise suspicion. Septic arthritis can be diagnosed by bursal aspiration and cultures.

Differential Diagnosis: Septic arthritis should be considered if there are fever and limited range of motion or if pain limits motion. Acute bursitis can be seen with gout and RA. Cellulitis or tendinitis may mimic bursitis with pain and erythematous skin changes.

Therapy: Antibiotics should be started soon after the initial bursal aspiration. Oral antibiotics are usually adequate. Although culture results are pending (usually 24–48 hours), the initial antibiotic should provide coverage for *S. aureus* until culture results can further guide therapy. Surgical drainage or bursal removal is rarely required.

Prognosis: Most patients recover completely without sequelae.

BIBLIOGRAPHY

Ho G, Su EY. Antibiotic therapy of septic bursitis: its implication in the treatment of septic arthritis. *Arthritis Rheum* 1981;24:905–911.

Pien FD, Ching D, Kim E. Septic bursitis: experience in a community practice. *Orthopedics* 1991;14:981–984.

SHOULDER PAIN

Definition: Pain referred to the shoulder is very common in the general population, particularly among the elderly. After back pain, it is the second most common acute musculoskeletal complaint in general practice. The prevalence of shoulder complaints among normal older persons is ~20%. With some forms of arthritis, such as RA, the prevalence of shoulder complaints exceeds 80%.

ICD-9 Code: 719.41.

DISEASES

Anatomic Considerations: Pain may originate from the shoulder joint or overlying structures or be referred from the neck, chest (e.g., Pancoast tumor), or even abdomen (e.g., gallbladder, hepatic, diaphragmatic lesions). The shoulder is an incomplete ball-and-socket type of joint, and thus the shoulder is less stable and is dependent on periarticular structures for support. The shoulder area defines a relatively narrow space through which many muscular, neurologic, and vascular structures must pass. Impingement of the rotator cuff, between the humeral head and the acromioclavicular arch, may occur with modest pathologic changes.

Etiology: Shoulder pain can derive from numerous structures in the area of the shoulder, including tendons, bursae, joints, nerves, ligaments, and muscles (see p. 25). Inciting stimuli for pain in these structures usually include inflammation, degeneration, trauma, and overuse.

The most common cause of shoulder pain is rotator cuff dysfunction (see p. 335), which may be affected in as many as 75% of patients with shoulder pain. Rotator cuff dysfunction represents a spectrum of conditions, from rota-

Table 42
Differential Diagnosis of Shoulder Pain

Bursitis/tendinitis
    Rotator cuff dysfunction (including tendinitis, tendon tears, impingement syndrome, frozen shoulder)
    Subacromial bursitis
    Bicipital tendinitis
Arthritis (degenerative or inflammatory, e.g., rheumatoid arthritis, gout, spondyloarthropathy)
    Glenohumeral arthritis
    Acromioclavicular joint arthritis
    Sternoclavicular joint arthritis
Bone disease
    Fracture
    Dislocation/separation
    Metastatic cancer
    Osteonecrosis (e.g., humeral head)
Neurologic/vascular
    Suprascapular nerve entrapment
    Thoracic outlet syndrome
    Brachial plexus injury (brachial plexopathy)
Other (including referred pain)
    Cervical spine disease
    Polymyalgia rheumatica
    Fibromyalgia
    Reflex sympathetic dystrophy (also known as shoulder-hand syndrome)
    Intrathoracic etiology (e.g., Pancoast tumor, myocardial infarction)
    Intraabdominal etiology (e.g., perihepatitis, cholecystitis)

tor cuff tendinitis to rotator cuff tear to frozen shoulder. Many patients have an associated subacromial bursitis.

Cardinal Findings: A focused history and physical examination often succeed in defining the cause of shoulder pain. Shoulder pain is often exacerbated by activity and is most prominent late in the day or at night. Many patients report an inability to sleep in a recumbent position, and many sleep upright or in a reclining chair. Any history of trauma should raise suspicion of fracture or rotator cuff damage. Acute shoulder pain may result from acute bursitis or tendinitis from overuse or rotator cuff damage. Less commonly, septic, inflammatory, or crystal-induced arthritis may cause acute shoulder pain. Causes of chronic shoulder pain include rotator cuff dysfunction, adhesive capsulitis, fibromyalgia, RA, and OA.

Testing for pain and range of motion on abduction, internal rotation, and external rotation of the humerus may establish rotator cuff dysfunction as the cause of the pain. Tenderness of the subacromial bursa will be apparent on direct palpation laterally below the acromion. Patients with glenohumeral arthritis often have substantial pain and resist any movement of the shoulder joint. Arthritis of other joints about the shoulder (acromioclavicular, sternoclavicular) can be elicited on palpation. Neurovascular function should be tested to rule out those structures as the cause of shoulder pain.

Diagnostic Tests: Laboratory testing is seldom useful. If radiculopathy is being considered, then nerve conduction studies may be indicated.

Imaging: Plain radiography can be used to detect fracture or arthritis (degenerative or inflammatory). Standard views include an anteroposterior view and an anteroposterior view with external rotation. The glenohumeral joint may also be viewed in an axillary view. MRI has largely replaced other imaging procedures for evaluation of persistent rotator cuff dysfunction. In skilled hands, the accuracy of ultrasonography approaches that of MRI.

Therapy: The goal of treatment is to relieve pain and optimize function and range of motion. In many cases, temporary rest followed by physiotherapy to optimize range of motion is indicated. For treatment of pain, many patients respond to NSAIDs or simple analgesics. Local injection with corticosteroids may be of value in subacromial bursitis, bicipital tendinitis, or monarticular arthritis of the shoulder. Surgery is most often considered with severe rotator cuff dysfunction or impingement syndrome. Common procedures include excision of the distal clavicle or acromioplasty (for impingement syndrome), glenohumeral synovectomy (e.g., RA), or total shoulder arthroplasty (replacement).

BIBLIOGRAPHY

Almekinders LC. Impingement syndrome. *Clin Sports Med* 2001;20:491–504.
Tallia AF, Cardone DA. Diagnostic and therapeutic injection of the shoulder region. *Am Fam Physician* 2003;67:1271–1278.

SJÖGREN'S SYNDROME

Synonyms: Keratoconjunctivitis sicca, sicca complex.

ICD-9 Codes: 710.2.

Definition: Sjögren's syndrome is a chronic autoimmune syndrome characterized by lymphocytic infiltration of lacrimal glands and salivary glands with
consequent dry eyes (xerophthalmia) and dry mouth (xerostomia). When it occurs without another autoimmune disorder, it is considered primary Sjögren's
syndrome. Secondary Sjögren's syndrome occurs in patients with preexisting
autoimmune disease, most commonly RA and scleroderma.

Etiology: The causative trigger is not known, although various viruses including Epstein-Barr virus and human T-cell lymphotropic virus type 1 have
been proposed as candidate agents. The high incidence in females suggests a
facilitating role for sex steroid hormones. HLA associations (HLA-B8, -DR3,
and -Dw52 in males) have been described, highlighting a genetic predisposition. Sex hormones may play a role because the condition is more common in
women and improved by androgen therapy.

Pathology: Salivary gland biopsies show benign lymphoepithelial infiltration
and proliferation in the exocrine (e.g., salivary, lacrimal, parotid) glands (see
labial salivary biopsy, p. 83). Adjacent areas of the gland may appear normal.
Helper (CD4$^+$) T cells predominate and most likely activate antibody production by infiltrating B lymphocytes, resulting in hypergammaglobulinemia and
circulating autoantibodies. Infiltrating lymphocytes mediate destruction and
dysfunction of the adjacent glandular tissue.

Demographics: Onset is usually in middle age, with a predominance of females.

Cardinal Findings: Dry mouth and eyes are the predominant presentation.
Xerostomia may be noticeable to the patient and may manifest as accelerated
dental caries in some. Inadequate saliva production may result in pharyngeal
dysphagia. Dry eyes may manifest as redness, conjunctival irritation, or the
sensation of sand in the eye. Patients may blink or rub their eyes excessively.
Parotid gland enlargement is found in a minority of patients. Musculoskeletal
features include fatigue and fibromyalgia in nearly 50% of patients. Fewer patients complain of arthralgias, and frank arthritis is rare.

Uncommon Manifestations: Lymphocytic infiltration into the kidney may
result in tubular dysfunction that is usually not clinically significant. Rarely,
such patients manifest a renal tubular acidosis with severe potassium wasting,
hypokalemia, and muscle weakness. CNS involvement (i.e., polyneuropathy,
cranial nerve neuropathy, multiple sclerosis–like symptoms, headaches, or altered mentation) occurs but is rare. Pulmonary involvement is subclinical in

most and rarely symptomatic. Pulmonary features include bronchitis, interstitial fibrosis, and lymphocytic alveolitis. GI features include dysphagia, atrophic gastritis, primary biliary sclerosis, and sclerosing cholangitis. A small subset of patients with Sjögren's syndrome may go on to develop malignant lymphoma. Hendytic anema, immune cytopenias, and vasculitis are rare.

Diagnostic Tests: Common laboratory testing abnormalities include an elevated ESR, polyclonal hypergammaglobulinemia, and an anemia of chronic disease. ANAs and RF are positive in 65% to 90% of patients, respectively. SSA antibodies are not specific for Sjögren's syndrome and can be seen in other autoimmune disorders. SSB antibodies tend to have a greater association with Sjögren's syndrome. Antibodies against SSA (anti-Ro) are seen in 70% to 80% of primary and in <10% of patients with secondary Sjögren's syndrome. Antibodies against SSB (anti-La) are seen in 50% to 75% of primary and <5% of patients with secondary Sjögren's syndrome.

The diagnosis of keratoconjunctivitis sicca can be further established with quantitative measures of tear production. The Schirmer test (see p. 98) uses adsorbent paper strips inserted into the lower palpebral fold to measure the amount of wetting or tear production. Alternatively, the ophthalmologist can facilitate the diagnosis by performing a Rose bengal test (see p. 97). Rose bengal is a vital stain that is taken up by dead or dying cells and is used to evaluate corneal abnormalities or suspected keratoconjunctivitis sicca. Biopsy of glandular tissue (i.e., minor salivary gland of the lip or parotid gland) may also reveal the characteristic lymphocytic infiltration diagnostic of Sjögren's syndrome.

Keys to Diagnosis: Xerostomia and xerophthalmia with parotid gland enlargement strongly suggests this diagnosis.

Differential Diagnosis: Infections (i.e., mumps) and infiltrative processes such as sarcoidosis may cause parotid gland enlargement. Parotid tumors are likely to be unilateral. Drugs (i.e., tricyclic antidepressants) and irradiation may cause dry eyes and mouth. A subset of HIV-positive patients develop xerostomia, parotid gland swelling, lymphadenopathy, lymphocytic pulmonary infiltrates, and negative tests for anti-Ro or anti-La (see DILS, p. 211).

Diagnostic Criteria: Recently proposed European Criteria are shown in Table 43.

Therapy: Sicca symptoms are treated with lubricating eyedrops and avoidance of aggravating factors such as hair dryers or drying medications. Wearing glasses outdoors may protect from the drying effects of the wind. Ophthalmic consultation is recommended for most. Punctal occlusion may improve tear retention and flow. Saliva substitutes are available and may be preferred by some patients. The use of sugar-free lemon hard candies may help stimulate salivary flow. Fastidious dental care is extremely important to avoid dental caries. The use of humidifiers at home or work may decrease symptoms significantly.

Table 43
Preliminary Criteria for the Classification of Sjögren's Syndrome[a]

1. Ocular symptoms: dry eyes, foreign body sensation in eyes, use of lubricants
2. Oral symptoms: dry mouth, swollen salivary glands, frequent fluid intake with food
3. Ocular signs: Schirmer or rose bengal tests
4. Characteristic histopathologic features: focus score $\geq$1 (labial minor salivary gland biopsy)
5. Salivary gland involvement documented by scintigraphy, sialography, or salivary flow
6. Autoantibodies: rheumatoid factor, antinuclear antibody, or anti-Ro (SSA) or anti-La (SSB)

The presence of 4 of 6 criteria has a sensitivity of 93.5% and specificity of 94%.

[a] Exclusions: lymphoma, acquired immunodeficiency syndrome, sarcoidosis, or graft versus host disease.

NSAIDs and analgesic agents may improve the arthralgias and myalgias. Corticosteroids should not be used for most and are only indicated for vasculitis, pleuropericarditis, or hemolytic anemia. Numerous second-line and immunosuppressive agents (including MTX, penicillamine, and cyclosporine) have been tried, and only hydroxychloroquine appears to have minimal benefit in patients with Sjögren syndrome. Investigational agents include bromhexine, interferon, and androgens. TNF inhibitors appear to be of no benefit.

Surgery: Diagnostic minor salivary gland biopsy may be performed by an oral surgeon. Parotid biopsy via a posterior approach to the subauricular portion of the gland is preferred to reduce the risk of facial nerve injury.

Prognosis: Most patients do well. Sicca problems may require prolonged eye care. High-grade lymphoma that may be resistant to chemotherapy is rare.

BIBLIOGRAPHY

Silver RM. Variant forms of scleroderma. In: Koopman WJ, ed. *Arthritis and allied conditions: a textbook of rheumatology.* Baltimore: Williams & Wilkins, 1996:1465–1480.
Vitali C, Bomardieri S, Moutsopoulos HM, et al. Preliminary criteria for the classification of Sjögren's syndrome: results of a prospective concerted action supported by the European Community. *Arthritis Rheum* 1993;36:340–347.

SLIPPED CAPITAL FEMORAL EPIPHYSIS

ICD-9 Code: 732.2.

Definition: Slipped capital femoral epiphysis is the most common disorder of the hip in adolescents.

Etiology: Etiology is unknown. Slipped capital femoral epiphysis is rarely occurs as a result of trauma. It occurs in either obese adolescents and those with skeletal maturational delay or a recent growth surge. For these reasons, slipped capital femoral epiphysis is postulated to be a consequence of growth-related hormonal change. Abnormalities of growth hormone, thyroid, pituitary, or sex hormones may alter the rate of skeletal growth, especially in the capital femoral epiphysis. Slipped capital femoral epiphysis can also occur as a complication of an underlying endocrine disorder such as hypothyroidism, pituitary disorders, and pseudohypoparathyroidism.

Pathogenesis: The hip is a ball-and-socket (femoral head and acetabulum) joint. The capital femoral epiphysis makes up most of the head. The growth and development of the acetabulum and femoral head are interdependent. Disproportionate changes in skeletal growth may lead to slippage in the weakest area of the physeal plate.

Demographics: Peak onset age is 12 to 15 years, with boys affected two to five times more frequently than girls. The incidence is 0.7 to 3.4 cases per 100,000 per year.

Cardinal Findings: Patients may have little or no pain and few physical findings. Slips are more common during adolescent growth, especially in obese children. Symptoms of pain in the hip, thigh, or knee (referred pain) are seen in less than half of patients. If the child cannot walk or bear weight, the slipped capital femoral epiphysis is said to be unstable. Stable slipped capital femoral epiphysis is more likely to be minimally symptomatic. In the unstable slipped capital femoral epiphysis, the physical examination is limited as a result of severe pain with any attempted hip motion. In a stable slipped capital femoral epiphysis, the patient may have an antalgic gait. Hip range of motion often demonstrates a lack of internal rotation and increased external rotation. Also because the hip is flexed, it becomes progressively externally rotated.

Complications: Slipped capital femoral epiphysis may be complicated by osteonecrosis and chondrolysis. Osteonecrosis or avascular necrosis occurs as a result of trauma to the retinacular vessels. Chondrolysis results in degeneration of the articular cartilage of the hip.

Diagnostic Tests: If indicated by history or examination, tests for an endocrinopathy may be needed.

Imaging: The earliest radiographic finding in slipped capital femoral epiphysis is widening and blurring of the femoral epiphysis. This is followed by slipping of the capital femoral epiphysis with resultant posteroinferior tilt of the femoral head in relation to the femur. This is best seen in lateral views. The femoral neck may rotate anteriorly, resulting in a varus deformity of the femoral head and neck. With unstable or advanced slipped capital femoral epiphysis, remodeling of the femoral head ensues. Scintigraphy is helpful in identifying ischemia and risk of osteonecrosis, especially in unstable slipped capital femoral epiphysis. However, MRI is superior to other modalities in demonstrating early changes and late complications.

Keys to Diagnosis: Adolescents, especially those who are obese, with nontraumatic anterior thigh or knee pain (referred pain), should be carefully evaluated for a slipped capital femoral epiphysis. If slipped capital femoral epiphysis occurs before puberty, an endocrine disorder (hypothyroidism, growth hormone deficiency) should be suspected.

Differential Diagnosis: Legg-Calvé-Perthes disease, fractures, osteonecrosis, overuse, osteomyelitis.

Therapy: The goals of treatment for slipped capital femoral epiphysis are to prevent further slippage and minimize complications. This is accomplished with surgical or interventional *in situ* pinning to stabilize the capital femoral epiphysis. Screw removal after capital femoral epiphysis closure is controversial. Advanced cases may also require rotational osteotomy as well.

BIBLIOGRAPHY

Lindsley CB, Asher MA, Olney BW. Legg-Perthes and other hip diseases in children. In: Hochberg MC, Silman AJ, Smolen JS, et al., eds. *Rheumatology,* 3rd ed. Edinburgh: Mosby, 2003;990–992.

SPINAL STENOSIS

ICD-9 Code: Unspecified, 724.0; lumbar, 724.02; thoracic, 724.01; cervical, 723.0.

Definition: Spinal stenosis refers to a narrowing of the lumen of the spinal canal. It occurs most commonly in the lumbar region but can also occur in the cervical spine. The characteristic clinical symptom of spinal stenosis is neurogenic claudication. Although it may be related in rare cases to developmental bony anomalies, the most common cause of spinal stenosis is degenerative change in the vertebrae (these nonspecific degenerative changes are also known as spondylosis).

Pathology: In most patients, a combination of factors contributes to the narrowing of the spinal canal. Anteriorly, degenerative changes of the intervertebral disc cause disc protrusion and extrusion into the spinal canal. Posteriorly, osteoarthritic changes of the facet (apophyseal) joints impinge directly on the spinal cord. Facet joint arthritis, very common among older persons, is also associated with hypertrophy of the ligamentum flavum, which is normally thin and lines the spinal canal. This further diminishes the area of the spinal canal. Degenerative changes of the facet joints may result in laxity and movement of one vertebral body in relation to others, either unilaterally (spondylolysis) or bilaterally (spondylolisthesis). This may result in further impingement of neural structures.

Demographics: Spinal stenosis is most common among the elderly, with a mean age at onset of approximately 60 years of age. Men are affected about twice as frequently as women. Many patients experience symptoms for months or even years before the correct diagnosis is established.

Cardinal Findings: Symptoms of neurogenic claudication (or pseudoclaudication) occur in >90% of patients. It is commonly described as an aching pain in the buttocks, posterior thigh, or calf (>90%) and is often provoked or aggravated by walking. However, it may also be described as numbness (~65%) or weakness (~40%) and is bilateral in ~70% of patients. Of note, the area of the lumbar spinal canal and neural foramina change with position. This space increases with flexion, and patients with spinal stenosis often report relief of symptoms when their backs are flexed (e.g., sitting, bending over, or sleeping in the fetal position). This may provide a useful clue to differentiating vascular from neurogenic claudication. Patients with vascular claudication are limited in their walking by vascular supply. Symptoms are relieved by stopping walking, and patients do not necessarily need to sit down or change position. In contrast, patients with neurogenic claudication find relief by sitting down or bending over. They may also have similar pain by standing erect without walking, and they can walk without limit if their spines are flexed (e.g., pushing a shopping cart or lawnmower).

On physical examination, most patients experience pain on straight leg raising. Many also have depressed lower extremity deep tendon reflexes. Muscle weakness or sensory defects are not common. Pulses are generally easily palpable, another potential point distinguishing neurogenic from vascular claudication.

Diagnostic Testing: Hematologic, chemical, and serologic studies are of no value in evaluating patients with spinal stenosis. Electrodiagnostic studies (e.g., nerve conduction velocity testing) may provide useful information. Such tests may exclude other conditions (e.g., neuropathies) and document the severity and extent of neurologic involvement from spinal stenosis.

Imaging: Plain radiographs are commonly used to evaluate patients with back pain, but their utility may be limited, particularly in spinal stenosis. Radiographs typically show degenerative changes of the lumbar spine. However, such changes provide no information regarding neurologic impingement and do not correlate with the severity of symptoms. Bony abnormalities and narrowing of the spinal canal are easily visualized by CT. However, CT must be combined with myelography for clear definition of bony impingement on the spinal cord or nerve roots. MRI, which allows definition of bone as well as soft and nerve tissue, is now the imaging procedure of choice for patients with spinal stenosis.

Differential Diagnosis: Vascular insufficiency, inflammatory SpA (e.g., AS), spinal metastases, disc disease, and Paget's disease should be considered.

Therapy: The most appropriate therapy depends on the extent and progression of symptoms. Conservative measures include physiotherapy (e.g., optimizing low back mechanics, muscle strengthening, enhancing flexibility) and analgesic medications.

Surgery: Patients with cauda equina syndrome (loss of bowel or bladder function, "saddle" [perineal] anesthesia) may require surgical decompression of the stenosed canal. Patients with progression of either neurologic defects (e.g., radiculopathy) or intractable pain likewise may benefit from surgical intervention. The type of surgery depends on the specific pathologic changes considered most responsible for the patient's symptoms. In most patients, laminectomy is the procedure of choice, although a few patients may benefit from foraminectomy or discectomy. Surgery is not required for all patients, and in some series, patients appear to have similar long-term outcomes with or without surgery.

Prognosis: The course of spinal stenosis is variable. For many patients, it is a chronic condition that may improve with intervention. Some patients experience relatively rapid progression from intermittent pain to excruciating persistent pain to neurologic defect.

BIBLIOGRAPHY

Hall S, Bartleson JD, Onofrio BM, et al. Lumbar spinal stenosis. *Ann Intern Med* 1985;103:271–275.
Moreland LW, Lopez-Mendez A, Alarcon GS. Spinal stenosis: a comprehensive review of the literature. *Semin Arthritis Rheum* 1989;19:127–149.
Swezey RL. Outcomes for lumbar stenosis. *J Clin Rheumatol* 1996;2:129–133.

SPONDYLOARTHROPATHY

Synonyms: SpA; seronegative SpA, incomplete SpA; HLA-B27-related SpA.

ICD-9 Codes: Spondyloarthropathy, 720.9; Codes for individual disorders: AS, 720.0; Reiter's syndrome, 099.3; psoriatic arthritis, 696.1.

Definition: SpA is a generic term applied to a constellation of clinical, radiographic, and immunogenetic features shared by a group of disorders that include AS (see p. 115), Reactive arthritis, psoriatic arthritis, and enteropathic arthritis. Because only a minority of patients manifest complete or classic findings of one of these individual disorders and most demonstrate incomplete or overlapping features, changes in nosology have been adopted to accommodate what is actually seen in clinical practice. This latter group is often designated as having an incomplete SpA or an HLA-B27-related SpA. The term SpA has gained popularity since 1990 when more liberal diagnostic criteria were proposed (Table 44).

Etiology: By virtue of their association with HLA-B27 and overlapping clinical and radiographic features, the disorders are presumed to share a similar etiopathogenesis. Most theories relate to unknown antigenic or infectious inciting events occurring in a genetically susceptible host, leading to either molecular mimicry or a chronic, antigen-driven reactive condition.

Demographics: This more liberally defined population is likely to be more prevalent than the individual subsets that they resemble. SpAs are more likely

Table 44

Diagnostic Criteria for the Spondyloarthropathies

ESSG Criteria for Spondyloarthropathy	Amor Criteria for the Spondyloarthropathies	Score
1. Inflammatory spinal pain *or* peripheral synovitis (asymmetric or lower limbs)	Lumbar pain at night or morning stiffness	1
	Asymmetric oligoarthritis	2
	Buttock pain (or bilateral or alternating buttock pain)	1
2. Plus ≥1 of the following:		
Alternate buttock pain		
Sacroiliitis	Sausage-like toe or digit(s)	2
Enthesopathy	Heel pain or enthesitis	2
Positive family history	Iritis	1
Psoriasis	Nongonococcal urethritis/cervicitis within 1 mo of onset	
Inflammatory bowel disease		
Urethritis or cervicitis or acute diarrhea occurring within 1 mo of the onset of arthritis	Psoriasis, balanitis, or inflammatory bowel disease	1
	Sacroiliitis (bilateral grade 2 or unilateral grade 3)	2
	HLA-B27 positive or positive family history of a spondyloarthropathy	2
	Rapid (<48 h) response to NSAIDs	2
	Diagnosis of a spondyloarthropathy requires a score ≥6	

ESSG, European Spondyloarthropathy Study Group.

to be seen in men. Women may tend to have milder disease that is more difficult to diagnose. Most patients present between the ages of 20 and 50 years.

Pathology: These disorders share a common pathologic profile, which includes a propensity for axial and peripheral inflammatory arthritis and inflammation involving the eye (conjunctivitis, uveitis), skin (psoriasis, nail changes), mucosal surfaces (oral and genital), and tendinous attachments to bone (enthesitis). Synovial membrane shows histologic inflammation similar to that seen with RA, with synovial proliferation and prominent infiltration with mononuclear cells in the sublining and perivascular areas. There is a greater propensity for fibrous ankylosis, osseous resorption, and heterotopic bone formation. Skin changes are compatible with keratoderma blenorrhagica or pustular psoriasis.

Cardinal Findings: The SpA share a constellation of characteristic clinical, radiographic, and immunogenetic manifestations that suggest a common or related etiopathogenesis (Table 44). Distinctive features include a propensity for axial arthritis (sacroiliitis and spondylitis); peripheral arthritis (often asymmetric and oligoarticular); inflammation at tendinous, ligamentous, or fascial insertions (enthesitis); and a familial pattern of inheritance based on the presence of the class I major histocompatibility complex antigen HLA-B27. These disorders can manifest extraarticular features that suggest a particular SpA. Extraarticular manifestations may involve periarticular structures (enthesitis), eyes (uveitis), GI tract (oral ulcerations, asymptomatic gut inflammation), genitourinary tract (urethritis), heart (aortitis, heart block), skin (keratoderma blennorrhagica), and nails (onycholysis). Occasionally, patients with overlapping features of more than one condition or with HLA-B27–positive unclassifiable disease may be encountered. Thus, approaching these conditions as a group of related disorders is important in understanding their pathologic consequences and in diagnosing them accurately.

Diagnostic Criteria: Criteria for the diagnosis of an SpA have been proposed by the European Spondyloarthropathy Study Group (Table 44). The criteria of Amor et al. perform equally well in population studies. These were devised because other disease-specific criteria (e.g., Rome criteria for AS) exclude many patients with SpA. Broader definitions used in these criteria allow earlier diagnosis and more liberal inclusion in clinical trials.

Imaging: Radiographic abnormalities are similar to those seen in AS and reactive arthritis. There is a propensity for sacroiliitis, spondylitis, peripheral arthritis with soft tissue swelling, juxtaarticular osteopenia, joint space narrowing, or ill-defined erosions. Areas of periostitis, reactive new bone formation, or osteitis are not uncommon.

Therapy: See sections on AS (p. 115) and reactive arthritis (p. 315) for guidance.

BIBLIOGRAPHY

Dougados M, van der Linden SM, Juhlin R, et al. The European Spondyloarthropathy Study Group preliminary criteria for the classification of spondyloarthropathy. *Arthritis Rheum* 1991;34:1218–1227.

Khan MA. Update on spondyloarthropathies. *Ann Intern Med* 2002;136:896–907.

Khan MA, van der Linden SM. A wider spectrum of spondyloarthropathies. *Semin Arthritis Rheum* 1990;20:107–113.

Miceli-Richard C, van der Heijde D, Dougados M. Spondyloarthropathy for practicing rheumatologists: diagnosis, indication for disease-controlling antirheumatic therapy, and evaluation of the response. *Rheum Dis Clin North Am* 2003;29:449–462.

STREPTOCOCCAL REACTIVE ARTHRITIS

Synonyms: Incomplete rheumatic fever, post-streptococcal arthritis.

ICD-9 Code: 711.0.

Etiology: Reactive arthropathy is caused by streptococcal infection (groups A and G).

Demographics: Streptococcal reactive arthritis is most common in children and young adults but also reported in adults.

Cardinal Findings: Onset follows streptococcal pharyngitis. Arthropathy (nonmigratory oligo- or polyarthritis) occurs within 2 weeks after a documented infection. Approximately one-third manifest episodic arthralgias or arthritis. Many develop systemic manifestations including fever, myalgias, prostration, and serositis.

Uncommon Findings: Few patients have developed carditis on long-term follow-up.

Diagnostic Tests: Most patients have an elevated antistreptolysin O or DNase B antibody titer.

Keys to Diagnosis: Streptococcal reactive arthritis is distinguished from ARF by a lack of sufficient features to meet the Jones criteria. Classic cutaneous, cardiac, and neurologic findings of ARF are absent.

Therapy: Therapy is similar to that of ARF, but whether subsequent antibiotic prophylaxis is necessary is controversial.

Course: Characteristically, response to therapy with salicylates or NSAIDs is slow or incomplete. The course is often benign with a good outcome.

BIBLIOGRAPHY

Deighton C. β-Hemolytic streptococci and reactive arthritis in adults. *Ann Rheum Dis* 1993;52:475–482.
Jansen TL, Janssen M, de Jong AJ, et al.. Post-streptococcal reactive arthritis: a clinical and serological description, revealing its distinction from acute rheumatic fever. *J Intern Med* 1999;245:261-267.

SUBSTANCE ABUSE: MUSCULOSKELETAL MANIFESTATIONS

Synonyms: Intravenous drug abuse–associated arthritis, brown heroin syndrome.

ICD-9 Code: Drug addiction, 304.9; vasculitis, 447.6; arthralgia, 719.4.

Definition: Various musculoskeletal syndromes are described among substance abuse patients. Symptoms are caused by the offending drug or adulterants within the drug. Implicated drugs include stimulants (e.g., methamphetamines, cocaine), narcotics (heroin), and hallucinogens (D-lysergic acid diethylamide, LSD). Although patients may admit to abusing a particular drug, abuse of multiple drugs is common.

Etiology: Causes vary, including immune complex-mediated disease, foreign body reactions, vessel spasm/toxicity, or other as-yet unidentified mechanisms.

Pathology: Pathology varies, depending on the syndrome. Vascular lesions may be similar to those seen in polyarteritis. Refractile particles caused by talc or other adulterants may be seen in small vessels by polarized microscopy.

Demographics: Those engaging in substance abuse are at risk.

Clinical Syndromes

—*Septic arthritis/osteomyelitis:* Substance abusers are at higher risk of septic arthritis, septic bursitis, and osteomyelitis. Commonly infected joints include the glenohumeral, sternoclavicular, knee, sacroiliac, and spinal (possibly with septic discitis) joints. Vertebral osteomyelitis and osteomyelitis of appendicular skeleton have been reported.

—*Drug withdrawal:* Myalgias and arthralgias, with or without fever, may be seen during drug withdrawal.

—*Intravenous drug abuse–induced angiitis:* Polyarteritis-like angiitis has been seen in those abusing methamphetamines, LSD, and cocaine. Patients have been described with fever, weight loss, arthralgia, myalgia, hypertension, abdominal pain, neuropathy, encephalopathy, pulmonary edema, leukocytosis, hemolysis, proteinuria, medium and large vessel vasculitis, and death.

—*Brown heroin:* Musculoskeletal manifestations have been described in those abusing brown heroin. Brown heroin gets its color from adulterants (procaine or papaverine) or impurities of the opium plant during manufacture. Symptoms arise days to months after use of brown heroin. Patients may complain of neck or low back pain, myalgia, or stiffness. Joint pain tends to be periarticular, affecting the knees, ankles, tarsus, wrist, elbow, or shoulder. Inflammatory synovitis is uncommon. Laboratory testing abnormalities include increased ESR and hypergammaglobulinemia. A minority test positive for ANA, RF, syphilis, or cryoglobulins. Antibiotics are of no value, but ASA or NSAIDs may be effective.

—*Cocaine vasculitis:* Cerebral vasculitis, Raynaud's phenomenon, myositis, rhabdomyolysis, and leukocytoclastic vasculitis have resulted from cocaine abuse. Such patients often have a very high ESR and an abnormal angiogram. Response to corticosteroids or cytotoxic therapy may be disappointing.

—*Barbiturate-related connective tissue disorders:* Patients using or abusing barbiturates (phenobarbital, primidone) are at low risk of developing arthralgias, Dupuytren contractures, or Peyronie disease. Bilateral rather than unilateral findings are common.

Also see Bacterial Endocarditis (p. 130), Bacterial Arthritis (p. 125), and Osteomyelitis (p. 273).

Infectious Associations: Because of nonsterile injection techniques, patients may be at risk of septic arthritis, osteomyelitis, septic thrombophlebitis, local and systemic candidiasis, and subacute bacterial endocarditis. Septic arthritis and osteomyelitis are more commonly caused by gram-positive infections (e.g., *S. aureus, S. pyogenes*), but gram-negative (e.g., *Pseudomonas, Serratia*) infections are seen. Septic arthritis commonly affects the large joints (e.g., knee) but may also involve the spine or sternoclavicular joint.

Cardinal Findings: Cutaneous needle tracks and other stigmata of substance abuse should be carefully sought. Cellulitis and cutaneous abscesses may be associated with intravenous or subcutaneous drug administration. (See above for clinical presentations.)

Comorbid Conditions: Chronic alcoholism, depression, drug withdrawal, infections (e.g., bacterial sepsis, pneumonia, subacute bacterial endocarditis, hepatitis, candidiasis, tuberculosis, HIV), pancreatitis, and schizophrenia are possible comorbid conditions.

Diagnostic Tests: Toxicologic screening may be necessary to identify the offending drug(s). Leukocytosis, with or without eosinophilia, may be seen. Selected visceral angiography may be useful in documenting vasculitis.

Therapy: Discontinuation of the offending agent may improve clinical outcome.

BIBLIOGRAPHY

Kak V, Chandrasekar PH. Bone and joint infections in injection drug users. *Infect Dis Clin North Am* 2002;6:681–695.

Lohr KM. Rheumatic manifestations of diseases associated with substance abuse. *Semin Arthritis Rheum* 1987;17:90–111.

Merkel PA. Drug-induced vasculitis. *Rheum Dis Clin North Am* 2001;27:849–862.

SWEET'S SYNDROME

Synonyms: Acute febrile neutrophilic dermatosis.

ICD-9 Code: 685.89.

Definition: Sweet's syndrome is a multisystem, febrile disorder accompanied by painful papules or plaques (with cutaneous neutrophilic infiltration), arthritis, and leukocytosis. Sweet's syndrome may occur in association with infection, neoplasms, or other systemic inflammatory disorders.

Etiology: The cause is unknown; a hypersensitivity reaction is proposed.

Pathology: Sweet's syndrome exhibits dense dermal infiltration with neutrophils, without vasculitic changes.

Demographics: Most patients are women between the ages of 30 and 60 years.

D
I
S
E
A
S
E
S

Cardinal Findings: Onset may follow upper respiratory infection. Systemic features include fever ($>38°C$ in $>80\%$ of patients), malaise, conjunctivitis, episcleritis, iridocyclitis, oral ulcers, proteinuria, arthralgias, myalgias, and arthritis. Skin lesions appear as tender red or violaceous papules, plaques, or pustules over the face, neck, and arms. Lesions typically resolve in 4 to 8 weeks but may recur. Self-limiting, asymmetric, oligo- or polyarthritis occurs in as many as 25% of patients. Arthritis tends to parallel skin lesions and usually affects the hands, wrists, ankles, or knees. Pulmonary features (cough, dyspnea, or pulmonary infiltrates) occur in $<10\%$ of patients.

Complications: Some (15% to 25%) develop a malignancy, particularly acute myelocytic leukemia, multiple myeloma, myelodysplasia, lymphoma, or solid tumors (e.g., prostate, ovarian, testicular, and breast cancer). Nearly 50% have other underlying conditions such as inflammatory bowel disease, pregnancy, or other connective tissue diseases (RA, SLE, relapsing polychondritis, sarcoidosis, Behçet's or Sjögren's syndrome).

Diagnostic Tests: Laboratory testing abnormalities include anemia and elevated ESR, WBC counts, and alkaline phosphatase. Proteinuria is seen in 15%. Positive P-ANCA test results have been reported.

Diagnostic Criteria: Major criteria are (a) abrupt-onset painful plaques or nodules and (b) neutrophilic infiltrates in the dermis without leukocytoclastic vasculitis. Minor criteria are (a) preceded by fever or infection; (b) accompanied by fever, arthralgia, conjunctivitis, or underlying malignant lesion; (c) leukocytosis; (d) good response to steroids but not antibiotics; and (e) increased ESR. Diagnosis requires that both major and two minor criteria be fulfilled.

Differential Diagnosis: Erythema elevatum diutinum, erythema nodosum, pyoderma gangrenosum, SLE, and Still's disease should be considered.

Therapy: Oral steroids (e.g., prednisone 40–60 mg/day) are effective. Steroids should be tapered over 4 to 6 weeks. Other therapies, including aspirin, NSAIDs, dapsone, colchicine, sulfapyridine, and potassium iodide, have had some success.

Comment: Onset of Sweet's syndrome underscores the need for a thorough history and physical examination to exclude an associated malignancy.

BIBLIOGRAPHY

Cohen PR, Kurzrock R. Sweet's syndrome: a review of current treatment options. *Am J Clin Dermatol* 2002;3:117–131.
Fett DL, Gibson LE, Su WPD. Sweets syndrome: systemic signs and symptoms. *Mayo Clin Proc* 1995;70:234–240.

SYSTEMIC LUPUS ERYTHEMATOSUS

Synonyms: Lupus, lupus erythematosus, SLE.

ICD-9 Codes: SLE, 710.0; discoid, 695.4; lupus anticoagulant, 286.5; drug in-duced, 695.4; nephritis, 583.81.

Definition: SLE is an autoimmune disease characterized by inflammation in many organ systems. Although some patients with SLE have relatively mild disease, others experience severe morbidity and accelerated mortality. The characteristic laboratory finding of SLE is the presence of autoantibodies that react with various components of the cell nucleus; antinuclear antibodies (ANA). The exact pathophysiologic role of most of these autoantibodies re-mains unknown. Much end-organ involvement in SLE involves deposition of immune complexes. The presence of specific autoantibodies correlates with particular organ involvement and prognosis.

Etiology: Etiology is unknown. Because of the female preponderance of SLE, sex steroids are presumed to play a key role in disease expression. Genetics play some role; monozygotic twins are concordant for SLE in ~30% of cases, whereas dizygotic twins and other siblings are concordant in 5%. This implies that other environmental risk factor(s) are superimposed on a susceptible ge-netic background. Certain major histocompatibility complex alleles (e.g., HLA-B8, DR2, DR3) are associated with a slightly greater risk of developing SLE. In addition, many patients with SLE have null alleles for complement protein C4. Although this may not be reflected in low serum C4 concentrations, it may af-fect the patient's ability to remove immune complexes effectively. Similarly, al-lelic differences in cell surface receptors for the Fc portion of IgG correlate with end-organ involvement in SLE.

Demographics: Peak incidence of SLE is between 15 and 40 years of age. In this age group, women are affected approximately 10 times as commonly as men. This female predominance decreases among older patients. There is a racial disparity: patients of African descent have both a greater incidence of SLE and a tendency toward more severe disease. The overall population preva-lence of SLE is approximately 25 to 50 per 100,000. Among some high-risk pop-ulations (e.g., young black women), the prevalence may be as high as four per 1,000.

Cardinal Findings: Characteristic clinical findings of SLE are shown in Table 45. The frequencies of end-organ involvement between populations and among patients with SLE differ substantially. This is relevant to the treatment of SLE, which is often guided by the particular constellation of clinical charac-teristics and the most severe end-organ involvement for a given patient. Some manifestations of SLE vary with race; for example, discoid skin lesions are more common and photosensitivity is less common among patients with SLE of African descent than others. Some manifestations are more typical of pa-tients with particular autoantibodies (e.g., renal disease in patients with anti-DNA antibodies). A number of patients with SLE have an overlap of signs and symptoms of other connective tissue diseases. Manifestations typical of sclero-derma (sclerodactyly, interstitial pulmonary disease, digital vasculitis) and in-flammatory myositis are commonly seen among patients with SLE.

DISEASES

Table 45
Clinical Manifestations of Systemic Lupus Erythematosus

Constitutional symptoms
  Fever, fatigue, malaise, anorexia, weight loss
Mucocutaneous
  Malar rash
  Discoid rash
  Other rashes
  Photosensitivity
  Oral/nasal ulcerations (typically painless at the onset),
  Xerophthalmia (dry eyes) and/or xerostomia (dry mouth) (these symptoms, sometimes called sicca symptoms, are consistent with Sjögren's syndrome)
  Alopecia (usually diffuse, in contrast to alopecia areata or male-pattern alopecia)
Musculoskeletal
  Arthritis
  Fibromyalgia
  Arthralgia
  Inflammatory myositis (with increased creatine kinase and proximal muscle weakness)
  Osteonecrosis (particularly with chronic corticosteroid use)
Renal/urologic
  Glomerulonephritis (WHO classification: I, normal; II, mesangial; III, focal proliferative glomerulonephritis; IV, diffuse proliferative glomerulonephritis; V, membranous glomerulonephritis; VI, diffuse sclerosis)
  Tubulointerstitial inflammation
  Lupus cystitis (*Note:* Hemorrhagic cystitis is a potential complication of cyclophosphamide therapy)
Hematologic
  Lymphopenia (absolute lymphocyte count < 1500/mm^3
  Leukopenia (WBC count < 4000/mm^3
  Thrombocytopenia (platelet count < 100,000/mm^3
  Hemolytic anemia (defined by positive Coombs test)
  Lymphadenopathy, splenomegaly
Neuropsychiatric
  Headache (particularly refractory migraine-like headaches)
  Seizures
  Psychosis
  Cerebral vascular accidents
  Peripheral neuropathy
  Cranial neuropathy
  Transverse myelitis
  Depression
  Cognitive dysfunction
Serosal
  Pleuritis (exudative pleural effusion)
  Pericarditis (exudative; rarely associated with hemodynamic compromise)
  Peritoneal inflammation (often presents with diffuse abdominal pain)
Vascular
  Raynaud's phenomenon
  Vasculitis
  Vasculopathy (vessel wall abnormalities with minimal inflammation or damage)
  Hypertension

Table 45 (continued)
Clinical Manifestations of Systemic Lupus Erythematosus

Clinical manifestations
   Myocarditis
   Endocarditis (e.g., Libman-Sacks lesions)
   Thromboembolic events (particularly in patients with systemic lupus erythematosus
     with anticardiolipin antibodies or the so-called lupus anticoagulant)
Immunologic laboratory testing
   Antineutrophil antibody [and other autoantibodies (see Table 46)]
   False-positive nonspecific tests for syphilis (e.g., VDRL), anticardiolipin antibodies
   Elevated serum concentrations of immune complexes
   Evidence of complement consumption (e.g., decreased serum concentrations of
     complement components C3 and C4, or increased concentrations of complement
     split products such as C4b, C5a, sC5b-9)
Miscellaneous
   Pulmonary (pulmonary hemorrhage, pulmonary hypertension, interstitial lung dis-
     ease)
   Ocular (cytoid bodies)
   Gastrointestinal (lupoid hepatitis, pancreatitis)

—*Skin:* Before the widespread availability of immunologic laboratory tests for SLE, dermatologic manifestations were perhaps the most characteristic finding of SLE. Indeed, before the early 1900s, SLE was considered a purely dermatologic disease. Lupus erythematosus refers to the red appearance of the malar rash, which was likened to a wolf bite. The malar rash, also known as the butterfly rash, is typically a maculopapular rash over the malar area of the cheeks. The rash tends to spare the nasolabial folds, in contrast to seborrheic dermatitis. Histopathologically, biopsy of a lupus rash reveals granular deposition of immune complexes and complement in a band-like pattern at the dermoepidermal junction (the so-called lupus band test). In acute lupus rashes such as the malar rash, clinically uninvolved skin also shows such deposits. In contrast, in discoid lupus skin lesions, immune deposits are only seen in involved skin. Unlike the malar rash and other dermatologic manifestations, discoid lupus may occur in the absence of systemic involvement. Another distinguishing feature of discoid lupus is that it tends to involve the supporting skin structures, such as hair follicles, and causes follicular plugging. When discoid lesions resolve, they often result in residual scarring or alopecia that can be disfiguring. By contrast, acute lupus lesions or subacute cutaneous lupus erythematosus lesions typically resolve without scarring. Subacute cutaneous lupus erythematosus refers to annular or papulosquamous lesions associated with antibodies to Ro (SS-A) and usually occurs in sun-exposed areas of the arms and trunk. Most lupus rashes tend to be exacerbated by sun exposure, and intense sun exposure may also precipitate a flare of systemic disease. The treatment of lupus rashes depends on their severity and extent. For many patients, topical corticosteroid preparations effectively control the lesions. In addition, the antimalarial hydroxychloroquine is effective for such lesions.

DISEASES

—*Renal:* Kidney involvement is very common in SLE and may be associated with substantial morbidity and mortality. Most patients with SLE have deposits of immune complexes and complement in the renal mesangium (Table 45). Although such lesions may require no specific intervention, they may progress to more serious lesions. Proliferative glomerular lesions, which may be characterized by subepithelial, subendothelial, and intramembranous immune complex deposits and diffuse glomerular inflammation, are of particular importance. Untreated, they often progress and cause renal failure. Membranous lesions that typically manifest with proteinuria may occur alone in combination with proliferative lesions. Patients with SLE with high titers of antibodies to double-stranded DNA (anti-DNA antibodies) are at greater risk of developing proliferative lupus nephritis. Evidence of active consumption of serum complement proteins (e.g., low concentrations of C3 or C4) is often seen in patients with active nephritis. Careful monitoring of the urine for signs of lupus activity (e.g., proteinuria, cellular casts, hematuria, pyuria) is an important part of the routine evaluation of patients with SLE. In addition, quantification of proteinuria (e.g., by a 24-hour urine collection) offers important information on the prognosis and response to therapy. For many patients, deciding how aggressively to treat lupus nephritis depends on its effects on the patient's renal function. Therefore, it is important to note that the serum creatinine level or the creatinine clearance estimated from a 24-hour collection may overestimate the glomerular filtration rate in patients with lupus nephritis. More accurate determinations of glomerular filtration rate (e.g., inulin clearance) may be of value in monitoring lupus nephritis. Therapy for lupus nephritis typically consists of corticosteroids in conjunction with cytotoxic medications. Many patients are begun on high-dose steroids (e.g., 1 mg/kg prednisone) at the time of diagnosis of lupus nephritis. Depending on the other organ systems involved, this may be tapered relatively rapidly. Occasionally, boluses of steroids (e.g., 1 g methylprednisolone on 3 successive days) are used to gain rapid control of disease activity. Based on the results of several prospective trials, cytotoxic drugs have become the standard therapy for lupus nephritis. At present, a typical regimen uses monthly boluses of cyclophosphamide (at a dose of approximately 750 mg/m²) for 6 months or longer, followed by additional boluses every 2 or 3 months for a total of at least 2 years. Patients treated with shorter courses tend to have relapses of their disease, and the ultimate length of treatment must be individualized based on the response. Treatment with intermittent boluses of cyclophosphamide is generally preferred to daily oral administration because it is associated with fewer adverse effects, particularly hemorrhagic cystitis. Azathioprine and mycophenolate mofetil have also been used successfully for the treatment of lupus nephritis, either as initial therapy or as maintenance therapy after intermittent pulse cyclophosphamide. For patients with lupus nephritis with a rapidly progressive course, plasmapheresis is sometimes used in conjunction with cytotoxic therapy. Drugs currently being evaluated for lupus nephritis include cyclosporine and the nucleoside analogue 2-CDA.

—*Neuropsychiatric:* Neuropsychiatric manifestations of SLE are very common, with a prevalence of ~50%. Signs and symptoms can be quite varied (Table 45). It is often difficult to pinpoint SLE as the definite cause of many of these symptoms. Thus, an important part of the diagnosis involves excluding other potential causes, including infections (e.g., bacterial meningitis, viral encephalitis), medications (including psychotropic medications, high-dose corticosteroids, and NSAIDs), metabolic causes (e.g., the CNS effects of uremia), other medical conditions (e.g., hypertensive encephalopathy), and primary psychiatric disorders. Confounding the diagnosis of neuropsychiatric SLE is the fact that there are no pathognomonic laboratory or imaging tests. Patients with CNS lupus may have elevated CSF protein (including CSF-derived or oligoclonal immunoglobulins) (see p. 55), elevated CSF cell counts, abnormal electroencephalograms, and various abnormalities on imaging studies (e.g., scattered high-intensity white matter lesions on MRI). Although such testing can help exclude other causes and can be consistent with a diagnosis of CNS lupus, no test definitively establishes the diagnosis. Treatment of neuropsychiatric SLE depends on the particular manifestations. Many patients, particularly those with severe involvement, receive corticosteroids or even cytotoxic agents. In addition, patients may benefit from therapies specific to their particular symptoms (e.g., antipsychotic medications for psychosis, antidepressants for depression, anticoagulants for thromboembolism).

—*Musculoskeletal:* Musculoskeletal manifestations of SLE affect almost 90% of patients. Although most patients have arthralgia, fewer demonstrate an inflammatory synovitis. The arthritis of SLE typically involves the small joints of the hands, wrists, and knees. In contrast to patients with RA, the arthritis is usually not associated with bony erosions observed on x-ray. Some patients with SLE develop changes in their joints that resemble those found in patients with RA (e.g., swan-neck deformity). However, unlike RA, in which there is joint destruction and tendon shortening, deformities in patients with SLE (known as Jaccoud's arthropathy) are correctable or reducible on physical examination. Treatment of arthritis in patients with SLE often includes NSAIDs and the antimalarial drug hydroxychloroquine. Although patients often respond to corticosteroids, attempts should be made not to use them long term solely for arthritis. In patients with SLE with severe arthritis, treatment is comparable with that for RA, and drugs such as MTX may be used. Patients with SLE with inflammatory myositis often require treatment with corticosteroids and other immunomodulatory drugs. Finally, osteonecrosis (e.g., hip, knee, shoulder) is seen among patients with SLE, particularly those treated with corticosteroids at high doses or for prolonged courses.

—*Vascular:* Vascular involvement is exceedingly common in SLE. Hypertension is among the most powerful predictors of patient survival in SLE. In addition, patients with SLE have excessive morbidity and mortality from atherosclerotic cardiovascular disease. Vasculitis with leukocytic infiltration and destruction of the involved vessel wall may be seen in skin lesions and in other organ systems. More commonly, a bland vasculopathy is seen. Such lesions have alterations to the vessel wall and impingement of the vessel lumen without frank vasculitic changes. These changes are commonly seen in the CNS and other organ systems. Another factor that may predispose to thromboembolism is the presence of ACL antibodies (see p. 343).

Uncommon Findings: A number of distinct clinical syndromes are seen in patients with SLE.

—*Drug-induced lupus (see p. 159):* Patients treated with some medications may develop signs and symptoms of SLE. Drug-induced lupus is also associated with development of positive ANA, particularly with reactivity to histones. Clinical features of drug-induced lupus typically include fever, arthritis, and serositis; lupus nephritis and CNS lupus are distinctly unusual in patients with drug-induced lupus. Agents strongly associated with drug-induced lupus include procainamide, hydralazine, and isoniazid. Others implicated include phenytoin, quinidine, tetracyclines, and TNF inhibitors.

—*Neonatal lupus:* Neonatal lupus arises in newborns of mothers with anti-Ro and/or anti-La antibodies. Although some mothers have SLE or Sjögren syndrome, many are asymptomatic. When the antibodies cross the placenta, they may bind cardiac tissue, resulting in heart block or myocarditis. Other manifestations may include rashes and thrombocytopenia. These are typically transient and resolve as the maternal antibody disappears from the infant's circulation.

Complications: Lupus is rarely complicated by TTP or Kikuchi's disease.

Diagnostic Tests: Around 1948, the observation of the LE cell (a leukocyte that had engulfed another leukocyte) provided the basis for the ultimate definition of ANAs as the laboratory testing hallmark of SLE. The LE cell, which depended on the presence of very high titers of ANA, was relatively specific but insensitive for the diagnosis of SLE and is only of historic interest currently. It was replaced by immunofluorescent tests that looked specifically for the presence of antibodies capable of binding various nuclear constituents. Initially, ANA tests were performed on rodent tissue sections. Of note, some nuclear antigens (e.g., Ro) are absent in rodents, and some organelles (e.g., nucleoli, centromeres) are present in limited numbers in normal tissue. Thus, in past years, there were patients who had clinical manifestations characteristic of SLE but were ANA negative. With the replacement of rodent tissues by the human HEp2 tumor cell as the standard substrate for ANA tests, the concept of ANA-negative lupus has largely disappeared. Although virtually all patients with SLE are positive for ANAs, the ANA test is not very specific. Many patients with other connective tissue diseases and even some healthy persons have ANAs, particularly at low titer.

Typically, positive ANA results are reported in terms of both titer and pattern. Higher titers are more consistent with, but not diagnostic of, SLE. Typically, titers of ≥1:160 are considered positive, whereas titers of ≤1:80 are equivocal and often nonspecific. Titers of positive ANAs do not generally correlate with disease activity, and there is little value in repeating an ANA test in a patient known to be positive.

The patterns of immunofluorescence observed may correlate with different antigen reactivity (Table 46). A speckled pattern of immunofluorescence is the most common but perhaps least specific. A speckled ANA is associated with various extractable nuclear antigens: Ro (SSA), La (SSB), Sm (anti-Smith), RNP, Scl-70, Jo-1, and many others. Anti-Ro and anti-La antibodies are also observed in patients with Sjögren syndrome (hence the designations SSA and SSB) and also may result in neonatal lupus. Anti-Sm is relatively specific for the diagnosis of SLE because it is seen infrequently in other diseases or in normal persons. Along with anti-RNP antibodies, patients with SLE with anti-Sm may be more prone to develop interstitial lung disease. Anti-RNP antibodies were also previously associated with MCTD (see p. 243). Anti-Scl-70 antibodies are associated with the diffuse form of systemic sclerosis.

A nucleolar pattern of the ANA is seen not only in SLE but also in inflammatory myositis and systemic sclerosis. A centromere pattern is associated with the limited form of systemic sclerosis (CREST syndrome). The homogeneous ANA is associated with antibodies to histones. Such antibodies are seen in SLE, and reactivity to specific histone proteins is characteristic of drug-induced lupus (see below).

A rim pattern of immunofluorescence is associated with antibodies to native or double-stranded DNA. Anti-DNA antibodies are useful for the diagno-

Table 46
Correlations between ANA Pattern, Antigen Specificity, and Clinical Disease

ANA Pattern	Antigen	Clinical Correlate
Diffuse	Deoxyribonucleoprotein	Low titer = nonspecific
	Histones	Drug-induced lupus, others
Peripheral	ds-DNA	50% of SLE (specific)
Speckled	U1-RNP	>90% of MCTD
	Sm	30% of SLE (specific)
	Ro (SSA)	Sjögren 60%, subacute cutaneous lupus erythematosus
		Neonatal LE, ANA-negative LE
	La (SSB)	50% of Sjögren, 15% SLE
	Scl-70	40% of PSS (diffuse disease)
	PM-Scl (PM-1)	Overlap scleroderma + myositis
	Jo-1	Myositis, lung disease, arthritis
Nucleolar	RNA polymerases	40% of PSS
Centromere	Kinetochore	75% CREST (limited disease)
Cytoplasmic (nonspecific)	Ro, ribosomal P,	Sjögren, SLE psychosis
	Cardiolipin,	Thrombosis, abortion, ↓Plts
	AMA, ASMA, tRNA synthetases	Primary biliary cirrhosis, chronic active hepatitis, Myositis, lung disease, arthritis

ANA, antinuclear antibody; ds-DNA, double-stranded DNA; LE, lupus erythematosus; SLE, systemic lupus erythematosus; MCTD, mixed connective tissue disease; PSS, progressive systemic sclerosis; AMA, anti-mitochondrial antibody; ASMA, anti–smooth muscle antibody; Plts, platelets SS-A and SS-B.

sis of SLE because they are seen uncommonly in other diseases. In addition, patients with high titers of anti-DNA antibodies are more prone to develop proliferative lupus nephritis. The titer of anti-DNA antibodies may vary with the activity of disease, particularly lupus nephritis, and sequential determination of anti-DNA is sometimes used to follow the activity of SLE. Specific determination of anti-DNA antibodies may be performed by several assays, including the *Crithidia luciliae* assay and the Farr test. Results from these various tests are reported in different units, and it is important to be familiar with the laboratory performing these tests.

Diagnosis: Classification criteria for SLE are shown in Table 47. A patient may be classified as having SLE if four or more of these 11 criteria are present at any time. Several relevant considerations affect the use of these criteria. First, they were developed to classify patients as having SLE rather than other autoimmune diseases such as scleroderma; therefore, some signs and symptoms that are very common not only among patients with SLE but also among patients with other autoimmune diseases (e.g., Raynaud phenomenon, alopecia) are not included. Second, they were developed in 1982, and some tests are no longer widely used (e.g., the LE cell preparation). Finally, they are ~95% sensitive and specific. Thus, a number of patients who actually have SLE will not have four or more of these criteria, and some patients having four or more criteria might actually have another disease process. The diagnosis of SLE can sometimes be aided by characteristic histopathologic findings (e.g., from renal or skin biopsy specimens). The most widely used diagnostic test for SLE is the ANA.

Therapy: Treatment depends on the particular manifestations for a given patient (see above). Patients with arthritis or serositis frequently respond to

Table 47

American College of Rheumatology Criteria for the Classification of Systemic Lupus Erythematosus[a]

1. Malar rash
2. Discoid rash
3. Photosensitivity
4. Oral ulcers
5. Arthritis
6. Serositis
7. Renal disorder [persistent proteinuria (>0.5 g/day) or cellular casts]
8. Neurologic disorder (seizures or psychosis)
9. Hematologic disorder (hemolytic anemia, leukopenia, lymphopenia, or thrombocytopenia)
10. Immunologic disorder (anti-DNA antibodies, anti-Sm antibodies, positive LE cell preparation)
11. Antinuclear antibody

[a]A patient may be classified as having systemic lupus erythematosus if ≥4 of the 11 criteria are present at any time.

NSAIDs. Antimalarials, particularly hydroxychloroquine, are effective for these same manifestations and are also used for SLE skin lesions. Despite concern about the adverse effects related to their use, corticosteroids are widely used for many manifestations of SLE. For skin disease, topical steroid preparations may suffice. For minor or moderate disease activity, doses of prednisone (≤0.5 mg/kg) are often of great benefit. For severe manifestations (nephritis, pneumonitis, cerebritis, severe cytopenias), high-dose steroids (1 mg/kg prednisone) may be required. In all instances, attempts should be made to taper steroids as rapidly as disease activity permits. Boluses of high doses (pulse dosing) of steroids (e.g., 250–1000 mg methylprednisolone daily for 3–4 days) have been used to gain rapid control of disease activity (e.g., cerebritis or nephritis). For patients who require high doses of steroids for long periods of time, immunosuppressive drugs such as azathioprine and cyclophosphamide may be used as steroid-sparing agents. Mycophenolate mofetil has been shown to be efficacious in managing lupus nephritis. Clinical trials are in progress to evaluate the efficacy of rituximab in the treatment of idiopathic thrombocytopenic purpura cytopenias and other refractory features of lupus. Refractory severe lupus skin disease may respond to thalidomide.

In addition to these immunomodulatory approaches, the optimal care of many patients with SLE also involves assiduous treatment of hypertension, treatment of clotting diatheses, and other general health measures.

BIBLIOGRAPHY

Boumpas DT, Austin HA 3rd, Vaughn EM, et al. Controlled trial of pulse methylprednisolone versus two regimens of pulse cyclophosphamide in severe lupus nephritis. *Lancet* 1992;340:741–745.

Karim MY, Alba P, Cuadrado MJ, et al. Mycophenolate mofetil for systemic lupus erythematosus refractory to other immunosuppressive agents. *Rheumatology* 2002;41:876–882.

Patel P, Werth V. Cutaneous lupus erythematosus: a review. *Dermatol Clin* 2002;20:373–385.

Sanna G, Bertolaccini ML, Mathieu A. Central nervous system lupus: a clinical approach to therapy. *Lupus* 2003;12:935–942.

Swale VJ, Perrett CM, Denton CP, et al. Etanercept-induced systemic lupus erythematosus. *Clin Exp Dermatol* 2003;28:604.

TARSAL TUNNEL SYNDROME

ICD-9 Code: 355.5.

Definition: To enter the foot, the posterior tibial nerve must pass through the tarsal tunnel beneath a flexor retinaculum located just below the medial malleolus of the ankle. Compression of the nerve at this location may lead to local pain or numbness.

Risk Factors: Local trauma (e.g., fracture), body habitus (e.g., valgus foot deformity), and repetitive use or injury are risk factors.

Demographics: Women are affected slightly more frequently than men.

Cardinal Findings: Patients typically present with numbness, burning pain, or paresthesias of the toes or the sole of the foot. Symptoms may be noted after a night's sleep or even awaken the patient. A positive Tinel test is suggested by repetitive tapping over the flexor retinaculum (posterior to the medial malleolus) to reproduce symptoms.

Diagnostic Tests: Definitive diagnosis may be made by demonstration of prolonged motor and sensory latencies on nerve conduction testing.

Differential Diagnosis: Other peripheral neuropathies (e.g., those related to diabetes mellitus and alcoholism) are in the differential diagnosis. In those conditions, symptoms and findings at examination more commonly affect the entire foot, in the so-called stocking-glove pattern typical of diffuse neuropathies.

Therapy: Initial treatment may involve conservative measures, such as selecting optimal footwear or orthoses. Some physicians use injections of corticosteroids directly into the flexor retinaculum in an attempt to decrease local swelling and thereby relieve the compression. In refractory patients, surgical decompression is indicated.

BIBLIOGRAPHY

Kuritz HM, Sokoloff TH. Tarsal tunnel syndrome. *J Am Podiatry Assoc* 1975;65:825–840.

TAKAYASU'S ARTERITIS

Synonyms: Aortic arch syndrome, pulseless disease, aortitis syndrome, occlusive thromboaortopathy.

ICD-9 Code: 446.7.

Definition: Takayasu's arteritis is a large vessel vasculitis of the aorta and its branches resulting in vascular ischemia.

Etiology: Takayasu's arteritis is associated with HLA Bw52 in >40% of afflicted individuals. Circulating antiarterial antibodies have been investigated as putative etiologic agents.

Pathology: Granulomatous panarteritis results in concentric vascular narrowing. Lymphoplasmacytic cell infiltrates may be seen throughout the vessel wall but are often localized toward the outer aspects of the vessel.

Demographics: Takayasu's arteritis occurs worldwide, but most reports come from Japan, India, and China. It is rare in whites (2.6 cases per million persons per year). It predominantly affects women, usually in their reproductive years.

Cardinal Findings: Variations in presenting manifestations often result in significant diagnostic delays. Fever develops in a minority of patients. Claudica-

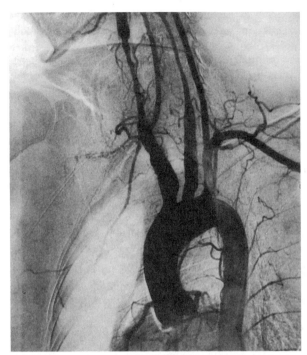

Figure 9. Schematic of subclavian angiogram showing stenosis. (From RM Gay, Ball GV. Vasculitis. In: Koopman WJ, ed. *Arthritis and allied conditions: a textbook of rheumatology,* 13th ed. Baltimore: Williams & Wilkins, 1997:1514, with permission.)

tion, more common in the upper than lower extremities, results from ischemia of affected limbs. The subclavian (90%) vessels are a preferred site of involvement, but other large vessels including the aorta (65%), carotid (60%), renal (40%), and vertebral (35%) arteries may be involved as well. Pulselessness and pressure discrepancies between the two arms are common. A bruit over an affected artery helps identify an area of stenosis and is the most common clinical finding. The aortic arch may be more commonly affected in Japanese patients than in Americans. Pulmonary artery involvement occurs in as many as 70% of patients, but frank pulmonary hypertension is much less common. Hypertension is present sometime during the disease course in 50% of patients and is often caused by renal artery stenosis. CNS symptoms such as light headedness, dizziness, and visual disturbances are well reported by >50% of patients. Musculoskeletal symptoms include chest wall pain, arthralgias, and myalgias and are seen in >50% of patients. Only 40% (30% at disease onset) of patients have constitutional symptoms such as fever, weight loss, and malaise. Stroke owing to vertebral or carotid ischemia or embolism has been described. Funduscopic findings of microaneurysms, venous dilation, and beading are noted early in the course of disease. Cardiac disease, including aortic regurgitation, angina, and pericarditis, is seen in almost 40% of cases. Skin lesions including erythema nodosum and hypersensitivity angiitis have been reported.

Uncommon Findings: Rare associations with other idiopathic inflammatory disorders such as inflammatory bowel disease and sarcoidosis have been reported.

Diagnostic Testing: The ESR is elevated in only ~30% of patients. However, the ESR is markedly increased in ~70% of patients with active disease. Vascular specimens at the time of surgical bypass reveal histologic evidence of active disease in ~40% of cases.

Imaging: Angiogram confirms a suspected vascular stenosis. Long-segment stenosis occurs almost four times more commonly than aneurysms. Magnetic resonance angiography is gaining prominence for visualizing vasculature, particularly of the aortic arch. The chest radiograph may demonstrate a widened aortic root or irregularities in other segments of the aorta.

Keys to Diagnosis: Look for pulselessness of an extremity, often in young women of Asian descent. Aortography and angiograms of other large vessels is highly diagnostic.

Diagnosis Criteria: The 1990 ACR Classification criteria include (a) age at onset 40 years or younger; (b) claudication of the extremities; (c) decreased brachial artery pressure; (d) blood pressure difference of >10 mm Hg between arms; (e) bruit over the subclavian artery or aorta; and (f) arteriogram abnormality. Criteria for Takayasu arteritis are met if at least three of these six are present (sensitivity, 90.5%; specificity, 97.8%).

Therapy: High-dose corticosteroids should be given when active disease is diagnosed. Addition of MTX or cytotoxic therapy (such as cyclophosphamide) both for disease control and as a steroid-sparing agent may improve outcome and result in fewer steroid complications. The use of TNF inhibitors is under investigation. Vascular bypass may be necessary if limb or organ ischemia appears threatening but is fraught with significant reocclusion problems.

Prognosis: The disease may be self-limiting in ~20% of cases. Approximately 25% of patients fail to achieve remission despite aggressive therapy. Half of the patients who respond to medical therapy later relapse. Arterial hypertension is an unfavorable prognostic indicator. Mortality is low (10%–20%), but considerable morbidity is related to organ and limb infarction (stroke, myocardial infarction, aortic dissection).

BIBLIOGRAPHY

Arend WP, Michel BA, Bloch DA, et al. The American College of Rheumatology 1990 criteria for the classification of Takayasu's arteritis. *Arthritis Rheum* 1990;33:1122–1128.
Kerr GS, Hallahan CW, Giordano J, et al. Takayasu arteritis. *Ann Intern Med* 1994;120:919–929.

TEMPORAL ARTERITIS

Synonyms: Giant cell arteritis (GCA), cranial arteritis.

ICD-9 Code: 446.5.

Definition: Temporal arteritis is a large vessel vasculitis preferentially affecting the superficial temporal artery and other branches of the external carotid artery system.

Etiology: The cause of temporal arteritis is unknown. There is an association with HLA-DR4 and particular HLA-DRB1 alleles. These alleles are similar to those associated with RA but involve polymorphisms in the second rather than the third hypervariable region. Research has focused on the unexplained increased prevalence in white people of northern European origin and possible seasonal variation, suggesting as-yet undetermined environmental agents as precipitating factors.

Pathology: Biopsy of an involved large vessel shows a mononuclear cell infiltrate with intimal hyperplasia and occasional giant cells focused along the internal elastic lamina. Disruption of the internal elastic lamina is characteristic. Vasculitis often occurs in a "skip" pattern, which underscores the need for a suitably large biopsy specimen (≥3 cm in length) with careful cross-sectional and longitudinal histopathologic examination to minimize the number of false-negative results. The disease has a particular predilection for blood vessels that contain large quantities of elastic lamina. This may explain a low incidence of intracranial complications because arteries lose their internal elastic lamina after passing through the dura matter.

Demographics: The prevalence of temporal arteritis is highest in elderly Caucasians from northern Europe and in the north central United States. Temporal arteritis is very uncommon in nonwhites. Incidence increases with advancing age and varies from 15 to 94 cases per 100,000 in people older than age 50. Women are afflicted twice as commonly as men.

Cardinal Findings: Onset may be abrupt or insidiously develop over weeks to months. Characteristically, patients have profound constitutional symptoms with fever, weight loss, and occasional night sweats. Moderate to severe headache, particularly in the temporal or occipital area, is reported by >90% of patients. Scalp tenderness is common, particularly in the temporal area. Headache may sometimes be reproduced by pressure over an affected artery. Visual symptoms of diplopia, blurred vision, or amaurosis fugax may antedate development of sudden unilateral blindness. Many patients describe a fullness or pressure sensation behind their eyes. Unfortunately, visual loss may be the presenting ophthalmologic symptom in some cases. Overall, 20% to 40% of patients experience vision loss. The most common cause of visual loss is ischemic

DISEASES

optic neuropathy. Jaw claudication with prolonged chewing results from vascular insufficiency to the muscles of mastication. Half of temporal arteritis cases are accompanied by polymyalgia rheumatic. Indeed, polymyalgia rheumatic and temporal arteritis may be varying manifestations of the same disorder, along a disease continuum. Seronegative synovitis may accompany temporal arteritis, with or without polymyalgia rheumatic. Tongue numbness or ulceration, cough, sore throat, dysphagia, hoarseness, and rare respiratory difficulties have all been described.

Uncommon Findings: Although the extracranial branches of the aorta supplying the eye and temporal area are preferentially affected, the aortic arch and subclavian vessels can be involved (10%) and lead to pulselessness, aortic dissection, or aortic valve insufficiency.

Complications: Neurologic complications appear uncommonly but may result from ischemia in the carotid or vertebral circulations. Transient ischemic attack or stroke has been reported in ~7% of cases. Peripheral neuropathies also have been reported.

Diagnostic Testing: Although biopsy-proven temporal arteritis with normal ESR is well documented, a markedly elevated ESR is seen in >95% of cases. CRP levels may be more sensitive to changes in disease activity and improvement with appropriate therapy. Anemia of chronic disease, decreased serum albumin, polyclonal gammopathy, and reactive thrombocytosis are also seen. Elevation in liver tests, particularly alkaline phosphatase, is common. Preliminary studies suggest a possible association of APL antibodies with temporal arteritis.

Biopsy/Imaging: A unilateral temporal artery biopsy is positive in ~80% of temporal arteritis cases, and the sensitivity for diagnosis increases to 90% with biopsy of both sides. Provided the disease remains active, the positive predictive value of the biopsy is only modestly influenced by previous short-term corticosteroid treatment. However, biopsy is best done as soon as possible when temporal arteritis is strongly suspected. If pulselessness, extremity claudication, angina, or symptoms of cerebrovascular ischemia are present, selective angiograms may be indicated.

Keys to Diagnosis: Look for markedly elevated ESR accompanied by headaches, significant constitutional symptoms, and polymyalgia rheumatica.

Diagnostic Criteria: The 1990 ACR classification criteria include (a) age at onset >50 years; (b) new headache; (c) temporal artery tender to palpation, enlarged, or with decreased pulsation; (d) elevated erythrocyte sedimentation rate; and (e) abnormal temporal artery biopsy. The presence of any three carries a sensitivity of 93.5% and a specificity of 91.2%.

Differential Diagnosis: Other causes of headaches and visual disturbances include classic migraines and intracranial mass lesions. A markedly elevated ESR and fever may suggest occult malignancies (such as lymphoma, myeloma), chronic infections (including bacteria endocarditis), polymyalgia rheumatica or other inflammatory disorders (other vasculitides). Takayasu arteritis affects similarly sized vessels such as the subclavian arteries; however, it develops almost exclusively in young women.

Therapy: Because of the risk of visual loss, high-dose corticosteroid (prednisone 60 mg/day) should be initiated immediately if clinical suspicion is high. With appropriate treatment, the chance of subsequent blindness is <20%. Once the symptoms and signs have stabilized (usually within 1 month) and levels of acute-phase reactants have declined, the prednisone dose is tapered rapidly at first (5–10 mg every 2–4 weeks) and subsequently more slowly (1 mg every 1–2 weeks when <10 mg/day). When weaning from corticosteroids, the patient's symptoms and ESR should be monitored closely. Limited data support the use of steroid-sparing agents, including weekly MTX or TNF inhibitors. NSAIDs may be added when the prednisone dose is <10 mg, particularly for symptoms of polymyalgia rheumatica. Angioplasty or vascular bypass may be required if large vessel involvement is producing claudication or other potentially treatable complications.

Prognosis: Although most patients successfully taper and discontinue corticosteroids within 2 years of disease onset, the relapse rate in the first year exceeds 60%. As a result, the mean requirement for corticosteroids exceeds 5 years. Consequently, the most devastating long-term complications from temporal arteritis commonly stem from corticosteroid-associated complications, particularly bone loss. As many as 60% of patients with temporal arteritis develop steroid toxicities, and steroid-associated fatalities may be as high as 21%.

BIBLIOGRAPHY

Hunder GH, Bloch DA, Michel BA, et al. The American College of Rheumatology 1990 criteria for the classification of giant cell arteritis. *Arthritis Rheum* 1990;33:1122–1128.

Huston KA, Hunder GH, Lie JT, et al. Temporal arteritis, a 25-year epidemiologic, clinical, and pathologic study. *Ann Intern Med* 1978;88:162–167.

Salvarani C, Cantini F, Boiardi L, et al. Polymyalgia rheumatica and giant-cell arteritis. *N Engl J Med* 2002;347:261–271.

THROMBOTIC THROMBOCYTOPENIC PURPURA

Synonyms: TTP.

ICD-9 Code: 446.6.

Definition: An acute, severe, occlusive thrombotic microangiopathy characterized by systemic platelet aggregation, vascular occlusion, organ ischemia, thrombocytopenia, and Coombs-negative hemolytic anemia with red blood cell fragmentation.

Etiology: Recent studies have demonstrated TTP to be associated with a deficiency in the von Willebrand factor–cleaving protease ADAMTS13. Deficiency is owing to a genetic/familial absence or an acquired deficiency from autoimmune inhibitors or drug effects. Lack of this protease leads to unusually large von Willebrand factor because ADAMTS13 normally cleaves hyperreactive unusually large von Willebrand factor multimers into smaller and less adhesive von Willebrand factor forms. Thus, the increase in adhesive unusually large von Willebrand factor multimers binds some platelet proteins and promotes aggregation and local thrombosis. Deficiency of ADAMTS13 distinguishes TTP from the hemolytic-uremic syndrome, wherein ADAMTS13 levels are normal. The gene for ADAMTS13 has been localized to chromosome 9 (q34). Drug-induced TTP (and ADAMTS13 deficiency) may be acute immune-mediated (ticlopidine, clopidogrel), dose-related (tacrolimus, penicillin, cyclosporine, oral contraceptives, bleomycin, mitomycin, cis platin) or may occur with quinine, which causes a hemolytic uremic–like syndrome. Other causes include pregnancy (often third trimester), post-partum, allogeneic bone marrow transplant, or autoimmune disorders (lupus, scleroderma) or HIV infection.

Pathology: Platelet-rich microthrombi occlude arterioles and capillaries (not venules), often with overlying endothelial proliferation. Incomplete occlusion leads to turbulent flow and red blood cell fragmentation and schistocytes. Vascular obliteration occurs systemically with prominent involvement of the kidneys, brain, pancreas, heart, spleen, adrenal glands, and, less commonly, the lung and GI tract.

Demographics: The median age at onset is 35 to 40 years, but it has been reported in infants and elderly. Female:male ratio ranges from 3:2 to 2:1. There is no racial preference. It is estimated there are 1,000 new cases per year.

Cardinal Findings: Initially, patients manifest malaise, fever (without chills), flu-like symptoms, weakness, or abdominal pains associated with nausea, vomiting, or diarrhea. Neurologic features include altered mental status, seizures, coma, or focal neurologic deficit. Some degree of renal impairment is seen in most, usually as microscopic hematuria, proteinuria, and, uncommonly, gross hematuria or rapid progression to acute renal failure. Although thrombocytopenia is profound (>20,000/mm^3) and petechiae common, frank bleeding (e.g., CNS, GI) is very uncommon.

Uncommon Findings: Cardiac involvement (congestive heart failure, arrhythmia), acute respiratory distress syndrome, pancreatitis.

Diagnostic Tests: Thrombocytopenia (<20,000 cells/mm^3), mild to moderate Coombs-negative anemia with evidence of hemolysis (schistocytes; increased lactate dehydrogenase, bilirubin, and reticulocytes; decreased haptoglobin) and occasional nucleated red blood cells. Mild to moderate leukocytosis (with left shift) is common. Renal studies may show proteinuria, hematuria, or oliguria. Bone marrow is seldom needed but typically shows a reactive picture with an increase in granulocytes and megakaryocytes. In contrast to disseminated intravascular coagulation, studies show normal prothrombin time, PTT, and fibrinogen levels.

Keys to Diagnosis: Thrombocytopenia (<20,000 cells/mm^3) with evidence of microangiopathic hemolysis (fragmented cells, schistocytes, elevated lactate dehydrogenase) and of organ ischemia.

Diagnostic Criteria: The classic pentad includes (a) microangiopathic hemolytic anemia, (b) thrombocytopenia, (c) neurologic abnormalities, (d) fever, and (e) renal dysfunction. The classic pentad is uncommon and is not required for the diagnosis.

Differential Diagnosis: TTP should be distinguished from sepsis (e.g., cytomegalovirus, Rocky Mountain spotted fever, meningococcemia), eclampsia, preeclampsia, HELLP syndrome, disseminated malignancy, hemolytic-uremic syndrome, Evan syndrome, malignant hypertension.

Therapy: Prompt use of plasma exchange is essential. Apheresis removes antibodies (to ADAMTS13), unusually large von Willebrand factors and replaces normal metalloproteinase activity. Platelet transfusion is not advised and may worsen the disorder. Adjunctive treatment with low-dose aspirin, ticlopidine, or steroids may be considered, especially when refractory to apheresis. Seldom patients may require the use of cyclophosphamide, vincristine, rituximab, intravenous gammaglobulin, protein A immunoadsorption column pheresis, or splenectomy.

Monitoring: Lactate dehydrogenase is a reliable daily measure of the degree of hemolysis.

Prognosis: In the prepheresis era, TTP carried a mortality rate in excess of 90%. When treated with plasma exchange or plasma infusion, 80% to 90% of patients survive acute TTP. Relapses may occur in 10% to 40% of patients, and a small subset may exhibit chronic TTP and require chronic intermittent plasma exchange.

BIBLIOGRAPHY

Nabhan C, Kwaan HC. Current concepts in the diagnosis and management of thrombotic thrombocytopenic purpura. *Hematol Oncol Clin North Am* 2003;17:177–199.
Tsai HM. Advances in the pathogenesis, diagnosis, and treatment of thrombotic thrombocytopenic purpura. *J Am Soc Nephrol* 2003;14:1072–1081.

TOXIC SYNOVITIS OF THE HIP

Synonyms: Transient synovitis of the hip, irritable hip.

Definition: Toxic (transient) synovitis of the hip is a self-limiting inflammatory process that affects young children with acute nontraumatic hip pain.

Etiology: Thought to be postviral, possibly reactive in nature.

Demographics: Peak onset age is 4 to 5 years but ranges from 6 months to 16 years. Males are more affected than females.

Cardinal Features: Acute or gradual onset of hip pain or limp, usually unilateral, with or without of hip, knee, or thigh pain. Bilateral in a minority. The child may be irritable with low-grade fever. There is pain on hip range of motion; hence, the hip is positioned flexed, abducted, or externally rotated to minimize discomfort. Episodes usually last days.

Uncommon Findings: Recurrent attacks in >15%. Chronic synovitis is less common. Rarely, patients with toxic synovitis of the hip will develop Legg-Calvé-Perthes disease.

Laboratory Tests: Modest elevations of WBCs, ESR, and CRP may be seen.

Imaging: Ultrasonography is effective at identifying hip effusions and can also be used for diagnostic aspiration.

Keys to Diagnosis: Limping or hip pain in a child with inflammatory indices, higher ESR, CRP, fevers, and neutrophil percentage (~90%) suggest septic arthritis rather than toxic hip synovitis.

Differential Diagnosis: Septic arthritis, Legg-Calvé-Perthes, juvenile pauciarticular spondylitis.

Treatment: Toxic synovitis of the hip is best managed with rest and antiinflammatory therapy. NSAIDs have been shown to reduce the duration of symptoms. Follow-up examination is also recommended to confirm diagnosis and maintenance of hip range of motion.

BIBLIOGRAPHY

Kermond S, Fink M, Graham K, et al. A randomized clinical trial: should the child with transient synovitis of the hip be treated with nonsteroidal anti-inflammatory drugs? *Ann Emerg Med* 2002;40:294–299.
Kim MK, Karpas A. The limping child. *Clin Pediatr Emerg Med* 2002;3:129–137.

TUBERCULOUS ARTHRITIS

Synonyms: TB, consumption, Pott's disease.

ICD-9 Code: 015.9 (711.4)

Definition: Tuberculous arthritis is a subacute, or occasionally chronic, arthritis secondary to *Mycobacterium tuberculosis* infection.

Etiology: Tuberculosis spreads from pulmonary sites to peripheral joints hematogenously or via lymphatic channels. Peripheral joints are usually infected by contiguous spread from adjacent tuberculous osteomyelitis. Spinal tuberculosis may originate from contiguous spread from the lungs or via blood or lymphatic routes. Because tuberculosis does not produce collagenase, joint destruction is slower than in bacterial arthritides.

Pathology: Synovial biopsy specimens may stain positively for the tuberculosis bacillus. Histologic findings include synovial proliferation, granulation tissue, and pannus.

Demographics: The prevalence of tuberculosis has declined considerably in the past 50 years, However, between 1985 and 1993, there was a resurgence of multidrug-resistant tuberculosis in the United States associated with the increase in AIDS (with a relative risk for tuberculosis 500 times that of the general population) and an increase in tuberculosis among some ethnic minorities and immigrants from underdeveloped countries. African Americans may be at higher risk of tuberculosis owing to both genetic and socioeconomic factors. Osteoarticular tuberculosis is seen in ≤5% of all patients with tuberculosis; 4- to 5-month delays in the diagnosis of osteoarticular tuberculosis are common in low-risk populations.

Cardinal Findings: After an insidious onset, the diagnosis of tuberculosis arthritis is often suggested by a chronic monarthritis (less commonly an oligoarthritis). Large weight-bearing joints may be preferentially affected in more endemic areas. Swollen joints may lack other manifestations of inflammation, such as warmth and erythema. Tuberculous spondylitis, or Pott disease, frequently begins in a thoracic disc space. It accounts for ~50% of osteoarticular tuberculosis. Spinal lesions may lead to severe kyphosis owing to vertebral destruction. Pulmonary disease is seldom active at the time of joint manifestations, although the chest radiograph remains abnormal in half of patients. Constitutional symptoms such as fever and weight loss are frequently present at the time of bone or joint disease.

Uncommon Findings: There are rare reports of tenosynovitis and fasciitis. Sacroiliac infection is present in ~7% of patients with skeletal tuberculosis. Poncet's syndrome describes a reactive polyarthritis of the hands and feet in patients with a current or past tuberculosis infection. Atypical mycobacteria may also cause arthritis or other musculoskeletal manifestations, particularly in patients with HIV infection. There are rare reports of reactive arthritis after intravesical bacille Calmette-Guérin immunotherapy.

Diagnostic Testing: Culture of *M. tuberculosis* from synovial fluid and/or synovial biopsy is positive in ~90% of cases. An acid-fast smear of synovial fluid alone has a yield of <10%. Improved culture techniques and the use of PCR may detect organisms in a much shorter time. Synovial biopsy demonstrating noncaseating granulomas by histopathology is a less specific diagnostic option. CT-guided needle biopsy of spinal lesions may prove diagnostic. Nonspecific synovial fluid findings include neutrophilic pleocytosis (total WBC count is usually 10,000–20,000 cells/mm^3), elevated protein, and low synovial fluid glucose (detected in >50% of patients). Some (90%) of people with osteoarticular disease exhibit a positive purified protein derivative test result.

Imaging: Radiographs of peripheral joints with late-stage tuberculous arthritis may reveal destructive arthropathy without significant reactive bone formation.

Keys to Diagnosis: Look for a chronic monarthritis in an at-risk host, with acid-fast bacilli identified on joint fluid culture or synovial biopsy.

Differential Diagnosis: Fungal arthritis, inflammatory OA, and pseudogout should be considered.

Therapy: Multi-drug regimens for osteoarticular tuberculosis are usually the same as those for pulmonary tuberculosis; however, at least 6 to 9 months (3 months beyond negative culture in non-AIDS hosts and 6 months beyond negative cultures in patients with AIDS) of treatment is required. Therapy is usually initiated with isoniazid (5 mg/kg to as much as 300 mg/day), pyrazinamide (15–30 mg/kg to as much as 2 g daily), and rifampin (10 mg/kg to as much as 600 mg orally daily). Pyrazinamide can be discontinued after 8 weeks. If the incidence of multidrug resistance is <4%, it is recommended that ethambutol (5–25 mg/kg) or streptomycin (15 mg/kg) be added until resistances are known. Treatment regimens are dictated by the resistance patterns in the community and the immune status of the host. Surgery may be necessary if extensive bone destruction has occurred or if the spinal cord is compromised in Pott disease.

Prognosis: If there is minimal bone involvement, articular disease is successfully managed with drug therapy alone. Pott's disease may result in neurologic damage, and in older series, mortality was as high as 20%. More recent reports suggest almost 80% resolution of even severe disease with appropriate drug therapy.

BIBLIOGRAPHY

American Thoracic Society, Centers for Disease Control and Prevention. Targeted tuberculin testing and treatment of latent tuberculosis infection. *Am J Respir Crit Care Med* 2000;161:S221–S247.
Harrington JT. Mycobacterial and fungal arthritis. *Curr Opin Rheumatol* 1998;10:335–338.

URTICARIA/ANGIODEMA

Synonyms: Hives.

ICD-9 Code: Urticaria, 708.9; angioedema, 995.1; hereditary angioedema, 277.6.

Definition: Urticaria are well-demarcated, evanescent skin reactions characterized by erythematous or blanched elevations of the upper layers of the dermis, usually associated with intense pruritus. A common distinction relevant to the etiology and treatment of this condition is duration: Acute urticaria is defined by symptom duration of <6 weeks, whereas chronic urticaria is present for >6 weeks. Angioedema, which often occurs along with urticaria, represents a similar process that primarily affects deeper subcutaneous tissue and is not usually associated with pruritus. Some conditions, such as the types of hereditary angioedema, are associated with angioedema without concomitant urticaria.

Etiology: There are numerous potential inciting stimuli for urticaria. However, even after thorough investigation, a substantial number of patients will have no cause found. A major advance in the understanding of chronic urticaria has been the demonstration of circulating IgG autoantibodies with reactivity to the α subunit of the high-affinity IgE receptor (Fc-epsiol-RI) or to IgE itself, which have been demonstrated in ~30% to 40% and 10% of patients with idiopathic urticaria, respectively. In addition to this autoimmune urticaria, physical causes of urticaria are also common, accounting for ~15% of cases of chronic urticaria. Subtypes of physical urticaria include dermatographism or pressure urticaria, delayed pressure urticaria, exercise-induced urticaria, cold-induced urticaria (including familial forms), solar-induced urticaria, aquagenic urticaria, and cholinergic urticaria (typically brought on by heat). Additional causes of urticaria include drugs, biological products, animal stings and bites, systemic diseases, hereditary diseases, and inhalants and contactants. Mechanistically, some of these represent true type I hypersensitivity, mediated by IgE antibodies (e.g., reactions foreign proteins such as insect venom), and some are caused by mast cell degranulation (e.g., reaction to radiocontrast dye); however, mechanisms are not known for many stimuli. Among drugs, NSAIDs are not an uncommon cause of urticaria and angioedema. Because they also inhibit the degradation of kinins, angiotensin-converting enzyme inhibitors may be associated with angioedema. SLE is among systemic diseases associated with urticaria, possibly related to enhanced activation of the complement cascade. Although similar in appearance to common urticaria, the lesions of urticarial vasculitis are distinct both clinically (owing to their persistence) and pathologically (with true vasculitis).

Hereditary angioedema and acquired angioedema are a group of conditions characterized by angioedema unassociated with urticaria and absent or dysfunctional C1 esterase inhibitor (see Complement, p. 58).

Pathology: Histopathologic examination of urticarial lesions reveals dilatation and engorgement of capillaries in the skin and a minimal perivascular infiltrate often composed of lymphocytes and eosinophils. In distinction to vasculitis, there is neither destruction of the vessel walls nor obliteration of the vascular lumen.

Demographics: Urticaria is common, and ~10% to 20% of the population will experience urticaria at some time. Acute urticaria is more common in children and young adults; chronic urticaria is more common in middle-aged women.

Diagnosis: Urticaria is a clinical diagnosis. Investigation into causes should be focused. Many inciting stimuli will be evident from a thorough history and physical examination supplemented by focused laboratory testing as appropriate. At present, tests for autoantibodies to Fc(RI) or IgE are not widely available. In the appropriate clinical setting, measurement of complement components may be of value (see section on Complement).

Treatment: For acute urticaria, removal of any offending agent and use of H^1 antihistamines (older agents: diphenhydramine, hydroxyzine, cyproheptadine, brompheniramine; newer nonsedating agents: chlorpheniramine, fexofenadine, loratadine, cetirizine) are the mainstay of therapy. For chronic urticaria, H^1 antihistamines are still an important part of the therapeutic regimen because pruritus is often the primary complaint, and excessive scratching can exacerbate the problem. In severe refractory cases, full doses of H^1 antihistamines with the addition of H^2 antihistamines have been recommended. Inhibitors of leukotrienes, such as montelukast, have also been reported to be useful. In autoimmune urticaria, corticosteroids have been used in short courses for patients with severe disease. Inhibitors of calcineurin such as cyclosporine have also been used, as has intravenous immunoglobulin. For patients with hereditary angioedema, attenuated androgens and plasma-derived C1 esterase inhibitor concentrates are used.

BIBLIOGRAPHY

Greaves M. Chronic urticaria. *J Allergy Clin Immunol* 2000;105:664–672.
Leung D, Boguniewicz M. Advances in allergic skin diseases. *J Allergy Clin Immunol* 2003;111: S805–S812.

UVEITIS

Synonyms: Iritis, iridocyclitis, anterior uveitis, posterior uveitis, chorioretinitis.

ICD-9 Codes: Acute uveitis, 364.0; chronic uveitis, 364.1.

Definition: Uveitis refers to any inflammatory disease that involves the uveal tract (or midportion of the eye, which includes the iris, ciliary body, and choroid layer). Between 20% and 40% of patients with uveitis have an associated systemic disease. Anterior uveitis may involve the iris (iritis) or iris and ciliary body (iridocyclitis) and may be associated with HLA-B27 and inflammatory joint disease (e.g., AS, Reiter syndrome, sarcoidosis). Posterior uveitis may involve the choroid (choroiditis), retina (retinitis), or vitreous near the macula and optic nerve. Posterior uveitis is commonly associated with infection. Sarcoidosis and Behçet disease are unique conditions that may involve either the anterior or posterior chamber.

Etiology: Uveitis may be isolated and idiopathic or result from a variety of infectious or immunologic conditions (Table 48). An association is seen with HLA-B27 positivity in nearly 60% of acute anterior uveitis patients.

Table 48
Systemic Conditions Associated with Uveitis

Viral	Human immunodeficiency virus, herpes simplex, herpes zoster, cytomegalovirus
Bacterial	Tuberculosis, leprosy, Lyme disease, syphilis, brucellosis
Parasitic	Toxoplasmosis, cysticercosis, amebiasis
Fungal	Histoplasmosis, coccidioidomycosis, candidiasis, aspergillosis, cryptococcus
Immunologic	Ankylosing spondylitis, Reiter syndrome, psoriatic arthritis, Behçet syndrome, Crohn disease, ulcerative colitis, sarcoidosis, relapsing polychondritis, systemic lupus erythematosus, vitiligo, vasculitis, interstitial nephritis, multiple sclerosis, Sjögren syndrome
Neoplastic (mistaken for uveitis)	Leukemia, lymphoma, retinoblastoma, retinitis pigmentosa

Pathology: Common findings include corneal edema, keratitic precipitates, and inflammatory changes in the anterior chamber. Posterior uveitis may show vitreal exudates, focal chorioretinal infiltrates, retinal vasculitis, or macular edema. Synechiae are fibrous scars (adhesions) that can be seen between the iris and lens or iris and cornea.

Demographics: Anterior uveitis is four times more prevalent than posterior uveitis. The incidence of anterior uveitis is 8.2 cases per 100,000 annually. Males and females are equally affected, unless the individual is HLA-B27 positive, wherein males predominate.

Cardinal Findings: Acute anterior uveitis usually has an acute onset, with deep eye pain, photophobia, and decreased visual acuity, with or without conjunctival injection. Corneal opacities (clouding) may be seen because of the inflammatory infiltrate in the anterior chamber. Synechiae may form between the lens and iris. Episodic or recurrent disease is not uncommon. Unilateral presentations are more common than bilateral. Bilateral uveitis has a greater association with systemic features and interstitial nephritis. Half of patients with acute anterior uveitis are positive for HLA-B27. HLA-B27-positive patients with uveitis are more likely to be male with younger age at onset, more synechiae, complications, and frequent association with an SpA (see p. 358). Chronic anterior uveitis is far less frequent and is seen in as many as 20% of children with juvenile arthritis.

Posterior uveitis tends to have an insidious onset with less discomfort (rather than pain), decreased visual acuity, and floating spots, usually affecting both eyes.

Complications: Permanent visual loss is a grave complication that may result from precipitates on the cornea or lens, secondary glaucoma, obstructive synechiae, cataracts, or, rarely, vasculitis, vascular occlusion, or retinal infarc-

DISEASES

tion. Topical ocular steroid therapy may be complicated by increased intraocular pressure and cataracts.

Diagnostic Tests: No specific laboratory test can diagnose uveitis. Investigations are often necessary to identify an underlying disorder (e.g., CBC, creatinine, urinalysis, ANA, ESR, VDRL, purified protein derivative, HLA-B27).

Imaging: Imaging procedures are not necessary to diagnose uveitis. In those with low back pain, radiographs may disclose evidence of sacroiliitis. Chest radiographs may be helpful in the diagnosis of suspected systemic disorders such as tuberculosis, sarcoidosis, or lymphoma.

Keys to Diagnosis: Patients suspected of having uveitis should have a slit lamp examination by an ophthalmologist.

Differential Diagnosis: Conjunctivitis, episcleritis, scleritis, keratitis, and acute angle-closure glaucoma must be differentiated.

Therapy: Most patients respond well to topical corticosteroids and mydriatics (i.e., homatropine hydrobromide 2% ophthalmic solution b.i.d.) that may retard development of synechiae. Prednisolone acetate 1% ophthalmic suspension is often given 2 drops every hour initially, then tapered to four times daily dosing. Chronic anterior uveitis may be more difficult to treat and may require systemic therapy. Posterior uveitis (not related to infection) may also require systemic therapy when vision is impaired. Infectious etiologies should be addressed with the appropriate antiinfective agent. Uveitis that is refractory to topical steroids may require systemic steroids, azathioprine, cyclosporine, chlorambucil, cyclophosphamide, or MTX.

BIBLIOGRAPHY

Petty RE, Smith JR, Rosenbaum JT. Arthritis and uveitis in children. A pediatric rheumatology perspective. *Am J Ophthalmol* 2003;135:879–884.
Rosenbaum JT. Uveitis: an internists view. *Arch Intern Med* 1989;149:1173–1176.
Tay-Dearney ML, Schwam BL, Lowder C, et al. Clinical features and associated systemic diseases of HLA-B27 uveitis. *Am J Ophthalmol* 1996;121:47–56.

WEGENER'S GRANULOMATOSIS

ICD-9 Code: 446.4.

Definition: Wegener's granulomatosis is a vasculitic syndrome associated with upper respiratory, pulmonary, and renal involvement. It is characterized histologically by necrotizing granulomatous vasculitis of small arteries and veins.

Etiology: Although it has long been suspected that Wegener's granulomatosis relates to exposure to some environmental agent, none has been implicated.

There is no evidence of immune complex disease. There are no other associated risk factors nor any genetic predisposition. It is unknown whether ANCA are pathogenic or epiphenomenal.

Pathology: Characteristic changes include granulomatous and vasculitic involvement of the upper and lower respiratory tract, sinuses, orbit, kidney, CNS, or heart. Vascular lesions involve small vessels with granuloma and multinucleated giant cells. Kidney lesions may present as pauci-immune rapidly progressive glomerulonephritis, focal necrotizing glomerulonephritis, crescentic glomerulonephritis, and less commonly, diffuse proliferative glomerulonephritis, or interstitial nephritis. Arteritis is seen in <8% of renal lesions. Vasculitis of the vasa nervorum is seen with mononeuritis multiplex.

Demographics: The mean age at onset is approximately 40 years, ranging from 8 to 80 years. Males are affected slightly more commonly than females. Wegener granulomatosis is uncommon, with a prevalence of approximately three cases per 100,000 population. Nearly 97% of patients are white and 2% are African American.

Cardinal Findings: Patients with Wegener's granulomatosis may present with a variety of manifestations. The most common symptoms reflect upper and lower respiratory tract involvement (see Table 49). Patients may also exhibit constitutional symptoms, such as fever, weight loss, and malaise. Others have no or minimal symptoms and have their disease discovered on a chest radiograph.

Although it can affect multiple organs, pulmonary, upper airway, and renal involvement are the most characteristic features. Approximately 25% of patients with Wegener's granulomatosis have the classic triad of involvement in these three organ systems. Others have more limited disease; ~20% have only upper and lower respiratory lesions, and ~17% each have renal involvement with either upper or lower respiratory tract involvement. The extent of lung and kidney disease usually determines therapy.

—*Upper respiratory tract:* Features include sinusitis, cough, rhinitis, nasal ulcers, serous otitis media, hearing loss, and, rarely, subglottic stenosis. Upper respiratory tract involvement in Wegener's granulomatosis is not typically life threatening. However, it can be a source of chronic and severe symptoms such as epistaxis, sinus tenderness, and purulent rhinorrhea. It can also destroy the nasal cartilage, leading to a "saddle nose" deformity. Many with Wegener's granulomatosis experience frequent bouts of infectious sinusitis, particularly with *S. aureus.* Sinus symptoms related to infection may be quite difficult to distinguish from those related to a flare of vasculitis. There also may be a causal relationship between infection and disease relapse.

—*Pulmonary:* Findings include dyspnea, cough, hemoptysis, and pleurisy. Bilateral pulmonary infiltrates (often nodular) are seen in half of patients and may eventually cavitate.

Table 49
Organ System Involvement in Wegener Granulomatosis

Organ System	At Presentation (%)	Involvement Ever (%)
Lungs	71	95
Sinuses	67	90
Kidneys	15	85
Joints	44	67
Nasal	33	64
Ears	25	61
Eyes	16	58
Skin	15	45

—*Renal:* Kidney involvement almost always follows upper and lower respiratory tract disease and may manifest as proteinuria, hematuria, red cell casts, or renal insufficiency. Hypertension is rarely seen. Glomerulonephritis is seen in a minority of patients at the onset but eventually develops in nearly 85% of cases. The typical renal lesion of Wegener's granulomatosis is a focal and segmental glomerulonephritis. This may progress to a diffuse necrotizing crescentic glomerulonephritis and may be associated with rapid onset of renal failure. However, end-stage renal disease is seen in <10% of patients.

—*Ocular:* Nearly half of patients have ocular findings, including proptosis (from retroorbital pseudotumor), conjunctivitis, dacryocystitis, scleritis, and cavernous sinus thrombosis.

Uncommon Findings: Less frequent manifestations of Wegener's granulomatosis include arthralgia (less commonly arthritis), cutaneous nodules, palpable purpura, granulomatous prostatitis, and parotitis. Mononeuritis multiplex is seen in <15% of patients. Other CNS findings include cranial neuropathy (II, V, VII, IX, XII) and polyneuropathy.

Complications: Complications may include saddle nose deformity, hearing loss, labyrinthitis, tracheal obstruction, pulmonary cavitation, end-stage renal disease (<10%), visual loss, amenorrhea, and therapy-related infection. Cyclophosphamide therapy may result in hemorrhagic cystitis and an increased risk of bladder cancer.

Diagnostic Tests: Most patients exhibit a normochromic, normocytic anemia, leukocytosis without eosinophilia, elevated ESR, hypergammaglobulinemia, and normal complement levels.

—*ANCA:* A major advance in the treatment of patients with Wegener granulomatosis was the description of antineutrophil cytoplasmic antibodies (ANCA) (see p. 39). These antibodies bind to proteinase-3, a cytoplasmic enzyme. Depending on disease activity, 50% to 90% of patients with Wegener granulomatosis have positive C-ANCA tests. This test is relatively specific because C-ANCA are uncommonly seen in other diseases. In the context of characteristic clinical findings, many physicians use the presence of C-ANCA as a diagnostic aid. The titer of C-ANCA may also vary with disease activity. Some patients have a decreased C-ANCA titer or even disappearance of C-ANCA with successful therapy, and an increased titer with a flare of disease activity; however, the activity of Wegener granulomatosis cannot be determined solely by following C-ANCA titers.

Differential Diagnosis: Other pulmonary/renal syndromes, such as Goodpasture's syndrome, subacute bacterial endocarditis, and SLE, are in the differential diagnosis. The upper respiratory tract involvement may resemble relapsing polychondritis and midline granuloma. Pulmonary manifestations of Wegener granulomatosis mimic sarcoidosis or vasculitides (e.g., Churg-Strauss syndrome), granulomatous infectious processes (e.g., tuberculosis, histoplasmosis, blastomycosis), and neoplastic diseases (e.g., lymphomatoid granulomatosis, lymphoma).

Diagnosis: Wegener's granulomatosis may be diagnosed by several means. Histopathologic definition of granulomatous vasculitis on respiratory tract biopsy specimen establishes the diagnosis in the correct clinical setting. Pulmonary biopsy specimens should be obtained by open lung biopsy rather than transbronchially because the latter has a lower diagnostic yield and may be associated with uncontrolled bleeding. Renal biopsy is seldom diagnostic or specific for Wegener's granulomatosis but may support the diagnosis depending on the other organ involvement. The ACR has formulated classification criteria that may help differentiate patients with Wegener's granulomatosis from those with other types of vasculitis (Table 50).

A patient may be classified as having Wegener's granulomatosis if two or more criteria are present (sensitivity, 88.2%; specificity, 92%).

Therapy: Before the use of immunomodulatory drugs, Wegener's granulomatosis was usually a fatal disease with a mean survival of approximately 6

Table 50
1990 American College of Rheumatology Classification Criteria for Wegener's Granulomatosis

Criterion	Definition
1. Nasal/oral inflammation	Oral ulcers or purulent or bloody nasal discharge
2. Abnormal chest x-ray	Chest x-ray with nodules, cavities, or fixed infiltrates
3. Hematuria	Microhematuria (>5 RBCs/hpf) or red cell casts
4. Granulomatous inflammation	Histologic changes on biopsy specimen showing granulomatous inflammation within the wall of an artery or in the perivascular area

RBCs/hpf, red blood cells per high-power field.

months and >80% 1-year mortality. Addition of prednisone prolonged the mean survival to approximately 1 year. Currently, the standard of care includes the use of cytotoxic drugs, particularly cyclophosphamide, and the long-term remission rate exceeds 90%. Therapy typically includes high-dose corticosteroids (e.g., 1 mg/kg/day prednisone) in conjunction with cyclophosphamide at doses of 1 to 2 mg/kg/day. Intermittent pulse intravenous cyclophosphamide does not appear as efficacious as daily oral dosing. When the manifestations of disease are under control, the dose of prednisone may be tapered. In general, cyclophosphamide is continued for at least a year after the disease is quiescent. For patients not responding to, or intolerant of, therapy with cyclophosphamide, MTX has been used with some success. In anecdotal reports, trimethoprim/sulfamethoxazole was reported to have possible value in treating Wegener's granulomatosis, especially when limited to the upper respiratory tract. Long-term treatment with this antibiotic decreases relapse of disease activity slightly. However, this therapy should not be considered a substitute for immunomodulatory therapy in patients with active Wegener's granulomatosis. The use of TNF inhibitors is under investigation.

Prognosis: Relapse is common in Wegener granulomatosis; ≥45% of successfully treated patients experience a relapse; median time to relapse is 42 months. The chance of cure is uncertain. Thus, all patients should be followed for relapse. The frequency of relapse and treatment exposure increases the risk of morbidity and mortality. Treatment-related morbidity may be significant and may include features related to corticosteroids (e.g., diabetes, fracture, osteonecrosis, cataracts) or cyclophosphamide (e.g., hair loss, hemorrhagic cystitis, bladder cancer, myelodysplasia). Death is usually related to renal disease, pulmonary disease, infection, or malignancy.

BIBLIOGRAPHY

Fauci AS, Haynes BF, Katz P, et al. Wegener's granulomatosis: prospective clinical and therapeutic experience with 85 patients for 21 years. *Ann Intern Med* 1983;98:76–85.
Hoffman GS, Kerr GS, Leavitt RY, et al. Wegener's granulomatosis: an analysis of 158 patients. *Ann Intern Med* 1992;116:488–498.
Langford CA. Wegener's granulomatosis: current and upcoming therapies. *Arthritis Res Ther* 2003;5:180–191.
Leavitt RY, Fauci AS, Bloch DA, et al. The American College of Rheumatology 1990 criteria for the classification of Wegener's granulomatosis. *Arthritis Rheum* 1990;33:1101–1107.
Regan MJ, Hellmann DB, Stone JH. Treatment of Wegener's granulomatosis. *Rheum Dis Clin North Am* 2001;27:863–886.
Talar-Williams C, Hijazi YM, Walther MM, et al. Cyclophosphamide-induced cystitis and bladder cancer in patients with Wegener granulomatosis. *Ann Intern Med* 1996;124:477–484.

WHIPPLE'S DISEASE

Synonyms: Intestinal lipodystrophy.

ICD-9 Code: 040.2.

Definition: Whipple disease is a multisystem infectious disorder characterized by inflammatory polyarthritis and small bowel colitis.

Etiology: Whipple disease is caused by infection with the gram-positive actinomycete *Trophermyma whippelii*. Intestinal or lymph node biopsy specimens may disclose periodic acid–Schiff staining deposits in macrophages, and electron microscopy may show rod-shaped bacilli.

Demographics: Whipple disease is most common in men (90%) older than 40 years of age.

Cardinal Findings: Diarrhea, steatorrhea, weight loss, fever, arthritis, serositis, and lymphadenopathy are seen. Arthralgia or arthritis frequently precedes the intestinal features. The inflammatory arthritis tends to be polyarticular, symmetric, and seronegative and may be chronic or transient.

Uncommon Findings: Iritis, vitreitis, ocular palsy, and progressive encephalitis have been described.

Diagnostic Tests: *T. whippelii* may be identified by PCR.

Keys to Diagnosis: A high index of suspicion is needed, especially in older men with seronegative RA-like polyarthritis, systemic features, and intestinal disease. Perform small bowel biopsy and a PCR test for the causative agent.

Therapy: Oral trimethoprim-sulfamethoxazole twice daily (or tetracycline 1 g/day) for 1 year is recommended.

BIBLIOGRAPHY

Fenollar F, Raoult D. Whipple's disease. *Curr Gastroenterol Rep* 2003;5:379–385.

WILSON'S DISEASE

Synonyms: Hepatolenticular degeneration.

ICD-9 Code: 275.1.

Definition: Wilson's disease is a multisystem disorder caused by copper accumulation.

Demographics: This unusual multisystem disorder is transmitted as an autosomal recessive gene and has an estimated prevalence of one in 30,000. Although manifestations may become apparent in childhood, approximately one-half of cases are not detected until after adolescence. It affects individuals between 6 and 40 years old.

Cardinal Findings: Deposition of excess copper can be observed in the cornea as the characteristic Kayser-Fleischer rings, which are diagnostic. The most common symptoms are movement disorders (from basal ganglia deposition), jaundice or hepatic dysfunction, liver abnormalities, and renal tubular damage.

Musculoskeletal manifestations seen in ≤50% adults (rare in children) manifest as premature OA with a polyarthropathy involving wrists, metacarpophalangeal joints, knees, and spine. Knee effusion may be seen with associated chondromalacia patellae or chondrocalcinosis. Significant osteoporosis is present in approximately one-half of all patients. Joint abnormalities are generally not as severe as those seen in hemochromatosis.

Diagnostic Tests: Ceruloplasmin levels may be low; renal tubular acidosis may appear.

Imaging: Radiographic findings include joint space loss, marked osteophytes, subchondral cysts, and chondrocalcinosis.

Keys to Diagnosis: Suspect this diagnosis in any patient younger than 40 years old with persistent, unexplained liver abnormalities. The diagnosis is confirmed by a low ceruloplasmin level with either Kayser-Fleischer rings or increased copper in a liver biopsy sample.

Therapy: Wilson disease is usually treated with penicillamine, which chelates copper. Initially, 1,000 mg/day is recommended; the dose can later be decreased to 750 mg/day. Early effective treatment with penicillamine ameliorates the arthritic manifestations.

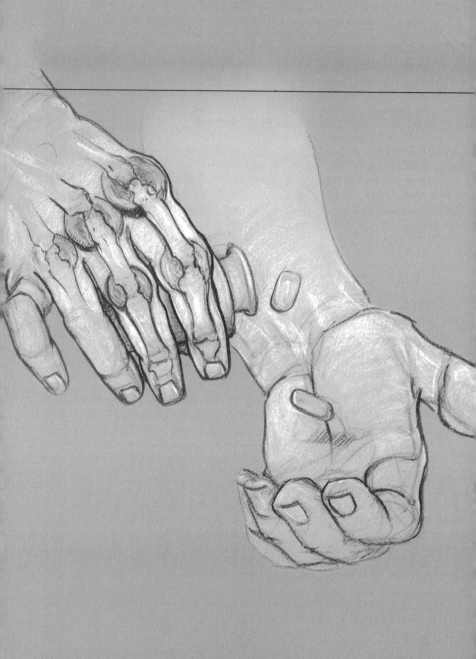

SECTION III.

PHARMACOPOEIA FOR THE RHEUMATIC DISEASES

This pharmacopoeia summarizes drugs commonly used in the treatment of patients with musculoskeletal diseases. The doses listed are provided as a guide for adult patients but need to be individualized according to clinical response and individual patients. Dose modifications may be required in particular patient populations such as the elderly and patients with impaired hepatic or renal function. The more common and clinically important adverse reactions and drug interactions are listed, but this information is not comprehensive.

Abbreviations used (also see p. xix–xxiii)
ACE—angiotensin-converting enzyme
AZA—azathioprine
CBC—complete blood count
CNS—central nervous system
COX—cyclooxygenase
CYP P-450—cytochrome P-450
DMARD—disease-modifying antirheumatic drug
FDA—U. S. Food and Drug Administration
g—gram
G6PD—glucose-6-phosphate dehydrogenase
GI—gastrointestinal
H_2 blocker—histamine type 2 receptor antagonist
IL—interleukin
i.m., i.v.—intramuscularly, intravenously
IU—international units
LFT—liver function test
MAOIs—monoamine oxidase inhibitors
microg—microgram
mg—milligram
ml—milliliter
MTX—methotrexate
NSAID—nonsteroidal antiinflammatory drug
OTC—over the counter
PDR—*Physicians' Desk Reference*
p.o.—by mouth
PPI—proton pump inhibitor
p.r.n.—as needed
RA—rheumatoid arthritis

DRUGS

RDA—recommended daily allowance
s.c.—subcutaneously
SLE—systemic lupus erythematosus
SSRI—selective serotonin reuptake inhibitor
TNF—tumor necrosis factor
WBCs—white blood cells

PRESCRIBING GUIDELINES

Indications

In this book, a listing in the Indications section does not imply that a particular drug has been approved by the FDA for a particular indication. In rheumatology, because many conditions are rare, trials for FDA approval may not have been performed and many patients are treated off label. In addition, because responses to established therapies for many conditions are often unsatisfactory, new drugs are sometimes tried, although there is only preliminary evidence to support their use, in patients who have failed other therapies.

Pregnancy Risk Category

The use of any drug in pregnancy represents a therapeutic decision reached after evaluating the potential risks and benefits to the mother and fetus. Drugs are classified into FDA-designated categories representing the risk of a particular drug being teratogenic. The pregnancy risk increases through categories A to D. Category X indicates drugs that are absolutely contraindicated in pregnancy. These categories are explained in Table 1.

Cost of Medication

The following key is used to indicate the relative cost of medication to the patient. The relative scale used is not meant to indicate a specific monetary value

Table 1
Pregnancy Risk Increases

Category	Drug Effects on Fetus
A	Controlled studies show no risk to the fetus, and possibility of fetal harm appears remote
B	Either (a) animal studies have not demonstrated a fetal risk, but there are no controlled studies in pregnant women or (b) animal studies have shown an adverse effect in pregnancy that was not confirmed in women in controlled studies
C	Either (a) animal studies demonstrate adverse effects on the fetus and there are no controlled studies in women or (b) studies in women and animals are not available
D	Positive evidence of human fetal risk but potential benefit may justify potential risk in certain circumstances
X	Contraindicated in women who are or may become pregnant

but rather to portray the range of possible cost of treatment to the individual. Unless otherwise noted, the cost represents the average cost of generic medication using a median effective dose.

$: Inexpensive (even for those with limited financial resources)

$$: Affordable to most patients (cost concerns are limited with such a drug)

$$$: Expensive (less expensive agents should be considered); agent may only be affordable when the cost of medication is subsidized by insurance programs

$$$$: Very expensive; cost limits use of this agent to those able to afford the high price of medication or those with "liberal" prescription programs

$$$$$: Cost prohibitive; should only be used if (a) the agent is absolutely indicated, (b) anticipated therapeutic benefits are sufficiently great, and (c) less expensive therapeutic options have been exhausted or are contraindicated; often the cost of such agents is not covered by medical insurance programs

Pitfalls in Prescribing

The clinician should be careful to avoid the following common mistakes in prescribing:

1. *Prescribing a drug when no drug is needed.* Alternative, nondrug methods of symptom control may be the appropriate intervention.
2. *Prescribing no drug when a drug is indicated.* Therapeutic nihilism or therapeutic ignorance may deny patients effective and necessary treatment.
3. *Prescribing a poorly chosen drug for the disease.* A drug that is ineffective, expensive, and potentially harmful (e.g., methotrexate to treat gout) should be avoided. Also common is the mistake of choosing a drug that has similar efficacy but is more expensive or has more side effects than the treatment of choice.
4. *Prescribing a poorly chosen drug for the patient.* The patient is a major determinant of rational prescribing. Children, the elderly, pregnant or lactating women, patients with renal or liver disease, and patients receiving other drugs all require special consideration.
5. *Prescribing a drug incorrectly.* A correct drug for the patient and the illness may be chosen, but the drug may be prescribed incorrectly. The dose, dose interval, duration of therapy, and route of administration must be considered. An example of this is the prolonged use of high-dose corticosteroids in RA (which should be tapered as soon as possible). Last, the prescriber should be familiar with the drug's indications, contraindications, proper dosing, common and uncommon side effects, precautions, drug interactions, mechanism(s) of action, and the drug's cost to the patient.
6. *Not providing a patient with essential information.* This is particularly important in long-term therapy with potentially dangerous drugs (e.g., cyclophosphamide) and drugs that must be taken in a particular way (e.g., alendronate).
7. *Failing to monitor appropriately.* Many drugs are potentially toxic, and appropriate long-term monitoring is essential. Assessing the patient's

clinical response and modifying therapy appropriately, in addition to laboratory monitoring, is important.

8. *Polypharmacy.* Many patients require long-term therapy with multiple drugs. Nonetheless, the requirement for ongoing medications should be thoughtfully reviewed.

9. *Illegibility.* Tragedies have occurred because of illegibility. Printing is preferable. Avoid abbreviations (e.g., MTX for methotrexate) when prescribing. Electronically generated prescriptions may lessen prescribing errors by both physicians and pharmacists.

Therapeutic Aims

Primary aims in the treatment of musculoskeletal illness are

1. To relieve pain and stiffness
2. To maintain and restore function and strength
3. To maintain or improve the quality of life
4. If possible, to prevent recurrence or progression of disease
5. If possible, to induce remission

Formulation of a Therapeutic Plan

Treatment of the various musculoskeletal conditions depends on the diagnosis, the severity of disease, and the individual patient's response to different forms of therapy. All these need to be evaluated before and during treatment. Treatment generally takes three major forms: (a) rehabilitation (including physical therapy, occupational therapy, splints), (b) drug therapy, and (c) surgery. A rational management plan is outlined below.

Key Steps in a Therapeutic Plan

Establish a diagnosis: A diagnostic consultation with a rheumatologist is more cost-effective than ordering numerous radiographs or an extensive rheumatology panel of laboratory tests.

Evaluate: Disease severity, aggravating factors, modifiable contributors, functional status, psychosocial status, and comorbidities must be evaluated.

Initiate the treatment plan: The plan should include patient education, appropriate physical and/or occupational therapy, appropriate drug or combination of drugs, and surgery, if indicated.

Monitor: Monitor the clinical status, complications, response to therapy, and toxicity from therapy. Employ measures to prevent toxicity.

Modify the treatment plan: Change therapy if unacceptable toxicity occurs or after an appropriate trial with inadequate efficacy; if the response is acceptable, evaluate maintenance doses or need for continued therapy.

In some rheumatic diseases (e.g., osteoarthritis, fibromyalgia) the efficacy of drug therapy may be modest, and nondrug therapies play an important adjunctive role. Few rheumatic diseases are cured by treatment; thus, the therapeutic plan for an individual patient is based on realistic treatment goals and may change over time as the illness evolves and new data become available. Management of RA, SLE, dermato-/polymyositis, and vasculitis is complex. Diagnostic and therapeutic issues may be clarified and complications or toxicities minimized by consulting a rheumatologist.

SPECIFIC AGENTS

ACETAMINOPHEN

Trade Names: Include Acephen, Aspirin-free Anacin, Tylenol, Tylenol Arthritis

Synonyms: Paracetamol

Drug Class: Analgesic/antipyretic

Preparations
Capsules: 325 and 500 mg (extra strength)
Tablets: 120, 160, 325, 500 mg; 650 mg (extended-release)
Suppositories: 80, 120, 325, 650 mg
Elixir, suspension, liquid, or syrup: 100 mg/mL and 160 mg/5 mL

Dose: Adults, 1–4 g/day in three to four divided doses; do not exceed 4 g/day

Indications: Pain, musculoskeletal pain, headache, fever; less likely to cause GI ulceration than NSAIDs

Mechanism of Action: Uncertain; may inhibit COX-2 and central prostaglandin synthesis

Contraindications: Hypersensitivity to acetaminophen

Precautions: Concomitant alcohol use, liver disease, and fasting may increase the risk of acetaminophen hepatotoxicity. Use lower doses in liver disease (usually <2 g/day). Avoid concomitant alcohol. May cause severe hepatotoxicity in overdose. Patient must avoid self-medication with OTC preparations that may also contain acetaminophen.

Pregnancy Risk: B

Adverse Effects: Rarely causes allergy, rash, or agranulocytosis. Hepatotoxicity is rare at therapeutic doses. Overdose (usually >8 g/day) causes delayed (48–72 hours) and potentially fatal hepatotoxicity. Some evidence links chronic use to increased risk of renal impairment.

DRUGS

Drug Interactions
Alcohol: Increases risk of hepatotoxicity
Warfarin: Acetaminophen ($>$2 g/day) may increase anticoagulant effect
Barbiturates, carbamazepine, hydantoins, and sulfinpyrazone may increase hepatotoxicity of acetaminophen

Patient Instructions: Do not exceed prescribed dose; do not take additional OTC or prescription medications that contain acetaminophen; do not drink alcohol.

Clinical Pharmacology: Rapid complete oral absorption; 95% metabolized in the liver (mainly conjugation). Duration of action is 4–6 hours. With overdose, a hepatotoxic metabolite accumulates.

Cost: $

ACETAMINOPHEN + OPIOID (CODEINE/HYDROCODONE/OXYCODONE/PROPOXYPHENE/TRAMADOL)

Trade Names
Acetaminophen + codeine: Capital and Codeine, Phenaphen with Codeine, Tylenol with Codeine
Acetaminophen + hydrocodone: Anexsia, Co-Gesic, Dolacet, Hydrocet, Lortab , Lorcet, Lorcet Plus, Vicodin, Vicodin ES
Acetaminophen + oxycodone: Percocet, Roxicet, Roxilox, Tylox
Acetaminophen + propoxyphene: Darvocet N-50, Darvocet N-100
Acetaminophen + tramadol: Ultracet

Drug Class: Analgesic/antipyretic with opioid analgesic

Preparations
Acetaminophen + codeine
Tablet: Acetaminophen with codeine #2, 15 mg codeine/300 mg acetaminophen; #3, 30/300 mg; #4, 60/300 mg
Capsules: Acetaminophen with codeine #2, 15 mg codeine/325 mg acetaminophen; #3, 30/325 mg; #4, 60/325 mg
Suspension: Acetaminophen with codeine, 12 mg codeine/120 mg acetaminophen per 5 mL.
Acetaminophen + hydrocodone
Tablet: Lortab 2.5/500 (2.5 mg hydrocodone/500 mg acetaminophen); Lortab 5/500; Lortab 7.5/500; Lorcet Plus (7.5/650); Lorcet 10/650, Vicodin (5/500); Vicodin ES (7.5/750)

Acetaminophen + oxycodone
  Capsule: Oxycodone 5 mg/acetaminophen 500 mg (Tylox)
  Tablet: Oxycodone 2.5 mg/acetaminophen 325 mg, 5/325 mg, 7.5/325 mg,
    10/325 mg (Percocet)
Acetaminophen + propoxyphene: Darvocet N-50 (50 mg propoxyphene and
  325 mg of acetaminophen); Darvocet N-100 (100/650 mg)
Acetaminophen + tramadol: Ultracet (37.5 mg tramadol and 325 mg aceta-
  minophen)

Dose

Do not exceed acetaminophen 4 g/day
Acetaminophen + codeine: Adult dose, one to two tablets containing acetaminophen 300 mg + codeine 15 or 30 mg q 4–6 h p.r.n.
Acetaminophen + hydrocodone: Adult dose, 500 to 750 mg acetaminophen +
  5 to 10 mg hydrocodone q 4–6 h p.r.n.
Acetaminophen + oxycodone: Adult dose, one to two tablets q 4–6 h p.r.n.
Acetaminophen + propoxyphene: Adult dose, 50 to 100 mg propoxyphene +
  325 to 650 mg acetaminophen q 4 h p.r.n. (maximum, 600 mg
  propoxyphene/day)
Acetaminophen + tramadol: Adult dose one to two tablets q 4–6 h p.r.n. (not
  to exceed eight tablets per day or 5 days of treatment)

Indications: Pain unresponsive to nonopioid regimens. Most studies show little benefit over nonopioid regimens in chronic musculoskeletal pain.

Mechanism of Action: Acetaminophen (uncertain) inhibits central prostaglandin synthesis. Opioids bind to opioid receptors in CNS and modify pain
perception.

Contraindications: Hypersensitivity reactions (commonly caused by opioids,
not acetaminophen); opioid or prescription drug abuse

Precautions: Concomitant alcohol use, liver disease, and fasting may increase
the risk of acetaminophen hepatotoxicity. Use lower doses in liver disease
(usually <2 g/day). Patient must avoid self-medication with OTC preparations that may also contain acetaminophen. Risk of psychological and physical
narcotic dependence should limit use. Avoid dose escalation. Limit dose and
duration of therapy if possible. One physician should prescribe all opioids for
a particular patient.

Pregnancy Risk: C

Adverse Effects: Acetaminophen rarely causes allergy, rash, or agranulocytosis. Hepatotoxicity is rare at therapeutic doses. Overdose (usually >10 g/day)
causes delayed (48–72 hours) and potentially fatal hepatotoxicity. Controversial evidence links chronic use of acetaminophen to increased risk of renal impairment.

DRUGS

Opioid toxicity (common): GI intolerance, constipation, and dependence are seen with chronic use. Less common are allergy, confusion, dizziness, nervousness, insomnia, and respiratory depression.

Drug Interactions
Alcohol: Increases risk of hepatotoxicity
Warfarin: Acetaminophen (>2 g/day) may increase the anticoagulant effect
CNS depressants: Effects may be potentiated by opioids

Patient Instructions: Do not exceed prescribed dose. Do not take additional OTC or prescription medications that contain acetaminophen. Do not drink alcohol. May cause drowsiness and constipation. Contains a narcotic and is addictive. Only take for pain.

Comment: Opioid/narcotic medications are seldom required in the treatment of inflammatory joint disease (i.e., RA, gout). In such conditions, control of inflammation usually controls the associated pain.

Clinical Pharmacology: Acetaminophen oral absorption is rapid and complete. It is 95% metabolized in the liver (mainly conjugation). In overdose, a hepatotoxic metabolite accumulates.

Codeine is methylmorphine, and 10% is metabolized to morphine by CYP2D6. Approximately 7% of people have an inactive CYP2D6 enzyme and have little or no analgesic response to codeine. Codeine undergoes hepatic metabolism and renal excretion. Duration of action is 4–6 hours.

Cost: $$

Aciphex (Rabeprazole; See Appendix C)
Actonel (See Risedronate)

ADALIMUMAB

Trade Names: Humira

Drug Class: DMARD, TNF antagonist

Preparations: 40-mg injection

Dose: 40 mg s.c. injection every 2 weeks. Lower doses appear to have less benefit. Dose escalation to weekly 40-mg s.c. injections appears to be necessary in 20% of patients, but such dose escalation has not been studied in clinical trials.

Indications: RA, psoriatic arthritis, ankylosing spondylitis, juvenile RA

Mechanism of Action: A human IgG_1 antibody against TNF-α that blocks the effects of the cytokine; does not bind TNF-β (lymphotoxin).

Contraindications: Hypersensitivity, untreated tuberculosis and other opportunistic infections, sepsis, active infection, chronic localized or recurrent infections, demyelinating disease, optic neuritis, or heart failure.

Precautions: Exclude latent tuberculosis with a skin test before starting therapy. In RA, 5 mm of induration indicates latent or active tuberculosis. Be aware that the risk of opportunistic infections is increased. Caution should be exercised if used in the debilitated or in those at high risk of infection. Avoid live virus vaccines. Influenza and pneumococcal vaccines appear to be unaffected by such therapy. Should not be used in combination with anakinra (increased risk of serious infection).

Monitoring: Monitor clinically for infection.

Pregnancy Risk: B

Adverse Effects

Common: Injection site reactions, positive antinuclear antibody, positive DNA antibody

Less common: Allergy, infection (bacterial, but particularly opportunistic infections such as tuberculosis, listeriosis, and histoplasmosis)

Rare: Lymphoma, hepatitis, demyelinating CNS disorders, optic neuritis, seizures, pancytopenia, drug-induced lupus

Drug Interactions: Concurrent use of high-dose steroids and other immunosuppressants may increase risk of infection.

Patient Instructions: Avoid live virus vaccines; avoid pregnancy; stop injections and call your doctor if an infection or fever develops that lasts more than a few days.

Comments: TNF antagonists are among the most effective treatments for RA. Patients respond quickly, usually within 4–6 weeks. However, not all patients respond. Combined therapy with MTX is more effective than either drug alone. The role of TNF antagonists in a range of diseases such as psoriasis, vasculitis, seronegative spondyloarthropathy, sarcoidosis, and inflammatory eye disease is being explored. The comparative risk of adverse effects such as tuberculosis, lymphoma, or demyelinating disease with individual TNF antagonists is not clear. Until this information is available, these side effects should be considered similar and regarded as a class effect. Patients may form antibodies to adalimumab that decrease its effect. Concurrent treatment with MTX may reduce the frequency of this.

Clinical Pharmacology: Half-life is 14 days. Biologic agents are not metabolized and thus have few drug interactions.

DRUGS

Cost: $$$$$

BIBLIOGRAPHY

Olsen NJ, Stein CM. New drugs for rheumatoid arthritis. *N Engl J Med* 2004;350:2167–2179.
Weinblatt ME, Keystone EC, Furst DE, et al. Adalimumab, a fully human anti-tumor necrosis factor alpha monoclonal antibody, for the treatment of rheumatoid arthritis in patients taking concomitant MTX: The ARMADA trial. *Arthritis Rheum* 2003; 48:35–45.

ALENDRONATE

Trade Names: Fosamax

Drug Class: Bisphosphonate

Preparations: 5-, 10-, 35-, 40-, 70-mg tablets

Dose/Administration
Osteoporosis: 5–10 mg p.o. daily or 70 mg once weekly
Paget's disease: 40 mg p.o. daily for 6 months. If disease relapses, retreatment can be considered.

Indications: Treatment and prevention of osteoporosis; treatment of Paget's disease

Mechanism of Action: Antiresorptive; localizes to areas of bone resorption and inhibits osteoclast activity without any effect on bone formation; increases bone mineral density and significantly reduces vertebral fracture rates; does not induce osteomalacia.

Contraindications: Hypersensitivity to alendronate, hypocalcemia, esophageal stricture, or dysmotility. Not recommended for patients with severe renal insufficiency (creatinine clearance <35 mL/min). Avoid use in patients who cannot stand or sit upright for 30 minutes after administration.

Precautions: If possible, avoid alendronate if esophageal problems or renal impairment are present. Ensure that patient understands how the drug should be taken.

Pregnancy Risk: C

Adverse Effects: Hypocalcemia (transient, mild), headache, mild GI disturbance (i.e., nausea, dyspepsia, dysphagia); rarely, severe erosive esophagitis, uveitis, altered taste, urticaria, or angioedema

Drug Interactions: GI adverse events are increased in patients taking NSAIDs and >10 mg/day alendronate.

Patient Instructions: Alendronate should be taken with a full glass of water on arising in the morning. Nothing other than water should be taken for at least 30 minutes after alendronate. Even coffee or fruit juice markedly reduce absorption. Delaying such intake for longer than 30 minutes (1–2 hours if possible) maximizes absorption. After taking alendronate, the patient must remain upright to reduce risk of esophageal irritation. Any other medications must be taken at least 30 minutes after alendronate.

Comments: Supplemental calcium and vitamin D are usually coadministered. Weekly dosing for osteoporosis is preferred.

Clinical Pharmacology: Oral bioavailability is very poor (<1%) and negligible if administered with or after food. Absorbed drug is renally excreted and not metabolized. Elimination half-life is several years, indicating localization and slow release from bone.

Cost: $$$$

BIBLIOGRAPHY

Delmas PD. Treatment of postmenopausal osteoporosis. *Lancet* 2002;359:2018–2026.
Delmas PD, Meunier PJ. The management of Paget's disease of bone. *N Engl J Med* 1997;336:558–566.

ALLOPURINOL

Trade Names: Zyloprim

Drug Class: Xanthine oxidase inhibitor; antigout agent

Preparations: 100- and 300-mg tablets

Dose: For prophylaxis of gout, initially use 100 mg/day, increased at 1- to 2-week intervals according to uric acid response. In the elderly, use <50 mg/day initially.

Usual maintenance dose is 200–300 mg/day. Patients with severe hyperuricemia and tophi may require higher doses. Maximum recommended dose is 800 mg/day. Doses >300 mg/day are given in divided doses.

In renal impairment, the dose is usually reduced to 25–200 mg/day (monitor closely for toxicity). If required in patients with renal failure, allopurinol dose is modified according to creatinine clearance; for example, if creatinine clearance is 10 mL/min, give 100 mg every second day; if 20 mL/min, then 100 mg daily; if 40 mL/min, then 150 mg daily; and if 60 mL/min, then 200 mg daily.

Indications: Prophylaxis of gout; treatment of chronic gout, uric acid nephropathy; prophylaxis of renal calculi, used to treat extreme hyperuricemia (e.g., renal failure, chemotherapy, tumor lysis)

Mechanism of Action: Inhibits formation of uric acid by inhibiting xanthine oxidase; has no antiinflammatory activity

DRUGS

Contraindications: Previous hypersensitivity to allopurinol

Precautions: Reduce dose in the elderly, patients on diuretics, and patients with renal impairment. Concurrent AZA or mercaptopurine requires major dose reduction of the cytotoxic drug.

Pregnancy Risk: C

Monitoring: Monitor CBC and liver and renal function periodically, particularly in the first few months of treatment. Uric acid level guides the allopurinol dose. Aim to reduce uric acid concentration to ≤6 mg/dL in tophaceous disease.

Adverse Effects
Common: Acute gout may occur with increased frequency after starting allopurinol; thus, it is not initiated during an acute gouty attack. If allergic rash is mild and not associated with other features of allopurinol hypersensitivity syndrome, discontinue and reintroduce cautiously but discontinue if rash recurs.

Rarely: Allopurinol hypersensitivity syndrome (exfoliative dermatitis/erythema multiforme, renal failure, hepatic impairment, vasculitis) is rare but may be fatal. Risk is increased in patients with impaired renal function or receiving diuretics. Desensitization has been tried in selected patients. Oxypurinol is sometimes tolerated by patients sensitive to allopurinol. Agranulocytosis and aplastic anemia are rare.

Drug Interactions
Azathioprine and mercaptopurine: Allopurinol decreases metabolism of these agents, leading to toxicity (bone marrow depression). If concurrent use cannot be avoided, the dose of AZA or mercaptopurine should be reduced to <25% of the usual dose and the CBC carefully monitored.
Warfarin: Anticoagulant effects potentiated
Cyclophosphamide: Increased potential for bone marrow suppression
Ampicillin/amoxicillin: Increased risk of rash
Thiazide diuretics and ACE inhibitors: Increased risk of allopurinol toxicity
Theophylline: Increased theophylline levels
Chlorpropamide: Increased chlorpropamide serum half-life
Alcohol: Decreases effectiveness

Patient Instructions: The drug needs to be taken every day (or as prescribed) to prevent gouty flares. It has no effect on the symptoms of gout and will not help when joints hurt. Discontinue drug and contact physician if rash develops. Do not drink alcohol.

Comments: Asymptomatic hyperuricemia should not routinely be treated; it is not necessary, especially when uric acid levels are <11 mg/dL. Allopurinol is used primarily to lower the uric acid level in patients with recurrent attacks of acute gout (more than one per year) or patients with tophaceous gout. Allopurinol is preferred over a uricosuric agent in patients with tophi, renal stones, and impaired renal function. Monitor serum uric acid and aim to decrease to 5–6 mg/dL. Failure to decrease uric acid often indicates poor compliance. Prevent acute attacks of gout with concurrent colchicine or NSAID treatment, particularly in first 3–6 months of therapy.

Clinical Pharmacology: Oral absorption is 90%; 70% is metabolized to the active metabolite oxypurinol. Excretion is largely renal as oxypurinol, and accumulation occurs if renal function is impaired. Half-life of allopurinol is 2 hours and 20 hours for oxypurinol. Reduction of uric acid is noted within days, and the level may normalize within weeks. If allopurinol is discontinued, uric acid concentrations return to pretreatment levels in weeks.

Cost: $

BIBLIOGRAPHY

Hande KR, Noone RM, Stone WJ. Severe allopurinol toxicity. Description and guidelines for prevention in patients with renal insufficiency. *Am J Med* 1984;76:47–56.
Rott KT, Agudelo CA. Gout. *JAMA* 2003; 289:2857–2860.
Terkeltaub RA. Clinical practice. Gout. *N Engl J Med* 2003;349:1647–1655.

Ambien (See Zolpidem)

AMITRIPTYLINE

Trade Names: Elavil, Vanatrip

Drug Class: Tricyclic antidepressant

Preparations: 10-, 25-, 50-, 75-, 100-, 150-mg tablets

Dose: Initially, 10 mg is taken 2 hours before bedtime. The dose can be increased, if tolerated, to a maximum of 300 mg/day. The usual maintenance dose for fibromyalgia is 10–75 mg taken 2 hours before bedtime.

Indications: Depression, fibromyalgia, insomnia; an adjunct for pain control (chronic or neuropathic); prophylaxis for migraines

Mechanism of Action: Increases synaptic concentrations of norepinephrine

Contraindications: Avoid in recovery period of myocardial infarction or if arrhythmias exist. Avoid for 14 days after patient has received an MAOI. Avoid in patients with narrow-angle glaucoma.

Precautions: Escalate dose slowly; it may cause drowsiness and affect the ability to drive or operate machinery; it aggravates symptoms of prostatism and keratoconjunctivitis sicca. It may precipitate acute glaucoma and may

DRUGS

lower seizure threshold. Long-term high doses should not be abruptly discontinued; use with caution in patients with a history of hyperthyroidism, renal or hepatic impairment, or cardiac conduction disturbances.

Pregnancy Risk: D

Adverse Effects

Common: Sedation and anticholinergic effects (dry eyes and mouth, blurred vision, constipation, difficulty with urination) are common; tolerance often occurs with continued use.

Less common: Postural hypotension, restlessness, tremor, parkinsonian syndrome, insomnia, rash

Rarely: Agranulocytosis, hepatic dysfunction, alopecia, arrhythmias, breast enlargement

Drug Interactions

Alcohol and CNS depressants: Effect of tricyclic is potentiated

Cimetidine, methylphenidate, many SSRIs, ritonavir, indinavir, diltiazem, verapamil: Inhibit metabolism of tricyclics; dose reduction (usually 20%–30%) may be required

MAOIs: Increased risk of hypertensive crises; deaths have been reported

Sympathomimetics: Tricyclics potentiate effect.

Clonidine: Amitriptyline inhibits hypotensive effects.

Warfarin: Prothrombin time may be prolonged.

Drugs that prolong QT interval: Increased risk of arrhythmia

Patient Instructions: Avoid alcohol use; may cause drowsiness

Clinical Pharmacology: Well absorbed, hepatic metabolism with renal excretion of metabolites; onset of antidepressant effects slow (2–4 weeks)

Cost: $

Amoxapine (Asendin; See Appendix D, p. 533)

ANAKINRA

Trade Names: Kineret

Drug Class: DMARD, IL-1 receptor antagonist

Preparations: 100-mg injection

Dose: 100 mg s.c. injection daily

Indications: RA

Mechanism of Action: Binds to IL-1 receptors and blocks the effects of the cytokine

Contraindications: Hypersensitivity; active infection

Precautions: Discontinue if patient develops an infection; do not use with TNF antagonists

Monitoring: Monitor clinically for infection; CBC monthly for 3 months, then every 3 months

Pregnancy Risk: B

Adverse Effects
Common: Injection site reactions (50%–80%)
Less common: Allergy, infection (primarily bacterial), leukopenia
Rare: Neutropenia, thrombocytopenia

Drug Interactions: Concurrent use of other immunosuppressants, particularly TNF antagonists, may increase risk of infection.

Patient Instructions: Avoid live virus vaccines. Avoid pregnancy. Stop injections if an infection or a fever develops that lasts more than a few days.

Comments: Anakinra appears less effective than TNF antagonists in clinical practice, but there are no head-to-head comparisons. Combination therapy with MTX is generally well tolerated and is more effective than monotherapy. Combination with TNF antagonists is avoided because of increased risk of infection.

Clinical Pharmacology: Half-life is 6 hours with renal excretion. Biologic agents are not metabolized and have few drug interactions.

Cost: $$$$$

BIBLIOGRAPHY

Cohen S, Hurd E, Cush J, et al. Treatment of rheumatoid arthritis with anakinra, a recombinant human interleukin-1 receptor antagonist, in combination with methotrexate: results of a twenty-four-week, multicenter, randomized, double-blind, placebo-controlled trial. *Arthritis Rheum* 2002;46:614–624.
Olsen NJ, Stein CM. New drugs for rheumatoid arthritis. *N Engl J Med* 2004;350:2167–2179.
Yang BB, Baughman S, Sullivan JT. Pharmacokinetics of anakinra in subjects with different levels of renal function. *Clin Pharmacol Ther* 2003;74:85–94.

Anaprox (See Naproxen)
Ansaid (See Flurbiprofen)
Antidepressants (See Appendix D, p. 533)

DRUGS

Arava (See Leflunomide)
Aredia (See Pamidronate)
Aristocort (See Corticosteroids, Intraarticular)
Aristospan (See Corticosteroids, Intraarticular)
Arthropan (See Choline Salicylate)
Arthrotec (See Diclofenac and Misoprostol)

ARTIFICIAL TEARS

Trade Names
Artificial tears: Liquifilm, Liquifilm Forte, Isopto Alkaline, Isopto Plain, Isopto Tears, Just Tears, Tears Naturelle, Tears Naturelle II
Artificial tears, preservative free: Celluvisc, Hypotears PF Refresh, Tears Naturelle Free
Ocular ointments: Duratears, Lacrilube
Ocular ointments, preservative free: Duolube, Refresh PM, Lacriserts

Synonyms: Hydroxypropyl methylcellulose

Drug Class: Ophthalmic protectant

Preparations
Hydroxypropyl methylcellulose ophthalmic solution
   0.3%: Bion Tears, Tears Naturelle, Tears Naturelle II, Tears Naturelle Free
   0.4%: Artificial Tears, Nature's Tears
   0.5%: Isopto Plain, Isopto Tears, Just Tears
   0.8%: Ocucoat, Ocucoat PF
   1%: Isopto Alkaline, Ultra Tears
   Hydroxypropyl cellulose ocular system: Lacrisert 5-mg insert

Dose: One drop of a 0.3%–1% tear solution applied topically to conjunctiva three to four times daily. In patients with keratoconjunctivitis sicca, drops should be applied regularly even if no symptoms are present. Some patients require more frequent application (every 2 hours). Hydroxypropyl cellulose 5-mg ophthalmic insert; use once or twice daily

Indications: Dry eyes

Mechanism of Action: Promotes corneal wetting by stabilizing and thickening the tear film

Contraindications: Hypersensitivity

Precautions: Use preservative-free preparations if preservative causes irritation.

Pregnancy Risk: C

Adverse Effects: Blurring of vision; eye irritation

Drug Interactions: None

Patient Instructions: Tears may be used as often as required. Regular use rather than waiting until symptoms are present is best. Do not instill with contact lens in place unless preparation is designed for use with contact lenses. Always wash hands before administration. Never touch tip of dropper to the eye surface.

Clinical Pharmacology: No systemic effects after ocular administration

Cost: $

Ascriptin (See Aspirin)

ASPIRIN

Trade Names
Plain aspirin: Bayer Aspirin, Empirin
Buffered aspirin: Ascriptin, Buffaprin, Buffasal, Buffinol, Bufferin, Alka-Seltzer
Enteric coated aspirin: Bayer Enteric, Ecotrin, Easprin, Genprin
Extended-release aspirin: 8-Hour Bayer Timed Release, Measurin, Zorprin

Synonyms: Acetylsalicylic acid, ASA

Drug Class: NSAID

Preparations
Chewable aspirin tablet: 81 mg
Tablets: 325 and 500 mg
Enteric coated tablets 81, 162, 325, 500, 650, 975 mg
Timed-/controlled-release tablets: 800 mg

Dose
Analgesic/antipyretic effect: 325–650 mg q 4–6 h (as high as 4 g/day)
Antiinflammatory effect: Divided doses of 3.6–5.4 g/day. In acute rheumatic fever, doses as high as 7.8 g/day have been used, but dose-related toxicity is common.
Antithrombotic effect: 81–325 mg/day

Indications: Treatment of pain, inflammation, and pyrexia and as antithrombotic prophylaxis; used in RA, osteoarthritis, rheumatic fever, Still's disease, Kawasaki disease, and inflammatory conditions such as bursitis; used for antithrombotic effect in myocardial infarction, anticardiolipin antibody syndrome, and transient ischemic attacks

Mechanism of Action: Nonselective COX inhibitor; decreases formation of prostaglandins and thromboxane from arachidonic acid

Contraindications: Hypersensitivity to aspirin (especially in those with asthma and nasal polyps), GI ulceration, hemorrhagic state, last trimester of pregnancy (may induce premature closure of ductus arteriosus), breastfeeding, children (risk of Reye syndrome), and G6PD deficiency (hemolysis)

Precautions: Fluid retention may aggravate heart failure and hypertension. Use with caution or avoid in patients at high risk of GI bleeding (i.e., previous GI bleeding, peptic ulcer, elderly, concurrent corticosteroid or warfarin treatment), but if prescribed, misoprostol or proton pump inhibitor prophylaxis is recommended. Administer with food. Use with caution in asthma, bleeding disorders, and hepatic or renal disease.

Monitoring: Monitor hematocrit, creatinine, and liver enzymes periodically (1 month after starting and then every 3–6 months). In patients at high risk of renal impairment (i.e., diuretics, receiving ACE inhibitors, edematous states, heart failure, renal failure, diabetes), monitor renal function more closely. Consider measuring salicylate levels if using high doses. Serum concentrations of 150–300 μg/mL are antiinflammatory. Salicylism (e.g., tinnitus) is common at levels >200 μg/mL.

Pregnancy Risk: C (D in third trimester of pregnancy)

Adverse Effects
Common: GI irritation (dyspepsia, esophageal reflux, epigastric pain); dose-related side effects at concentrations >200 μg/mL (tinnitus/deafness)
Less common: GI ulceration or hemorrhage, minor elevations of liver enzymes, hypersensitivity (asthma; urticaria; angioedema, particularly in patients with nasal polyps); impaired renal function, acidosis with overdose, and high serum concentrations (>400 μg/mL), especially in the elderly

Drug Interactions
Antacids: Decreased salicylate levels through increased elimination in alkaline urine
Anticoagulants: Activity of warfarin increased; increased hemorrhagic risk with other anticoagulants and thrombolytics
NSAIDs: Increased risk of GI side effects if aspirin is used with other NSAIDs. Coadministration of traditional NSAIDs such as ibuprofen or naproxen (but

not COX-2–selective NSAIDs) may antagonize the long-term antiplatelet effect of aspirin.
MTX: May increase levels of MTX (however, with the doses of MTX used in RA, this is usually clinically insignificant); may potentiate MTX toxicity with high doses
Lithium: Increased levels
Valproic acid: Aspirin may enhance toxicity
Probenecid: Aspirin may antagonize effects

Patient Instructions: Take with food. Discontinue and seek medical advice if unusual bleeding develops.

Comments: With high doses, metabolic pathways become saturated, and a small dose increase can result in large increases in plasma concentrations. Enteric coated or delayed-release formulations of aspirin are better tolerated than regular aspirin.

Clinical Pharmacology: Rapidly and well absorbed after oral administration. Hydrolyzed to salicylate with hepatic metabolism and renal excretion of conjugated metabolites. Urinary pH alters elimination (alkaline urine increases elimination). Wide variation in plasma concentrations exists in individuals receiving the same dose. Half-life varies with dose (2–3 hours with low doses, >20 hours with high therapeutic doses). At high doses, the elimination pathway is saturated, and a small increase in dose can lead to a large increase in serum concentration.

Cost: $

ASPIRIN + OPIOIDS (CODEINE/ HYDROCODONE/OXYCODONE/ PROPOXYPHENE)

Trade Names
Aspirin + codeine: Empirin with Codeine
Aspirin + hydrocodone: Azdone, Lortab ASA
Aspirin + oxycodone: Percodan, Roxiprin
Aspirin + propoxyphene: Darvon with aspirin
Aspirin + pentazocine: Talwin compound

Drug Class: Analgesic/antiinflammatory with opioid analgesic

Preparations: Tablets
Aspirin + codeine: Aspirin with codeine #2, 325 mg aspirin/15 mg codeine; Aspirin codeine #3, 325 mg/30 mg; Aspirin with codeine #4, 325 mg/60 mg
Aspirin + hydrocodone: 5 mg hydrocodone/500 mg aspirin

Aspirin + oxycodone: Aspirin 325 mg/oxycodone 4.5 mg (*Percodan*)
Aspirin + propoxyphene: 65 mg propoxyphene/325 mg of aspirin
Aspirin + pentazocine: 12.5 mg pentazocine/325 mg of aspirin

Dose
Aspirin + codeine: Adult dose, one to two tablets q 4 h p.r.n.
Aspirin + hydrocodone: Adult dose, one to two tablets q 4–6 h p.r.n.
Aspirin + oxycodone: Adult dose, one tablet q 4–6 h p.r.n.
Aspirin + propoxyphene: Adult dose, 1 tablet q 4–6 h p.r.n.
Aspirin + pentazocine: Adult dose, two caplets q 6–8 h p.r.n.

Indications: Pain is unresponsive to nonopioid regimens. Most studies show little benefit over nonopioid regimens in chronic musculoskeletal pain.

Mechanism of Action: Aspirin inhibits prostaglandin synthesis. Opioids bind to opioid receptors in CNS and modify pain perception.

Contraindications: Hypersensitivity reactions to opioids or aspirin; opioid or prescription drug abuse

Precautions
Aspirin: Fluid retention may aggravate heart failure and hypertension. Consider misoprostol or proton pump inhibitor prophylaxis in patients at high risk of GI bleeding (prior GI bleeding, peptic ulcer, elderly, concurrent corticosteroid or warfarin treatment). Administer with food. Use with caution in asthma, bleeding disorders, and hepatic or renal disease.
Opioids: Risk of psychologic and physical narcotic dependence should limit use. Avoid dose escalation. Limit dose and duration of therapy if possible. One physician should prescribe all opioids for a particular patient.

Pregnancy Risk: C

Adverse Effects: (see Aspirin above). Opioid toxicity: (common) GI intolerance, constipation, dependence with chronic use; (less common) allergy, confusion, dizziness, nervousness, and insomnia

Drug Interactions: See Aspirin above; effects of CNS depressants may be potentiated by opioids.

Patient Instructions: Do not exceed prescribed dose. Do not drink alcohol. May cause drowsiness or constipation. Contains a narcotic and is addictive. Only use for pain.

Clinical Pharmacology: See individual drugs

Cost: $$

AURANOFIN (ALSO SEE APPENDIX B, P. 529)

Trade Names: Ridaura

Synonyms: Oral gold

Drug Class: DMARD

Preparations: 3-mg capsule

Dose: Adults, 6 mg p.o. daily as single or divided dose. If no response after 3 months, it can be increased to 9 mg/day (in 3 divided doses). If no response after a further 3 months, discontinue and consider an alternative DMARD.

Indications: Active RA, psoriatic arthritis, and other inflammatory arthritides

Mechanism of Action: Unknown; has several immunomodulatory effects, primarily affecting macrophages, including inhibition of phagocytosis

Contraindications: Hypersensitivity to gold; prior blood dyscrasias; severe renal impairment

Precautions: May exacerbate or cause exfoliative dermatitis. Use caution in hepatic or renal impairment.

Monitoring: CBC (WBC count with differential, hemoglobin, and platelet count) and urinalysis before, 1–2 weeks after starting treatment, and then monthly. In patients who have tolerated auranofin well for ≥12 months, the frequency of monitoring can often safely be decreased to every 2–3 months.
    Discontinue use if significant rash, proteinuria, or decrease in blood elements develops.

Pregnancy Risk: C

Adverse Effects
Common: Diarrhea, rash, itching, mouth ulcers, proteinuria, conjunctivitis
Less common: Leukopenia, thrombocytopenia, agranulocytosis, aplastic anemia, hepatotoxicity, peripheral neuropathy, angioedema

Drug Interactions: Toxicity of other DMARDs (penicillamine, antimalarials, cytotoxic agents, immunosuppressants) may be increased if used in combination therapy.

Patient Instructions: Avoid sunlight because photosensitivity may occur. Regular monitoring of urine and blood count is required. Discontinue if rash develops. It may take as long as 3 months for benefits to appear.

DRUGS

Comments: Onset of antirheumatic action is slow, over several months. Auranofin is seldom prescribed but is occasionally useful for patients with early and mild disease. The combination of auranofin with MTX did not increase efficacy but did increase side effects.

Clinical Pharmacology: Oral absorption is 25%. Renal excretion is the major route of elimination. The plasma half-life is 26 days.

Cost: $$$

BIBLIOGRAPHY

American College of Rheumatology Committee on Rheumatoid Arthritis Guidelines. Guidelines for the management of rheumatoid arthritis: 2002 update. *Arthritis Rheum* 2002;46:328–346.

Williams HJ, Ward JR, Reading JC, et al. Comparison of Auranofin, methotrexate, and the combination of both in the treatment of rheumatoid arthritis. *Arthritis Rheum* 1992;35:259–269.

AZATHIOPRINE (ALSO SEE APPENDIX B, P. 529)

Trade Names: Imuran

Drug Class: Immunosuppressive, purine antagonist, DMARD

Preparations: Tablets: 50 mg, scored

Dose: Adult, 1.0–2.5 mg/kg/day (given once or twice daily)

Indications: Refractory RA; SLE; dermatomyositis/polymyositis; used as a steroid-sparing agent in a wide range of autoimmune disorders when the disease requires prolonged high doses of corticosteroids

Mechanism of Action: The active metabolite is 6-mercaptopurine, which is a purine analogue that interferes with purine synthesis and thus with DNA synthesis.

Contraindications: Hypersensitivity, concomitant allopurinol, lactation, or pregnancy

Precautions: Consider genetic testing for thiopurine methyltransferase deficiency (see Comments). Use caution in hepatic or renal impairment. If creatinine clearance is 10–50 mL/min, use 75% of usual dose; if <10 mL/min, use ≤50% of usual dose. AZA is carcinogenic in animals and increases the risk of malignancy, primarily lymphoma and leukemia, in humans.

Monitoring: CBC and platelet count every 1–2 weeks for the first 2 months or after a dose increase, then monthly on stable dose. Do LFTs every 1–3 months.

Pregnancy Risk: D

Adverse Effects

Common: Fever, chills, GI symptoms (vomiting, diarrhea, nausea), dose-related effects on bone marrow (thrombocytopenia, leukopenia)

Less common: Herpes zoster, hepatotoxicity, pancreatitis, pneumonitis, hypersensitivity, stomatitis, rash, secondary infection, increased risk of lymphoma/leukemia, hepatic venoocclusive disease

Drug Interactions

Allopurinol: Increased accumulation of 6-mercaptopurine and thus toxicity. Avoid concurrent treatment if possible; if necessary, reduce dose of AZA to 25% (or less) of usual dose and monitor frequently.

Sulfasalazine: Increased leukopenia

Immunosuppressants: Concurrent use with other immunosuppressants increases the risk of infection and long-term risk of malignancy.

Live vaccines: Replication of the attenuated virus may occur because of immunosuppression.

Patient Instructions: Use contraception to avoid pregnancy. Do not exceed prescribed dose. Regular monitoring of blood count is essential. Report to physician if persistent sore throat, unusual bleeding, bruises, or fatigue develops.

Comments: Rather than starting with a high maintenance dose, it is advisable to start at a low dose, usually 50 mg/day and increase by 25-mg increments at 1- to 2-week intervals. Onset of action is delayed, so reduce dose at first sign of a large or persistent ($<3,000/mm^3$) decrease in WBCs or platelets ($<100,000/mm^3$). A complete genetic deficiency of the enzyme thiopurine methyltransferase occurs in one in 300 persons and partial deficiency in 10%. Complete thiopurine methyltransferase deficiency is associated with severe, life-threatening myelosuppression because of impaired metabolism; thus, AZA should be avoided if possible. Partial deficiency is associated with increased side effects and lower doses are indicated. Genetic testing for thiopurine methyltransferase deficiency is available, and it is prudent to check before starting therapy.

GI tolerability may improve with split (twice daily) dosing.

Response in RA may not occur for several months. AZA is not more effective than other DMARDs, but adverse effects are more common. Combination studies on RA show that MTX + AZA is more effective than AZA alone, but the MTX + AZA combination is not more effective than MTX alone and may have added toxicity. Uncontrolled studies suggest possible efficacy of MTX + AZA + antimalarial combination therapy. Combination therapy should not be undertaken routinely.

Clinical Pharmacology: AZA is well absorbed orally and largely biotransformed to 6-mercaptopurine and 6-thioinosinic acid; it is further metabolized by xanthine oxidase and renally excreted as metabolites. Half-life is 5 hours (drug and active metabolites), but immunosuppressive action is prolonged for

DRUGS

weeks because of the intracellular accumulation of active thioguanine nucleotides.

Cost: $$$

BIBLIOGRAPHY

Kerstens PJ, Stolk JN, De Abreu RA, et al. Azathioprine-related bone marrow toxicity and low activities of purine enzymes in patients with rheumatoid arthritis. *Arthritis Rheum* 1995;38:142–145.

Stein CM. Immunoregulatory drugs. In: Harris ED, Ruddy S, Sledge CB, eds. *Kelley's Textbook of Rheumatology*, 7th ed. Philadelphia: WB Saunders, 2004.

Willkens RF, Urowitz MB, Stablein DM, et al. Comparison of azathioprine, methotrexate, and the combination of both in the treatment of rheumatoid arthritis. *Arthritis Rheum* 1992;35:849–856.

Azulfidine (See Sulfasalazine)

Benemid (See Probenecid)

Bextra (See Valdecoxib)

BOSENTAN

Trade Names: Tracleer

Drug Class: Endothelin receptor antagonist

Preparations: Tablets: 62.5 and 125 mg

Dose: Initially 62.5 mg twice daily for a month; if tolerated, increase to 125 mg twice daily in adults weighing >40 kg.

Indications: Primary pulmonary hypertension, pulmonary hypertension associated with connective tissue diseases

Mechanism of Action: Blocks endothelin A and B receptors and prevents vasoconstriction

Contraindications: Hypersensitivity, pregnancy, use of glyburide or cyclosporine.

Precautions: Avoid with hepatic impairment. Obtain baseline LFTs. Exclude pregnancy. Ensure adequate contraception.

Monitoring: Monitor LFTs at least monthly. Stop bosentan if transaminases have increased and there are any symptoms of clinical hepatic injury (fatigue, jaundice, nausea); decrease dose or interrupt therapy and monitor carefully (at least every 2 weeks) if a modest (two to four times) increase in transaminases and no clinical symptoms of liver injury. Stop drug if transaminases are markedly elevated (five times or greater). Perform a monthly pregnancy test. Monitor hemoglobin monthly for 3 months, then every 3 months.

Pregnancy Risk: X. Teratogenic; contraindicated in pregnancy

Adverse Effects
Common: GI side effects, headache, anemia, increased transaminases
Less common: Fatigue, flushing, edema, liver injury, rash

Drug Interactions
Increased bosentan levels: ketoconazole, cyclosporine, and likely other CYP3A inhibitors
Increased hepatotoxicity: glyburide
Decreased levels of other drugs: Bosentan decreases levels of cyclosporine, and because it induces CYP2C9 and CYP3A, it may decrease levels of a range of other drugs including hormonal contraceptives.

Patient Instructions: Do not become pregnant. Report nausea, vomiting, and orange-yellow discoloration of eyes, skin, or urine.

Comments: Bosentan is only prescribed by physicians expert in the management of pulmonary hypertension, generally cardiologists or pulmonologists with a special interest in pulmonary hypertension. Access to the drug is limited and obtained through the Tracleer access program (1-866-228-3546). In subset analysis of a clinical trial, stabilization of 6-minute walk distance occurred in patients with scleroderma with pulmonary hypertension treated with bosentan. There are case reports of digital ulcers improving.

Clinical Pharmacology: Bioavailability, 50%; half-life, 5 hours; hepatic metabolism by CYP3A and 2C9

Cost: $$$$$

BIBLIOGRAPHY
Rubin LJ, Badesch DB, Barst RJ, et al. Bosentan therapy for pulmonary arterial hypertension. *N Engl J Med* 2002;346:896–903.

Bupropion (Wellbutrin; See Appendix D, p. 533)
Butazolidin (See Phenylbutazone)
Calcimar (See Calcitonin)

DRUGS

CALCITONIN

Trade Names
Injectable: Calcimar (salmon), Cibacalcin (human)
Nasal spray: Miacalcin (salmon)

Synonyms: Salmon calcitonin, human calcitonin

Drug Class: Hormone

Preparations
Salmon calcitonin: Injection 200 U/mL (2 mL)
Nasal spray 2 mL bottle, 200 IU/spray
Human calcitonin: Injection 0.5 mg/vial

Dose: Salmon calcitonin injection: Skin test 0.1 mL of a 10-IU/mL solution injected intradermally and observed for 15 minutes; appearance of more than mild erythema or a weal is a positive response, and the drug should not be used. For osteoporosis and Paget's disease, use 50–100 IU s.c. or i.m. daily or alternate days. For hypercalcemia, use 4 IU/kg q 12 h i.m. or s.c. (increase dose if necessary as high as 8 IU/kg q 12 h).

Salmon calcitonin nasal: One spray (200 IU) daily; use alternate nostrils.

Human calcitonin: Paget disease: 0.5 mg/day s.c. initially. Dose required varies from 0.25 to 0.5 mg two to three times weekly to 0.25 mg daily.

Indications
Injectable calcitonin: Treatment and prevention of osteoporosis, treatment of
    Paget's disease, and adjunctive treatment for hypercalcemia
Nasal calcitonin: Osteoporosis

Mechanism of Action: Calcitonin inhibits osteoclastic bone resorption and promotes renal excretion of calcium.

Contraindications: Hypersensitivity to salmon protein

Precautions: Perform skin test before administering salmon calcitonin injection. Have epinephrine available to treat anaphylaxis. Skin testing should be considered before nasal calcitonin for patients with suspected sensitivity, but allergic reactions are less frequent than with the injectable form.

Monitoring: Serum electrolytes (especially calcium) and alkaline phosphatase or 24-hour urinary hydroxyproline concentrations or other bone turnover markers at 3- to 6-month intervals are useful for measuring response in Paget disease. Repeated measurement of bone density at 1- to 2-year intervals may be useful as a guide to treatment of osteoporosis.

Pregnancy Risk: C

Adverse Effects
Common: Flushing, headache, nausea, diarrhea, injection site reaction
Less common: Chills, tingling, rash, hypersensitivity. Nasal calcitonin seldom causes the above systemic side effects, but rhinitis and nasal irritation are common.

Drug Interactions: None of significance

Patient Instructions: Teach the patient the injection technique. For nasal spray, use alternate nostrils. Discontinue if nasal ulceration or bleeding occurs.

Comments: Antibody formation occurs more commonly to salmon calcitonin, and 5%–10% of patients may become resistant to treatment after long-term use. In contrast to bisphophonates, a decrease in both vertebral and hip fracture rate is not well established with calcitonin. Thus, bisphosphonates are the preferred drugs for osteoporosis. Adequate calcium (1,000–1,500 mg elemental calcium/day) and vitamin D (400 IU/day) intake is recommended when using calcitonin.

Clinical Pharmacology: Short half-life (1–2 hours), rapid metabolism by kidneys. Absorption of nasal spray is poor (10%–25%).

Cost: $$$

BIBLIOGRAPHY

Delmas PD. Treatment of postmenopausal osteoporosis. *Lancet* 2002;359:2018–2026.
Delmas PD, Meunier PJ. The management of Paget's disease of bone. *N Engl J Med* 1997;336:558–566.

Calcitriol (See Vitamin D)

CALCIUM SALTS

Trade Names
Calcium carbonate: Alka-Mints, Calci-Chew, Caltrate, Os-Cal, Oyst-Cal 500, Rolaids Calcium Rich, Titralac, Tums, Tums E-X Extra Strength
Calcium citrate: Citracal
Calcium glubionate: Neo-Calglucon
Calcium lactate: Generic
Calcium phosphate dibasic: Generic
Calcium phosphate tribasic: Posture

Drug Class: Calcium supplement

DRUGS

Preparations

Calcium carbonate: Tablets: 500, 650, 667 mg; 1.25 and 1.5 g; chewable tablets: 420, 500, 750 mg

Calcium citrate: Tablets 950 mg; effervescent tablets: 2,376 mg

Calcium glubionate: Syrup 1.8 g/5 mL

Calcium lactate: Tablets 325 and 650 mg

Calcium phosphate dibasic: 500-mg tablet

Calcium phosphate tribasic: 300- and 600-mg tablets

Dose: Prevention and treatment of osteoporosis in adults requires at least 1–1.5 g of elemental calcium/day. Various salts contain

Calcium carbonate: 400 mg elemental calcium/g

Calcium citrate: 220 mg elemental calcium/g

Calcium glubionate: 64 mg elemental calcium/g

Calcium lactate: 130 mg elemental calcium/g

Calcium phosphate dibasic: 115 mg elemental calcium/g

Calcium phosphate tribasic: 400 mg elemental calcium/g

Indications: Prevention of osteoporosis, hypocalcemia

Mechanism of Action: Calcium supplement helps prevent osteoporosis in patients with inadequate intake. Calcium in bone is in exchange with calcium in plasma, so bone stores are depleted if intake is inadequate.

Contraindications: Renal calculi, hypercalcemia, digoxin toxicity, or renal failure

Precautions: Use care in patients with arrhythmias.

Monitoring: Serum calcium before treatment and annually

Pregnancy Risk: C, but problems are unlikely; used in pregnancy to supplement calcium intake

Adverse Effects

Common: Constipation, flatulence

Uncommon: Nausea, hypercalcemia, renal stones

Drug Interactions

Calcium channel antagonists: Doses of calcium that increase serum calcium concentrations may antagonize the effects of calcium channel antagonists.

Digoxin: Doses of calcium that increase serum calcium concentrations may increase the risk of cardiac arrhythmias.

Iron supplements: Oral absorption is decreased if taken together.

Tetracyclines: Oral absorption is decreased if taken together.

Patient Instructions: Best taken with a large glass of water before or during a meal. Do not take calcium within 1–2 hours of taking another medication (may impair absorption).

Table 1
Calcium Tablets and Costs

	Elemental Calcium (mg)	Vitamin D (IU)	Tablets/Day[a,b]	Cost[c]
Calcium carbonate, generic price	600	200	2	$3.59
Caltrate + D (Lederle)	600	200	2	$5.99
Os-Cal 500 (SK Beecham)	500	200	2	$5.25
Tums 500 (SK Beecham)	500		2	$4.49
Calcium citrate				
Citracal + D (Mission)	315	200	3	$8.24
Calcium Citrate + D (Nature Made)	315	200	3	$8.99
Calcium phosphate				
Posture-D (Selfcare)	600	125	2	$5.99

[a]Amount of elemental calcium and Vitamin D per tablet are shown

[b]Needed to provide 1,000–1,200 mg elemental calcium daily.

[c]Cost for a 30-day supply from an internet pharmacy.

Modified and reproduced with permission from *Med Lett* 2000;42:29–31.

Comments: Most studies show that calcium and vitamin D do not increase bone density. In subjects with inadequate calcium intake, they may slow bone loss. Calcium and vitamin D supplements are therefore only part of the treatment of established osteoporosis (see p. 278).

Clinical Pharmacology: Poor absorption; 20% is eliminated renally and 80% appears in the stool. Vitamin D is required for absorption.

Cost: $ (see Table 1)

BIBLIOGRAPHY

Anonymous. Calcium supplements. *Med Lett* 1996;38:108–109.

Caltrate (See Calcium)

CAPSAICIN

Trade Names: Zostrix, Capsin, Theragen, Trixaicin, Capsagel, Dolorac

Drug Class: Topical analgesic

Preparations
Cream: 0.025% (45- and 90-g tube); 0.075% (30- and 60-g tube)
Gel: 0.025% (15 and 30 g)
Lotion: 0.025% (59 mL), 0.075% (59 mL)
Roll-on: 0.075% (60 mL)

D R U G S

Dose: Apply to affected area three to four times daily. Less frequent application is less effective.

Indications: Postherpetic neuralgia, RA, osteoarthritis, diabetic neuropathy, chronic neuralgic pain

Mechanism of Action: Depletes peripheral sensory neurons of substance P, a mediator of pain.

Contraindications: Hypersensitivity to capsaicin

Precautions: Avoid contact with eyes, mucous membranes, genitalia, or open wounds. Wash hands immediately after applying.

Pregnancy Risk: C

Adverse Effects
Common: Transient sensation of burning when first applied that diminishes with use.
Less common: Erythema

Drug Interactions: None

Patient Instructions: For external use only. Do not apply to broken skin. Wash hands after use or use gloves. Avoid contact with eyes. Regular use is required for effect. Effect is slow; clinical benefits may take weeks or months. There is a transient sensation of burning when first applied.

Comments: The transient burning that occurs in most patients initially has made it difficult to perform true double-blind studies to assess efficacy. In practice, few patients derive clinically useful benefit from capsaicin in the treatment of pain owing to arthritis. Most suitable are patients with a few affected joints. The requirement for regular and frequent application and the slow onset of action over several weeks are disadvantages.

Clinical Pharmacology: Not known

Cost: $

BIBLIOGRAPHY

Zhang WY, Po ALW. The effectiveness of topically applied capsaicin. A meta-analysis. *Eur J Clin Pharmacol* 1994;46:517–522.

CARISOPRODOL

Trade Names: Rela, Soma

Drug Class: Skeletal muscle relaxant

Preparations
Tablet: 350 mg
Compound tablet: Carisoprodol 200 mg and aspirin 325 mg
Dose: Adults: 350 mg two to four times daily or 350 mg at night

Indications: Treatment of painful muscle spasm; useful in some patients with fibromyalgia

Mechanism of Action: Unknown; has a sedative effect and may modify pain perception

Contraindications: Hypersensitivity to carisoprodol; acute intermittent porphyria

Precautions: Use caution in renal or hepatic dysfunction.

Pregnancy Risk: C

Adverse Effects
Common: Drowsiness
Uncommon: Allergy, anaphylaxis, psychologic dependence and drug abuse, flushing, rash, nausea, fever, paradoxical stimulation, tremor, hematologic abnormalities

Drug Interactions
CNS depressants: Increased CNS depression
Increased toxicity: Alcohol, CNS depressants, phenothiazines, clindamycin, MAOIs

Patient Instructions: Avoid alcohol. It may cause drowsiness.

Comments: Nighttime sedative effect is sometimes useful in improving sleep and pain control in fibromyalgia.

Clinical Pharmacology: Rapid oral absorption, hepatic metabolism, renal excretion

Cost: $$

Celebrex (See Celecoxib)

CELECOXIB (ALSO SEE APPENDIX A)

Trade Names: Celebrex

Drug Class: COX-2 selective NSAID

Preparations
Capsules: 100 and 200 mg
Dose: 100–200 mg once or twice daily

DRUGS

Clinical Pharmacology: Well absorbed after oral administration; hepatic metabolism (CYP2C9) and renal excretion of metabolites; half-life 11 hours

Cost: $$$

Comments: COX-2 selective NSAIDs are no more effective than traditional NSAIDs that inhibit both COX-1 and COX-2, but they are less likely to cause GI complications. How a traditional NSAID with a proton pump inhibitor compares with a COX-2 selective NSAID as regards GI risk is not known. Either is a reasonable strategy for patients who have a high risk of GI complications and are unable to do without an NSAID. Therapy with low-dose aspirin and a COX-2–selective drug may abrogate the GI benefits of the COX-2 selectivity. Celecoxib is avoided if possible in patients allergic to sulfonamides. Fluconazole and other drugs that inhibit CYP2C9 increase concentrations of celecoxib.

See NSAIDs for Indications, Mechanism of Action, Contraindications, Precautions, Monitoring, Pregnancy Risk, Adverse Effects, Interactions, and Patient Instructions.

BIBLIOGRAPHY

FitzGerald GA, Patrono C. The coxibs, selective inhibitors of cyclooxygenase-2. *N Engl J Med* 2001;345:433–442.
Silverstein FE, Faich G, Goldstein JL, et al. Gastrointestinal toxicity with celecoxib vs non-steroidal anti-inflammatory drugs for osteoarthritis and rheumatoid arthritis: the CLASS study: a randomized controlled trial. Celecoxib Long-Term Arthritis Safety Study. *JAMA* 2000;284:1247–1255.

CellCept (See Mycophenolate)

CEVIMELINE

Trade Names: Evoxac

Drug Class: Cholinergic agent

Preparations: 30-mg capsule

Dose: 30 mg three times daily

Indications: Xerostomia, Sjögren's syndrome

Mechanism of Action: Stimulates muscarinic receptors to increase saliva production

Contraindications: Hypersensitivity to pilocarpine, iritis, uncontrolled asthma

Precautions: Asthma, GI ulceration, cardiovascular disease, urinary tract obstruction, gallstones

Pregnancy Risk: C

Adverse Effects
Common: Sweating
Less common: Nausea, rash, flushing, tachycardia, dizziness
Rare: Arrhythmia, cytopenias

Drug Interactions
Beta-blockers: Increased risk of cardiac conduction defects
Anticholinergic drugs: Decreased effect
Increased levels with CYP2D6 inhibitors (quinidine, fluoxetine, paroxetine, and others) and CYP3A inhibitors (erythromycin, azole antifungals, diltiazem, verapamil,

Patient Instructions: Expect increased sweating. It make take several weeks for response to occur. It may decrease visual acuity, particularly for night vision.

Clinical Pharmacology: Half-life 5 hours; hepatic metabolism CYP2D6 and CYP3A4

Cost: $$$

CHLORAMBUCIL

Trade Names: Leukeran

Drug Class: Alkylating agent

Preparations: 2-mg tablet

Dose: 0.05–0.2 mg/kg/day; usual dose range, 4–8 mg/day, with dose adjusted according to WBC count

Indications: Immunosuppressant, usually as an alternative for patients who cannot tolerate cyclophosphamide

Mechanism of Action: Alkylation and cross-linking of DNA strands interfering with DNA replication

Contraindications: Hypersensitivity, bone marrow suppression

Precautions: Teratogenic; can cause severe immunosuppression; carcinogenic; caution in renal impairment

DRUGS

Monitoring: CBC, platelet count, serum uric acid, and LFTs 1–2 weeks after initiation, then every 4 weeks

Pregnancy Risk: D

Adverse Effects
Common: Myelosuppression, rash, GI intolerance, oral ulceration
Less common: Confusion, seizures, sterility, pulmonary fibrosis, liver necrosis, drug fever, secondary malignancy

Drug Interactions
Immunosuppressants: Concurrent use of chlorambucil increases risk of myelosuppression and infection.

Patient Instructions: Avoid live virus vaccines. Avoid pregnancy. Regular monitoring is required.

Comments: When possible, AZA and MTX are used in preference to alkylating agents because the risk of secondary neoplasms is lower.

Clinical Pharmacology: Well absorbed; food decreases absorption 20%. Half-life 2 hours; hepatic metabolism and renal excretion of metabolites

Cost: $$$

BIBLIOGRAPHY
Steinberg AD. Chlorambucil in the treatment of patients with immune-mediated rheumatic diseases. *Arthritis Rheum* 1993;36:325–328.

Chloroquine (See Hydroxychloroquine)

CHLORZOXAZONE

Trade Names: Parafon Forte

Drug Class: Skeletal muscle relaxant, centrally acting

Preparations: 500-mg caplet; 250-mg tablet

Dose: Usual dose, 250–500 mg three to four times daily; to as high as 750 mg three to four times daily

Indications: Relief of muscle spasm. Questionable efficacy and potentially serious adverse effects limit indications.

Mechanism of Action: Acts via spinal cord and subcortical regions to decrease muscle tone

Contraindications: Hypersensitivity to chlorzoxazone, impaired liver function

Monitoring: LFTs periodically with long-term use

Pregnancy Risk: C

Adverse Effects
Common: Drowsiness, lightheadedness, allergy, rash, nausea, cramps
Less common: Hematologic toxicity (aplastic anemia, leukopenia), unpredictable fatal hepatotoxicity

Drug Interactions: CNS depressants have increased effect.

Patient Instructions: It may cause drowsiness. Avoid alcohol.

Clinical Pharmacology: Rapid absorption; hepatic metabolism and renal excretion of metabolites

Cost: $$

BIBLIOGRAPHY

Anonymous. Chlorzoxazone hepatotoxicity. *Med Lett* 1996;38:46.

CHOLINE MAGNESIUM TRISALICYLATE (ALSO SEE APPENDIX A, P. 527)

Trade Names: Trilisate, Tricosal

Drug Class: Nonacetylated salicylate, NSAID

Preparations
Liquid: 500 mg/5 mL
Tablets: 500, 750, 1000 mg

Dose: Adult: 500 mg to 1.5 g, two or three times daily; usual maintenance dose, 1.0–4.5 g/day

Indications: RA, osteoarthritis

Mechanism of Action: Weak inhibitor of prostaglandin synthesis

Contraindications: Hypersensitivity to salicylates

Precautions: Administer with food. Use caution in asthma, bleeding disorders, and hepatic or renal disease.

DRUGS

Monitoring: Monitor hematocrit, creatinine, LFTs periodically (1 month after starting and then every 3–6 months). Periodically check serum magnesium with high-dose therapy or in the presence of impaired renal function.

Pregnancy Risk: C/D third trimester

Adverse Effects
Common: GI irritation (dyspepsia, reflux, epigastric pain)
Less common: GI ulceration or hemorrhage; minor elevations of liver enzymes; hypersensitivity (asthma, urticaria, angioedema, particularly in patients with nasal polyps). Cross-sensitivity occurs between NSAIDs, but hypersensitivity is less common with the nonacetylated salicylates. Dose-related side effects include tinnitus and deafness.

Drug Interactions
Antacids: Decreased salicylate levels because of increased elimination in alkaline urine
Anticoagulants: Activity of warfarin is increased

Patient Instructions: Take with food. Discontinue and seek medical advice if unusual bleeding occurs.

Comments: Magnesium may accumulate in patients with renal impairment. Serum salicylate concentrations of 150–300 μg/mL are antiinflammatory. Nonacetylated salicylates have little effect on platelet function and cause less GI toxicity than classical NSAIDs, which are more potent inhibitors of prostaglandin synthesis.

Clinical Pharmacology: See Aspirin

Cost: $

CHOLINE SALICYLATE

Trade Names: Arthropan

Drug Class: Nonacetylated salicylate, NSAID

Preparations: Liquid, 870 mg/5 mL

Dose: Adult: 5–10 mL (870–1,740 mg) up to four times daily

Indications: RA, osteoarthritis in patients who cannot swallow tablets

Mechanism of Action: Weak inhibitor of prostaglandin synthesis

Contraindications: Hypersensitivity to salicylates

Precautions: Administer with food. Use caution in asthma, bleeding disorders, and hepatic or renal disease.

Monitoring: Monitor hematocrit, creatinine, liver enzymes periodically (1 month after starting and then every 12 months).

Cost: $

See Choline Magnesium Trisalicylate for Pregnancy Risk, Adverse Effects, Drug Interactions, Patient Instructions, Clinical Pharmacology, Comments.

Cimetidine (Tagamet; See Appendix C)

CISAPRIDE

Trade Names: Propulsid

Drug Class: Gastric motility stimulant

Preparations
Tablets: 10 and 20 mg
Suspension: 1 mg/mL

Dose: 10 mg 15 minutes before meals and before bedtime; some patients may require up to 20 mg per dose.

Indications: Refractory gastroparesis, gastroesophageal reflux disease, bowel hypomotility in scleroderma. Withdrawn from market in 2000, available through limited access protocol only

Mechanism of Action: Local release of acetylcholine

Contraindications: Hypersensitivity to cisapride; mechanical bowel obstruction; concomitant therapy with drugs that inhibit CYP P4503A (ketoconazole, fluconazole, itraconazole, miconazole, erythromycin, clarithromycin, troleandomycin, nefazodone, protease inhibitors and others); QT prolongation, therapy with drugs that prolong QT interval; uncorrected electrolyte disorder, cardiovascular disease

Precautions: Baseline ECG and electrolytes, evaluate risks and benefits carefully

Pregnancy Risk: C

Adverse Effects
Common: Rash, abdominal cramps, diarrhea, flatulence
Less common: Ventricular arrhythmias (torsade des pointes) particularly with overdose or concomitant use of drugs that inhibit metabolism (see Contraindications above).

DRUGS

Drug Interactions: Concomitant therapy with drugs that inhibit CYP3A (see Contraindications) increases concentrations of cisapride and increases risk of fatal arrhythmias

Patient Instructions: Cisapride may cause fatal arrhythmias. Do not exceed dose, do not start any new medication without checking with you physician

Comments: Potentially fatal arrhythmias and many drug interactions have resulted in the removal of cisapride from the general market.

Clinical Pharmacology: Bioavailability, 40%; metabolized (CYP3A substrate) to norcisapride and eliminated in urine; half-life 6–12 hours.

Cost: $$$$

BIBLIOGRAPHY

Sjogren RW. Gastrointestinal motility disorders in scleroderma. *Arthritis Rheum* 1994;37: 1265–1282.
Wysowski DK, Corken A, Gallo-Torres H, et al. Postmarketing reports of QT prolongation and ventricular arrhythmia in association with cisapride and Food and Drug Administration regulatory actions. *Am J Gastroenterol* 2001;96:1698–1703.

Clinoril (See Sulindac)

CODEINE (ALSO SEE ACETAMINOPHEN + OPIOIDS)

Synonyms: Codeine sulfate, codeine phosphate

Drug Class: Narcotic analgesic

Preparations
Tablets: 15, 30, 60 mg
Oral solution: 15 mg/5 mL

Dose: 15–30 mg q 4–6 h (maximum dose should not exceed 360 mg/24 h)

Indications: Pain not controlled by nonopioid drugs

Mechanism of Action: Binds to opioid receptors in CNS

Contraindications: Hypersensitivity to codeine; substance abuse

Precautions: Use caution in patients with hypersensitivity to other opioids, respiratory disease, or renal or hepatic impairment. Decrease dose if hepatic or renal impairment.

Monitoring: Make sure drug is used to control pain.

Pregnancy Risk: C; D in high doses

Adverse Effects
Common: Drowsiness, constipation, dysphoria, nausea
Less common: Rash, CNS stimulation, insomnia, seizures

Drug Interactions: Increased toxicity occurs with other CNS depressants. Avoid with MAOIs.

Patient Instructions: Drug is metabolized to morphine and is addictive. Use only to control pain. Do not use with alcohol or other CNS depressants.

Comments: Patients with low CYP2D6 activity (approximately 8% of the population) have a genetic inability to form morphine from codeine and derive no therapeutic effect from the drug. Codeine is commonly administered as an acetaminophen/codeine combination (see Acetaminophen + Opioid).

Clinical Pharmacology: Oral absorption; hepatic metabolism to morphine; urinary elimination as metabolites

Cost: $$

BIBLIOGRAPHY

Cherny NI. Opioid analgesics. Comparative features and prescribing guidelines. *Drugs* 1996;51:713–737.

COLCHICINE

Drug Class: Antigout agent

Preparations
Tablets: 0.5 and 0.6 mg
Injection: 0.5 mg/mL

Dose
Acute gout
Oral: 0.5 or 0.6 mg every 1–2 hours until pain is relieved, nausea/diarrhea develops, or maximum of 4 mg is administered
Intravenous: See Comment
Prophylaxis of gout: 0.5 or 0.6 mg once or twice daily

Indications: Treatment of acute gout and prophylaxis of acute gout; also used in the treatment of familial Mediterranean fever and amyloidosis

Mechanism of Action: Decreases leukocyte migration and phagocytosis

Contraindications: Hypersensitivity to colchicine; significant renal or hepatic impairment

Precautions: Use caution in renal or hepatic impairment; dose reduction is required.

Pregnancy Risk: C/D

Adverse Effects
Common: Nausea, vomiting, GI cramps, diarrhea
Less common: Neuropathy, myopathy, rash, bone marrow suppression, hepatic damage, alopecia

Drug Interactions
Cyclosporine: Increased risk of nephrotoxicity and myopathy
Cimetidine, erythromycin, tolbutamide: Increased colchicine concentrations

Patient Instructions: Discontinue if nausea or vomiting occurs.

Comments: In treatment of acute gout, colchicine is more effective if used early in the attack. Intravenous use of colchicine has been associated with fatalities and should generally be avoided. Depot corticosteroids (intramuscular or intraarticular) are safer and more effective than intravenous colchicine in patients in whom NSAIDs are contraindicated.

Clinical Pharmacology: Time to onset of action in gout is slow (6–12 hours); peak effect is 24–48 hours after first oral dose. Hepatic biotransformation (CYP3A substrate) and renal and hepatic elimination; high degree of tissue uptake, with only 10% of dose eliminated from the body in 24 hours.

Cost: $

BIBLIOGRAPHY

Moreland L, Ball GV. Colchicine and gout. *Arthritis Rheum* 1991;34:782–785.
Rott KT, Agudelo CA. Gout. *JAMA* 2003;289:2857–2860.
Terkeltaub RA. Clinical practice. Gout. *N Engl J Med* 2003;349:1647–1655.

CORTICOSTEROIDS

Trade Names
Oral
    Prednisone: Deltasone, Orasone
    Prednisolone: Delta-Cortef
    Methylprednisolone: Medrol
    Dexamethasone: Decadron, Dexone
Parenteral
    Methylprednisolone sodium succinate: Solu-Medrol

Hydrocortisone: Solu-Cortef
Dexamethasone: Decadron
Intraarticular
    Prednisolone tebutate suspension: Hydeltra TBA.
    Methylprednisolone acetate suspension: Depo-Medrol
    Triamcinolone acetonide suspension: Kenalog
    Triamcinolone diacetate suspension: Aristocort Forte
    Triamcinolone hexacetonide suspension: Aristospan Intra-articular

Drug Class: Glucocorticoid

Preparations
Oral
    Prednisone: 1-, 2.5-, 5-, 10-, 20-, 50-mg tablets
    Prednisolone: 2-, 4-, 8-, 16-, 24-mg tablets
    Dexamethasone: 0.25-, 0.5-, 0.75-, 1-, 1.5-, 2-, 4-, 6-mg
Parenteral
    Methylprednisolone sodium succinate injection: 40, 125, 500, 1,000,
        2,000 mg
    Hydrocortisone injection: 50, 100, 250, 500 mg
    Dexamethasone: 0.25, 0.5, 0.75, 1, 1.5, 2, 4, 6 mg
Intraarticular
    Methylprednisolone acetate suspension: 20, 40, 80 mg/mL
    Prednisolone tebutate suspension: 20 mg/mL
    Triamcinolone acetonide suspension: 10 and 40 mg/mL
    Triamcinolone diacetate suspension: 40 mg/mL
    Triamcinolone hexacetonide suspension: 20 mg/mL

Dose: Varies according to the indication. For serious inflammatory disease, give 1 mg/kg/day of prednisone or equivalent initially and titrate down according to response. (Adult dose ranges from 5 to 80 mg/day in divided doses.)

    Approximate equivalent doses for glucocorticoid efficacy: 0.75 mg dexamethasone = 4 mg methylprednisolone = 5 mg prednisone or prednisolone = 20 mg hydrocortisone. Intraarticular doses of depot steroid depend on the size of the joint.

Indications: Antiinflammatory or immunosuppressant therapy in a wide range of diseases including inflammatory arthritis, inflammatory muscle disease, vasculitis, SLE, and RA.

Mechanism of Action: A wide range of effects on numbers of inflammatory cells, their migration, and production of inflammatory mediators

Contraindications: Known hypersensitivity to a glucocorticoid preparation

Precautions: Use caution in diabetes, atherosclerosis, immunosuppression, hypertension, osteoporosis, infection, peptic ulcer, and cirrhosis.

DRUGS

Because of dose-related adverse effects, the minimum effective dose should be used. After prolonged glucocorticoid therapy, acute adrenal insufficiency may occur if the glucocorticoid is discontinued abruptly. After discontinuation of glucocorticoid therapy, the hypothalamus-pituitary-adrenal axis may remain suppressed for as long as a year, so supplementary doses of glucocorticoid are required during acute stress such as surgery.

Monitoring: Monitor for adverse effects with long-term therapy: potassium and glucose concentrations and bone density measurement and osteoporosis prophylaxis or treatment (with long-term use).

Pregnancy Risk: C

Adverse Effects: Most are dose related. Almost all patients on high doses for more than a few weeks experience adverse effects, including cushingoid appearance, weight gain, skin fragility, bruising, edema, hypertension, diabetes, hypokalemia, atherosclerosis, cataracts, infection, insomnia, mood swings, psychosis, GI ulceration with NSAIDs, myopathy, osteoporosis, and fractures. Suppression of the hypothalamus-pituitary-adrenal axis and acute adrenal insufficiency may occur if therapy is discontinued suddenly or with severe physiologic stress (major surgery) after therapy has been discontinued.

Drug Interactions
Hepatic enzyme inducers (rifampin, phenytoin, phenobarbitone): Decreased effect of corticosteroids
Diuretics: Increased potassium depletion

Patient Instructions: Corticosteroids should not be discontinued suddenly. Before a procedure or surgery, notify your surgeon or doctor that you are receiving corticosteroids. Careful attention to diet is necessary to avoid significant weight gain.

Comments: Marked leukocytosis and neutrophilia occur after even a single dose of glucocorticoid, and if the cause is not recognized, an unnecessary infection workup results.

Adverse effects are related to dose and duration of therapy. Once disease control has been established, high doses of steroids may be tapered relatively rapidly with 5- to 10-mg decrements at doses between 40 and 60 mg. Lower doses require a more gradual taper. Between 20 and 40 mg, taper in 5-mg decrements; between 10 and 20 mg, taper in 2.5-mg decrements, and <10 mg, taper in 1-mg decrements. A common error is tapering high doses too slowly and low doses too fast, resulting in adverse effects and disease flare, respectively.

Triamcinolone hexacetonide is the least soluble intraarticular preparation and has the longest duration of action. Triamcinolone or other fluorinated corticosteroid preparations should not be used for injection of soft tissue or bursae because marked atrophy of soft tissue may result. Methylprednisolone/ prednisolone preparations can be used for such soft tissue injections.

Clinical Pharmacology: Prednisone is inactive until metabolized to prednisolone. Hepatic conversion is rapid and complete. Plasma half-life of prednisone/prednisolone is 3–4 hours, but the biologic effect lasts 18–36 hours.

Dexamethasone has almost no mineralocorticoid effect. It is more potent than prednisone/prednisolone but more difficult to titrate clinically.

Depot injection preparations, either intraarticularly or intramuscularly, provide low plasma concentrations of steroid for 2–4 weeks.

Cost: $

BIBLIOGRAPHY

American College of Rheumatology ad hoc Committee on Glucocorticoid-Induced Osteoporosis. Recommendations for the prevention and treatment of glucocorticoid-induced osteoporosis: 2001 update. *Arthritis Rheum* 2001;44:1496–1503.
McCarthy GM, McCarty DJ. Intrasynovial corticosteroid therapy. *Bull Rheum Dis* 1994;43:2–4.
Stein CM, Pincus T. Glucocorticoids. In: Kelley WN, Harris ED, Ruddy S, et al., eds. *Textbook of Rheumatology,* 5th ed. Philadelphia: WB Saunders, 1997:787–803.

Cuprimine (See Penicillamine)

CYCLOBENZAPRINE

Trade Names: Flexeril

Drug Class: Muscle relaxant

Preparations: 10-mg tablet

Dose: 20–40 mg/day in two divided doses (maximum dosing should not exceed 60 mg/day)

Indications: Muscle spasm, fibromyalgia

Mechanism of Action: Centrally acting skeletal muscle relaxant; related to tricyclic antidepressants

Contraindications: Hypersensitivity to cyclobenzaprine. Do not use within 14–21 days of an MAOI.

Precautions: As for tricyclics: heart failure, arrhythmias, urinary obstruction

Pregnancy Risk: B

Adverse Effects
Common: Anticholinergic effects (dry mouth, difficulty urinating), drowsiness
Less common: Dizziness, blurred vision, weakness, allergy, GI symptoms, headache, confusion, arrhythmias

D
R
U
G
S

Drug Interactions
Tricyclic antidepressants: Additive toxicity
CNS depressants (alcohol, benzodiazepines): Increased effect
MAOIs: Hypertensive crisis

Patient Instructions: Causes drowsiness; may impair ability to drive

Comments: Sedative effect is useful at night.

Clinical Pharmacology: Rapid, complete oral absorption; hepatic metabolism and renal elimination of metabolites

Cost: $$

CYCLOPHOSPHAMIDE (ALSO SEE APPENDIX B)

Trade Names: Cytoxan, Neosar

Synonyms: CTX, CYT

Drug Class: Cancer chemotherapeutic; alkylating agent

Preparations
Tablets: 25 and 50 mg
Powder for injection: 100, 200, 500 mg; 1 and 2 g

Dose: Varies according to indication and patient response
Oral dose: 50–100 mg/m^2/day or 1–3 mg/kg/day
Intravenous infusion: Pulse dose of 500–1,000 mg/m^2 repeated every 21–28 days. Adjust dose according to clinical response and WBC nadir and recovery. In SLE nephritis, after 6–12 months of monthly infusions, the frequency of infusions may be gradually decreased to every 3 months.

Indications: Vasculitis, rheumatoid vasculitis, SLE with organ involvement, polymyositis/dermatomyositis refractory to treatment

Mechanism of Action: Interferes with DNA synthesis by alkylating and cross-linking DNA strands

Contraindications: Hypersensitivity to cyclophosphamide; pregnancy

Precautions: Bone marrow suppression, active infection; decrease dose in renal/hepatic impairment, avoid live virus vaccines, consider dose reduction if renal or hepatic function impaired

Monitoring: Frequent monitoring of CBC and platelets is required. Nadir of WBC occurs 10–14 days after a single dose. A WBC nadir of 3,000/mm³ is used as a target for intravenous pulses.

With long-term use, monitor urinalysis for blood. During and after long-term oral use, monitor for bladder cancer with urinalysis, cytology, and (if needed) cystoscopy.

Pregnancy Risk: D.

Adverse Effects: Dose and duration dependent; myelosuppression (WBC more than platelets), infections (usual bacterial and viral infections and opportunistic organisms). Hemorrhagic cystitis is more common with daily oral regimens. Gonadal suppression and permanent infertility occur. Risk of ovarian failure is greater with oral regimens and increases in frequency with increased age of female patients. GI symptoms increase with dose. Pulmonary fibrosis, rashes, hypersensitivity, and fluid retention occur. Long-term risk of secondary malignancy: bladder, lymphoma, leukemia, and skin cancers.

Drug Interactions
Allopurinol: Increases myelosuppression of cyclophosphamide
Thiazide diuretics: May cause prolonged leukopenia
Immunosuppressants: Concurrent therapy increases risk of myelosuppression and infection
Digoxin: Cyclophosphamide may decrease serum digoxin levels

Patient Instructions: Take as a single dose in the morning and drink lots of liquids to keep urine diluted. Empty bladder frequently. Report blood in urine. Avoid live virus vaccines. Regular follow-up is essential. Report any significant fever. Use reliable contraception.

Comments: Life-threatening complications may occur with cyclophosphamide treatment. Titrate dose according to WBC count. Oral regimens are preferred by many for vasculitis, and the less toxic monthly intravenous regimen is preferred for SLE. Duration of cyclophosphamide therapy is empirical, but after disease remission, the frequency of infusions can often be decreased to every 3 months. Premedicate with antiemetic regimen and continue antiemetic prophylaxis for 24–48 hours.

Mesna (see Mesna) intravenously initially and then orally may be used with intravenous regimens to protect against hemorrhagic cystitis.

Clinical Pharmacology: Good rapid oral absorption; hepatic metabolism to several active metabolites including 4-hydroxycyclophosphamide. Plasma half-life is 2–10 hours. Metabolites are eliminated in the urine. Acrolein is the urinary metabolite thought to cause hemorrhagic cystitis.

Cost: $$$$

DRUGS

BIBLIOGRAPHY

Fraiser LH, Kanekal S, Kehrer JP. Cyclophosphamide toxicity-characterizing and avoiding the problem. *Drugs* 1991;42:781–795.

Stein CM. Immunoregulatory drugs. In: Harris ED, Ruddy S, Sledge CB eds. *Kelley's textbook of Rheumatology*, 7th ed. Philadelphia: WB Saunders, 2004.

Steinberg AD, Gourley M. Cyclophosphamide in lupus nephritis. *J Rheumatol* 1995;22: 1812–1815.

CYCLOSPORINE (ALSO SEE APPENDIX B, P. 529)

Trade Names: Sandimmune, Neoral

Synonyms: Cyclosporin A, CyA, CSA

Drug Class: Immunosuppressant, DMARD

Preparations
Soft gelatin capsules: 25, 50, 100 mg
Oral liquid: 100 mg/mL
Injection: 50 mg/mL

Dose: Starting dose in autoimmune disease is 2.5 mg/kg/day orally in divided doses. Calculate dose according to approximate ideal body weight in obese patients. After 8–12 weeks, the dose may be increased monthly by 0.5 mg/kg/day to maximum of 4 mg/kg/day. The risk of renal disease increases with doses >4 mg/kg/day. Minimum effective dose is between 2 and 3 mg/kg/day. The dose of the two preparations available (Neoral and Sandimmune) is similar. However, if switching from Sandimmune to Neoral, lower doses of Neoral may be required.

Indications: RA refractory to standard DMARD treatment; also approved for use in psoriasis; anecdotal reports of efficacy in psoriatic arthritis, SLE, myositis, Behçet syndrome, and pyoderma gangrenosum

Mechanism of Action: Inhibits production of IL-2; immunomodulator

Contraindications: Hypersensitivity to cyclosporine; immunodeficiency; renal failure

Precautions: Avoid if past or present malignancy, uncontrolled hypertension, or renal or hepatic dysfunction. Avoid live virus vaccines.

Monitoring: Monitor blood pressure and creatinine every 2 weeks for first 2–3 months and then monthly if stable. If creatinine rises by >30% above baseline values, reduce dose of cyclosporine by 0.5 mg/kg/day and check again in a week. Continue dose reduction until the creatinine concentration is back within 30% of baseline. Elevations of creatinine level (>30% of baseline), even if within the normal range, require action. Monitor potassium and uric acid levels, and hepatic enzymes every 1–3 months.

Pregnancy Risk: C

Adverse Effects
Common: Hypertension, increased creatinine, hirsutism, nausea, cramps, tremor, gingival hypertrophy, hyperkalemia, hypomagnesemia, hyperuricemia
Less common: Seizures, headache, muscle cramps, allergy, myositis, pancreatitis, infection, lymphoma

Drug Interactions
Increased concentrations of cyclosporine: Grapefruit juice, azithromycin, clarithromycin, erythromycin, ketoconazole, fluconazole, itraconazole, diltiazem, verapamil, nicardipine, protease inhibitors, and others
Decreased cyclosporine concentrations: rifampicin, phenytoin, phenobarbital, carbamazepine, isoniazid
K^+-sparing diuretics: hyperkalemia
Lovastatin: increased risk of myopathy, rhabdomyolysis, acute renal failure
Nephrotoxic drugs: increased nephrotoxicity

Patient Instructions: Avoid sunlight (skin cancer). Regular blood monitoring is required.

Comments: Neoral is a newer microemulsion formulation of cyclosporine that gives a more favorable pharmacokinetic profile with higher peak levels and less inter- and intraindividual variability in levels. Efficacy and toxicity of Neoral and Sandimmune are similar.
     There is limited long-term safety data for cyclosporine in RA. Cyclosporine as a single agent in RA is no more effective than other available drugs. The combination of MTX and cyclosporine is more effective than MTX alone, but limited safety data exist for this combination. The use of NSAIDs is permitted in patients with RA taking cyclosporine, and in many studies, they have been used together. However, NSAIDs may be stopped if renal function declines while taking cyclosporine. Monitoring blood levels of cyclosporine is a poor predictor of efficacy and toxicity in autoimmune disease and is seldom indicated (e.g., assessing compliance, absorption, drug interaction).

Clinical Pharmacology: Cyclosporine is variably and erratically absorbed. The Neoral formulation has more predictable bioavailability. Hepatic metabolism is by CYP3A enzymes, which is the source of the multiple drug interactions with cyclosporine. Renal excretion of metabolites.

Cost: $$$$

DRUGS

BIBLIOGRAPHY

American College of Rheumatology Committee on Rheumatoid Arthritis Guidelines. Guidelines for the management of rheumatoid arthritis: 2002 update. *Arthritis Rheum* 2002;46:328–346.

Panayi G, Tugwell P. The use of cyclosporin A in rheumatoid arthritis: conclusions of an international review. *Br J Rheumatol* 1994;33:967–969.

Stein CM. Immunoregulatory drugs. In: Harris ED, Ruddy S, Sledge CB eds. *Kelley's textbook of Rheumatology*, 7th ed. Philadelphia: WB Saunders, 2004.

Cytotec (See Misoprostol)
Cytoxan (See Cyclophosphamide)

DANAZOL

Trade Names: Danocrine

Drug Class: Attenuated androgen-gonadotropin inhibitor

Preparations: 50-, 100-, 200-mg capsules

Dose: Hereditary angioedema, 400–600 mg/day in two or three divided doses; decrease if favorable response

Indications: Hereditary angioedema prophylaxis, fibrocystic breast disease, endometriosis, SLE, or idiopathic thrombocytopenic purpura with refractory thrombocytopenia

Mechanism of Action: Prevents attacks of angioedema by increasing concentrations of C1 esterase inhibitor and thus C4; suppresses ovarian production of pituitary gonadotropins and ovarian hormone production; has weak androgenic effects

Contraindications: Hypersensitivity, pregnancy, significant renal or hepatic impairment, undiagnosed vaginal bleeding, androgen-dependent tumors

Precautions: Thromboembolic disease, hepatic or renal dysfunction, seizure disorders, migraines, cardiac disease

Pregnancy Risk: X

Adverse Effects
Common: Androgenic effects (hirsutism, irregular menstrual cycles, intercycle menstrual bleeding, weight gain); fluid retention
Less common: Cholestatic jaundice or liver dysfunction, pancreatitis, leukopenia, thrombocytopenia, rashes, benign intracranial hypertension

Drug Interactions: Increased effects of warfarin, carbamazepine, hypoglycemics, cyclosporine, tacrolimus. Rhabdomyolysis with statins.

Patient Instructions: Nonhormonal contraception is recommended. Avoid sunlight because of photosensitivity.

Clinical Pharmacology: Hepatic metabolism and renal excretion; half-life 4–6 hours

Cost: $$$$

Danocrine (See Danazol)

DANTROLENE SODIUM

Trade Names: Dantrium

Synonyms: Dantrolene

Drug Class: Antispasticity agent

Preparations
Capsules: 25, 50, 100 mg
Injection: 20 mg powder for injection

Dose: Orally, initially 25 mg/day, increased at weekly intervals to a maximum of 100 mg two to four times daily

Indications: Muscle spasticity associated with upper motor neuron lesions; prevention and treatment of malignant hyperthermia

Mechanism of Action: Acts on the sarcoplasmic reticulum of muscle to inhibit release of calcium

Contraindications: Hepatic dysfunction

Precautions: Use caution if cardiac or pulmonary function is impaired.

Monitoring: LFTs before and at intervals during therapy

Pregnancy Risk: C

Adverse Effects
Common: Drowsiness, dizziness, fatigue, rash, GI symptoms such as diarrhea, cramps, and vomiting
Less common: Pleural or pericardial effusion, seizures, respiratory depression, speech and visual disturbances, hepatotoxicity (especially in women older than 30 taking estrogens). Hepatotoxicity may occasionally be fatal.

Drug Interactions
Hepatotoxic medications: Increased risk of hepatotoxicity
Estrogens: Increased hepatotoxicity

DRUGS

CNS depressant effects: Additive depressant effect
Additional drug interactions: MAOIs, phenothiazines, clindamycin, verapamil, warfarin, clofibrate, and tolbutamide

Patient Instructions: Avoid alcohol and CNS depressants; may cause drowsiness.

Comments: Baclofen is usually tried first.

Clinical Pharmacology: Poor absorption from GI tract; hepatic metabolism;
half-life 9 hours

Cost: $$$$

DAPSONE

Trade Names: Avlosulfon

Drug Class: Sulfone bacteriostatic

Preparations: 25- and 100-mg tablets

Dose: 50 mg/day initially, increased by 25- to 50-mg increments to as high as
200 mg/day

Indications: Skin lesions of systemic or discoid lupus erythematosus, urticarial vasculitis, and pyoderma gangrenosum; has been used in relapsing polychondritis and RA. Nonrheumatologic uses include leprosy, malaria, prophylaxis of *Pneumocystis carinii,* and dermatitis herpetiformis.

Mechanism of Action: Immunomodulatory mechanism unknown; has sul-
fonamide-like action competing for p-aminobenzoic acid and preventing bacterial synthesis of folic acid

Contraindications: Hypersensitivity to dapsone

Precautions: Use caution in patients allergic to sulfonamides, G6PD deficiency, and severe anemia.

Monitoring: Determine G6PD status before treatment of patients from ethnic
groups at greater risk. Monitor CBC in all patients initially weekly, then
monthly, and then every 2–3 months. Monitor LFTs at intervals.

Pregnancy Risk: C

Adverse Effects
Common: Rash, dose-related hemolysis, and methemoglobinemia

Less common: GI intolerance, leukopenia, agranulocytosis, exfoliative dermatitis, hepatitis, cholestatic jaundice

Drug Interactions
Rifampin: Decreased effect of dapsone
Folic acid antagonists (trimethoprim, sulfonamides): Increased toxicity

Patient Instructions: Regular blood monitoring is required. May cause photosensitivity.

Comments: The incidence of hemolytic anemia can be reduced by using concomitant antioxidant therapy (vitamin E or C).

Clinical Pharmacology: Well absorbed; acetylated in the liver. Acetylator phenotype (slow or fast) does not affect clinical use. CYP P-450–mediated hydroxylation; renal elimination of metabolites; half-life 30 hours

Cost: $$

BIBLIOGRAPHY

Stein CM. Immunoregulatory drugs. In: Harris ED, Ruddy S, Sledge CB eds. *Kelley's textbook of Rheumatology,* 7th ed. Philadelphia: WB Saunders, 2004.

Darvocet (See Acetaminophen + Opioid)
Daypro (See Oxaprozin)
Demerol (See Meperidine)
Depen (See Penicillamine)
Depo-Medrol (See Corticosteroids, Intraarticular)
Desyrel (See Trazodone)
Dexamethasone (See Corticosteroids)

DICLOFENAC (SEE APPENDIX A)

Trade Names: Cataflam (immediate release), Voltaren (enteric coated, extended release), Voltaren XR, Arthrotec (diclofenac + misoprostol)

Drug Class: NSAID

Preparations
Tablets: 25, 50, 75 mg; diclofenac/misoprostol: 50 mg/200 µg or 75 mg/200 µg
Sustained-release tablet (XR): 100 mg

Dose: 100–200 mg/day in two to four divided doses (100 mg/day of sustained release)

Clinical Pharmacology: Well absorbed after oral administration; hepatic metabolism and renal excretion of metabolites; half-life 2–3 hours.

Cost: $$$

See NSAIDs for Indications, Mechanism of Action, Contraindications, Precautions, Monitoring, Pregnancy Risk, Adverse Effects, Interactions, and Patient Instructions.

See Misoprostol for details regarding that component of Arthrotec (diclofenac + misoprostol).

Didronel (See Etidronate)

DIFLUNISAL

Trade Names: Dolobid

Drug Class: NSAID

Preparations: 250- and 500-mg tablets

Dose: 500–1,500 mg/day in two to three divided doses

Clinical Pharmacology: Well absorbed after oral administration; hepatic metabolism and renal excretion of metabolites; half-life 8–12 hours

Cost: $$$

See NSAIDs for Indications, Mechanism of Action, Contraindications, Precautions, Monitoring, Pregnancy Risk, Adverse Effects, Interactions, and Patient Instructions.

Disalcid (See Salsalate)
DMARDs/SAARDs/SMARDs (See Appendix B)
Dolobid (See Diflunisal)
Doxepin (Sinequan; See Appendix D)
Duragesic (See Fentanyl)
Easprin (See Aspirin)
Ecotrin (See Aspirin)

EDROPHONIUM CHLORIDE

Trade Names: Tensilon, Enlon, Reversol

Drug Class: Short-acting cholinesterase inhibitor

Preparations: Injection, 10 mg/mL (1 mL)

Dose: Diagnostic test for myasthenia gravis: 2 mg i.v. over 15–30 seconds; then, if no response is seen, 8 mg 45 seconds later

Indications: Diagnostic test for myasthenia gravis; used to differentiate cholinergic crisis from myasthenic crisis

Mechanism of Action: Increases acetylcholine concentrations by inhibiting its breakdown by acetylcholinesterase

Contraindications: Hypersensitivity to edrophonium or sulfites; GI or genitourinary obstruction

Precautions: May worsen weakness if this is caused by overtreatment (cholinergic crisis); intravenous atropine must be available to treat cholinergic symptoms. Use with caution in patients with asthma or those receiving cardiac glycosides.

Monitoring: Must be administered under medical supervision with resuscitation facilities on hand.

Pregnancy Risk: C

Adverse Effects
Common: Cholinergic symptoms: nausea, vomiting, cramps, diarrhea, salivation, sweating, small pupils, lacrimation
Less common: Bradycardia, seizures, hypersensitivity, bronchospasm, laryngospasm

Drug Interactions: Anticholinesterases neostigmine and physostigmine show increased effect.

Clinical Pharmacology: Onset of action is within 60 seconds; duration of effect is 10 minutes.

Cost: $$$

Elavil (See Amitriptyline)
Enbrel (See Etanercept)

DRUGS

Equagesic (See Meprobamate and Aspirin)
Esomeprazole (Nexium; See Appendix C)

EPOPROSTENOL

Trade Names: Flolan

Synonyms: Prostacyclin, PGI2

Drug Class: Prostaglandin

Preparations: Injection: 0.5- and 1.5-mg vials

Dose: Administered by a pump as a continuous intravenous infusion through a central line. The usual starting dose is 2 ng/kg/min, and the dose is titrated up depending on clinical response and adverse effects.

Indications: Primary pulmonary hypertension, pulmonary hypertension associated with connective tissue diseases

Mechanism of Action: Prostacyclin is a potent vasodilator and also decreases platelet aggregation.

Contraindications: Hypersensitivity, heart failure with severe left ventricular systolic dysfunction

Precautions: Sudden discontinuation of drug can cause rebound pulmonary hypertension.

Monitoring: Monitor closely for clinical response, adverse effects, pump dysfunction, status of central line and adherence to therapy.

Pregnancy Risk: B

Adverse Effects
Common: Flushing, tachycardia, GI side effects (nausea, vomiting, diarrhea, cramps), dizziness, headache, jaw pain, tremor
Less common: Hypotension, syncope, angina, edema, rash, anemia, central line infection

Drug Interactions: May potentiate the hypotensive effects of other vasodilators or antihypertensive drugs

Patient Instructions: Therapy requires care of a central line, wearing a pump, and self-administration of drug. Dose titration is required. Do not discontinue the drug suddenly.

Comments: Epoprostenol is only prescribed by physicians expert in the management of pulmonary hypertension, generally cardiologists or pulmonologists with a special interest in pulmonary hypertension. In clinical trials, the 6-minute walk distance improved in patients with scleroderma with pulmonary hypertension treated with epoprostenol. There are reports of digital ulcers or digital ischemia improving.

Clinical Pharmacology: Rapidly hydrolyzed in blood, half-life 5 minutes

Cost: $$$$$

BIBLIOGRAPHY

Badesch DB, Tapson VF, McGoon MD, et al. Continuous intravenous epoprostenol for pulmonary hypertension due to the scleroderma spectrum of disease. A randomized, controlled trial. *Ann Intern Med* 2000;132:425–434.

ETANERCEPT

Trade Names: Enbrel

Drug Class: DMARD, TNF antagonist

Preparations: 25-mg injection

Dose: 25 mg by subcutaneous injection twice weekly or 50 mg once weekly

Indications: RA, psoriatic arthritis, ankylosing spondylitis, juvenile RA

Mechanism of Action: Etanercept is a dimer of p75 TNF receptors fused to the Fc portion of IgG1. The addition of IgG1 increases the half-life. Etanercept binds TNF-α and TNF-β and blocks its ability to bind with its receptor on the cell.

Contraindications: Hypersensitivity, untreated tuberculosis or other opportunistic infections, sepsis, active infections, chronic localized or recurrent infections, demyelinating disease, optic neuritis or heart failure

Precautions: Exclude latent tuberculosis with a skin test before starting therapy. In RA, 5 mm of induration indicates latent or active tuberculosis. Be aware that the risk of opportunistic infections is increased. Caution should be exercised if used in the debilitated or in those at high risk of infection. Avoid live virus vaccines. Influenza and pneumococcal vaccines appear to be unaffected by such therapy. It should not be used in combination with anakinra (increased risk of serious infection).

Monitoring: Monitor clinically for infection.

DRUGS

Pregnancy Risk: B

Adverse Effects

Common: Injection site reactions, positive antinuclear antibody, positive DNA antibody

Less common: Allergy, infection (bacterial, but particularly opportunistic infections such as tuberculosis, listeriosis, and histoplasmosis)

Rare: Lymphoma, hepatitis, demyelinating CNS disorders, optic neuritis, seizures, pancytopenia, drug-induced lupus

Drug Interactions: Concurrent use of other immunosuppressants may increase risk of infection.

Patient Instructions: Avoid live virus vaccines. Avoid pregnancy. Stop injections if an infection develops that requires antibiotics or a fever develops that lasts more than a few days.

Comments: TNF antagonists are among the most effective treatments for RA. Patients respond quickly, usually within 4–6 weeks. However, not all patients respond. Combined therapy with MTX is more effective than either drug alone. The role of TNF antagonists in a range of diseases such as psoriasis, vasculitis, seronegative spondyloarthropathy, sarcoidosis, and inflammatory eye disease is being explored. The comparative risk of adverse effects such as tuberculosis, lymphoma, and demyelinating disease with individual TNF antagonists is not clear. Until this information is available, these side effects should be considered similar and regarded as a class effect.

Clinical Pharmacology: Half-life is 4–5 days. Biologic agents are not metabolized and thus have few drug interactions.

Cost: $$$$$

BIBLIOGRAPHY

Bathon JM, Martin RW, Fleischmann RM, et al. A comparison of etanercept and methotrexate in patients with early rheumatoid arthritis. *N Engl J Med* 2000;343:1586–1593.

American College of Rheumatology Subcommittee on Rheumatoid Arthritis Guidelines. Guidelines for the management of rheumatoid arthritis: 2002 update. *Arthritis Rheum* 2002;46:328–346.

Mease PJ, Goffe BS, Metz J, et al. Etanercept in the treatment of psoriatic arthritis and psoriasis: a randomised trial. *Lancet* 2000;356:385–390.

Olsen NJ, Stein CM. New drugs for rheumatoid arthritis. *N Engl J Med* 2004;350:2167–2179.

Weinblatt ME, Kremer JM, Bankhurst AD, et al. A trial of etanercept, a recombinant tumor necrosis factor receptor:Fc fusion protein, in patients with rheumatoid arthritis receiving methotrexate. *N Engl J Med* 1999;340:253–259.

ETIDRONATE

Trade Names: Didronel

Synonyms: Disodium etidronate, sodium etidronate

Drug Class: Bisphosphonate

Preparations
Tablets: 200 and 400 mg
Injection: 50 mg/mL (6 mL)

Dose
Newer bisphosphonates preferred (see Comments)
Paget's disease: 5 mg/kg/day orally for as long as 6 months
Osteoporosis: 400 mg for 14 days every 3 months; calcium (1 g/day) and vitamin D (400 U/day) supplementation is usual

Indications: Paget's disease, hypercalcemia of malignancy, heterotopic calcification after hip replacement, osteoporosis

Mechanism of Action: Adsorbs onto hydroxyapatite crystals and blocks their aggregation and growth

Contraindications: Hypersensitivity to bisphosphonates; severe renal impairment; osteomalacia; Paget's disease with lytic lesions that have a risk of fracture

Precautions: Reduce dose in mild renal impairment.

Monitoring: In Paget's disease, alkaline phosphatase and urinary hydroxyproline are monitored as mea .res of response to treatment.

Pregnancy Risk: B

Adverse Effects
Common: Nausea, diarrhea, metallic taste
Less common: Increased bone pain in Paget's disease, osteomalacia with increased risk of fractures, constipation, hypocalcemia, hypersensitivity, seizures

Drug Interactions
Antacids: Decreased bioavailability of etidronate
Calcium: If taken together, decreased bioavailability of etidronate

Patient Instructions: Take on an empty stomach (2 hours before meals). Supplement calcium and vitamin D intake.

Comments: Alendronate and risedronate are FDA approved for treatment of osteoporosis; etidronate is not. The newer bisphosphonates are less likely to cause osteomalacia than etidronate, are more potent, and are generally favored over etidronate.

Clinical Pharmacology: Absorption 1%–5%; no metabolism; renal excretion. Half of absorbed dose is eliminated in 24 hours; the rest binds to calcium phosphate surfaces and is eliminated over months to years.

DRUGS

Cost: $$$

ETODOLAC (ALSO SEE APPENDIX A, P. 527)

Trade Names: Lodine, Lodine XL

Synonyms: Etodolic acid

Drug Class: NSAID

Preparations
Capsules: 200 and 300 mg
Tablets: 400 and 500 mg
Tablets, extended release (XL): 400, 500, 600 mg

Dose: 200–400 mg two or three times daily; maximum daily dose 20 mg/kg for patient weighing <60 kg. Extended release 400–1,000 mg once daily.

Clinical Pharmacology: Well absorbed after oral administration; hepatic metabolism and renal excretion of metabolites; half-life 7 hours

Comments: Compared with traditional, older NSAIDs, somewhat COX-2 "preferential" and some evidence suggesting less GI toxicity

Cost: $$$

See NSAIDs for Indications, Mechanism of Action, Contraindications, Precautions, Monitoring, Pregnancy Risk, Adverse Effects, Interactions, and Patient Instructions.

Evoxac (See Cevimeline)
Famotidine (Pepcid; See Appendix C)
Feldene (See Piroxicam)

FENOPROFEN (ALSO SEE APPENDIX A)

Trade Names: Nalfon

Synonyms: Fenoprofen calcium

Drug Class: NSAID

Preparations
Capsules: 200 and 300 mg
Tablet: 600 mg

Dose: 300–600 mg three to four times daily; maximum dose not to exceed 3.2 g/day

Clinical Pharmacology: Well absorbed after oral administration; hepatic metabolism and renal excretion of metabolites; half-life 3 hours

Cost: $$

See NSAIDs for Indications, Mechanism of Action, Contraindications, Precautions, Monitoring, Pregnancy Risk, Adverse Effects, Interactions and Patient Instructions

FENTANYL

Trade Names: Duragesic, Sublimaze

Drug Class: Opioid analgesic

Preparations: Transdermal system: 25 μg/h (10 cm^2), 50 μg/h (20 cm^2), 75 μg/h (30 cm^2), 100 μg/h (40 cm^2)

Dose: For adult pain control, initially use the transdermal 25 μg/h system and titrate according to response. Most patients require application every 72 hours. Apply to dry, nonhairy skin on trunk or upper arms.

Indications: Chronic intractable pain

Mechanism of Action: Binds to opioid receptors in CNS.

Contraindications: Hypersensitivity to fentanyl; substance abuse

Precautions: Use caution in patients with hypersensitivity to other opioids, respiratory disease, or renal or hepatic impairment. Decrease dose if hepatic or renal impairment.

Monitoring: Ensure that drug is used to control pain.

Pregnancy Risk: B (D in high doses)

Adverse Effects
Common: Drowsiness, constipation, dysphoria, nausea, hypotension, bradycardia
Less common: CNS stimulation, insomnia, seizures, respiratory depression, dependence, itching, hives

Drug Interactions
CNS depressants: Increased toxicity
MAOIs: Risk of hypertensive crisis

D
R
U
G
S

Patient Instructions: Drug is addictive. Use only to control pain. Do not use with alcohol or other CNS depressants.

Comments: The respiratory depressant effect may last longer than the analgesic effect. Absorption from the patch increases in patients with fever. Patch is suitable for continuous pain, but its slow onset of action makes it unsuitable for immediate pain control.

Clinical Pharmacology: Slow absorption from transdermal preparation; hepatic metabolism and urinary elimination as metabolites. After application of a new dose, evaluate analgesic effect after 24 hours.

Cost: $$$$

BIBLIOGRAPHY

Cherny NI. Opioid analgesics. Comparative features and prescribing guidelines. *Drugs* 1996;51:713–737.

Jeal W, Benfield P. Transdermal fentanyl. A review of its pharmacological properties and therapeutic efficacy in pain control. *Drugs* 1997;53:109–138.

Ferrous Sulfate, Ferrous Gluconate (See Iron Preparations)

Flexeril (See Cyclobenzaprine)

Flolan (See Epoprostenol)

FLURBIPROFEN

Trade Names: Ansaid

Drug Class: NSAID

Preparations: 50- and 100-mg tablets

Dose: 200–400 mg/day in two to four divided doses

Clinical Pharmacology: Well absorbed after oral administration; renal elimination; half-life 4 hours

Cost: $$

See NSAIDs for Indications, Mechanism of Action, Contraindications, Precautions, Monitoring, Pregnancy Risk, Adverse Effects, Interactions, and Patient Instructions.

Fluoxetine (Prozac; See Appendix D)

FOLIC ACID

Trade Names: Folvite

Synonyms: Folate, pteroylglutamic acid

Drug Class: Vitamin

Preparations
Tablets: 0.1, 0.4, 0.8, 1 mg
Injection: 5 and 10 mg/mL

Dose: For prophylaxis of MTX adverse effects, 1–2 mg/day

Indications: Used to prevent adverse effects caused by MTX (oral ulcers, GI intolerance, hematologic)

Mechanism of Action: May inhibit effects of MTX in some cells; does not affect MTX control of RA

Contraindications: Vitamin B_{12} deficiency. Folate may obscure the diagnosis of pernicious anemia. Neurologic deficit may progress while anemia improves.

Precautions: If patient is macrocytic, check vitamin B_{12} level before folate supplementation.

Pregnancy Risk: A

Adverse Effects: Uncommon: flushing, rash

Comments: Patients treated with MTX should usually receive folic acid. Some evidence suggests elevated homocysteine levels are a risk factor for coronary heart disease. Folic acid lowers homocysteine levels.

Cost: $

BIBLIOGRAPHY

Dijkmans BA. Folate supplementation and methotrexate. *Br J Rheumatol* 1995;34:1172–1174.
van Ede AE, Laan RF, Rood MJ, et al. Effect of folic or folinic acid supplementation on the toxicity and efficacy of methotrexate in rheumatoid arthritis: a forty-eight week, multicenter, randomized, double-blind, placebo-controlled study. *Arthritis Rheum* 2001;44:1515–1524.

FOLINIC ACID

Trade Names: Wellcovorin

Synonyms: Leucovorin calcium, citrovorum factor, tetrahydrofolate

Drug Class: Vitamin

Preparations
Injection: 3 mg/mL
Powder for injection: 25–50, 100, 350 mg
Tablets: 5, 15, 25 mg

Dose: After high-dose MTX, inadvertent overdose, or prolonged MTX concentrations in patients with renal failure, use folinic acid 10 mg/m² i.v. q 6 h for 72 hours until MTX concentrations decrease to $<1 \times 10^{-8}$ mol/L. Extremely high concentrations of MTX may require higher doses of folinic acid. (Dosing graphs are available in the package insert to further delineate dose.) With routine MTX use, 5 mg folinic acid is given post-dose to lessen side effects.

Indications: MTX toxicity

Mechanism of Action: Replaces the folinic acid whose synthesis is inhibited by MTX

Monitoring: In MTX overdose or toxicity, measurement of MTX concentrations is a useful guide to therapy.

Pregnancy Risk: C

Comments: Folinic acid has been used to prevent minor adverse effects owing to MTX, but the data supporting the use of folic acid are stronger, folic acid is cheaper, and there is concern that folinic acid may antagonize the antiinflammatory effects of MTX.

Cost: $$$

BIBLIOGRAPHY

Dijkmans BA. Folate supplementation and methotrexate. *Br J Rheumatol* 1995;34:1172–1174.
van Ede AE, Laan RF, Rood MJ, et al. Effect of folic or folinic acid supplementation on the toxicity and efficacy of methotrexate in rheumatoid arthritis: a forty-eight week, multicenter, randomized, double-blind, placebo-controlled study. *Arthritis Rheum* 2001;44:1515–1524.

Forteo (See Teriparatide)
Fosamax (See Alendronate)

γ-GLOBULIN

Trade Names: Gamimune, Gammagard, Iveegam, Polygam, Sandoglobulin

Synonyms: Intravenous immunoglobulin

Drug Class: Immunoglobulin

Preparations
Gamimune: 10, 50, 100 mL (5%, 50 mg/mL) and 10% (100 mg/mL)
Gammagard and Polygam: 0.5, 2.5, 5, 10 g
Sandoglobulin: 1 g, 3 g, 6 g

Dose
Administered intravenously at the rate specified by the manufacturer's instructions; generally start at a slow rate 0.5–1.0 mL/min and increase.
Primary immunodeficiencies: 200–400 mg/kg every 4 weeks
Kawasaki disease: 2 g/kg in one dose, 800 mg/kg/day for 2 days, or 400 mg/kg/day for 4 days. Concomitant aspirin therapy is indicated.
Chronic idiopathic thrombocytopenic purpura: 400 mg/kg/day for 5 days or 1 g/kg/day for 1–2 days; repeated at 10- to 21-day intervals according to platelet count
Inflammatory myositis: 1 g/kg/day for 2 days once monthly
Other autoimmune disease: 400 mg/kg for 1–4 days per month

Indications: Primary immunodeficiencies associated with hypogammaglobulinemia or agammaglobulinemia; also used in idiopathic thrombocytopenic purpura, Kawasaki disease, Guillain-Barré syndrome, and chronic inflammatory demyelinating polyneuropathy. Uncontrolled reports suggest efficacy in autoimmune disease refractory to other treatment.

Mechanism of Action: In primary immunodeficiencies, intravenous immunoglobulin replaces IgG; in autoimmune disease, mechanism unknown. Theories include blockade of Fc receptors, T cell inhibition, and solubilization of immune complexes.

Contraindications: Hypersensitivity to immunoglobulin. In patients with profound IgA deficiency (serum IgA <5 mg/dL), many intravenous immunoglobulin products containing larger amounts of IgA are contraindicated as they may cause anaphylactic reactions.

Precautions: Patients with profound IgA deficiency may develop anaphylactic reactions. If intravenous immunoglobulin is required in these patients, use an IgA-deficient preparation.

Monitoring: For autoimmune disease, intravenous immunoglobulin is usually administered in the hospital on an outpatient basis, with monitoring of vital signs.

Pregnancy Risk: C

Adverse Effects
Common: Flushing, tachycardia, chills, dyspnea all usually respond to slowing the rate of infusion
Less common: Hypotension, anaphylaxis, aseptic meningitis, nephritic syndrome. Transmission of viral infection is uncommon. In the past, rare cases

DRUGS

of transmission of hepatitis C have occurred with inadequately treated preparations.

Drug Interactions: May interfere with the action of live virus vaccines

Comments: Prepared from pooled plasma. Few controlled trials exist to guide appropriate use of intravenous immunoglobulin in the rheumatic diseases.

Cost: $$$$$

BIBLIOGRAPHY

Dalakas MC, Illa I, Dambrosia JM, et al. A controlled trial of high dose intravenous immuno-globulin infusion as treatment for dermatomyositis. *N Engl J Med* 1993;329:1993–2000.
Dwyer JM. Manipulating the immune system with immune globulin. *N Engl J Med* 1992;326:107–116.
Nydegger UE, Sturzenegger M. Adverse effects of intravenous immunoglobulin therapy. *Drug Saf* 1999;21:171–185.

GLUCOSAMINE

Trade Names: Sold in health food stores as a dietary supplement under many brand names, often in conjunction with chondroitin sulfate.

Synonyms: Glucosamine sulfate

Drug Class: Dietary supplement

Preparations
Tablets: 250, 500, 750 mg alone and in combination with chondroitin
Dose: Usual dose is 500 mg three times daily or 750 mg twice daily

Indications: Osteoarthritis

Mechanism of Action: Unknown; hypothesized to incorporate into cartilage and stimulate proteoglycan synthesis

Contraindications: Hypersensitivity; unstable diabetes

Precautions: Caution in patients allergic to shellfish

Pregnancy Risk: Unknown

Adverse Effects: Uncommon: GI side effects (gas, loose stools, cramps)

Comments: Because it is a dietary supplement and not a drug, glucosamine has not been subjected to the usual rigorous evaluation applied to new drugs by the FDA. Uncontrolled and some controlled studies have reported modest beneficial effects on OA symptoms and possible slowing of radiologic loss of cartilage in the knees. Moreover, the effects of glucosamine on osteoarthritis of the hands, hips, or spine have not been studied. However, the robustness of the evidence supporting the use of glucosamine for treating osteoarthritis is debated and large-scale controlled trials are in progress to define whether this approach has symptomatic and "chondroprotective" effects. The differential benefit of glucosamine versus chondroitin sulfate is unknown but is being studied in an ongoing National Institutes of Health trial. Animal studies raised concern that glucosamine might impair glucose tolerance, but a study in diabetic patients found no change in hemoglobin A1c.

Clinical Pharmacology: Little information available

Cost: $

BIBLIOGRAPHY

McAlindon T. Why are clinical trials of glucosamine no longer uniformly positive? *Rheum Dis Clin North Am* 2003;29:789–801.

GOLD, INJECTABLE PREPARATIONS

Trade Names: Aurothioglucose, Solganal; gold sodium thiomalate, Aurolate, Myochrysine (availability varies)

Drug Class: DMARD

Preparations
Aurothioglucose: 50 mg/mL (10 mL)
Gold sodium thiomalate: 10, 25, 50 mg/mL

Dose: 10 mg i.m. test dose first week, 25 mg i.m. the next week, and 50 mg/wk i.m. thereafter until response or a cumulative dose of 1 g. Once response is obtained, decrease frequency of injections to every 2 weeks for 2 months, then decrease frequency and maintain on 50 mg i.m. every 3–4 weeks. Most patients receive a maintenance dose of 50 mg monthly (every 4 weeks).

Indications: RA, juvenile RA, psoriatic arthritis

Mechanism of Action: Unknown; probably interferes with normal macrophage function

Contraindications: Hypersensitivity to gold, severe renal or hepatic disease, blood dyscrasias

Precautions: Regular monitoring is required. Administer first few doses under medical supervision with facilities to treat anaphylaxis.

Monitoring: Perform baseline CBC, creatinine, and LFTs. Check CBC, platelets, and urinalysis before each injection and LFTs periodically. Discontinue gold if there is a rapid fall in any blood parameter or if WBC is <4,000, granulocytes <1,500, or platelets <100,000. If mild rash occurs, decrease frequency of injections. If severe rash occurs, discontinue. If there is persistent proteinuria (>300 mg/24 h), discontinue.

Pregnancy Risk: C

Adverse Effects

Common: Rash, itching, painful mouth ulcers, altered taste, proteinuria

Less common: Anaphylaxis, exfoliative dermatitis, glomerulonephritis, nephrotic syndrome, blue/black skin discoloration. Blood dyscrasias (aplastic anemia, agranulocytosis, thrombocytopenia) should be looked for because they may be severe, precipitous, and fatal. Hepatotoxicity, pulmonary fibrosis, and peripheral neuropathy are uncommon. Gold sodium thiomalate preparations have uncommonly been associated with a nitritoid reaction (flushing, sweating, dizziness) after the injection.

Drug Interactions: Potentially increased toxicity with other DMARDs

Patient Instructions: Frequent monitoring is essential. Do not become pregnant. Notify physician of rash and mouth sores.

Comments: Onset of response is slow (6–12 weeks). If no response by 24 weeks, consider stopping. If there is a poor response after 1 g total dose, discontinue. A minority of patients with RA respond very well to intramuscular gold and tolerate it long term. Less than 20% of patients initiating gold therapy will still be receiving it 3–5 years later. Toxicity is common. Largely obsolete and replaced by newer DMARDs.

Clinical Pharmacology: Injectable gold is only given intramuscularly. Absorption is slow and erratic. Most is renally excreted. Plasma half-life is ~30 days, but gold is present in tissues months to years later.

Cost: $$ (Medication is relatively inexpensive, but the cost of weekly administration and laboratory work increases the total cost.)

BIBLIOGRAPHY

American College of Rheumatology Ad Hoc Committee on Clinical Guidelines. Guidelines for monitoring drug therapy in rheumatoid arthritis. *Arthritis Rheum* 1996;39:723–731.

American College of Rheumatology Committee on Rheumatoid Arthritis Clinical Guidelines. Guidelines for the management of rheumatoid arthritis: 2002 update. *Arthritis Rheum* 2002;46:328–346.

Gold: Oral Preparation (See Auranofin)

Humira (See Adalimumab)

Hyalgan (See Hyaluronan injections)

HYALURONATE INJECTIONS

Trade Names: Hyalgan: sodium hyaluronate; Synvisc: Hylan GF 20; *Orthovisc:* high molecular weight hyaluronan

Synonyms: Viscosupplements, hyaluronic acid

Drug Class: Viscosupplement

Preparations
Synvisc injection: 2 mL preloaded syringe
Hyalgan injection : 2 mL vial or 2 mL preloaded syringe
Orthovisc: 2 ml preloaded syringe

Dose
Synvisc: Intraarticular injection 2 mL once weekly for 3 weeks
Hyalgan: 2 ml intraarticular injection once weekly for 5 weeks. Some patients
    benefit after 3 injections
Orthovisc: Intraarticular injection 2 ml once a week for 3 or 4 weeks

Indications: Osteoarthritis of the knee

Mechanism of Action: Unknown; initially thought to improve viscosity of synovial fluid but because the duration of clinical effects can far exceed the time the drug is present in the joint, other mechanisms of action are likely.

Contraindications: Hypersensitivity, joint or skin infection, allergy to birds, eggs, or bird prodcuts

Precautions: Strict aseptic technique, do not inject extraarticularly.

Pregnancy Risk: Unknown; do not use in pregnancy.

Adverse Effects
Common: Pain and swelling in the injected knee
Less common: Rash, flushing, hypersensitivity
Comments: Most trials have found efficacy greater than placebo. Efficacy
    equivalent to that of intraarticular corticosteroid injection but of longer duration has been reported. The clinical benefit is on average modest, but it may last many months. Injection reactions in the treated knee are usually minor but can resemble septic arthritis.

Cost: $$$

BIBLIOGRAPHY

Brandt KD, Block JA, Michalski JP, et al. Efficacy and safety of intraarticular sodium hyaluronate in knee osteoarthritis. ORTHOVISC Study Group. *Clin Orthop* 2001; 130–143.
Brandt KD, Smith GN Jr, Simon LS. Intraarticular injection of hyaluronan as treatment for knee osteoarthritis: what is the evidence? *Arthritis Rheum* 2000;43:1192–1203.

DRUGS

Hydeltra (See Corticosteroids, Intraarticular)
Hydrocodone (See Acetaminophen + Opioids)
Hydrocortisone (See Corticosteroids)

HYDROXYCHLOROQUINE AND CHLOROQUINE PHOSPHATE

Trade Names: Hydroxychloroquine, Plaquenil; chloroquine, Aralen

Drug Class: Antimalarial, DMARD

Preparations
Hydroxychloroquine: 200-mg tablet (base 155 mg)
Chloroquine: 250-mg tablet (150-mg base), 500-mg tablet (300-mg base)

Dose
Hydroxychloroquine: 5 mg/kg lean body weight. The usual initial dose is 400 mg/day (once daily or in divided doses). The dose may be reduced to 200–300 mg/day once a clinical response is achieved.
Chloroquine: As much as 4 mg/kg lean body weight; usually 250 mg daily

Indications: RA, SLE, discoid lupus erythematosus, palindromic rheumatism, psoriatic arthritis. In RA, it is used as a single agent for mild or early disease. With more severe disease, it may be used in combination with other DMARD regimens. In SLE, it is particularly useful for skin and joint manifestations; generally not thought to be effective in controlling renal, CNS, or hematologic manifestations of SLE.

Hydroxychloroquine is the preferred antimalarial because it is less toxic to the eye. Chloroquine is sometimes tolerated by patients who do not tolerate hydroxychloroquine.

Mechanism of Action: Unknown; theories include interference with macrophage presentation of antigen to T cells

Contraindications: Hypersensitivity to hydroxychloroquine, chloroquine, or 4-aminoquinolines

Precautions: Use caution in hepatic disease, psoriasis, and porphyria. Reports suggest that antimalarials may exacerbate psoriasis, but they are often safely used to treat psoriatic arthritis.

Monitoring: Ophthalmologic (retinal and visual field) testing should be performed at baseline or soon after drug initiation and then every 6 months. Risks of retinal toxicity with hydroxychloroquine increase with a cumulative dose

>800 g, age >70 years, daily dose >6.0 mg/kg, and impaired hepatic or renal function.

Pregnancy Risk: C

Adverse Effects
Common: GI irritation, headache, rash, itch, blurred vision owing to ciliary muscle dysfunction
Less common: Yellow/orange is more common than blue/black discoloration of skin; also uncommon are reversible corneal opacities, irreversible retinal toxicity, neuromyopathy, blood dyscrasias, ototoxicity, emotional changes, and hemolysis with G6PD deficiency.

Drug Interactions: Penicillamine: increased toxicity

Comments: Retinal toxicity is very rare, and some maintain it almost never occurs with a hydroxychloroquine dose of ≤5 mg/kg/day and normal liver and renal function. When it does occur, retinal toxicity usually occurs after many years of use and is slow in onset and irreversible. Baseline ophthalmologic monitoring can be deferred until the patient has been on the drug for a few months and seems likely to continue on it.

Clinical Pharmacology: Good oral absorption, may be taken with food, partial hepatic metabolism and renal elimination; extensive tissue deposition with tissue concentrations 300 times that of plasma. Only 10% of a dose is excreted in 24 hours, and hydroxychloroquine remains in tissues for months.

Cost: $$$

BIBLIOGRAPHY

American College of Rheumatology Committee on Rheumatoid Arthritis Guidelines. Guidelines for the management of rheumatoid arthritis: 2002 update. *Arthritis Rheum* 2002;46:328–346.
Maksymowych W, Russel AS. Antimalarials in rheumatology: efficacy and safety. *Semin Arthritis Rheum* 1987;16:206–221.
Wallace D. Antimalarial agents and lupus. *Rheum Dis Clin North Am* 1994;20:243–263.

IBUPROFEN

Trade Names: Advil (OTC), Genpril, Ibuprin, Motrin, Nuprin (OTC), Rufen

Drug Class: NSAID

Preparations
Tablets: 300, 400, 600, 800 mg
Suspension (oral): 100 mg/5 mL
Drops: 40 mg/mL
OTC: 200 mg

Chewable tablets: 50 and 100 mg

Dose: 400–800 mg three to four times daily; maximum of 3.2 g/day

Clinical Pharmacology: Well absorbed after oral administration; hepatic metabolism and renal excretion of metabolites; half-life 2–4 hours

Cost: $

See NSAIDs for Indications, Mechanism of Action, Contraindications, Precautions, Monitoring, Pregnancy Risk, Adverse Effects, Interactions, and Patient Instructions.

Imipramine (Tofranil; See Appendix D)
Imuran (See Azathioprine)
Indocin (See Indomethacin)

INDOMETHACIN

Trade Names: Indocin, Indocin-SR, Indameth, Indochron ER

Drug Class: NSAID

Preparations
Capsules: 25 and 50 mg
Capsule, sustained release: 75 mg
Suspension oral: 25 mg/5 mL
Suppository: 50 mg

Dose
25–50 mg orally or rectally two to three times daily (1–2 mg/kg/day); maximum, 200 mg/day
Sustained-release capsule (75 mg) administered one or two times

Clinical Pharmacology: Well absorbed after oral administration; hepatic metabolism and renal excretion of metabolites; half-life 4–5 hours

Comments: Indomethacin may be more likely to cause CNS side effects (headaches, somnolence, cognitive dysfunction), particularly in the elderly.

Cost: $

See NSAIDs for Indications, Mechanism of Action, Contraindications, Precautions, Monitoring, Pregnancy Risk, Adverse Effects, Interactions, and Patient Instructions.

INFLIXIMAB

Trade Names: Remicade

Drug Class: DMARD, TNF antagonist

Preparations: 100-mg injection

Dose: 3 mg/kg by slow intravenous infusion (at least 2 hours) at 0, 2, and 6 weeks and then repeated every 8 weeks. The maintenance dose required ranges from 3 to 10 mg/kg every 4–8 weeks. Dose escalations over time (5–10 mg/kg or at 4- to 6-week intervals) may be necessary to control disease in a minority of patients with aggressive disease.

Indications: RA, psoriatic arthritis, ankylosing spondylitis, juvenile RA, Crohn's disease

Mechanism of Action: A chimeric monoclonal antibody to TNF that blocks the effects of the cytokine TNF-α and TNF-β and blocks its ability to bind with its receptor on the cell.

Contraindications: Hypersensitivity or severe infusion reactions, untreated tuberculosis or other opportunistic infections, sepsis, active infections, chronic localized or recurrent infections, demyelinating disease, optic neuritis or heart failure

Precautions: Exclude latent tuberculosis with a skin test before starting therapy. In RA, 5 mm of induration indicates latent or active tuberculosis. Be aware that risk of opportunistic infections is increased. Caution should be exercised if used in the debilitated or in those at high risk of infection. Avoid live virus vaccines. Influenza and pneumococcal vaccines appear to be unaffected by such therapy. Should not be used in combination with anakinra (increased risk of serious infection).

Monitoring: Monitor vital signs during infusion. Monitor clinically for infection.

Pregnancy Risk: B

Adverse Effects

Common: Infusion reactions (rash, hives, itching, tachycardia, fever, nausea) are usually mild to moderate and can usually be controlled with acetaminophen and antihistamines and slowing the rate of infusion. These may be more common in patients not receiving background MTX or DMARD therapy. Also common, but clinically insignificant, are the development of positive antinuclear antibody and double-stranded DNA antibody and antiinfliximab antibodies

D R U G S

Less common: Serious infusion reactions occur in <2% of patients and may manifest as severe rashes, hypotension, hemodynamic instability, chest tightness, severe dyspnea, or a feeling of impending doom. Cessation and aggressive treatment may require intravenous corticosteroids and hemodynamic support. Serious infection (bacterial, but particularly opportunistic infections such as tuberculosis, listeriosis, and histoplasmosis) may occur, particularly in those with advanced disease, comorbidities, and steroid therapy.

Rare: Anaphylaxis, lymphoma, hepatitis, demyelinating CNS disorders, optic neuritis, seizures, pancytopenia, and drug-induced lupus

Drug Interactions: Concurrent use of high-dose corticosteroids and other immunosuppressants may increase the risk of infection

Patient Instructions: Avoid live virus vaccines. Avoid pregnancy. Stop injections and call the doctor if an infection or fever develops that lasts more than a few days.

Comments: TNF antagonists are among the most effective treatments for RA. Patients respond quickly, usually within 4–6 weeks. However, not all patients respond. Combined therapy with MTX is more effective than either drug alone. The role of TNF antagonists in a range of diseases such as psoriasis, vasculitis, seronegative spondyloarthropathy, sarcoidosis, and inflammatory eye disease is being explored. The comparative risk of adverse effects such as tuberculosis, lymphoma, and demyelinating disease with individual TNF antagonists is not clear. Until this information is available, these side effects should be regarded as a class effect. Patients may form antibodies to infliximab that decrease its effect. Concurrent MTX treatment is used to reduce the frequency of this. In patients who are unable to take MTX, infliximab has been combined with another immunosuppressant such as leflunomide to decrease the formation of antibodies against infliximab; however, little information is available about this.

Clinical Pharmacology: Half-life is 9 days. Biologic agents are not metabolized and thus have few drug interactions.

Cost: $$$$$

BIBLIOGRAPHY

American College of Rheumatology Committee on Rheumatoid Arthritis Guidelines. Guidelines for the management of rheumatoid arthritis: 2002 update. *Arthritis Rheum* 2002; 46:328–346.

Lipsky PE, van der Heijde DM, St Clair EW, et al. Infliximab and methotrexate in the treatment of rheumatoid arthritis. Anti-Tumor Necrosis Factor Trial in Rheumatoid Arthritis with Concomitant Therapy Study Group. *N Engl J Med* 2000;343:1594–1602.

Olsen NJ, Stein CM. New drugs for rheumatoid arthritis. *N Engl J Med* 2004;350:2167–2179.

St Clair EW, Wagner CL, Fasanmade AA, et al. The relationship of serum infliximab concentrations to clinical improvement in rheumatoid arthritis: results from ATTRACT, a multicenter, randomized, double-blind, placebo-controlled trial. *Arthritis Rheum* 2002;46:1451–1459.

Intravenous Immunoglobulin (See γ-Globulin)

IRON PREPARATIONS (ORAL)

Trade Names: Ferrous fumarate: Femiron, Feostat, Ferro-Sequels
Ferrous gluconate: Fergon
Ferrous sulfate: Feosol, Feratab, Fer-iron, Slow FE

Drug Class: Antianemia agent (iron supplement)

Preparations
Ferrous fumarate (elemental iron 33%)
  Tablets: 63 mg (Femiron), 195 mg, 200 mg, 300 and 325 mg
  Chewable tablet: 100 mg (Feostat)
  Oral suspension: 100 mg/5 mL (Feostat)
Ferrous gluconate (elemental iron 11.6%)
  Capsule: 325 mg (generic)
  Tablets: 300, 320, 325 mg
  Elixir: 300 mg/5 mL (Fergon)
Ferrous sulfate (elemental iron 20%)
  Tablets: 195, 300, 325 mg
  Extended-release tablet: 325 mg, 525 mg
  Extended-release capsules: 150 and 250 mg
  Oral solution: 125 mg/mL
  Enteric coated tablets: 300 and 325 mg
Ferrous sulfate dried preparations (elemental iron 32%)
  Capsules: 159 mg (Feosol), 190 mg (Fer-In-Sol)
  Tablet: 200 mg (Feosol)
  Extended-release tablet: 160 mg (Slow Fe)

Dose
Treatment of iron deficiency anemia : 60–100 mg of elemental iron twice
  daily
Prophylaxis of iron deficiency: 10–15 mg of elemental iron daily

Indications: Prevention and treatment of iron deficiency anemia

Mechanism of Action: Replaces deficient iron stores

Contraindications: Hypersensitivity to iron preparations; hemochromatosis

Precautions: Tablets/capsules may be corrosive to the bowel. In patients with
dysphagia, liquid preparations are preferred.

DRUGS

Monitoring: Hemoglobin and reticulocyte count to monitor response

Pregnancy Risk: A; oral iron preparations are often required in pregnancy

Adverse Effects
Common: GI cramps, nausea, constipation, dark stools
Less common: Diarrhea, GI ulceration

Drug Interactions
Tetracyclines: Decreased absorption of tetracycline and iron
Antacids, histamine blockers and proton pump inhibitors; decreased iron absorption
Penicillamine: Decreased absorption of iron and penicillamine
Fluoroquinolones: Decreased absorption of antibiotic

Patient Instructions: Take regularly. May cause blackish/dark green stools or guaiac-positive tests for occult blood. Keep out of reach of children.

Comments: Many patients with inflammatory rheumatic disease have a hypochromic microcytic anemia that is not due to iron deficiency but to chronic disease. This anemia does not respond to iron therapy. Failure of an iron deficiency anemia to respond to oral therapy usually signals an incorrect diagnosis or poor compliance. Once the hemoglobin concentration has been corrected, continue prophylactic doses of iron for 3–6 months to load body iron stores.

Clinical Pharmacology: Oral absorption of iron is increased to 30% in iron deficiency anemia. Absorption is decreased by gastrectomy and achlorhydria. Absorbed iron is stored in the body and is eliminated in small amounts by cellular shedding. After starting treatment, onset of reticulocytosis is rapid (3–5 days), and hemoglobin increases within 2–4 weeks.

Cost: $

IRON DEXTRAN (PARENTERAL)

Trade Names: InFeD, Dexferrum

Drug Class: Antianemia agent (iron supplement)

Preparations: Injection, 50 mg/mL (2 mL, 10 mL)

Dose: Test dose 0.5 mL i.v. or i.m. Observe for at least 1 hour before administering dose. Calculate dose by referring to the treatment nomogram in the package insert.
    Intravenous injection must be slow. Dilute in 250–1,000 mL normal saline and infuse over 1–6 hours. Infuse very slowly initially, and observe for allergy

or anaphylaxis. Intramuscular regimen requires daily injections (maximum at one site is 2 mL).

Indications: Treatment of iron deficiency anemia in patients unable to take oral medication

Mechanism of Action: Replaces deficient iron stores

Contraindications: Hypersensitivity to iron preparations; hemochromatosis

Precautions: Administer under medical supervision with facilities available to treat anaphylaxis. Administer test dose first. If administered by intramuscular injection, it must be by a deep intramuscular injection, using a Z-track technique, in the upper outer quadrant of the buttock (not in upper arm).

Monitoring: Monitor for allergy/anaphylaxis during administration. Use hemoglobin and reticulocyte count to monitor response.

Pregnancy Risk: C

Adverse Effects
Common: Dizziness, fever, sweating, nausea, vomiting, metallic taste, discolored urine, staining skin at site of injection, leukocytosis
Less common: Anaphylaxis, cardiovascular collapse, urticaria. Onset of arthralgia, sweating, urticaria, and dizziness may be delayed 1–2 days after administration.

Cost: $$$ (includes cost of administration)

Kenalog (See Corticosteroids, Intraarticular)

KETOPROFEN

Trade Names: Orudis, Oruvail (sustained release), Orudis KT (OTC), Actron (OTC)

Drug Class: NSAID

Preparations
Capsules: 25, 50, 75 mg
Capsules, sustained release: 100 and 200 mg
OTC: 12.5 mg

Dose: 50–75 mg three to four times daily; maximum 300 mg/day. Sustained release, 200 mg once daily

Clinical Pharmacology: Well absorbed after oral administration; hepatic metabolism and renal excretion of metabolites. Half-life is 1–4 hours.

Cost: $$

See NSAIDs for Indications, Mechanism of Action, Contraindications, Precautions, Monitoring, Pregnancy Risk, Adverse Effects, Interactions, and Patient Instructions.

KETOROLAC

Trade Names: Toradol

Drug Class: NSAID

Preparations
Tablet: 10 mg
Injection: 15 mg/mL (1 mL), 30 mg/mL (1 mL, 2 mL)

Dose
Tablet: 10 mg three to four times daily; maximum 40 mg/day; maximum 5
    days administration
Injection: 30 mg then 15–30 mg every 6 hours as needed for 5 days maximum

Indications: Short-term management of acute pain

Comments: Only use for short-term control of pain.

Clinical Pharmacology: Well absorbed after oral administration; hepatic metabolism; renal excretion of 60% of drug unchanged. Half-life of 2–8 hours is increased in elderly persons.

Cost: $$$

See NSAIDs for Indications, Mechanism of Action, Contraindications, Precautions, Monitoring, Pregnancy Risk, Adverse Effects, Interactions, and Patient Instructions.

BIBLIOGRAPHY
Gillis JC, Brogden RN. Ketorolac. A re-appraisal of its pharmacodynamic and pharmacokinetic properties and therapeutic use in pain management. *Drugs* 1997;53:139–188.

Lansoprazole (Prevacid; See Appendix C)

LEFLUNOMIDE

Trade Names: Arava

Drug Class: Antimetabolite, DMARD

Preparations: 10-, 20-, 100-mg tablets

Dose: Leflunomide is often initiated with a loading dose of 100 mg daily for 3 days followed by 20 mg/day. Many rheumatologists omit or decrease the loading dose to minimize GI side effects. A maintenance dose of 10 mg/day (20 mg every 2 days) may be effective in patients who cannot tolerate 20 mg/day. When used in combination with MTX, a starting dose of 10 mg/day (for 4–8 weeks) pending the results of clinical and laboratory monitoring.

Indications: RA and possibly psoriatic arthritis.

Mechanism of Action: Inhibition of dihydroorotate dehydrogenase and pyrimidine synthesis

Contraindications: Hypersensitivity to leflunomide, liver disease, hepatitis B or C infection, alcoholism, and pregnancy.

Precautions: The patient must understand the risks and benefits of treatment and the requirement for monitoring. Pregnant women must not receive leflunomide. Counsel regarding risk, and ensure that contraceptive methods are in place in both men and women before starting therapy. Women of childbearing age who discontinue therapy should take cholestyramine 8 g three times daily for 11 days to reduce plasma levels to <0.02 mg/L. Without this elimination procedure, it could take as long as 2 years to reach these plasma concentrations. Although drug levels are higher in patients with impaired renal function, it appears that leflunomide can be used cautiously in such patients. Leflunomide is not dialyzed.

Monitoring
Baseline: CBC, platelets, LFTs, creatinine. Check for hepatitis B and C infection.
Maintenance: Initially or with dose increases, check CBC and LFTs every 4 weeks for 3 months; then if LFTs are stable, every 6–8 weeks. Dose reduction is indicated for minor increases in liver enzymes. Discontinue leflunomide in patients with persistent liver test abnormalities.

Pregnancy Risk: X (teratogen). Leflunomide is teratogenic in animals. Ensure that women are not pregnant before starting treatment and ensure reliable contraception during treatment. When women of childbearing age discontinue leflunomide treatment, use the cholestyramine protocol described under Precautions to speed elimination of the drug.

Adverse Effects
Common: Diarrhea, GI cramps, reduced uric acid
Less common: Hypertension, hair loss, rash, nausea, vomiting, weight loss, minor LFT abnormalities
Uncommon: Allergy, interstitial pneumonitis, leukopenia, liver failure, peripheral neuropathy, increased risk of infection

DRUGS

Rare: Stevens-Johnson syndrome or toxic epidermal necrolysis. The risk of death from hepatocellular necrosis is estimated to be one per 50,000 prescriptions.

Drug Interactions
Rifampin: Increased concentrations of the active form of leflunomide
Warfarin: Case reports of increased warfarin effect
Activated charcoal and cholestyramine: enhance elimination of the drug by interfering with enterohepatic recycling

Patient Instructions: Do not become pregnant. Do not drink alcohol.

Comments: Leflunomide is as effective as MTX and is useful for patients who cannot tolerate MTX. Its long half-life and teratogenicity make it less suitable for women of childbearing age. The combination of leflunomide and MTX is more effective than monotherapy but carries a greater risk of liver toxicity and careful monitoring is needed. The loading dose is sometimes omitted or decreased in clinical practice to improve GI tolerability. Minor toxicities can be managed by holding or lowering the dose and brief use of cholestyramine 8 g three times daily for 1–2 days to lower plasma concentrations by nearly 50%. Serious toxicities require drug cessation and a full-dose drug elimination (see Precautions).

Clinical Pharmacology: Well absorbed and rapidly converted to the active M1 metabolite (A77 1726). Hepatic metabolism with enterohepatic recycling. Half-life 15 days.

Cost: $$$$

BIBLIOGRAPHY

American College of Rheumatology Committee on Rheumatoid Arthritis Guidelines. Guidelines for the management of rheumatoid arthritis: 2002 update. *Arthritis Rheum* 2002; 46:328–346.
Olsen NJ, Stein CM. New drugs for rheumatoid arthritis. *N Engl J Med* 2004;350:2167–2179.

Lodine (See Etodolac)

Lortab (See Acetaminophen + Opioids)

Magnesium Choline Salicylate (See Choline Magnesium Salicylate)

Maprotiline (Ludiomil; See Appendix D)

MECLOFENAMATE SODIUM

Trade Names: Meclomen

Drug Class: NSAID

Preparations: 50- and 100-mg capsules

Dose: 200–400 mg/day in three to four divided doses

Clinical Pharmacology: Well absorbed after oral administration; hepatic metabolism and renal excretion of metabolites; analgesic effect lasts 4–6 hours.

Cost: $$

See NSAIDs for Indications, Mechanism of Action, Contraindications, Precautions, Monitoring, Pregnancy Risk, Adverse Effects, Interactions, and Patient Instructions.

Meclomen (see Meclofenamate Sodium)

MELOXICAM

Trade Name: Mobic

Drug Class: NSAID

Preparations: 7.5- and 15-mg capsules

Dose: 7.5–15 mg once daily

Clinical Pharmacology: Hepatic metabolism and renal excretion of metabolites; half-life 15 hours

Cost: $$$

Comments: Compared with traditional, older NSAIDs, somewhat COX-2 "preferential" and some evidence suggesting less GI toxicity
See NSAIDs for Indications, Mechanism of Action, Contraindications, Precautions, Monitoring, Pregnancy Risk, Adverse Effects, Interactions, and Patient Instructions.

MEPERIDINE

Trade Names: Demerol

Synonyms: Meperidine hydrochloride, pethidine

Drug Class: Narcotic analgesic, opioid

DRUGS

Preparations
Tablets: 50 and 100 mg
Syrup: 50 mg/5 mL (500 mL)
Injection: 10, 50, 100 mg/mL

Dose: Oral, intramuscular, intravenous, or subcutaneous: 50–100 mg/dose every 3–4 hours (50–75 mg of meperidine is roughly equivalent to 10 mg morphine). The oral dose is less potent than the intramuscular dose.

Indications: Pain not controlled by nonopioid drugs. Morphine is generally preferred. Do not use to treat chronic pain.

Mechanism of Action: Binds to opioid receptors in the CNS

Contraindications: Hypersensitivity to meperidine; substance abuse; patients receiving MAOIs in the previous 14 days; renal failure

Precautions: Use caution in patients with hypersensitivity to other opioids, seizure disorder, respiratory disease, renal or hepatic impairment. Decrease the dose if there is hepatic or renal impairment. The metabolite normeperidine accumulates in patients with impaired renal function and causes CNS stimulation and seizures. Meperidine is not suitable for long-term use. Use the lowest dose necessary to control pain. Escalate dose only with uncontrolled pain.

Monitoring: Monitor blood pressure and respiration if used parenterally.

Pregnancy Risk: B; D in high doses

Adverse Effects
Common: Drowsiness, constipation, dysphoria, nausea, hypotension
Less common: Rash, CNS stimulation, insomnia, twitchiness, seizures, respiratory depression, dependence, histamine release

Drug Interactions
CNS depressants: Increased toxicity
MAOIs: Avoid because risk of hypertensive crisis.
SSRIs: Avoid fluoxetine and other drugs in this class because of increased toxicity of meperidine.
Cimetidine: Increased meperidine levels

Patient Instructions: Drug is a narcotic and addictive. Use only to control pain. Do not use with alcohol or other CNS depressants.

Comments: Meperidine offers little advantage over morphine and has a worse adverse effect profile, particularly the increased risk of seizures owing to normeperidine. Meperidine is often given intravenously along with intramuscular hydroxyzine (Vistaril, 25–50 mg) to decrease nausea.

Clinical Pharmacology: Onset of action within 10 minutes, duration of effect is 2–4 hours; hepatic metabolism; urinary elimination as metabolites. Half-life of meperidine is 3–4 hours, but that of the toxic metabolite normeperidine is 15–30 hours and depends on renal function.

Cost: $

MEPROBAMATE AND ASPIRIN

Trade Names: Equagesic

Drug Class: Analgesic (aspirin) combined with anxiolytic (meprobamate)

Preparations: 200 mg meprobamate + 325 mg aspirin

Dose: One tablet three to four times daily as needed

Indications: Pain with anxiety, tension headache, muscle spasm

Mechanism of Action: Combination of an NSAID and CNS depressant acting through unknown mechanisms

Contraindications: Hypersensitivity to meprobamate or aspirin

Precautions: Same as for aspirin (see Aspirin). Meprobamate may result in physical or psychologic dependence and abuse. Use the lowest dose necessary to control pain. Escalate dose only with uncontrolled pain.

Monitoring: Monitor for continued need for drug, physical dependence, or abuse. Perform CBC periodically.

Pregnancy Risk: D

Adverse Effects: Aspirin (see Aspirin), meprobamate
Common: Drowsiness, dizziness, rash, diarrhea
Less common: Allergy, edema, paradoxical excitement, confusion, purpura, thrombocytopenia, leukopenia, agranulocytosis, renal failure

Drug Interactions: Same as aspirin (see Aspirin)
    CNS depressants: Increased effect of meprobamate

Patient Instructions: May cause drowsiness. Addictive. Avoid with alcohol. Risk of GI bleeding exists.

Comments: The use of meprobamate is largely obsolete as its side effect profile is worse than that seen with the benzodiazepines.

Clinical Pharmacology: Same as Aspirin (see Aspirin)

DRUGS

Meprobamate: Hepatic metabolism, renal elimination. Half-life is 10 hours.

Cost: $$

MESNA

Trade Names: Mesnex

Drug Class: Thiol compound

Preparations: Injection, 100 mg/mL (2, 4, 10 mL); tablet, 400 mg

Dose

Intravenous: Administer mesna to a total of 60%–120% of the cyclophosphamide dose (milligram for milligram) divided into several doses, given 15 minutes before cyclophosphamide and 3, 6, 9, and 12 hours after cyclophosphamide. For intravenous infusions, mesna is diluted in normal saline (concentration 1–20 mg/mL) or D5W and administered over 15–30 minutes.

Oral: Administer mesna equivalent to 40% of the cyclophosphamide dose (milligram for milligram) for first dose before cyclophosphamide and two doses at 3- to 4-hour intervals after cyclophosphamide (total dose, 120% of cyclophosphamide dose). Intravenous mesna is recommended over oral therapy, particularily for initial dose and if patient vomits.

Indications: Prophylaxis of hemorrhagic cystitis caused by cyclophosphamide or ifosfamide

Mechanism of Action: Binds and detoxifies with urotoxic metabolites such as acrolein (seen with cyclophosphamide therapy)

Contraindications: Hypersensitivity to mesna

Pregnancy Risk: B

Adverse Effects

Common: Bad taste, headache, diarrhea, nausea, musculoskeletal pain
Uncommon: Allergic rash, hives

Comments: Most rheumatologists prefer intravenous cyclophosphamide protocols to the oral form because there is less hemorrhagic cystitis. Some rheumatologists use mesna routinely, others reserve it for patients experiencing hemorrhagic cystitis with intravenous or oral cyclophosphamide therapy.

Clinical Pharmacology: Peak plasma levels 2–3 hours after oral administration; rapidly oxidized in the blood to mesna disulfide; excreted by glomerular filtration. Half-life of mesna disulfide is 1.2 hours.

Cost: $$$

METHOCARBAMOL

Trade Names: Robaxin

Drug Class: Skeletal muscle relaxant

Preparations
Tablets: 500 and 750 mg
Injection: 100 mg/mL (10 mL)

Dose: Oral: 4 g/day in three to six divided doses (the intravenous preparation is rarely indicated in the treatment of musculoskeletal disorders)

Indications: Treatment of painful muscle spasm; useful in some patients with fibromyalgia

Mechanism of Action: Reduces spinal nerve traffic to skeletal muscle

Contraindications: Hypersensitivity to methocarbamol; renal impairment

Precautions: Use caution in hepatic and renal dysfunction and patients with seizures. Avoid extravasation of intravenous solution, which is hypertonic.

Pregnancy Risk: C

Adverse Effects
Common: Drowsiness; dizziness, although methocarbamol is less sedating
  than other muscle relaxants
Uncommon: Allergy, flushing, rash, nausea, leukopenia. Urine may turn dark
  when left to stand.

Drug Interactions
Increased toxicity of CNS depressants

Patient Instructions: Avoid alcohol; may cause drowsiness

Comments: Nighttime sedative effect is sometimes useful in improving sleep in fibromyalgia.

Clinical Pharmacology: Rapid oral absorption; hepatic metabolism; renal excretion. Half-life is 1–2 hours.

Cost: $$

DRUGS

METHOTREXATE

Trade Names: Rheumatrex, Trexall

Synonyms: MTX

Drug Class: Antimetabolite and cytotoxic (at high doses); DMARD, antiinflammatory (at low doses)

Preparations
Tablet: 2.5 mg; dose packs of four cards (with two, three, four, five, or six tablets each); one card is taken on the same day each week.
Injection: 25 mg/mL (2 mL vial)

Dose: MTX is typically initiated in a dose of 7.5 mg once weekly (all taken on the same day). Start elderly patients with 5 mg/wk. Most patients start on oral tablets. Dose may be increased after 4–8 weeks if clinical benefit is not achieved. If necessary, increase dose by 2.5–5 mg (one to two tablets) every 4–8 weeks to 15 mg/wk. Higher doses are occasionally used in RA (to as much as 20 or 25 mg/wk), based on limited evidence of incremental efficacy. Doses of 20–25 mg/wk may be necessary to control cutaneous psoriasis or inflammatory muscle disease.

If nausea, diarrhea, or mucositis occurs, the clinician has several options: (a) lower the dose or temporarily suspend therapy (for 1–2 weeks); (b) initiate vitamin A 8,000–10,000 U/day; (c) divide the total weekly dose and administer two doses at 12-hour intervals; (d) premedicate with antiemetics (e.g., promethazine); or (e) switch to weekly intramuscular or subcutaneous injections for an improved side effect profile and more reliable absorption (patients can be taught to self-administer weekly subcutaneous injections); (f) increase dose of folate to 2 mg/day.

The injectable form is 80%–90% cheaper than the tablets and is the preferred alternative for those of limited financial resources. The injectable (parenteral) form may be administered intramuscularly, subcutaneously, or orally (diluted in water or fruit juice). Patients must be taught how to draw up the proper amount of parenteral MTX accurately and that 0.1 mL of the parenteral form equals 2.5 mg (or one tablet) of MTX.

All patients should receive concomitant folate (1 mg/day) to lessen the incidence of serious toxicities, especially hepatic, pulmonary, and marrow toxicity.

Indications: RA, psoriasis, psoriatic arthritis, juvenile RA, inflammatory myositis, maintenance in vasculitis (after control achieved with cyclophosphamide), SLE, Reiter's syndrome, inflammatory arthritis

Mechanism of Action: The cytotoxic action is based on inhibition of dihydrofolate reductase by MTX, but this does not appear to be the mechanism of action with the doses typically used in rheumatic diseases. Thus, concomitant folate administration will not negate the clinical effects of MTX. Postulated mechanisms underlying its antiinflammatory effects include inhibition of methylation reactions and increased adenosine release.

Contraindications: Hypersensitivity to MTX, liver disease, alcoholism, pregnancy, or renal impairment. Most rheumatologists avoid its use in patients with marked leukopenia, human immunodeficiency virus, or hepatitis B or C infection.

Precautions: The patient must understand the risks and benefits of treatment and the requirement for monitoring. Pregnant women must not receive MTX. Contraceptive methods should be reviewed and strongly advised (in both men and women) before starting MTX therapy, during MTX therapy, and for at least 3 months after discontinuing MTX. Patients should wait at least 3 months after discontinuing MTX before becoming pregnant.

    MTX toxicity is more common in those with renal impairment, Down syndrome, or folate deficiency and those receiving high-dose aspirin (4–6 g/day).

Monitoring

Baseline: CBC, platelets, LFTs, creatinine, chest x-ray (within the past year). Check for hepatitis B and C infection; if at risk, exclude human immunodeficiency virus infection.

Maintenance: CBC and creatinine 2 weeks after initiating treatment; then CBC, LFTs (including albumin, AST, ALT), and creatinine every 4 weeks until efficacy and stable dose are achieved. Patients on a stable dose with no previous WBC or LFT abnormalities may have the laboratory testing interval gradually increased to every 4–8 weeks. Dose reduction is indicated for minor increases in liver enzymes. Inquire whether the patient is receiving other hepatotoxic agents (e.g., alcohol, NSAIDs). If minor elevations persist, a liver biopsy or discontinuation of MTX should be considered. The chest x-ray should only be repeated if there is a suspicion of MTX pneumonitis or if it is otherwise indicated. Detailed guidelines on monitoring MTX use in RA have been established and are outlined in Table 2.

Pregnancy Risk: X (teratogen). Ensure that women are not pregnant before starting treatment, ensure reliable contraception during treatment, and avoid conception for 3 months after discontinuing MTX.

Adverse Effects

Common: Oral ulcers, postdose (1–2 days) nausea or diarrhea

Less common: Worsening of rheumatoid nodules (MTX nodulosis), fatigue, somnolence, photosensitivity, reversible hair loss, vomiting

Uncommon: Pneumonitis (MTX lung), impotence, elevated uric acid level, bone marrow suppression (primarily leukopenia or pancytopenia), osteoporosis (with long-term high-dose MTX), increased risk of infection, irreversible hepatic fibrosis, lymphoma (sometimes reversible on stopping MTX)

Table 2
Recommendations for Monitoring for Hepatic Safety in Patients with Rheumatoid Arthritis Receiving Methotrexate

A. Baseline
   1. Tests for all patients
      a. Liver blood tests (aspartate aminotransferase, alanine aminotransferase, alkaline phosphatase, albumin, bilirubin), hepatitis B and C serologic studies
      b. Other standard tests, including complete blood cell count and serum creatinine determination (avoid methotrexate if creatinine abnormal)
   2. Pretreatment liver biopsy (Menghini suction-type needle) only for patients with
      a. Previous excessive alcohol consumption
      b. Persistently abnormal baseline aspartate aminotransferase values
      c. Chronic hepatitis B or C infection
B. Monitor aspartate aminotransferase, alanine aminotransferase, albumin at 4- to 8-week intervals
C. Perform liver biopsy if
   1. Five of 9 determinations of aspartate aminotransferase within a given 12-month interval (6 of 12 if tests are performed monthly) are abnormal (i.e., above the upper limit of normal)
   2. Serum albumin level falls below the normal range (in the setting of well-controlled rheumatoid arthritis)
D. If results of liver biopsy are
   1. Roenigk grade I, II, or IIIA, resume methotrexate and monitor as in B, C1, and C2 above
   2. Roenigk grade IIIB or IV, discontinue methotrexate
E. Discontinue methotrexate in patients with persistent liver test abnormalities as defined in C1 and C2 above who refuse liver biopsy

Reproduced with permission from Kremer JM, Alarcon GS, Lightfoot RW, et al. *Arthritis Rheum* 1994;37:316–328.

Drug Interactions

Trimethoprim/sulfamethoxazole: Increased marrow toxicity of MTX
Immunosuppressants: additive toxicities
NSAIDs: Minor increases in MTX levels (seldom of clinical significance with RA doses of MTX)
Probenecid: Increased risk of MTX toxicity

Patient Instructions: Take MTX only once weekly. Never increase the dose by yourself. Do not become pregnant. Do not drink alcohol. Avoid prolonged exposure to direct sunlight.

Comments: MTX has become the most widely used first-line drug for the treatment of RA in the United States, primarily because of its ease of use, relatively rapid onset of action (4–8 weeks), and durable responses. Approximately 40% to 50% of patients are still taking it after 5 years. Folic acid supplementation (1 mg/day) decreases side effects and is used routinely by many rheumatologists. Impaired renal function is the most important cause of serious MTX toxicity.

Studies of MTX used in combination with cyclosporine or sulfasalazine and hydroxychloroquine or anti-TNF antagonists, or anakinra suggest increased benefit in patients not controlled with MTX alone.

MTX is not a first-line drug in the treatment of vasculitis but has been used after control is achieved with cyclophosphamide in conditions such as Wegener's granulomatosis. Similarly, in SLE and inflammatory myositis, MTX has been used as a steroid-sparing agent.

Clinical Pharmacology: Most administered MTX is eliminated unchanged in urine. Some is metabolized in the liver to 7-hydroxymethotrexate. Plasma half-life is approximately 10 hours. Intracellular MTX forms polyglutamates, which increase the biologic effect and toxicity of MTX beyond that expected from the plasma half-life. Cellular toxicity is related to concentration but more importantly to duration of exposure. Accumulates in pleural effusions and ascites and can cause toxicity.

Cost: Parenteral form, $; oral tablets, $$$

BIBLIOGRAPHY

American College of Rheumatology Committee on Rheumatoid Arthritis Guidelines. Guidelines for the management of rheumatoid arthritis: 2002 update. *Arthritis Rheum* 2002;46:328–346.

American College of Rheumatology Ad Hoc Committee on Clinical Guidelines. Guidelines for monitoring drug therapy in rheumatoid arthritis. *Arthritis Rheum* 1996;39:723–731.

Bannwarth B, Labat L, Moride Y, et al. Methotrexate in rheumatoid arthritis. An update. *Drugs* 1994;47:25–50.

Cronstein BN. Molecular therapeutics. Methotrexate and its mechanism of action. *Arthritis Rheum* 1996;39:1951–1960.

Miacalcin (See Calcitonin)

MINOCYCLINE

Trade Names: Minocin, Dynacin

Synonyms: Minocycline hydrochloride

Drug Class: Tetracycline antibiotic

Preparations
Capsules: 50 and 100 mg
Injection: 100 mg

Dose: Effective dose in RA is 200 mg/day (100 mg b.i.d.)

Indications: RA (see PDR for infectious indications and doses)

DRUGS

Mechanism of Action: Unknown; RA effects are probably related to down-regulation of intraarticular metalloproteinases rather than antibacterial effects.

Contraindications: Hypersensitivity to minocycline; children younger than 9 years old; pregnancy

Precautions: Renal impairment

Pregnancy Risk: D

Adverse Effects
Common: Diarrhea, nausea, photosensitivity, discoloration of teeth in children
Less common: Allergy, rash, increased intracranial pressure, pericarditis, dysphagia, enterocolitis, drug-induced lupus, pseudotumor cerebri, vertigo, hyperpigmentation particularly affecting the face with long-term use

Drug Interactions
Antacids: Decreased absorption of minocycline
Oral contraceptive: decreased contraceptive efficacy
Warfarin: Increased effect

Patient Instructions: Avoid sunlight. Do not take with antacids or milk.

Comments: Clinical effect in RA is small; may be most suitable for patients with mild or early disease.

Clinical Pharmacology: Well absorbed after oral administration; renal elimination. Half-life is 15 hours.

Cost: $$$

BIBLIOGRAPHY
American College of Rheumatology Committee on Rheumatoid Arthritis Guidelines. Guidelines for the management of rheumatoid arthritis: 2002 update. *Arthritis Rheum* 2002; 46:328–346.
Tilley BC, Alarcon GS, Heyse SP, et al. Minocycline in rheumatoid arthritis. A 48-week, double blind, placebo-controlled trial. *Ann Intern Med* 1995;122:81–89.

MISOPROSTOL

Trade Names: Cytotec, Arthrotec (misoprostol + diclofenac)

Synonyms: Synthetic prostaglandin E1

Drug Class: Synthetic prostaglandin, protects against NSAID gastropathy

Preparations: 100- and 200-μg tablets

Dose: Prophylaxis of NSAID-induced gastropathy 100–200 μg four times daily. Efficacy best demonstrated for 200 μg four times daily, but lower doses (200 μg b.i.d. or 100 μg q.i.d.) are better tolerated and may be nearly as effective.

Indications: Prevention of NSAID-induced gastropathy (see Comments)

Mechanism of Action: Substitutes for endogenous prostaglandins (necessary to stimulate gastric mucous and bicarbonate secretion) whose synthesis is inhibited by NSAIDs

Contraindications: Hypersensitivity to misoprostol, pregnancy

Precautions: Safety in children is not established. Ensure that women are not pregnant before starting treatment, and ensure reliable contraception while receiving misoprostol.

Pregnancy Risk: X (abortifacient and teratogenic)

Adverse Effects
Common: Diarrhea, abdominal cramps
Less common: Headaches, vaginal bleeding, miscarriage

Patient Instructions: Do not consider becoming or become pregnant while on misoprostol. May cause diarrhea. Take with food.

Comments: Misoprostol reduces serious GI complications caused by NSAIDs by 40%. Prophylactic therapy should be considered in patients at high risk of NSAID-induced GI complications (those with previous GI bleeding or previous peptic ulcer, the elderly, those on combination NSAID and corticosteroid therapy) if therapy with an NSAID is necessary. Proton pump inhibitors are better tolerated. Prophylaxis in unselected NSAID users is not cost-effective. Misoprostol does not prevent GI pain (indigestion, dyspepsia) associated with NSAID use.

Clinical Pharmacology: Rapidly absorbed and metabolized to the free acid. Plasma concentrations are highest within 30 minutes of dosing. Half-life is 20–40 minutes.

Cost: $$$

BIBLIOGRAPHY

Levine JS. Misoprostol and nonsteroidal anti-inflammatory drugs: a tale of effects, outcomes and costs. *Ann Intern Med* 1995;123:309–310.
Silverstein FE, Graham DY, Senior JR, et al. Misoprostol reduces serious gastrointestinal complications in patients with rheumatoid arthritis receiving nonsteroidal anti-inflammatory drugs. A randomized, double-blind, placebo-controlled trial. *Ann Intern Med* 1995; 123:241–249.

DRUGS

Mobic (See Meloxicam)
Motrin (See Ibuprofen)

MYCOPHENOLATE

Trade Names: CellCept

Synonyms: Mycophenolate mofetil

Drug Class: Immunosuppressant

Preparations
Tablet: 500 mg
Capsule: 250 mg
Injection: 500 mg

Dose: Usually started at 500 mg twice daily and, if tolerated, increased to 1 g twice daily. Preliminary studies suggest that 1.5 g twice daily is more effective for lupus.

Indications: Prevention of organ rejection; treatment of SLE, vasculitis, inflammatory muscle disease, RA

Mechanism of Action: Inhibits guanine and *de novo* purine synthesis; inhibits T and B lymphocyte proliferation

Contraindications: Hypersensitivity to mycophenolate

Precautions: The patient must understand the risks and benefits of treatment and the requirement for monitoring. Pregnant women must not receive mycophenolate. Contraceptive methods should be reviewed and be in place before starting therapy. Because mycophenolate may affect the efficacy of estrogen contraceptives, two methods of contraception are recommended. Avoid live virus vaccines.

Monitoring
CBC, platelets, LFTs, creatinine at baseline; check CBC after 2 weeks and then CBC and LFTs every 4–8 weeks.

Pregnancy Risk: C.

Adverse Effects
Common: Nausea, GI cramps, diarrhea, headache
Less common: Vomiting, leukopenia, elevated liver enzymes, hypertension, edema, rash, hyperglycemia, tremor, increased risk of infection and skin cancer, herpes zoster

Drug Interactions
Antacids and cholestyramine: Decreased serum concentrations
Azathioprine: Increased toxicity, avoid this combination

Patient Instructions: Never increase the dose by yourself. Do not become pregnant. Protect skin from the sun.

Comments: The role of mycophenolate mofetil in rheumatic diseases is under investigation, and its role is not clearly established. It shows promise in lupus nephritis (see Bibliography) and has been tried in other conditions as an alternative to AZA.

Clinical Pharmacology: Rapidly and completely absorbed, rapidly deesterified to mycophenolic acid, the active drug, which is glucuronidated and excreted in the urine. Plasma half-life of mycophenolic acid is 16 hours.

Cost: $$$$$

BIBLIOGRAPHY

Chan TM, Li FK, Tang CS, et al. Efficacy of mycophenolate mofetil in patients with diffuse proliferative lupus nephritis. Hong Kong-Guangzhou Nephrology Study Group. *N Engl J Med* 2000;343:1156–1162.
Conteras G, Pardo V, Leclerq B, et al. Sequential therapies for proliferative lupus nephritis. *N Engl J Med* 2004;350:971–980.
Stein CM. Immunoregulatory drugs. In: Harris ED, Ruddy S, Sledge CB, eds. *Kelley's textbook of Rheumatology,* 7th ed. Philadelphia: WB Saunders, 2004.

Myochrysine (See Gold)

NABUMETONE

Trade Names: Relafen

Drug Class: NSAID

Preparations: 500- and 750-mg tablets

Dose: 1,000 mg/day in a single or divided doses. Dose may be increased to 1,500–2,000 mg/day in divided doses.

Comments: Some data suggest that nabumetone may have less GI toxicity than other commonly used non-selective NSAIDs.

Clinical Pharmacology: Well absorbed after oral administration. Nabumetone is an inactive prodrug that is metabolized to the 6-methoxy-2-naphthyl acetic acid. Hepatic metabolism. Half-life is 20–30 hours (even longer in the elderly).

DRUGS

Cost: $$$

See NSAIDs for Indications, Mechanism of Action, Contraindications, Precautions, Monitoring, Pregnancy Risk, Adverse Effects, Interactions, and Patient Instructions.

Nalfon (See Fenoprofen)
Naprosyn (See Naproxen)

NAPROXEN

Trade Names: Aleve (OTC), Anaprox, EC-Naprosyn, Naprelan, Naprosyn

Synonyms: Naproxen sodium

Drug Class: NSAID

Preparations
Tablets: 250, 375, 500 mg
Tablets (enteric coated): 375 and 500 mg
Tablets, as sodium (Anaprox): 275 mg (250 mg base), 550 mg (500 mg base).
OTC: 220 mg (200 mg base)
Oral suspension: 125 mg/5 mL

Dose: 500–1,000 mg/day in two divided doses

Clinical Pharmacology: Well absorbed after oral administration; hepatic metabolism; renal elimination. Half-life is 13 hours.

Cost: OTC (low dose), $; generic, $$

See NSAIDs for Indications, Mechanism of Action, Contraindications, Precautions, Monitoring, Pregnancy Risk, Adverse Effects, Interactions, and Patient Instructions.

Neoral (See Cyclosporine)
Nexium (Esomeprazole; See Appendix C)

NITROGLYCERIN OINTMENT

Trade Names: Nitro-Bid Ointment, Nitrol Ointment

Synonyms: Nitropaste, NTG, glyceryl trinitrate

Drug Class: Nitro vasodilator

Preparations: 2% ointment

Dose: For angina, use 2–5 cm (15–30 mg) applied to skin two to three times daily. For digital ulcers, smaller amounts are applied to the fingertips.

Indications: Severe Raynaud's syndrome with digital ulceration

Mechanism of Action: Nitric oxide donor. Nitric oxide acts through cyclic guanosine 3',5'-monophosphate to relax vascular smooth muscle.

Contraindications: Hypersensitivity to nitroglycerin, concommitant use of sildenafil (Viagra)

Pregnancy Risk: C

Adverse Effects
Common: Flushing, headache, dizziness, rash

Comments: Use small amounts on tips of fingers. Efficacy is uncertain

Clinical Pharmacology: Systemic absorption occurs transdermally, and this preparation is used to treat angina. Duration of action is 2–12 hours.

Cost: $

Nizatidine (Axid; See Appendix C)

Norflex (See Orphenadrine)

NORTRIPTYLINE

Trade Names: Aventyl, Pamelor

Drug Class: Antidepressant

Preparations: Capsules: 10, 25, 50, 75 mg

DRUGS

Dose

Depression (adults): 25 mg three to four times daily (to as much as 150 mg/day)

Fibromyalgia: Initiate with 10–25 mg at bedtime, can often be given as a single 10- to 75-mg dose at night

Indications: Depression, chronic pain, fibromyalgia

Mechanism of Action: Increases synaptic concentrations of neurotransmitters such as norepinephrine and serotonin by blocking their reuptake.

Contraindications: Hypersensitivity to tricyclic antidepressants; narrow-angle glaucoma, urinary retention, pregnancy, use of MAOI within 14 days

Precautions: Use caution in cardiac disease, renal or hepatic impairment, hyperthyroidism

Monitoring: Blood pressure and pulse at scheduled visits

Pregnancy Risk: D

Adverse Effects

Common: Dizziness, drowsiness, anticholinergic effects (dry mouth, constipation, urinary retention, blurred vision), weight gain

Less common: Postural hypotension, arrhythmias, confusion, parkinsonism, tremor, anxiety, seizures, hepatitis, hematologic abnormalities, worsening of psychosis in schizophrenics

Overdose signs: Confusion, restlessness, agitation, vomiting, fever, rigidity, hyperreflexia, abnormal electrocardiogram, hypotension, seizures, respiratory depression

Drug Interactions

CNS depressants: Additive action

MAOIs: Hypertensive crisis, fever, hyperpyrexia, tachycardia

Warfarin: Increase in anticoagulation effect

Sympathomimetics: Potentiates effects of norepinephrine and epinephrine

Cimetidine: Reduces metabolism

Patient Instructions: Avoid alcohol. May cause drowsiness. May discolor urine. Dry mouth often improves after a few weeks.

Clinical Pharmacology: Hepatic metabolism (CYP2D6 substrate); eliminated largely as metabolites in the urine. Half-life is 30 hours.

Cost: $$

NONSTEROIDAL ANTIINFLAMMATORY DRUGS (ALSO SEE INDIVIDUAL DRUGS AND APPENDIX A)

Indications: RA, juvenile RA, osteoarthritis, ankylosing spondylitis, spondyloarthropathy, gout, pain

Mechanism of Action: Antiinflammatory and antiplatelet properties are mediated by the inhibition of COX enzymes and decreased production of prostaglandins. Drugs that inhibit COX-2 are antiinflammatory because they decrease the formation of prostaglandins by activated cells. Drugs that inhibit COX-1 decrease the production of thromboxane and thus decrease platelet activation. Because COX-1 contributes to the maintenance of gastric mucosa, blocking COX-1 increases the risk of peptic ulceration. NSAIDs are classified according to whether they inhibit both COX-1 and COX-2 (nonselective NSAIDs) or whether they are more selective for COX-2 and spare COX-1 (COX-2 selective NSAIDs or coxibs). Nonacetylated salicylates such as salsalate are weak inhibitors of COX, and their mechanism of action is poorly understood.

Contraindications: Hypersensitivity to NSAIDs, GI ulceration, hemorrhagic state, and last trimester of pregnancy (risk of premature closure of ductus arteriosus)

Precautions: Fluid retention may aggravate heart failure and hypertension. Use with caution or avoid in patients at high risk of GI bleeding (i.e., previous GI bleeding, peptic ulcer, elderly, concurrent corticosteroid or warfarin treatment); if benefit outweighs risk, a nonselective NSAID with misoprostol or proton pump inhibitor prophylaxis or a COX-2 selective drug should be used. Administer with food. Use with caution in asthma, bleeding disorders, and hepatic or renal disease.

Monitoring: Monitor hematocrit, creatinine, liver enzymes periodically (1 month after starting and then every 3–6 months). In patients at high risk of renal impairment (diuretics, receiving ACE inhibitors, edematous states, heart failure, renal failure, diabetes), monitor renal function more closely after starting treatment.

Pregnancy Risk: Most NSAIDs category B, but category D in third trimester Arthrotec-category X because of misoprostol

Adverse Effects
Common: GI irritation (dyspepsia, reflux, epigastric pain), rash, fluid retention
Less common: GI ulceration, hemorrhage, or gastric outlet obstruction; hepatitis with elevations of liver enzymes; hypersensitivity (anaphylaxis, asthma,

urticaria, angioedema particularly in patients with nasal polyps, exfoliative dermatitis); hematologic toxicity (agranulocytosis, anemia, leukopenia, thrombocytopenia); renal toxicity (interstitial nephritis, proteinuria, nephrotic syndrome, acute renal failure, hypertension, hyperkalemia); CNS toxicity (drowsiness, insomnia, nervousness)

Drug Interactions
Anticoagulants: Increased hemorrhagic risk with anticoagulants and thrombolytics
NSAIDs: Increased risk of GI side effects if combinations of NSAIDs used
Aspirin: A nonselective NSAID such as ibuprofen taken before aspirin blunted the long-term antiplatelet effects of aspirin perhaps because ibuprofen blocked the access of aspirin to its binding site on the COX-1 enzyme. If patients took aspirin first and then ibuprofen, the long-term antiplatelet effects of aspirin were not altered. A COX-2 selective drug did not affect the antiplatelet effect of aspirin, irrespective of whether it was taken before or after aspirin. The clinical implications of these findings are unclear.
MTX: Increased levels of MTX with many NSAIDs, but with the MTX doses used in RA, usually not of clinical importance
Cyclosporine: May increase risk of nephrotoxicity.
Diuretics: Decreased effects of thiazides and furosemide; increased renal toxicity with diuretics; increased risk of hyperkalemia with K$^+$-sparing diuretics
Lithium: Increased lithium levels
Antihypertensive agents: Antihypertensive effect reduced

Patient Instructions: Take with food. Discontinue and seek medical advice if unusual bleeding occurs.

BIBLIOGRAPHY

FitzGerald GA, Patrono C. The coxibs, selective inhibitors of cyclooxygenase-2. *N Engl J Med* 2001;345:433–442.

Omeprazole (Prilosec; See Appendix C)
Ophthalmic Solutions (See Artificial Tears)

ORPHENADRINE CITRATE

Trade Names: Norflex

Drug Class: Muscle relaxant

Preparations
Tablet: 100 mg

Dose: 100 mg twice daily

Indications: Treatment of muscle spasm

Mechanism of Action: Central atropine-like action is thought to induce skeletal muscle relaxation.

Contraindications: Hypersensitivity to orphenadrine; myasthenia gravis, bowel obstruction, glaucoma

Precautions: Use caution with cardiac arrhythmias.

Pregnancy Risk: C

Adverse Effects
Common: Drowsiness, blurred vision, dizziness
Less common: Tachycardia, rash, anticholinergic effects, nausea, constipation, flushing

Drug Interactions
Anticholinergics: Additive anticholinergic effects

Patient Instructions: May cause drowsiness. Avoid alcohol.

Clinical Pharmacology: Hepatic metabolism and renal excretion. Half-life is 14–16 hours.

Cost: $$$

Orudis (See Ketoprofen)
Oruvail (See Ketoprofen)
Oscal (See Calcium)

OXAPROZIN

Trade Names: Daypro

Drug Class: NSAID

Preparations: 600-mg tablet

Dose: 600–1,200 mg/day once daily. Do not exceed maximum dose of 1,800 mg/day or 26 mg/kg (whichever is lower).

Clinical Pharmacology: Well absorbed after oral administration. Half-life is 40–50 hours.

Cost: $$$

See NSAIDs for Indications, Mechanism of Action, Contraindications, Precautions, Monitoring, Pregnancy Risk, Adverse Effects, Interactions, and Patient Instructions.

OXYCODONE

Trade Names: Roxicodone, OxyIR, Oxycontin (controlled release)

Drug Class: Narcotic analgesic

Preparations
Tablets: 5, 15, 30 mg
Tablets (controlled release): 10, 20,40, 80 mg
Oral suspension: 5 mg/5 mL

Dose: 5–10 mg three to four times daily; may divide and convert total dose to every 12 hours sustained release.

Indications: Pain not controlled by nonopioid drugs

Mechanism of Action: Binds to opioid receptors in CNS

Contraindications: Hypersensitivity to oxycodone; substance abuse

Precautions: Use caution in patients with hypersensitivity to other opioids, respiratory disease, or renal or hepatic impairment. Decrease dose with hepatic or renal impairment.

Monitoring: Use the lowest dose necessary to control pain. Escalate dose only for uncontrolled pain.

Pregnancy Risk: D

Adverse Effects
Common: Drowsiness, dizziness, constipation, dysphoria, nausea
Less common: Rash, CNS stimulation, insomnia, hypotension

Drug Interactions: Increased toxicity with other CNS depressants. Avoid with MAOIs.

Patient Instructions: Drug is addictive. Use only to control pain. Do not use with alcohol or other CNS depressants. Do not crush slow-release tablets.

Comments: 30 mg oxycodone p.o. is approximately equivalent in opioid effect to 10 mg morphine i.m.

Clinical Pharmacology: Oral absorption and hepatic metabolism; urinary elimination as metabolites. Half-life is 3 hours. Duration of effect is 3–4 hours.

Cost: $$

Oxycodone and Acetaminophen (See Acetaminophen + Opioids)

Oxycodone and Aspirin (See Aspirin + Opioids)

Pamelor (See Nortriptyline and Appendix D)

PAMIDRONATE

Trade Names: Aredia

Drug Class: Bisphosphonate

Preparations: Powder for injection: 30, 60, 90 mg

Dose
Paget's disease: 30 mg as a dilute intravenous infusion over 4 hours for 3 days.
Hypercalcemia of malignancy: 60–90 mg as a slow infusion over 4–24 hours; may need to be repeated at 2- to 3-week intervals

Indications: Hypercalcemia of malignancy, Paget's disease

Mechanism of Action: Localizes to areas of bone resorption and inhibits osteoclast activity

Contraindications: Hypersensitivity to pamidronate or other bisphosphonates

Precautions: Use caution in renal impairment.

Monitoring: Monitor serum electrolytes periodically.

Pregnancy Risk: C

Adverse Effects
Common: Fever, hypocalcemia, hypokalemia, hypomagnesemia, nausea, diarrhea, bone pain, dyspnea, thrombophlebitis at infusion site
Less common: Rash, hypersensitivity, leukopenia

Drug Interactions
Diuretics: Increased risk of electrolyte abnormalities

Comments: Alendronate is more commonly used for the treatment of Paget's disease. Supplemental calcium and vitamin D are usually administered when bisphosphonates are used to treat Paget's disease.

Clinical Pharmacology: Oral bioavailability is very poor; renal excretion. Plasma half-life is short (2–3 hours), but bone half-life is 1 year, indicating localization and release from bone.

Cost: $$

BIBLIOGRAPHY

Delmas PD, Meunier PJ. The management of Paget's disease of bone. *N Engl J Med* 1997; 336:558–566.
Fitton A, McTavish D. Pamidronate: a review of its pharmacological properties and therapeutic efficacy in resorptive bone diseases. *Drugs* 1991;41:289–318.

Pantoprazole (Protonix; See Appendix C)
Parafon Forte (See Chlorzoxazone)
Paroxetine (Paxil; See Appendix D)

PENICILLAMINE

Trade Names: Cuprimine, Depen

Synonyms: D-Penicillamine

Drug Class: Chelating agent, DMARD

Preparations
Capsules: 125 and 250 mg
Tablet: 250 mg

Dose: For RA, use 125 mg daily initially. Increase by 125-mg increments at 1- to 3-month intervals until usual maintenance dose of 375–750 mg/day is reached. Do not exceed maximum dose of 1.5 g/day.

Indications: RA, Felty syndrome, scleroderma, primary biliary cirrhosis, Wilson's disease, cystinuria, lead poisoning

Mechanism of Action: In RA, mechanism is unknown but may be related to inhibition of T cell function.

Contraindications: Hypersensitivity to penicillamine

Precautions: Cross-sensitivity to penicillin is possible. Penicillamine has a high frequency of adverse effects, and most patients experience an adverse drug reaction.

Monitoring: CBC, differential, platelets, and urinalysis (for protein) should initially be done within 1–2 weeks and then monthly until therapeutic effect and a stable dose are achieved. The frequency of laboratory testing may be changed to every 4–12 weeks if the laboratory indices remain stable on repeat testing.

Pregnancy Risk: D

Adverse Effects
Common: Rash, hives, itching, altered (metallic) taste, proteinuria, arthralgia
Less common: Fever, hematologic toxicity (agranulocytosis, thrombocytopenia, leukopenia, aplastic anemia), glomerulonephritis, myasthenia gravis, Goodpasture syndrome, optic neuritis, hepatitis, lymphadenopathy, drug-induced lupus, pemphigus, inflammatory myositis

Drug Interactions: Antacids/iron/food: Significantly decreased absorption of penicillamine

Patient Instructions: Take on an empty stomach. Altered taste may occur. Regular laboratory monitoring is required. Do not become pregnant.

Comments: Penicillamine has largely been replaced by MTX and other DMARDs for the treatment of RA. Most patients who take penicillamine for RA discontinue it within 1–2 years because of lack of efficacy or toxicity. Data suggesting benefits of penicillamine in scleroderma are largely based on retrospective studies, and its efficacy for this indication remains unproven. A controlled study found no difference between 125 mg on alternate days (a placebo substitute dose) and 750–1,000 mg/day.

Clinical Pharmacology: Absorption is 50%. Half-life is 2–3 hours. Elimination is primarily renal as unchanged drug.

Cost: $$$

BIBLIOGRAPHY

American College of Rheumatology Committee on Rheumatoid Arthritis. Guidelines for the management of rheumatoid arthritis: 2002 update. *Arthritis Rheum* 2002;46:328–346.
Clements PJ, Furst DE, Wong WK, et al. High-dose versus low-dose D-penicillamine in early diffuse systemic sclerosis: analysis of a two-year, double-blind, randomized, controlled clinical trial. *Arthritis Rheum* 1999;42:1194–1203.
Taylor HG, Samanta A. Penicillamine in rheumatoid arthritis. A problem of toxicity. *Drug Saf* 1992;7:46–53.

Percocet (See Acetaminophen + Codeine)
Percodan (See Aspirin + Codeine)

DRUGS

PHENYLBUTAZONE

Trade Names: Butazolidin, Butazone

Drug Class: NSAID

Preparations: 100-mg tablet

Dose: 100 mg three to four times daily

Indications: Ankylosing spondylitis refractory to other NSAIDs

Comments: Phenylbutazone is no longer widely available commercially. Phenylbutazone is rarely used because of hematologic toxicity (agranulocytosis, thrombocytopenia) and should only be used in patients with ankylosing spondylitis when other NSAIDs have failed to control active disease. The drug should not be given to elderly persons because they are at greatest risk of hematologic toxicity. Its use should be restricted to rheumatologists. The potential risks and benefits must be evaluated with the patient before prescribing phenylbutazone.

Clinical Pharmacology: Rapid absorption; hepatic metabolism; renal elimination. Half-life is 50–100 hours.

Cost: Not available

See NSAIDs for Indications, Mechanism of Action, Contraindications, Precautions, Monitoring, Pregnancy Risk, Adverse Effects, Interactions, and Patient Instructions.

PILOCARPINE

Trade Names: Salagen

Drug Class: Cholinergic agent

Preparations: 5-mg tablet

Dose: 5 mg three times daily; titrate to as high as 10 mg three times daily if needed

Indications: xerostomia, Sjögren's syndrome

Mechanism of Action: Stimulates muscarinic receptors to increase saliva production

Contraindications: Hypersensitivity to pilocarpine, iritis, uncontrolled asthma

Precautions: Asthma, GI ulceration, cardiovascular disease, urinary tract obstruction

Pregnancy Risk: C

Adverse Effects
Common: Sweating
Less common: Nausea, rash, flushing, tachycardia

Drug Interactions
Beta-blockers: Increased risk of cardiac conduction disturbances
Parasympathomimetics: Additive effects
Anticholinergics (atropine, ipratropium): Antagonize effects

Patient Instructions: Expect increased sweating. It may take several weeks for response to occur.

Clinical Pharmacology: Half-life is 1 hour; duration of action 3–5 hours.

Cost: $$$

PIROXICAM

Trade Names: Feldene

Drug Class: NSAID

Preparations: 10- and 20-mg capsules

Dose: 10–20 mg/day as a single dose

Clinical Pharmacology: Well absorbed after oral administration. The drug undergoes hepatic metabolism and renal elimination. Half-life is 50 hours.

Cost: $$

See NSAIDs for Indications, Mechanism of Action, Contraindications, Precautions, Monitoring, Pregnancy Risk, Adverse Effects, Interactions, and Patient Instructions.

Plaquenil (See Hydroxychloroquine)

PLASMAPHERESIS

Indications: Plasmapheresis can be effective in a number of rheumatologic and immunologic disorders, including Goodpasture syndrome, myasthenia gravis, Guillain-Barré syndrome, hyperviscosity syndrome (e.g., with Waldenström macroglobulinemia), cryoglobulinemia (particularly with renal involvement), thrombotic thrombocytopenic purpura, idiopathic demyelinating polyneuropathy, rapidly progressive glomerulonephritis, and refractory autoimmune hemolytic anemia or posttransfusion purpura. In addition to thrombotic thrombocytopenic purpura, plasmapheresis may be of benefit in other disorders associated with microangiopathic hemolytic anemia, including hemolytic-uremic syndrome, SLE presenting with thrombotic thrombocytopenic purpura–like features, disseminated intravascular coagulation, and the catastrophic antiphospholipid syndrome. Plasmapheresis may be of benefit in other conditions, e.g., SLE with transverse myelitis or other CNS or peripheral nervous systems manifestations. However, the evidence is anecdotal at best. For SLE nephritis, several studies showed that in unselected groups of patients, plasmapheresis is of no benefit. Whether plasmapheresis is indicated in some instances (e.g., SLE nephritis with a rapidly deteriorating course, in conjunction with high-dose cyclophosphamide) is still controversial. Plasmapheresis is not indicated in RA or dermatomyositis/polymyositis.

Mechanisms of Action: Plasmapheresis nonspecifically removes plasma constituents, including immunoglobulins and other plasma proteins. Removal of particular antibodies or immune complexes presumably underlies its effect in most diseases. In thrombotic thrombocytopenic purpura, some of the benefit also derives from infusion of normal plasma.

Comments: There are few adequate controlled trials in rheumatic diseases. Plasmapheresis should usually be used in conjunction with immunosuppressive therapy to prevent rebound increase in antibody production. Evidence suggests little benefit in RA or polymyositis/dermatomyositis. Plasmapheresis alone has no benefit in lupus nephritis, but plasmapheresis with pulse cyclophosphamide has anecdotally been shown to be beneficial.

Cost: $$$$$. An important consideration in the use of plasmapheresis is its cost, which runs upward of several thousand dollars for a treatment. Although generally well tolerated, it may also be associated with transient hypocalcemia and bleeding diathesis.

BIBLIOGRAPHY

Braun-Moscovici Y, Furst DE. Plasmapheresis for rheumatic diseases in the twenty-first century: take it or leave it? *Curr Opin Rheumatol* 2003;15:197–204.

Euler HH, Schroeder JO, Harten P, et al. Treatment-free remission in severe systemic lupus erythematosus following synchronization of plasmapheresis with subsequent pulse cyclophosphamide. *Arthritis Rheum* 1994;37:1784–1794.

von Baeyer H. Plasmapheresis in immune hematology: review of clinical outcome data with respect to evidence-based medicine and clinical experience. *Ther Apher Dial* 2003;7:127–140.

Prednisolone (See Corticosteroids)
Prednisone (See Corticosteroids)

PROBENECID

Trade Names: Benemid

Drug Class: Uricosuric

Preparations: 500-mg tablet

Dose: Initially, 250 mg twice daily for the first week, then increase to 500 mg twice daily, and, if needed, to a maintenance dose of 1–3 g/day in divided doses

Indications: Hyperuricemia is associated with gout in patients who excrete <800 mg of urate in a 24-hour urine collection have normal renal function, no tophi, and no history of renal calculi.

Mechanism of Action: Inhibits renal tubular reabsorption of uric acid

Contraindications: Hypersensitivity to probenecid, renal impairment, nephrolithiasis. Do not administer to patients with either acute gout or chronic tophaceous gout.

Precautions: Use caution with peptic ulcer. It inhibits excretion of penicillins, and toxic levels may accumulate in patients with impaired renal function.

Monitoring: Monitor uric acid periodically

Pregnancy Risk: B

Adverse Effects
Common: Nausea, vomiting, headache
Less common: Rash, itch, allergy, precipitation of an acute attack of gout, leukopenia, aplastic anemia, urate nephropathy, nephrotic syndrome

Drug Interactions
Salicylates (high dose): Antagonize uricosuric effect
β-Lactams (penicillins, cephalosporins) and quinolones: Increased plasma levels of antibiotics
MTX: Increased MTX toxicity
Antivirals: Reduced excretion of acyclovir and zidovudine

Patient Instructions: Drink plenty of fluids. Avoid aspirin or other salicylates (may antagonize the uricosuric effect).

Comments: To prevent acute attacks of gout, chronic colchicine or NSAID therapy is coadministered for the first 3–12 months of probenecid therapy. In patients with tophi or renal stones, allopurinol is preferred.

Clinical Pharmacology: Rapid, complete absorption; hepatic metabolism and renal excretion. Half-life is 6–12 hours.

D
R
U
G
S

Cost: $

BIBLIOGRAPHY

Rott KT, Agudelo CA. Gout. *JAMA* 2003;289:2857–2860.
Terkeltaub RA. Clinical practice. Gout. *N Engl J Med* 2003;349:1647–1655.

Propulsid (See Cisapride)
Protonix (Pantoprazole; See Appendix C)
Rabeprazole (Aciphex; See Appendix C)

RALOXIFENE

Trade Names: Evista

Drug Class: Selective estrogen receptor modulator

Preparations: 60-mg tablet

Dose/Administration: Osteoporosis: 60 mg p.o. daily

Indications: Treatment and prevention of osteoporosis in postmenopausal women

Mechanism of Action: Acts on some estrogen receptors and blocks others; acts on bone to prevent bone loss

Contraindications: Pregnancy or planned pregnancy (not intended for use in premenopausal women), hypersensitivity, active thromboembolism

Precautions: Thromboembolism, previous arterial or venous clots, history of carcinoma of cervix or uterus, renal or hepatic impairment

Pregnancy Risk: X

Adverse Effects
Common: Hot flashes, arthralgia
Less Common: Fever, migraine, insomnia, myalgia, cramps, thromboembolism, thrombophlebitis, pulmonary embolism, hypertriglyceridemia

Drug Interactions
Ampicillin and cholestyramine: decreased raloxifene concentrations

Comments: Selective estrogen receptor modulators such as raloxifene preferentially act on estrogen receptors outside the uterus and breast. Raloxifene, unlike estrogens, does not increase the risk of breast cancer; in fact, in preliminary reports, it reduced the risk. Unlike hormone replacement therapy, hot flashes do not improve; they may get worse.

Clinical Pharmacology: Oral bioavailability is poor. Extensive hepatic metabolism; half-life 30 hours.

Cost: $$$$

Ranitidine (Zantac; See Appendix C)
Refresh (See Artificial Tears)
Relafen (See Nabumetone)
Remicade (See Infliximab)
Rheumatrex (See Methotrexate)
Ridaura (See Auranofin)

RISEDRONATE

Trade Names: Actonel

Drug Class: Bisphosphonate

Preparations: 5-, 30-, 35-mg tablets

Dose/Administration
Osteoporosis: 5 mg p.o. daily or 35 mg once weekly
Paget disease: 30 mg p.o. daily for 2 months. If disease relapses, retreatment
   can be considered.

Indications: Treatment and prevention of osteoporosis; treatment of Paget's disease

Mechanism of Action: Antiresorptive; localizes to areas of bone resorption and inhibits osteoclast activity without any effect on bone formation; increases bone mineral density and significantly reduces vertebral fracture rates; does not induce osteomalacia

Contraindications: Hypersensitivity to risedronate, hypocalcemia, esophageal stricture, and dysmotility; not recommended for patients with severe renal insufficiency (creatinine clearance <35 mL/min). Avoid use in patients who cannot stand or sit upright for 30 minutes after administration.

Precautions: If possible, avoid use if esophageal problems or renal impairment are present. Ensure that patient understands how the drug should be taken.

DRUGS

Pregnancy Risk: C

Adverse Effects: Hypocalcemia (transient, mild), headache, mild GI disturbance (i.e., nausea, dyspepsia, dysphagia); rarely, severe erosive esophagitis, uveitis, altered taste, urticaria or angioedema

Drug Interactions: GI adverse events are increased in patients taking NSAIDs

Patient Instructions: Risedronate should be taken with a full glass of water on arising in the morning. Nothing other than water should be taken for at least 30 minutes after risedronate. Even coffee or fruit juice markedly reduce absorption. Delaying such intake for >30 minutes (1–2 hours if possible) maximizes absorption. After taking risedronate, the patient must remain upright to reduce risk of esophageal irritation. Any other medications must be taken at least 30 minutes after risedronate.

Comments: Supplemental calcium and vitamin D are usually coadministered. Weekly dosing for osteoporosis is preferred.

Clinical Pharmacology: Oral bioavailability is very poor (<1%) and negligible if administered with or after food. Absorbed drug is renally excreted and not metabolized. Terminal half-life exceeds 10 days, but the drug localizes in bone and is slowly released for years.

Cost: $$$$

BIBLIOGRAPHY

Delmas PD. Treatment of postmenopausal osteoporosis. *Lancet* 2002;359:2018–2026.

Rituxan (See Rituximab)

RITUXIMAB

Trade Names: Rituxan

Drug Class: A chimeric monoclonal antibody against the CD-20 antigen on B lymphocytes

Preparations: Injection: 10 mg/mL (10 and 50 mL)

Dose: Refer to individual protocols. The representative lymphoma dose is 375 mg/m^2 every week for 4 weeks slowly administered at an initial infusion rate of 50 mg/h. In RA protocols, the regimen calls for 1,000 mg i.v., given as two doses 2 weeks apart. The need for premedication with high-dose corticosteroids or background MTX or cyclophosphamide has not been conclusively defined.

Indications: Lymphoma, autoimmune thrombocytopenia. There are no established rheumatologic indications for rituximab, but its use is being explored in RA, Sjögren's syndrome, vasculitis, lupus, and a wide range of other conditions.

Mechanism of Action: Binds to antigen on CD-20 positive cells and lyses them

Contraindications: Hypersensitivity to murine proteins; breast feeding

Precautions: Do not administer as intravenous push; administer slowly per protocols outlined in package insert. Infusion reactions are common and may respond to slowing or temporary discontinuation of infusion or premedication with acetaminophen and diphenhydramine.

Monitoring: Monitor for infusion reactions during infusion and monitor CBC frequently thereafter.

Pregnancy Risk: C

Adverse Effects
Common: Infusion reactions (40%–80%); allergy, angioedema, headache, nausea, leukopenia, urticaria
Less common: Hypotension, vomiting, thrombocytopenia, neutropenia, red cell aplasia, arrhythmia

Comments: The place of rituximab in the therapy of rheumatic diseases is under investigation and has not been clearly established.

Clinical Pharmacology: Half-life is 50–200 hours; can be detected in serum several months after administration; B cell recovery begins approximately 6 months after treatment.

Cost: $$$$

BIBLIOGRAPHY

Silverman GJ, Weisman S. Rituximab therapy and autoimmune disorders: prospects for anti-B cell therapy. *Arthritis Rheum* 2003;48:1484–1492.

Robaxin (See Methocarbamol)
Rocaltrol (See Vitamin D)

ROFECOXIB (ALSO SEE APPENDIX A)

Trade Names: Vioxx

Drug Class: COX-2 selective NSAID

DRUGS

Preparations
Capsules: 12.5, 25, 50 mg

Dose: Osteoarthritis and RA 12.5–25 mg daily
Acute pain: 50 mg daily for no more than 5 days

Clinical Pharmacology: Hepatic metabolism and renal excretion of metabolites; half-life 17 hours

Cost: $$$

Comments: COX-2–selective NSAIDs are no more effective than traditional NSAIDs that inhibit both COX-1 and COX-2, but they are less likely to cause GI complications. How a traditional NSAID with a proton pump inhibitor compares with a COX-2–selective NSAID as regards GI risk is not known. Either is a reasonable strategy for patients at high risk of GI complications and unable to do without an NSAID. Therapy with low-dose aspirin and a COX-2–selective drug may abrogate the GI benefits of the COX-2 selectivity. Hypertension and edema are more common with the 50-mg dose, which is not approved for long-term use. In the VIGOR study, there were more myocardial infarctions in patients receiving rofecoxib than in those receiving naproxen. It is unclear whether this represents a chance finding, a protective effect of naproxen, or a deleterious effect of this dose of rofecoxib (50 mg) in this population (RA). Many studies examining the 25-mg dose show no increased risk of myocardial infarction.

See NSAIDs for Indications, Mechanism of Action, Contraindications, Precautions, Monitoring, Pregnancy Risk, Adverse Effects, Interactions, and Patient Instructions.

BIBLIOGRAPHY

Bombardier C, Laine L, Reicin A, et al. Comparison of upper gastrointestinal toxicity of rofecoxib and naproxen in patients with rheumatoid arthritis. VIGOR Study Group. *N Engl J Med* 2000;343:1520–1528.
FitzGerald GA, Patrono C. The coxibs, selective inhibitors of cyclooxygenase-2. *N Engl J Med* 2001;345:433–442.

SALSALATE

Trade Names: Argesic-SA, Disalcid, Salflex

Synonyms: Disalicylic acid, salicylsalicylic acid

Drug Class: Nonacetylated salicylate, NSAID

Preparations
Capsule: 500 mg
Tablets: 500 and 750 mg

Dose: Adult: 3 g/day in two or three divided doses

Indications: RA, osteoarthritis, pain

Mechanism of Action: Weak inhibitor of prostaglandin synthesis

Contraindications: Hypersensitivity to salicylates

Precautions: Administer with food. Use caution in asthma, bleeding disorders, anticoagulant use, or hepatic or renal disease.

Monitoring: Monitor hematocrit, creatinine, liver enzymes periodically (1 month after starting and then every 3–6 months). Serum salicylate levels may be assayed periodically, if necessary.

Pregnancy Risk: C

Adverse Effects
Common: GI irritation (dyspepsia, reflux, epigastric pain)
Less common: GI ulceration or hemorrhage; minor elevations of liver enzymes; hypersensitivity (asthma, urticaria, angioedema, particularly in patients with nasal polyps); cross-sensitivity occurs between NSAIDs, but hypersensitivity is less common with the nonacetylated salicylates; dose-related side effects include tinnitus and deafness.

Drug Interactions
Antacids: Decreased salicylate levels through increased elimination in alkaline urine
Anticoagulants: Activity of warfarin increased
Uricosurics: Decreased uricosuric effect

Patient Instructions: Take with food. Discontinue and seek medical advice if fainting, vomiting of blood, or unusual bleeding develops.

Comments: Nonacetylated salicylates have little effect on platelet function and cause less GI toxicity than classic NSAIDs, which are more potent inhibitors of prostaglandin synthesis. In practice, the antiinflammatory effect of salsalate is less than that of classic NSAIDs.

Clinical Pharmacology: Rapidly and well absorbed after oral administration; hepatic metabolism and renal excretion of conjugated metabolites. Urinary pH alters elimination (alkaline urine increases elimination). Wide variation in plasma concentrations in individuals receiving the same dose. Half-life varies with dose (2–3 hours with low doses, ≥20 hours with high doses). At high doses, the salicylate elimination pathway is saturated, and a small increase in dose can lead to a large increase in serum concentrations.

Cost: $

DRUGS

Salagen (See Pilocarpine)

Sandimmune (See Cyclosporine)

Sertraline (Zoloft; See Appendix D)

Solganol (See Gold)

Soma (See Carisoprodol)

Sucralfate (Carafate; See Appendix C)

SULFASALAZINE

Trade Names: Azulfidine, Azulfidine EN-tabs

Synonyms: Salazopyrin; 5-aminosalicylic acid plus sulfapyridine

Drug Class: Sulfonamide/salicylate congener, DMARD

Preparations
Tablet: 500 mg
Tablet, enteric coated: 500 mg

Dose: In rheumatic diseases, 2–3 g/day in two or three divided doses. Initial dose of 500 mg daily is increased by 500-mg increments weekly as tolerated. Usual maintenance dose is 2–3 g/day. Higher doses may be associated with greater GI toxicity.

Indications: RA, juvenile RA, Reiter's syndrome, ankylosing spondylitis, psoriatic arthritis, inflammatory bowel disease

Mechanism of Action: Unknown; the sulfonamide component is thought to be more active in the treatment of rheumatic diseases than the 5-aminosalicylic component.

Contraindications: Hypersensitivity to sulfonamides or salicylates, porphyria, GI/genitourinary obstruction

Precautions: Use caution in impaired renal function; it may cause hemolysis in G6PD deficiency.

Monitoring: Hematologic adverse effects are most likely in the first 6 months. CBC every 2–3 weeks for first 3 months, then gradually decrease frequency to every 3 months. Periodic LFTs (3- to 6-month intervals) should be done.

Pregnancy Risk: B (D at term)

Adverse Effects

Common: GI side effects (nausea, vomiting, diarrhea, cramps), rash, itch, dizziness, headache

Less common: Reversible oligospermia, neutropenia, aplastic anemia, agranulocytosis, hemolysis, Stevens-Johnson syndrome, photosensitivity, SLE-like syndrome, nephrotic syndrome, orange-yellow discoloration of urine, hepatitis

Drug Interactions

Warfarin: Resistance to warfarin described, monitor international normalized ratio for change

MTX: Increased MTX toxicity (see Comments)

Patient Instructions: May cause orange-yellow discoloration of skin, urine, and contact lenses. Beware of photosensitive reactions to prolonged sunlight exposure.

Comments: GI intolerance is often prominent when starting treatment. Thus, start with a low dose and work up. Some evidence indicates that the enteric coated tablets are better tolerated. Efficacy in RA appears similar to that of MTX, but there may be more minor side effects and less serious toxicity. Widely used in Europe as a first-line DMARD for RA; more recently, used in combination with MTX and hydroxychloroquine in patients with RA not responding to MTX alone. Efficacy in ankylosing spondylitis, Reiter's syndrome, and psoriatic arthritis is variable and probably greatest in those with peripheral arthropathy (rather than axial disease alone). It may cause folate deficiency (consider supplementation with folate, 1 mg/day).

Clinical Pharmacology: The azo bond joining 5-aminosalicylic and sulfapyridine is broken by bacteria in the colon. Approximately 15%–30% is absorbed; hepatic metabolism; renal excretion. Half-life is 6–10 hours. Slow acetylators have higher sulfapyridine blood levels and perhaps more minor side effects, but acetylator status need not be routinely determined.

Cost: Generic, $$; enteric coated, $$$

BIBLIOGRAPHY

American College of Rheumatology Committee on Rheumatoid Arthritis Guidelines. Guidelines for the management of rheumatoid arthritis: 2002 update. *Arthritis Rheum* 2002; 46:328–346.

O'Dell JR, Haire CE, Erikson N, et al. Treatment of rheumatoid arthritis with methotrexate alone, sulfasalazine and hydroxychloroquine, or a combination of all three medications. *N Engl J Med* 1996;334:1287–1291.

Rains CP, Noble S, Faulds D. Sulfasalazine. A review of its pharmacological properties and therapeutic efficacy in the treatment of rheumatoid arthritis. *Drugs* 1995;50:137–156.

DRUGS

SULFINPYRAZONE

Trade Names: Anturane

Drug Class: Uricosuric

Preparations
Tablet: 100 mg
Capsule: 200 mg

Dose: 100–200 mg twice daily; maximum daily dose 800 mg

Indications: Hyperuricemia associated with gout in patients who excrete ≤800 mg of urate/24 h, have normal renal function, no tophi, and no renal calculi.

Mechanism of Action: Decreases renal reabsorption of filtered uric acid

Contraindications: Hypersensitivity to sulfinpyrazone; renal failure, gouty nephropathy, bone marrow depression, hyperuricemia of cancer, chemotherapy

Precautions: Caution with renal impairment, peptic ulcer disease

Monitoring: Monitor uric acid periodically.

Pregnancy Risk: C/D

Adverse Effects
Common: Nausea, vomiting, cramps
Less common: Rash, dizziness, anemia, leukopenia, hepatitis, nephrotic syndrome

Drug Interactions
Salicylates: Decreased uricosuric effect
Theophylline: Decreased theophylline levels
Verapamil: Decreased verapamil levels
Anticoagulants: Effect of warfarin enhanced
Antidiabetics: Sulfonylurea effects enhanced

Patient Instructions: Drink plenty of fluids and take with food. Avoid large doses of aspirin or other salicylates.

Clinical Pharmacology: Well absorbed; hepatic metabolism and renal excretion; half-life 4 hours

Cost: $$

SULINDAC

Trade Names: Clinoril

Drug Class: NSAID

Preparations: 150- and 200-mg tablets

Dose: 150–200 mg twice daily

Comments: Sulindac may be safer than other NSAIDs in patients at high risk of renal impairment. Such benefits may only apply to short-term use (<6 weeks), and claims that sulindac is renal sparing are based on limited and controversial evidence.

Clinical Pharmacology: Well absorbed after oral administration, sulindac is a prodrug. After ingestion, there is hepatic metabolism to an active sulfide metabolite, which later undergoes renal elimination. Half-life of parent drug is 7 hours and half-life of metabolite is 18 hours.

Cost: Generic, $$

See NSAIDs for Indications, Mechanism of Action, Contraindications, Precautions, Monitoring, Pregnancy Risk, Adverse Effects, Interactions, and Patient Instructions.

Synvisc (See Hyaluronan injections)
Tears, Artificial (See Artificial Tears)
Tensilon (See Edrophonium)

TERIPARATIDE

Trade Names: Forteo

Synonyms: Human recombinant parathyroid hormone (1-34)

Drug Class: Hormone

Preparations: Prefilled injection pen 750 μg/3 mL (28-day supply)

Dose: 20 μg daily by subcutaneous injection

Indications: Osteoporosis with high risk of fracture failed alternative therapies; safety beyond 2 years has not been studied; until additional information is available, treatment for >2 years is not recommended.

DRUGS

Mechanism of Action: Mimics action of parathyroid hormone and stimulates new bone formation

Contraindications: Hypersensitivity; increased risk of osteosarcoma (Paget's disease, previous irradiation), skeletal malignancy, open epiphyses, children, hypercalcemia

Precautions: Renal stones, unexplained increase in alkaline phosphatase, digoxin therapy

Monitoring: Monitoring of serum calcium level periodically may be prudent.

Pregnancy Risk: C

Adverse Effects: Causes osteosarcoma in rats; the significance of this as regards risk in humans not established
Common: Transient increase in serum calcium concentration 4–6 hours after injection; dizziness, leg cramps
Uncommon: Orthostatic hypotension 4–6 hours after injection

Drug Interactions
Digoxin: Increased serum calcium may predispose to toxicity
Alendronate: Impairs ability of teriparatide to increase bone density

Patient Instructions: Refrigerate (do not freeze) the injection pen. Follow manual of instructions that comes with the pen.

Comments: Carries a "black box" warning that it causes osteosarcoma in rats and should only be prescribed for patients for whom benefits outweigh risk. Antiresorptive drugs such as bisphosphonates impair the anabolic effects of teriparatide.

Clinical Pharmacology: Good rapid absorption, half-life 1 hour after subcutaneous injection

Cost: $$$$

BIBLIOGRAPHY

Finkelstein JS, Hayes A, Hunzelman JL, et al. The effects of parathyroid hormone, alendronate, or both in men with osteoporosis. *N Engl J Med* 2003;349:1216–1226.
Neer RM, Arnaud CD, Zanchetta JR, et al. Effect of parathyroid hormone (1-34) on fractures and bone mineral density in postmenopausal women with osteoporosis. *N Engl J Med* 2001;344:1434–1441.

Thalomid (See Thalidomide)

THALIDOMIDE

Trade Names: Thalomid

Drug Class: Immunomodulator

Preparations: Capsule: 50 mg

Dose: 100–300 mg daily in divided doses; must only be administered in compliance with the STEPS program

Indications: Erythema nodosum leprosum. Small, mostly uncontrolled reports have suggested possible benefit in graft versus host disease, aphthous ulcers in human immunodeficiency virus, mucocutaneous lesions of Behçet's disease, lupus skin disease, sarcoidosis, systemic onset juvenile RA, and pyoderma gangrenosum. Trials in myeloma are in progress.

Mechanism of Action: Unknown; may inhibit angiogenesis and TNF

Contraindications: Pregnancy, hypersensitivity to thalidomide, childbearing potential and noncompliance with contraception, neutropenia

Precautions: May only be prescribed by physicians registered in the System for Thalidomide Education and Prescribing Safety (STEPS) program (see FDA Web site http:/www.fda.gov/cder/news/thalinfo/thalomid.htm). If possible, avoid in women of childbearing potential; if not possible, ensure contraception for 4 weeks before and 4 weeks after therapy and a negative pregnancy test within 24 hours of beginning treatment.

Monitoring: Monthly pregnancy tests, monthly assessment for peripheral neuropathy, consider electrophysiologic testing to monitor for neuropathy, monitor CBC periodically

Pregnancy Risk: X, highly teratogenic

Adverse Effects
Common: Peripheral neuropathy that may be permanent; this can occur after short-term use. Postural hypotension, dizziness, sleepiness. If used during pregnancy, causes birth defects such as phocomelia
Less common: Neutropenia, Stevens-Johnson syndrome, seizures, edema, rash, deep vein thrombosis

Drug Interactions: Increased sedation with sedatives

Patient Instructions: Do not share the medication. Use two forms of contraception if a women and a latex condom if a man. This drug causes birth defects; do not become pregnant. Report changes in sensation in your hands and feet. Can cause sleepiness and dizziness on standing. Do not donate blood.

Comments: This agent has limited potential for long-term use owing to frequent side effects, teratogenicity, lack of proven efficacy in rheumatic diseases, and the relapse of disease after discontinuation. Strategies to prevent fetal exposure to thalidomide are outlined in the STEPS program. The drug can only be prescribed by program-approved physicians.

DRUGS

Clinical Pharmacology: Peak concentrations at 4 hours; elimination half-life is 5 hours, largely through nonenzymatic hydrolysis

Cost: $$

BIBLIOGRAPHY

Stein CM. Immunoregulatory drugs. In: Harris ED, Ruddy S, Sledge CB, eds. *Kelley's Textbook of Rheumatology,* 7th ed. Philadelphia: WB Saunders, 2004.

Tolectin (See Tolmetin)

TOLMETIN

Trade Names: Tolectin

Synonyms: Tolmetin sodium

Drug Class: NSAID

Preparations: 200-, 400-, 600-mg tablets

Dose: 600–1,800 mg daily in three or four divided doses

Clinical Pharmacology: Well absorbed after oral administration; hepatic metabolism and renal elimination; half-life 2–5 hours

Cost: $$

See NSAIDs for Indications, Mechanism of Action, Contraindications, Precautions, Monitoring, Pregnancy Risk, Adverse Effects, Interactions, and Patient Instructions.

Tracleer (See Bosentan)
Toradol (See Ketorolac)

TRAMADOL

Trade Names: Ultram

Drug Class: Opioid analgesic

Preparations: 50-mg tablet

Dose: Adults: 50–100 mg every 4–6 hours (not to exceed 400 mg/day)

Indications: Pain not controlled by nonopioid analgesics

Mechanism of Action: Binds to μ-opioid receptors; inhibits uptake of norepinephrine and serotonin

Contraindications: Hypersensitivity to tramadol or opioids; drug abuse

Precautions: Seizure risk is increased in patients also receiving tricyclic antidepressants and structurally related drugs (cyclobenzaprine, promethazine), MAOIs, SSRIs. Renal and hepatic impairment decreases clearance of tramadol.

Monitoring: Use the lowest dose necessary to control pain. Escalate dose only with uncontrolled pain.

Pregnancy Risk: C

Adverse Effects
Common: Dizziness, nausea, constipation, headache, sleepiness, itch
Less common: Respiratory depression, seizures, dependence, increased hepatic
   enzymes

Drug Interactions
Antidepressants, MAOIs, opioids: Increased seizure risk
Quinidine: Increased tramadol concentrations
Carbamazepine: Decreased tramadol concentrations

Patient Instructions: Drug is addictive and must only be used to control pain. Do not drink alcohol. It may cause drowsiness.

Comments: Efficacy seems similar to that of other weak opioids; it is thought to have less potential for abuse.

Clinical Pharmacology: Bioavailability 70%; hepatic metabolism by CYP P-450 2D6 to M1 metabolite. Half-life is 5 hours.

Cost: $$$

BIBLIOGRAPHY

Dayer P, Collart L, Desmeules J. The pharmacology of tramadol. *Drugs* 1994;47(Suppl 1):3–7.

TRAZODONE

Trade Names: Desyrel

Drug Class: Antidepressant

Preparations: 50-, 100-, 150-, 300-mg tablets

Dose

Depression: Initially 150 mg/day in three divided doses; increase dose by 50 mg/day every week, if needed, to maximum of 600 mg/day.

Fibromyalgia: As a sleep aid, the usual starting dose is 25–50 mg nightly. This can be increased by 50 mg per week (to as much as 150 mg) until maximum improvement in sleep is achieved without causing morning somnolence.

Indications: Treatment of depression or sleep disturbance in fibromyalgia

Mechanism of Action: Inhibits presynaptic uptake of norepinephrine and serotonin

Contraindications: Hypersensitivity to trazodone

Precautions: Sedating but little anticholinergic effect. Concomitant MAOI therapy is potentially dangerous. Allow a 14-day washout between trazodone and MAOI therapy. Use caution in cardiac, renal, and hepatic disease.

Monitoring: Plasma levels are not routinely measured and may not correlate with efficacy.

Pregnancy Risk: C

Adverse Effects

Common: Sedation, nausea, bad taste, dry mouth, dizziness, weight gain

Less common: Weakness, diarrhea, constipation, nightmares

Uncommon: Rash, orthostatic symptoms (tachycardia, postural dizziness), arrhythmias, heart block, agitation, seizures, extrapyramidal effects, priapism, urinary retention

Drug Interactions

CNS depressants: Increased CNS depression

Phenytoin: Increased phenytoin levels reported

Increased toxicity: MAOI (serotonin syndrome)

Patient Instructions: May cause drowsiness; avoid alcohol. Keep medication away from children.

Comments: Maximum effect may be delayed for 4 weeks. Sometimes used for sedative effect to correct sleep disorders caused by SSRIs.

Clinical Pharmacology: Well absorbed; 90% protein bound; hepatic metabolism with half-life of 5–9 hours

Cost: $

Tricyclic Antidepressants (See Appendix D)

Trilisate (See Choline Magnesium Salicylate)

Tums (See Calcium)

Tylenol (See Acetaminophen)

Tylenol #3 (See Acetaminophen + Opioids)

Tylox (See Acetaminophen + Opioids)

Ultracet (See Acetaminophen + Opioids)

Ultram (See Tramadol)

VALDECOXIB (ALSO SEE APPENDIX A)

Trade Names: Bextra

Drug Class: COX-2 selective NSAID

Preparations: 10- and 20-mg capsules

Dose: 10 mg daily

Clinical Pharmacology: Well absorbed after oral administration; hepatic metabolism and renal excretion of metabolites; half-life 10 hours

Cost: $$$

Comments: COX-2–selective NSAIDs are no more effective than traditional NSAIDs, which inhibit both COX-1 and COX-2, but they are less likely to cause GI complications. How a traditional NSAID with a proton pump inhibitor compares to a COX-2 selective NSAID as regards GI risk is not known. Either are reasonable strategies for patients who have a high risk of GI complications and are unable to do without an NSAID. Therapy with low-dose aspirin and a COX-2–selective drug may abrogate the GI benefits of the COX-2 selectivity. Avoid in patients with sulfonamide allergy.

See NSAIDs for Indications, Mechanism of Action, Contraindications, Precautions, Monitoring, Pregnancy Risk, Adverse Effects, Interactions and Patient Instructions

BIBLIOGRAPHY

FitzGerald GA, Patrono C. The coxibs, selective inhibitors of cyclooxygenase-2. *N Engl J Med* 2001;345:433–442.
Pavelka K, Recker DP, Verburg KM. Valdecoxib is as effective as diclofenac in the management of rheumatoid arthritis with a lower incidence of gastroduodenal ulcers: results of a 26-week trial. *Rheumatology* 2003;42:1207–1215.

DRUGS

Venlafaxine (Effexor; See Appendix D)
Vicodin (See Acetaminophen + Opioids)
Vioxx (See Rofecoxib and Appendix A)

VITAMIN D (ERGOCALCIFEROL, CALCITRIOL)

Trade Names: Ergocalciferol, Calciferol; calcitriol, Rocaltrol

Synonyms: Ergocalciferol, vitamin D_2; calcitriol, 1,25-dihydroxycholecalciferol

Drug Class: Vitamin

Preparations
Ergocalciferol: Capsule 50,000 U (1.25 mg), multiple OTC preparations containing 400 U/tablet
Calcitriol: 0.25- and 0.5-μg capsules

Dose
Ergocalciferol: Dietary supplement/prevention of osteoporosis, 400 U/day; treatment of osteomalacia, 1,000–5,000 U/day.
Calcitriol: Renal failure, individualize dose to maintain serum calcium level; usual dose, 0.25 μg daily or alternate days. Higher doses may be required.

Indications: Most often used as a dietary supplement with calcium to ensure adequate intake of calcium and vitamin D in the prophylaxis and treatment of osteoporosis. Vitamin D is also used to treat rickets/osteomalacia, and calcitriol is used to treat hypocalcemia associated with renal failure.

Mechanism of Action: Promotes absorption of calcium from GI tract and stimulates calcium reabsorption from the renal tubule

Contraindications: Hypercalcemia, vitamin D toxicity

Precautions: Adequate calcium intake required; avoid hypercalcemia

Monitoring: With dietary supplementation using doses in the range of the RDA (400 U/day) of vitamin D_2, serum calcium may be monitored occasionally. With higher doses of vitamin D or use of the more potent calcitriol preparation, close monitoring of serum calcium level is prudent.

Pregnancy Risk: A, but D in doses above the RDA

Adverse Effects: Doses of vitamin D_2 in the RDA range have minimal side effects. The more potent calcitriol preparation has more often been associated with hypercalcemia, hypercalciuria, and renal stones.

With any vitamin D preparation, dose-related hypercalcemia may occur, resulting in weakness, anorexia, polyuria, thirst, constipation, nausea, myalgia, irritability, and psychosis.

Drug Interactions: Increased serum calcium with thiazide diuretics

Comments: The effect of vitamin D preparations on osteoporosis is controversial. Generally, vitamin D is supplemented in the treatment and prophylaxis of osteoporosis in doses that ensure a daily intake that meets the RDA. The risk/benefit balance of using a more potent vitamin D preparation such as calcitriol or alphacidol in osteoporosis is controversial, and they are not widely used for this purpose.

Clinical Pharmacology: Cholecalciferol (vitamin D_3) and ergocalciferol (vitamin D_2) are activated in the liver to calcifediol (25-hydroxycholecalciferol) and then in the kidneys to calcitriol (1,25-dihydroxycholecalciferol). Vitamin D is fat soluble and is stored in the liver and fat; thus, effects are prolonged.

Cost: $$$

BIBLIOGRAPHY

Orcel P. Calcium and vitamin D in the prevention and treatment of osteoporosis. *J Clin Rheumatol* 1997;3:S52–S56.

Voltaren (See Diclofenac)

ZOLPIDEM

Trade Names: Ambien

Drug Class: Sedative-hypnotic

Preparations: 5- and 10-mg tablets

Dose: Usual dose, 5–10 mg before bedtime (elderly use 5 mg)

Indications: Treatment of insomnia

Mechanism of Action: Not a benzodiazepine but binds to the benzodiazepine 1 subtype of the γ-aminobutyric acid receptor

Contraindications: Hypersensitivity to zolpidem

Precautions: May cause impaired cognitive and motor performance, particularly in the elderly. There is decreased elimination with impaired hepatic function; decrease dose to 5 mg in such patients. It may exacerbate sleep apnea.

Pregnancy Risk: B

Adverse Effects
Common: Headache, drowsiness, rash, nausea
Less common: Confusion, falls, amnesia, allergy, paradoxical agitation

Drug Interactions: CNS depressants have increased effect

Patient Instructions: Causes drowsiness; avoid alcohol; keep away from children.

Comments: Limit use to short periods of time.

Clinical Pharmacology: Rapid absorption; 70% first-pass extraction; 90% protein bound; hepatic metabolism (CYP3A substrate) to inactive metabolites. Half-life is 2–4 hours.

Cost: $$$

BIBLIOGRAPHY
Kupfer DJ, Reynolds CF. Management of insomnia. *N Engl J Med* 1997;336:341–346.

Zorprin (See Aspirin)
Zostrix (See Capsaicin)
Zyloprim (See Allopurinol)

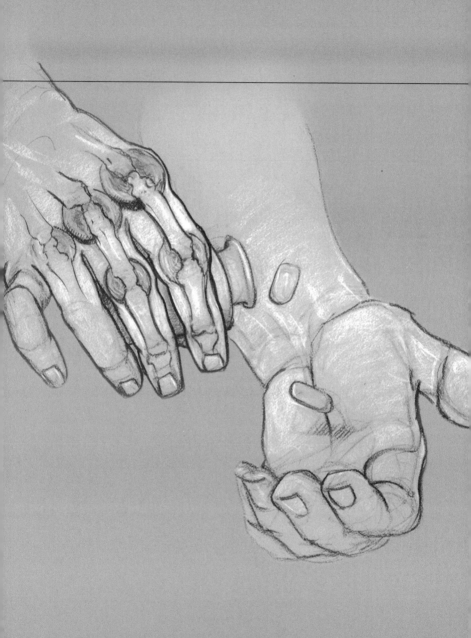

APPENDICES

COMPARISON OF NONSTEROIDAL ANTI-INFLAMMATORY DRUGS

Generic Name	Trade Name(s)	Strength (mg)	Daily Frequency	Daily Dose range (mg)	Other Preparations
Very Cheap–Cheap (generic form: $5–40/mo)					
Aspirin	Ecotrin, Easprin, Bufferin	325, 500, 650, 975	3–4	2,000–6,000	Supp EC
Ibuprofen	Motrin	200, 400, 600, 800	2–4	1,200–3,200	Susp
Indomethacin	Indocin	25, 50	3–4	75–200	Susp supp
Naproxen	Naprosyn,	250, 375, 500	2–3	500–1,500	Liquid EC
Diclofenac	Voltaren	25, 50, 75	2–4	150–225	Supp oph
Etodolac	Lodine	200, 300, 400, 500	2–4	600–1,200	—
Fenoprofen	Nalfon	200, 300, 600	3–4	1,200–3,200	—
Meclo-fenamate	Meclomen	50, 100	3–4	300–400	—
Piroxicam	Feldene	10, 20	1–2	10–20	—
Salsalate	Disalcid	500, 750	2–3	2,000–4,500	—
Sulindac	Clinoril	150, 200	1–2	200–400	—
Tolmetin	Tolectin	200, 400, 600	3–4	1,200–1,800	—
Intermediate (generic form, $40–80/mo)					
Ketorolac	Toradol	10	1–4	10–40	Parenteral
Choline Mg salicylate	Trilisate	500, 750,1,000	3–4	2,000–4,000	Susp
Diclofenac	Voltaren XR, Cataflam	50, 100	1–2	100–200	—
Diflunisal	Dolobid	250, 500	2–3	1,000–1,500	—
Etodolac	Lodine XL	400, 500, 600	1–2	800–1,200	—
Flurbiprofen	Ansaid	50, 100	2–4	200–400	Oph
Indometh-acin- SR	Indocin-SR	75	1–2	75–150	—
Ketoprofen	Orudis	25, 50, 75	2–3	150–300	—
Ketoprofen-SR	Oruvail	100, 150, 200	1	100–200	—
Nabumetone	Relafen	500, 750	1–2	1,000–2,000	—
Naproxen-SR	Naprelan	375, 500	1	500–1,500	—
Oxaprozin	Daypro	600	1–2	1,200–1,800	—
Very Expensive ($80–100/mo)					
Diclofenac/ Misoprostol	Arthrotec	50/200, 75/200	1–2	50–150	—
Meloxicam	Mobic	7.5, 15	1	7.5–15	—
Celecoxib	Celebrex	100, 200	1–2	200–400	—
Rofecoxib	Vioxx	12.5, 25 50	1	12.5–50	Susp
Valdecoxib	Bextra	10, 20	1	10–20	—

SR, sustained release formulation; Supp, suppository; EC, enteric coated; Oph, opthalamic solution; Susp, suspension; mg, magnesium.

SECOND-LINE DRUGS FOR THE TREATMENT OF RHEUMATOID ARTHRITIS

Drug	Mechanisms of Action	Common Adverse Effects	Usual Dosing Regimens
Disease-Modifying Antirheumatic Drugs			
Injectable gold Aurothioglucose Gold sodium thiomalate	Inhibits macrophage function Inhibits angiogenesis Inhibits protein kinase C	Mucocutaneous eruptions Proteinuria Thrombocytopenia	50 mg/wk i.m. to a total dose of 1,000 mg; then 50 mg i.m. q 2–4 wk
Oral gold Auranofin	Inhibits macrophage function Inhibits PMN function	Diarrhea Mucocutaneous eruptions	3 mg p.o., b.i.d.
Antimalarials Hydroxychloro- quine	Inhibits cytokine secretion Inhibits lysosomal enzymes Inhibits macrophage function	Rash Visual disturbance	400 mg p.o., q.d.
D-Penicillamine	Inhibits helper T cell function Inhibits angiogenesis	Mucocutaneous eruptions Proteinuria Thrombocytopenia	500–1,000 mg p.o., q.d.
Sulfasalazine	Inhibits B cell responses Inhibits angiogenesis	Nausea, abdominal pain, diarrhea Rash	1,000 mg p.o., b.i.d. or t.i.d.
Methotrexate	Dihydrofolate reductase inhibitor Antiinflammatory via induction of adenosine release Inhibits chemotaxis	Mucocutaneous eruptions Bone marrow Nausea, diarrhea Hepatic abnormalities	7.5–25 mg/wk, p.o., (may also be administered parenterally SC or IM)
Leflunomide	Inhibits pyrimidine synthesis Hepatic abnormalities	Hepatic abnormalities Diarrhea, nausea	20 mg/day, p.o., (initial loading dose of 100 mg/day for 3 days)
Anakinra	IL-1 receptor antagonist	Injection site reactions Infection	100 mg s.c. injection daily

Adalimumab	TNF antibody (human)	Injection site reactions Opportunistic infections	40 mg s.c. injection q 14 days
Infliximab	TNF antibody (chimeric)	Infusion reactions Opportunistic infections	3 mg/kg i.v. slow infusion wk 0, 2, 6, then every 8 wk
Etanercept	Soluble TNF receptor	Injection site reactions Opportunistic infections	25 mg s.c. injection twice weekly or 50 mg/wk s.c.
Systemic immunosuppressives			
Cyclosporine	Inhibits synthesis of IL-2 and other T cell cytokines	Hypertension Renal insufficiency Hirsutism	2.5–4 mg/kg p.o., q.d.
Azathioprine	Inhibits DNA synthesis	Bone marrow suppression	1–2 mg/kg p.o., q.d.
Mycophenolate	Inhibits lymphocyte Proliferation	GI, leukopenia Nausea Hepatic abnormalities	1.0–1.5 g p.o. b.i.d..
Cyclophosphamide	Crosslinks DNA and inhibits cellular proliferation	Nausea, emesis Bone marrow suppression Ovarian failure Hemorrhagic cystitis ↑ Risk of cancer	1-2 mg/kg p.o., q.d.

i.m., intramuscularly; q, every; PMN, polymorphonucleocyte; p.o., by mouth; q.d., everyday b.i.d., twice daily; t.i.d., three times daily; IL, interleukin; s.c., subcutaneously; TNF, tumor necrosis factor; GI, gastrointestinal.

DRUGS USED TO TREAT AND PREVENT PEPTIC ULCER DISEASE

Drug	Dose
H$_2$-receptor antagonists	
Cimetidine (Tagamet)	400 mg twice daily
Famotidine (Pepcid)	20 mg twice daily
Nizatidine (Axid)	150 mg twice daily
Ranitidine (Zantac)	150 mg twice daily
Proton pump inhibitors	
Lansoprazole (Prevacid)	30 mg once or twice daily
Omeprazole (Prilosec)	20 mg once or twice daily
Esomeprazole (Nexium)	20 mg once or twice daily
Rabeprazole (Aciphex)	20 mg once or twice daily
Pantoprazole (Protonix)	40 mg once or twice daily
Miscellaneous drugs	
Misoprostol (Cytotec)	200 μg 4 times daily
Sucralfate (Carafate)	1 g 4 times daily

Note: H$_2$-receptor antagonists are often used in lower doses for maintenance after ulcer healing. H$_2$-receptor antagonists and proton pump inhibitors are most often used to treat peptic ulcers and reflux esophagitis. Cimetidine inhibits cytochrome P-450 drug metabolism, and clinically important interactions occur with warfarin, theophylline, phenytoin, quinidine, and propranolol. Proton pump inhibitors are particularly useful in reflux esophagitis associated with scleroderma. Misoprostol or proton pump inhibitors are most often used to prevent nonsteroidal antiinflammatory drug–related gastrointestinal complications. Frequency of proton pump inhibitor dosing depends on whether utilized for acute gastroesophageal reflux disease/ulceration (twice daily) or chronic prevention (once daily).

COMPARISON OF COMMON ANTIDEPRESSANTS

Drug	Daily Dose Range[a] (mg/day)	Anticholinergic	Drowsiness	Arrhythmias
First-generation Antidepressants (tricyclics)				
Amitriptyline (Elavil)	75–300	++++	++++	+++
Doxepin (Sinequan)	75–300	++++	++++	++
Imipramine (Tofranil)	75–200	+++	+++	+++
Nortriptyline (Pamelor)	50–100	++	++	+++
Second-generation antidepressants				
Amoxapine (Asendin)	100–400	++	++	++
Maprotilene (Ludiomil)	100–225	++	+++	++
Trazodone (Desyrel)	150–400	+	+++	+
Bupropion (Wellbutrin)	200–450	0/+	0/+	+
Third-generation antidepressants				
SSRIs				
Fluoxetine (Prozac)	10–40	0	0	0
Paroxetine (Paxil)	20–50	0/+	0	0
Sertraline (Zoloft)	50–150	0	0	0
Citalopram (Celexa)	20–60	0	0	0
Escitalopram (Lexapro)	10–20	0	0	0
Norepinephrine/SSRIs				
Venlafaxine (Effexor)	75–225	+	+	0

[a] Usual dose ranges for depression are expressed as total daily dose. For many drugs, this is administered in two or three divided doses. Initial doses and doses for other indications (e.g., insomnia, pain control) may be much lower than maintenance doses for depression. Monoamine oxidase inhibitors are not included and should only be prescribed by experts in the treatment of depression.

SSRIs, selective serotonin reuptake inhibitors.

DERMATOMAL MAPS

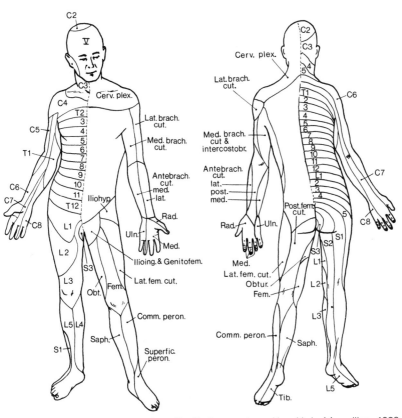

(Reproduced from Gilroy J, Holliday PL. Basic neurology. New York: Macmillan, 1982, with permission.)

VASCULITIS: CLASSIFICATION AND COMPARISONS

Diagnosis (by vessel size)	Demographic Features	Local Findings	Systemic Findings	Diagnostic Test(s)[a]	Treatment
Small vessel vasculitis					
Leukocytoclastic (hypersensitivity) vasculitis	M = F; all ages can be affected	Palpable purpura; superficial erosions, bullae, urticaria	Associated with HSP, cryo-globulinemia, RA, SLE, PAN, Wegener's, Churg-Strauss, PBC, ulcerative colitis, drugs, infection (gonococcus, mening-ococcus, staphylococcus, SBE, HBV, HCV, CMV, EBV), neoplasia (Hodgkin's, lymphoma, leukemia, myeloma)	Skin Bx is diagnostic	Treat under-lying disorder; seldom requires the use of steroids, colchicine, or dapsone
Henoch-Schönlein purpura	M = F; children (2-11 years), adults (30-70 years)	Palpable purpura of the lower extremities and buttocks; diarrhea, cramping, intussusception	Renal failure, arthralgia, arthritis, fever	IgA deposition on skin, GI or renal Bx	Self-limiting in most and will only require supportive care; steroids are not effective and are reserved for CNS, testicular, intestinal, or joint disease

Diagnosis (by vessel size)	Demographics Features	Local Findings	Systemic Findings	Diagnostic Test(s)[a]	Treatment
Hypocomplementemic urticarial vasculitis	F > M; usually young adults (range, 20-60 years)	Recurrent or chronic urticaria, palpable purpura	Arthralgias, arthritis, abdominal pain, N/V, fever, lymphadenopathy	Dx by skin Bx; low C3, C4, CH50; ↑ ESR, RF negative, some have low-titer ANA	Most are treated with NSAIDs or prednisone; hydroxychloroquine or cytotoxic therapy is seldom needed
Microscopic polyangiitis	M > F; middle-aged and elderly adults (range, 40-60 years)	Palpable purpura, hemoptysis, abdominal pain, hematochezia, neuropathy, crescentic GN	Arthralgia, myalgia, fever	Dx by tissue Bx; 40% cANCA +; 60% pANCA +; ↑ ESR	↑ High dose prednisone and CTX
Small and medium-size vasculitis					
Wegener's granulomatosis	M > F; middle-aged and elderly Caucasians	Sinusitis, otitis media, cough, hemoptysis, dyspnea, proteinuria, hematuria, renal failure	Fever, weight loss, malaise, arthralgia, mononeuritis multiplex, polyneuropathy	Dx by tissue(nasal, pulmonary, renal) Bx (granulomatous vasculitis), 90% cANCA+, ↑ ESR	CTX + prednisone; SMX/TMP for localized disease
Polyarteritis nodosa	M > F (2:1); age 40-60 years	Renal failure, proteinuria, mononeuritis multiplex, abdominal pain, GI hemorrhage, bowel infarction, livedo reticularis, skin ulcers	Hypertension, fever, malaise, weight loss, arthralgias, myalgias, back pain	Dx by angiogram or tissue (nerve, muscle, testicle, kidney)Bx; ↑ ESR, leukocytosis, anemia, low C4 or C3, hepatitis B or C positive in some	↑ High dose prednisone and CTX or azathioprine

Churg-Strauss angiitis (allergic angiitis)	M > F; middle-aged adults (range 15-70 years)	Asthma, pulmonary infiltrates, rhinitis, cardiac (CHF) involvement	Arthralgia, fever, mono-neuritis multiplex	Eosinophilia, necrotizing vasculitis with eosinophils and granuloma, 70% pANCA+	↑ High dose prednisone
Rheumatoid vasculitis	M > F; with longstanding, severe seropositive RA	Splinter hemorrhages, skin ulcers, peripheral neuropathy, palpable purpura, visceral arteritis	Weight loss, splenomegaly, nodules	Dx by tissue (skin, rectal, , nerve) Bx or angiogram; ↑ titer RF, ↑ ESR, low C3 or C4, anemia	↑ High dose prednisone; some may require oral or IV CTX
Large vessel vasculitis					
Giant cell arteritis	F > M; elderly (>60 years) Caucasians	Headache, diplopia, blindness, scalp tenderness, jaw claudication	PMR symptoms (girdle muscle pain and stiffness), fever, weight loss	Extreme ↑ ESR; temporal artery Bx positive 80-90% of patients	↑ High dose prednisone
Takayasu arteritis	>90% F; young/middle-aged adults; common in Japan, China, India; rare in whites	Arm claudication, bruits, pulselessness and pressure difference	Hypertension, arthralgias, myalgias, fever, weight loss	Dx by angiogram; ↑ ESR in 70%	↑ High dose prednisone; may require MTX or CTX in resistant patients
Primary CNS angiitis	M > F; adults 20-60 years	Headache, confusion, cognitive dysfunction, seizure, cranial neuropathy	Uncommon: arthralgia, myalgia, fever	Dx by angiogram or lepto-meningeal Bx; ↑ ESR	↑ High dose prednisone ± CTX

M, male; F, female; HSP, Henoch-Schönlein purpura; RA, rheumatoid arthritis; SLE, systemic lupus erythematosus; PAN, polyarteritis nodosa; PBC, primary biliary cirrhosis; SBE, subacute bacterial endocarditis; HBV, hepatitis B virus; HCV, hepatitis C virus; CMV, cytomegalovirus; EBV, Epstein-Barr virus; Bx, biopsy; GI, gastrointestinal; N/V, nausea and vomiting; ESR, erythrocyte sedimentation rate; RF, rheumatoid factor; ANA, antinuclear antibody; Dx, diagnosis; CTX, cyclophosphamide; MTX, methotrexate; SMX/TMP, sulfamethoxazole-trimethoprim; CHF, congestive heart failure; IV, intravenous; PMR, polymyalgia rheumatica.

[a]List of those tests most helpful in establishing the diagnosis.

INDICATIONS FOR SURGERY

Orthopedic surgical procedures can dramatically improve the quality of life for patients with various types of arthritis. Progress in the development of surgical interventions has been among the most important advances in the care of arthritis patients during the past century.

Types of Surgery

Commonly available types of orthopedic procedures include (1) synovectomy or tenosynovectomy (i.e., removing synovial tissue from joints or tendons), (2) ligament or tendon reconstruction (e.g., repair of torn or fraying tendons), (3) osteotomy (cutting of bone to optimize mechanics), (4) arthrodesis (intentional fusion of joints), and (5) arthroplasty (joint replacement surgery).

Joint replacement surgery has been particularly useful for severe arthritis of the hip and knee joints. Many patients can have successful results for 10 to 20 years or more after surgery; therefore, joint replacement is often the preferred procedure for the hips or knees. Other joints that may be considered for joint replacement include the metacarpophalangeal, shoulder, and first carpometacarpal joints. Osteotomy is a more limited procedure than joint replacement. It may be useful in some instances (e.g., unilateral knee osteoarthritis) in which realignment may optimize joint mechanics and thereby improve pain and function. Arthrodesis is considered for joints for which the results of joint replacement have not been so promising (e.g., wrists, ankles). It should be noted that repeated attempts to replace the same joint are often more difficult and less successful than the first procedure.

Indications: The main indications for joint surgery include (1) intractable or refractory pain, (2) significant functional limitation, and (3) objective evidence of progressive damage (by examination or imaging). When considering referring patients to an orthopedic surgeon, it should be clear that either the pain and/or the impairment in functional status are directly related to damage to, or destruction of, the affected joint. For example, a person with advanced degenerative changes on x-ray who experiences severe pain both with activity and at rest should be considered a potential candidate for surgical intervention. On the other hand, if a patient has severe pain but no evidence of joint damage, other etiologies for the pain should be considered (e.g., neuropathic pain, fibromyalgia). In addition, before undertaking surgery, other interventions should be tried. For example, simple analgesics are the first step in managing pain, and assistive devices can help optimize functional status.

Tenosynovectomy and tendon or ligament repairs are generally less extensive surgical procedures than joint replacement. Indications for these procedures include (1) rupture or impending rupture and (2) severe, refractory localized synovitis.

Contraindications: Contraindications to joint surgery include active infection and uncontrolled bleeding diathesis. Because postoperative rehabilitation is crucial to a good outcome after joint replacement, many of the relative contraindications to this surgery include conditions that could interfere with rehabilitation potential (e.g., decreased mobility unrelated to the involved joint, morbid obesity, lack of motivation, severe comorbid diseases). Younger age is also a relative contraindication to joint replacement surgery because (1) patients who are extremely physically active after joint replacement may experience failure of the prosthesis sooner than those with normal activity and (2) repeat procedures are often associated with a poorer outcome.

Complications: The risk of an infected prosthesis after joint replacement is ≤ 2%.

Cost: The cost of total joint arthroplasty (hip or knee) is usually between $25,000 and $35,000.

SUBJECT INDEX

Page numbers followed by *f* indicate figures; page numbers followed by *t* indicate tables.

A

Acanthocytes, 51
ACE, 31
  inhibitors
    for high blood pressure, 347
  with Loefgren syndrome, 341
Acephen, 403–404
Acetaminophen (Paracetamol), 403–404
  for fibromyalgia, 181
  pregnancy, 306
Acetaminophen + Opioids (Codeine/
    Hydrocodone/Oxycodone/
    Propoxyphene/Tramadol),
    404–406
Acetylsalicylic acid (ASA), 415–417
  for Henoch-Schonlein purpura, 203
Achilles tendinitis, 263
Achilles tendonitis, 166–168
Acid maltase deficiency, 250
Acipciphex, 531
Aciphex, 531
ACL
  antibodies, 43–45
  antibody test, 121
  syndrome, 119–122
Acne arthritis, 338
Acne-associated SpA, 338
Acquired angioedema
  complement, 60*t*
ACR. *See* American College of
    Rheumatology (ACR)
Acromegalia, 107–108
Acromegaly, 107–108
Acromioplasty, 351
Acropachy, 215–217
Activated charcoal
  interacting with leflunomide, 476
Activity, 6
Actonel, 505–506
Actron, 527
Acute arthritis
  with hepatitis, 206
Acute febrile neutrophilic dermatosis,
    363–364
Acute gout, 188, 190, 193–194
Acute-phase reactants, 32–34
Acute rheumatic fever (ARF), 108–110
Adalimumab (Humira), 406–408, 530

Adams-Baker cyst, 262–263
Adult-onset Still disease (AOSD), 110–112
Advil, 467–468
Aerobic exercise
  for osteoarthritis, 271
Albumin, 99
Alcaptonuria, 112–113
Alcohol
  interacting with acetaminophen, 404
  interacting with allopurinol, 410
  interacting with amitriptyline, 412
Aldolase (ALD), 34–35
Alendronate (Fosamax), 408–409
  interacting with teriparatide, 514
Aleve, 490–491
Algodystrophy, 319–321
Allergic angiitis, 149–150
Allopurinol (Zyloprim), 409–411
  for acute gout, 194, 195
  interacting with azathioprine, 421
  interacting with cyclophosphamide,
    443
Alpha globulins, 99
AMAS, 38–39
Ambien, 521–522
  for fibromyalgia, 181
Amblyomma americanum, 237
American College of Rheumatology
    (ACR)
  classification criteria, 70–73
    fibromyalgia, 180*t*
    juvenile rheumatoid arthritis, 225*t*
    rheumatoid arthritis, 71*t*
    Wegener's granulomatosis, 391*t*
5-aminosalicylic acid plus sulfapyridine,
    510–511
Amitriptyline (Elavil, Vanatrip), 411–412,
    533
  for fibromyalgia, 181
Amoxapine (Asendin), 533
Amoxicillin
  for Lyme disease, 241*t*
Ampicillin
  interacting with allopurinol, 410
  interacting with raloxifene, 504
Amyloidosis, 113–114
  with familial recurrent polyserositis, 172
  syndromes of, 113*t*